Psychology in the Physical and Manual Therapies

For Churchill Livingstone:

Publishing Director: Mary Law
Project Development Manager: Mairi McCubbin
Project Manager: Gail Wright
Senior Designer: Judith Wright
Illustration Manager: Bruce Hogarth

Psychology in the Physical and Manual Therapies

Edited by

Gregory S. Kolt BSc BAppSc(Phty) PhD GradDipEd GradDipBehavHlthCare

Professor of Health Science and Associate Dean (Research), Faculty of Health, Auckland University of Technology, Auckland, New Zealand

and

Mark B. Andersen BA(Psych) MSc(Psych) PhD(Psych)

Associate Professor, School of Human Movement, Recreation and Performance, Faculty of Human Development, Victoria University, Melbourne, Australia

Foreword by

Katherine F. Shepard PhD PT FAPTA

Professor and Director, PhD Program in Physical Therapy, Department of Physical Therapy, College of Allied Health Professions, Temple University, Philadelphia, PA, USA

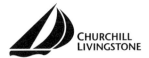

CHURCHILL
LIVINGSTONE

EDINBURGH   LONDON   NEW YORK   OXFORD   PHILADELPHIA   ST LOUIS   SYDNEY   TORONTO   2004

CHURCHILL LIVINGSTONE
An imprint of Elsevier Limited

First published 2004

ISBN 0 443 07352 X

British Library Cataloguing in Publication Data
A catalogue record for this book is available from the British Library

Library of Congress Cataloging in Publication Data
A catalog record for this book is available from the Library of Congress

Notice
Medical knowledge is constantly changing. Standard safety precautions must be followed, but as new research and clinical experience broaden our knowledge, changes in treatment and drug therapy may become necessary or appropriate. Readers are advised to check the most current product information provided by the manufacturer of each drug to be administered to verify the recommended dose, the method and duration of administration, and contraindications. It is the responsibility of the practitioner, relying on experience and knowledge of the patient, to determine dosages and the best treatment for each individual patient. Neither the Publisher nor the editors and contributors assumes any liability for any injury and/or damage to persons or property arising from this publication.

Neither the Publisher nor the editors and contributors will be liable for any loss or damage of any nature occasioned to or suffered by any person acting or refraining from acting as a result of reliance on the material contained in this publication.

The Publisher

Printed in China

Contents

Contributors

Mark B. Andersen BA(Psych) MSc(Psych) PhD(Psych)
Associate Professor, School of Human Movement, Recreation and Performance, Faculty of Human Development, Victoria University, Melbourne, Australia

Esther K. Black BSc(Hons)(Psych)
Trainee Clinical Psychologist, Department of Psychological Medicine, Academic Centre, Gartnavel Royal Hospital, Glasgow, UK

Britton W. Brewer PhD
Associate Professor of Psychology, Department of Psychology, Springfield College, Springfield, MA, USA

Melainie Cameron BAppSc(Ost) MHSc(Research)
Registered Osteopath
Lecturer, Osteopathic Medicine Unit, Victoria University, Melbourne, Australia

Allen Cornelius MA PhD
Associate Director and Commissioner of Research, National Football Foundation Center for Youth Development through Sport, Springfield College, Springfield, MA, USA

Beth L. Dinoff PhD
Postdoctoral Fellow, Spain Rehabilitation Center, Birmingham, AL, USA

Helen Graham BA MPhil
Retired, Market Drayton, UK

Stephen A. Gudas BSc MS PhD
Associate Professor, Department of Anatomy and Neurobiology and Physical Therapist, Cancer Rehabilitation Program, Virginia Commonwealth University/Medical College of Virginia, Richmond, VA, USA

Urban Johnson PhD
Assistant Professor in Psychology, Halmstad University, Halmstad, Sweden

Robert M. Kaplan PhD
Professor and Chair, Family and Preventive Medicine, University of California, San Diego, La Jolla, CA, USA

Gregory S. Kolt BSc BAppSc(Phty) PhD GradDipEd GradDipBehavHlthCare
Professor of Health Science and Associate Dean (Research), Faculty of Health, Auckland University of Technology, Auckland, New Zealand

Lynda M. Mainwaring BA(Psych) BHK(Hon) MHK PhD CPsych
Associate Professor, Faculty of Physical Education and Health, University of Toronto; Adjunct Assistant Professor, Faculty of Human Kinetics, University of Windsor, Windsor; Research Scientist, Hospital for Sick Children, Toronto, Canada

Rona Moss-Morris BSc MHSc(Hons) PhD
Senior Lecturer in Health Psychology, Department of Health Psychology and Practitioner Development Unit, Faculty of Medical and Health Sciences, The University of Auckland, Auckland, New Zealand

Rosemary A. Payne BSc(Hons)(Psych) MCSP
Private Practitioner, Cardiff, UK

Al Petitpas
Professor of Psychology and Director of the National Football Foundation Center for Youth Development through Sport, Springfield College, Springfield, MA, USA

J. Scott Richards PhD
Professor of Physical Medicine and Rehabilitation, Spain Rehabilitation Center, Birmingham, AL, USA

Joseph H. Ricker PhD ABPP (CN RP)
Associate Director, Neuropsychology Laboratory,
Kessler Medical Rehabilitation Research and Education
Corporation, West Orange, NJ; Associate Professor,
Department of Physical Medicine and Rehabilitation,
University of Medicine and Dentistry of New Jersey,
West Orange, NJ, USA

Pia B. Santiago BA MS
Doctoral Student in Clinical Psychology, Joint Doctoral
Program in Clinical Psychology, San Diego State
University/University of California, San Diego, CA,
USA

Craig A. White BSc(Hons)(Psych) ClinPsyD
PostgradCert(Cognitive Therapy)
Macmillan Consultant Clinical Psychologist (Cancer
and Palliative Medicine), Ayrshire and Arran Primary
Care NHS Trust, Ayr, UK

Diane M. Wiese-Bjornstal PhD
Associate Professor of Kinesiology, School
of Kinesiology, University of Minnesota, Minneapolis,
MN, USA

Wendy Wrapson MA(Hons)
PhD Student, Department of Health Psychology and
Practitioner Development Unit, Faculty of Medical and
Health Sciences, The University of Auckland, Auckland,
New Zealand

Foreword

When students in a physical therapy or manual therapy curriculum are given a choice between attending an anatomy course or a psychology of illness and wellness behavior course, there would be no doubt in students' minds that anatomy was the most important course. The faculty in any such curriculum would generally agree with the students' choice. Even though we work with humans, the lack of social and behavioral science information in our professional curricula is obvious. To student therapists, whose focus is on learning to use their hands and other tools in patient care, a course on human psychology pertinent to healthcare seems either valued as a "break" from the real "science courses" or devalued as "useless, because it is all common sense". To faculty, information in the social and behavioral sciences is often relegated to prerequisite courses or is "integrated" into the health professional curricula by faculty describing client circumstances that interfere with treatment progress. After all, time is a precious commodity and academic and clinical instructors work hard to ensure students can "hit the ground running" with specific hands-on skills when they enter clinical practice.

However, ask experienced clinicians what they wish they had had more of in their academic curricula and the answer would not be anatomy. Rather, clinicians yearn for information and skills related to increasing their ability to work with the many clients they see whose anxiety, fear of pain, depression, or "lack of motivation" interferes with their return to or commitment to a healthy, productive life.

There are several reasons for this vast difference in perceptions between those who labor in the academic life and those who labor in the clinical life. One is that healthcare curricula reflect Western medicine's approach to separating the mind from the body. Another is the perception that physical and other manual therapies are only physical, and that psychosocial factors "belong" to psychologists or social workers. Another, sadly, is poor academic experiences with psychology courses that give students a great deal of information regarding research with lower forms of life (e.g., pigeons and rats) and little in the way of information helpful to human–human interactions.

Thus, *Psychology in the Physical and Manual Therapies* is a most welcome addition to the literature that will be of extraordinary help to therapists who feel puzzled and somewhat helpless when having difficulty in assisting patients to achieve improved heath and wellness. The editors have done a masterful job of identifying authors on three continents who can write concise, clear, well-documented accounts of theory and related practice ideas for therapists. They have provided enough evidence-based practice and theory to satisfy the scientific mind, and sufficient easily related useful approaches to client care to satisfy the busy clinician.

The underlying premise of the authors is the importance of building a therapeutic partnership and "walking beside" clients. The book therefore focuses on identifying and working with the common psychological aspects of recovery as well as on knowing when clients need referral to other practitioners such as to psychologists for assistance in facilitating clients' self-management of pain, or to dietitians for assistance with those who exhibit eating disorders.

The presentation of useful clinical practice techniques in this book follows one or other of two forms. One is the identification of personal traits that can help practitioners better understand the client as well as themselves. See, for example, the excellent chapter on "Transference and counter-transference" (Chapter 6). The second is the description of specific techniques which engage the mind part of the mind–body difficulties clients bring with them to the clinical setting. Some of the mind–body connectedness is obvious, such as working with post-traumatic stress disorders. Other mind–body connections are less obvious, such as clients who have difficulty in concentrating on tasks due to underlying depression. Whatever the connection, any physical or manual therapist can save time and improve the therapeutic outcome by understanding and responding to how the psychological, social, and spiritual aspects of life accompany the patho-physiological and physical dysfunction aspects of life.

Some of the therapeutic techniques presented in *Psychology in the Physical and Manual Therapies* which use the mind to enhance work with the body, such as relaxation exercises and imagery, are known to be often underutilized by physical and manual therapists. Relearning these techniques will be easy for readers of this book. Actually using these techniques as common therapeutic tools will take conscious effort and convincing oneself that progress into health is not a muscle–joint problem but a human existence problem. Other therapeutic techniques presented, such as the use of principles of cognitive behavior therapy, may be new to readers. However, therapists will find a clear and logical presentation of this psychological approach in this book and will realize that the use of even one or two of the cognitive behavior therapy principles with clients may represent a turning point in clients' commitment to their own health.

One cautionary note: The reader should remember that personality and character disorders identified in this text are to help practitioners understand and work more effectively with clients, not to predict behavior or place a disheartening label on a person. For example, people who crave attention may or may not have a narcissistic personality disorder. In this text, techniques are presented for working with dependent self-centered clients whether or not they are identified as having a personality disorder.

In summary, *Psychology in the Physical and Manual Therapies* will offer:

- Extraordinary assistance to experienced physical and manual therapists in improving their effectiveness with clients.
- A model for faculty on how to present to students an ongoing integration of the physical and psychological aspects of healthcare. For a good example, see the chapter "Injury from sport, exercise, and physical activity" (Chapter 16).
- Clear examples for students about the always present mind–body relationships of clinical practice
- Hope for clients to learn how to embrace and self-manage healthy lives.

Katherine F. Shepard

Preface

This book, *Psychology in the Physical and Manual Therapies*, has evolved over 2 years, but only after many years of discussion with our colleagues, students, and clients. The common theme arising from this dialogue has been, "If only those in the physical and manual therapies could pay more attention to the person and not just to the injury or illness." Far too often in clinical settings do we hear comments such as, "When you've finished seeing that ankle, can you start with the patellar dislocation in the next room." Being able to work with the person, and not just parts of their anatomy or their illnesses, is integral to client-centered healthcare. It is not until relatively recently that training programs in the physical and manual therapies have incorporated relevant aspects of psychology and behavioral sciences into standard curricula. Both research and anecdotal evidence have indicated that professionals working in the physical and manual therapies feel they would benefit from additional training in psychological aspects of healthcare. Almost on a daily basis, practitioners encounter clients who present with symptoms both physical and psychological, and often these symptoms are entangled. Working with the client on reducing the physical symptoms alone is often not enough. To be effective as a healthcare practitioner, one must incorporate several approaches to the issues that clients present. Knowing about the psychological aspects of a variety of conditions with which physical and manual therapists work (e.g., stroke and head injury, spinal cord injury, cardiorespiratory conditions, injury from sport, exercise, and physical activity, the arthritides, functional somatic syndromes, terminal illness) is integral to adequate client care. Being able to recognize psychopathologies and personality disorders in clients can greatly assist practitioners in their understanding of why clients react to treatment and rehabilitation in particular ways. Topics such as managing pain, practitioner–client relationships, and terminating therapeutic relationships are crucial to the understanding of client care. For physical and manual therapists, to have a basic understanding of a variety of cognitive and behavioral interventions that they can incorporate with their more physical skills, provides them with a more holistic approach to client care, and one that considers more than just the injury or illness.

In this book we have provided a contemporary and, wherever possible, evidence-based coverage of a variety of psychological topics relevant to physical and manual therapists. Authors from across the world, and in a variety of relevant disciplines, have contributed in their expert areas. We hope the ideas and practices in this book will help practitioners offer quality care to their clients.

Gregory S. Kolt

Auckland and Melbourne 2004   *Mark B. Andersen*

Acknowledgments

In completing this book and making it a success, a large number of people have contributed in a variety of ways. Elsevier has put a great team of people onto this project. Mary Law, the Publishing Director, is always encouraging, efficient, and full of positive and constructive feedback. She saw a place for this book and gave us the opportunity to work on it. Mairi McCubbin, our Project Development Manager, is thanked for her efficiency, publishing advice, and for keeping us to time – no small task for a book with 21 contributors from 6 countries. Gail Wright took the book through the production stages with attention to detail and a high level of commitment. Many of my colleagues at Auckland University of Technology and elsewhere around the world have provided important input and support for this book. Rachael Stewart provided invaluable administrative support for the project and Nicola Dose undertook much of the time-consuming literature searching, proofreading, and formatting for the project. The late Professor Rob Kirkby (my academic mentor and friend) was instrumental in shaping my professional life, and in many ways indirectly responsible for me completing a project such as this. Finally, I want to thank my family: Emma, Daisy Chayne, and Satchel have provided a balance in my life over this period and a great reason to hurry up and finish the book, while my parents never stop giving me encouragement to pursue whatever I think worthwhile.

Gregory S. Kolt

First of all, I would like to express gratitude and thanks to Greg Kolt for asking me along on this journey. It has not all been smooth sailing, but Greg has been a patient and skilled captain. A big part of the motivation to complete this project came from students in my psychology of rehabilitation graduate class. More motivation came from my big sister, Brittony Thomas, a tremendous physical therapist doing great work in Colorado. Coming from a family of helpers (Mom, an exemplary nurse; Dad, the most therapeutic accountant I know; little sister Sal, a fine educator) has colored my life, and they remain great strengths on whom I draw every day. I must also thank the School of Human Movement, Recreation, and Performance, and specifically my Head of School, Professor Terence Roberts, for giving me time to complete this project. His support has helped me develop as an academic and as a psychologist. My Dean, Professor Carol Morse, has also been a strong source of support and encouragement in this endeavor. Dr. Harriet Speed (such a great name for a sport psychologist) is a great friend, and a source of endless laughter. Her support has been at least as good as psychotherapy. Finally, I want to thank my partner, Jeffrey Armstrong, for his support, his feedback on my writing, and his love.

Mark B. Andersen

SECTION 1

Injury, illness, and rehabilitation: psychological principles

Chapter 1

Using psychology in the physical and manual therapies

Gregory S. Kolt, Mark B. Andersen

INTRODUCTION

Having both taught in rehabilitation and physical therapy programs over many years, we have identified a clear need for a psychology text designed for advanced-level students and practitioners. A review of educational programs in the physical and manual therapies has revealed a small but growing number of institutions offering more substantial training in the psychological aspects of client care. The fields of health and rehabilitation psychology are relative newcomers in applied service delivery, but have the potential to contribute significantly to practitioners' quality of care.

Numerous rehabilitation and health psychology texts are available, and have much to offer professionals in the physical and manual therapies. To date, however, this is the first comprehensive psychology text aimed at integrating theories, principles, and applications with the more physical aspects of client care. Specifically, this text focuses on professions where touch plays an integral role in the management of injury and illness. Such professions include physical therapy (physiotherapy), rehabilitation medicine, osteopathy, massage and soft tissue therapy, chiropractic, athletic training (in North America), podiatry, and nursing. Throughout many of the chapters, references will be made to the psychological aspects of touch, and the role physical contact plays in the healing process.

Studies in the physical and manual therapies have indicated that practitioners would have liked to have had a greater amount of psychology in their training programs (Frances et al 2000, Gordon et al 1991, Ninedek & Kolt 2000). The contents of this book provide a foundation from which one can explore the intersections of psychological care and the physical and manual therapies.

TERMINOLOGY

In the physical and manual therapies, practitioners use a variety of terms to describe the people they work with. The terms *clients* and *patients* are commonly used, and often interchangeably. Usage of one term or another often depends on the country the practitioner is working in or the specific health discipline that they work in. For example, traditionally, physical therapists have used the term *patient*, however, many are now using *client*. In psychology, the norm has been to use *client*. The word *patient* shares the same Latin root as the words "passive" and "suffering" and implies that treatment is a one-way street moving from therapist to patient. *Client*, however, is usually used to reflect a more equal and collaborative relationship with the therapist. As this book has contributions from a variety of practitioners from several countries, and is aimed at a variety of healthcare professionals, both the terms *clients* and *patients* will be used interchangeably. Regardless of terminology, in the models of care we present in this book, treatment is viewed as a collaborative effort that is worked out between (at least) two people. Stemming from George Kelly's work, Beck used the term "collaborative empiricism" to describe the process of psychotherapy (see Beck et al 1979). What he meant is that two people are working together to answer some questions, figure out something, and understand experiences. We think the term fits well in the physical and manual therapies.

HOLISTIC MODELS OF MANAGEMENT

"Once you've finished with that shoulder please take a look at the knee in examination room five." Experience tells us that most practitioners in the physical and manual therapies would recognize that this manner of speech, when referring to clients, is not uncommon. This example of how language is used to describe clients speaks volumes about the way in which practitioners view treatment and care. Many practitioners from the "old school" are pathology oriented, and treat knees and shoulders with little attention paid to the individuals who own those body parts. More recent models of client care emphasize that attention to the whole person is at least as important as the treatment of

their pathology. For example, a practitioner may work with a client who, through a work-related accident, has sustained significant trauma to her lumbar spine. Her future in her chosen work field is highly uncertain, and she is showing signs of depression. Recognizing these signs is paramount to successful rehabilitation and return to former level of functioning. If the practitioner treats only the lumbar spine and associated musculature, rehabilitation progress may be limited. The uncertainty, sadness, and depressed mood of the client may interfere with several aspects of rehabilitation (e.g., adherence to home exercise, effort, perceived efficacy of rehabilitation tasks). An astute practitioner will recognize the signs and discuss them with the client to establish whether they are a normal reaction to injury or whether they require more formal attention by a qualified psychologist.

We are not advocating that physical and manual therapists take over the roles of psychologists. Rather, what we would like to see in the professions is practitioners who have a solid grounding in psychology, who can recognize psychological problems that may benefit from treatment, and who can teach some basic psychological skills (e.g., relaxation, imagery) to their clients. For example, it is almost always a good idea to have some goals in rehabilitation, but how to set goals in a way that would be motivating and helpful is not exactly an intuitive act. There are several principles from cognitive-behavior therapy that would be wise to follow in terms of formulating short-, medium-, and long-term goals (e.g., flexible, challenging, realistic). Goal setting is actually quite a complex collaborative process if done correctly (see Chapter 8). Besides goal setting, there are several other psychological avenues to pursue with clients. It would be hard to think of a situation in the physical and manual therapies where the client would not gain some measure of benefit from learning how to relax. Using imagery in healthcare has quite a long history (see Graham 1995). Learning self-hypnotic techniques, such as autogenic training, can help clients change blood flow patterns and relax them too (Shultz & Luthe 1969). All of these interventions are therapeutic and psychology based, but practitioners in the physical and manual therapies are not doing psychotherapy, nor would they be expected to provide such a service. In terms of service delivery, it comes down to what we know and what we do not know. One should practice what one knows, and with supervision, practice what one is learning. For example, if an osteopath has a good background in autogenic training, then by all means she should teach it to clients where it might be beneficial. If she has only read about it in a book, then trying to teach it to someone else becomes problematic. A little knowledge is a dangerous thing.

REFERRAL NETWORK

Most physical and manual therapists can handle many of the common psychological aspects of rehabilitation (e.g., anxiety over recovery, fear of pain, boredom, frustration) through listening, empathy, genuineness, and just being there with the client. There are times when the client presents with a concern that is outside the therapist's area of competence, and that is when a referral may be necessary. We suggest to students and practitioners that they begin to cultivate a referral network as early as possible that includes a wide range of practitioners, both in and outside the field of practice (e.g., physicians, psychologists, psychiatrists, dieticians, fitness instructors). For example, eating disorders are quite common in the general population, and the chances of working in rehabilitation with someone who is bulimic or anorexic is quite high. Sensitive referrals to a physician (to assess physical and physiological damage), a dietician (to get the person on a good healthy diet), and a psychologist (to explore what is maintaining the behavior) would be the team approach to an extremely complicated disorder. Treating people with eating disorders is difficult, but the goals in such situations are similar to goals in many other cases: taking care of the person, not just the knee. That care can be accomplished through a team approach, as in working with someone with an eating disorder, or through just "checking in" with the client on how other parts of their lives are functioning.

CURRENT PSYCHOLOGICAL EDUCATION IN THE PHYSICAL AND MANUAL THERAPIES

In going through several university and college catalogs, we found that there was some psychology in virtually all programs in the physical and manual therapies. The depth and breadth of what was offered in psychology, however, was highly variable, ranging from an introduction to psychology course to some basic counseling and cognitive

behavioral skills. It is apparent that over the past 10 years or so, many physical and manual therapy programs are increasing the amount and breadth of psychology training at both undergraduate and postgraduate levels. Not only is this content being taught as separate coursework within a program, but also in an integrated fashion with other more physical-based rehabilitation coursework. This relatively new approach is what we are advocating in this text.

HAVE YOU HAD A PATIENT LIKE THIS?

All practitioners in the physical and manual therapies have run into clients who manifest difficulties in psychological or behavioral realms. For example, a client comes to a practitioner for postsurgical rehabilitation of an anterior cruciate ligament reconstruction. Prior to this surgery the client and the practitioner had met to discuss the rehabilitation process. For that consultation, the client was 20 minutes late and did not bother to apologize. The history taken at that consult indicated that he had shopped around for a surgeon and was not pleased with several of them. They were not "good enough." He also expressed doubts that his current surgeon was going to meet his special needs. He was somewhat angry and resentful that all this was happening to him. Postsurgery, the client complains that the whole thing is unfair, that this is going to slow down his big plans for success, and that the practitioner needs to give him extra consideration. The client is also very defensive when asked about adherence to home exercises and activity restrictions. What is going on here? From this brief description of the client, it appears that he has many of the diagnostic criteria for narcissistic personality disorder (NPD). People with NPD are insensitive to others (no apology for being late), have fantasies of fame (his big plans for success), crave attention (he needs extra consideration), become very defensive when challenged, and believe that they are special. People with narcissistic personalities are difficult to work with and are also at risk of dropping out of rehabilitation because they are not getting the special treatment they believe they deserve, or because their therapist is not becoming an admiring ally. Treatment of NPD is long, complicated, and often unsuccessful, and we would never expect a physical or manual therapist to go down that path. There are, however, ways to work with someone with NPD that will make it more likely that the client will stay in rehabilitation (see Chapter 7).

Here is another example that many practitioners will recognize. A physically active 45-year-old woman has just received a diagnosis of osteoarthritis of the hip. She is the head of her own business, works hard, watches her diet extremely carefully, and is quite a fitness junkie. She is surprised that she has been diagnosed with osteoarthritis and cannot understand how it has happened, given her activity and diet. One of her first questions to the practitioner is "OK, now what do I have to do to get rid of this?" For the first couple of weeks the client religiously shows up for appointments, is enthusiastic, and is optimistic. In the third week, however, the client comes in, and even though she tries to hide it, the same manual techniques used in the previous week are now causing a great deal of pain. In talking with the client, the practitioner discovers that she is overdoing her home exercises. Her thinking is that if ten repetitions are good, then 20 are twice as good. What may be going on here? The client here has many features similar to people with perfectionistic and obsessive-compulsive tendencies, as evidenced by her rigid diet and gym routine. The problem with such clients is not getting them to adhere to home exercise and cryotherapy routines; it is making sure they do not overdo it, end up causing more damage, and setting back the rehabilitation. Taking time to get a feel for the psychological state, personality, and style of the client may help practitioners adjust their own service in ways that will work better.

INTEGRATING PSYCHOLOGICAL THEORY AND APPLICATION

Psychological theory forms the groundwork for each of the chapters in the book. Whenever two people get together psychological principles of that social encounter begin to operate. It would probably be useful for practitioners to have a firm grasp of what some of those psychological sequelae of being in treatment with another person are. Also practitioners are in a good position to use psychological theory and techniques to better their client care. Again, we are not trying to turn physical and manual therapists into psychologists, but if, for example, a physical therapist has been trained in delivering relaxation, then there is no reason why that service should not be delivered. For example,

several manual techniques may temporarily increase pain levels (e.g., joint mobilization). A way to help clients through the treatment might be to teach them how to use diaphragmatic breathing to relax and distract them from what is happening (see Chapter 9).

Physical and manual therapists, like psychologists, are the members of the healthcare professions who probably spend more time with their clients than any other service delivery provider. In clinical and counseling psychology there is considerable research and discussion on what happens in therapy when two people start talking. Much of what is written in that counseling psychology literature has direct application to people in the physical and manual therapies (see Chapters 5 and 6).

EVIDENCE FOR PSYCHOLOGICAL CARE

How do physical and manual therapists know if their treatments have been helpful to clients? How do psychologists know if their psychotherapeutic care has brought about salubrious change? These epistemological questions go to the heart of all healthcare professions and service delivery. For many decades, the gold standard for determining (knowing) a treatment is efficacious in the biomedical and psychological fields has been the use of randomized clinical trials (RCTs; see Chambless & Hollon 1998). An RCT design, in its simplest (and possibly most common) form, involves the random assignment of participants to either a treatment or a control group, and then they are measured pre- and post-treatment to test for any differences between groups on some dependent variable(s) of choice (e.g., range of motion, happiness, serum cortisol, neuroticism). This type of treatment efficacy research has very strong internal validity due to the use of control groups, random assignment to groups, and the standardization of treatments. RCTs do, however, have some problems. Although RCTs may have strong internal validity, their external validity (do they reflect what is going on in the real world outside the RCT?) is often tenuous. In the real world, clients are never randomly assigned to treatments, treatments are never really standardized, and interventions are designed in idiosyncratic manners. Outcomes of real world interventions depend on interactions among a huge variety of variables that RCTs cannot logistically embrace. These variables include the personality of the client, the personality of the therapist, the social climate of the clinic, the social environment of the client, the gender of both parties, and a whole host of other variables. Looking at what works in the real world is called examining treatment effectiveness, in contrast to treatment efficacy (RCTs). In this book, the authors of the chapters will be reviewing the evidence for treatment efficacy by reporting studies from the literature that represent this paradigm of knowing what works. Many authors in this book will also draw from the effectiveness research and report on what practitioners out in the real world have found to be effective treatments. For more arguments on efficacy versus effectiveness research, see Goldfried & Wolfe (1998).

A WALK THROUGH *PSYCHOLOGY IN THE PHYSICAL AND MANUAL THERAPIES*

Health and rehabilitation psychology bring together a variety of models of service delivery with input from a range of psychological theories. When applying such models of psychology to the physical and manual therapies, an understanding of physical therapy models of care should be considered. If physical and manual therapists are to integrate psychological approaches and interventions with their physical rehabilitation protocols they need to be able to apply skills in a way that their clients will consider as usual and expected parts of rehabilitation. To produce a text that will assist physical and manual therapists in taking a holistic psychology-based approach to client care it was important to bring together a group of authors from a variety of healthcare areas. The chapter authors in this book represent a range of health disciplines including physical therapy, occupational therapy, health psychology, rehabilitation psychology, clinical psychology, counseling psychology, neuropsychology, sport and exercise psychology, consulting psychology, osteopathy, exercise science, and statistics and research design. The vast majority of authors are involved in both practice and research, with many also involved in teaching at undergraduate and postgraduate levels.

Psychology in the Physical and Manual Therapies is divided into three sections. Section 1, Injury, Illness, and Rehabilitation: Psychological Principles, covers three aspects of injury and illness and how psychological principles can be integrated with usual physical care. Chapter 1, Using Psychology in the Physical and Manual Therapies, outlines the importance of adopting more holistic approaches to healthcare that are based on the integration of psychological principles and physical techniques. This chapter also deals with the current psychology education in physical and manual therapy academic programs, and the need for a strong evidence base to support the psychological approaches that are used by physical and manual therapists. Chapter 2, Psychological Antecedents to Injury and Illness, focuses on a range of psychosocial factors that influence the onset of illness and injury. In particular, models of injury risk are evaluated in light of current research. This chapter also covers injury and illness prevention through interventions aimed at psychological risk factors. Chapter 3, Psychological Responses to Injury and Illness, covers responses to injury and illness including adjustment disorders, depression, anxiety, and diminished self-efficacy. Theoretical models addressing the psychosocial sequelae to injury and illness are also presented. Chapter 4, Psychological Aspects of Rehabilitation, outlines literature on adherence to rehabilitation, the link between rehabilitation adherence and outcome, and methods of enhancing adherence. In addition, this chapter discusses the client–practitioner relationship with reference to communication and perception, as well as psychological readiness to return to preinjury/illness activity.

Section 2, Psychological Care in the Physical and Manual Therapies: An Integrated Approach, addresses several topics of importance to practitioners for effective and comprehensive client care. Chapter 5, Practitioner–client Relationships: Building Working Alliances, focuses on the dynamics of practitioner–client interactions. Specifically, models of the client–practitioner interactions are discussed, and the importance of the therapeutic relationship for rehabilitation success is emphasized. Psychological characteristics and interpersonal qualities such as acceptance, empathy, genuineness, communication, and attending are outlined. Chapter 6, Transference and Countertransference, takes principles from psychodynamic theory to demonstrate how past interpersonal histories of both practitioner and client can influence current functioning and interaction within a therapeutic relationship. Chapter 7, Recognizing Psychopathology, outlines a variety of psychopathological conditions that clients present with in the physical and manual therapies. These include depression, anxiety disorders, disordered eating, and exercise dependence. The emphasis in this chapter is on practitioner recognition of these disorders, sensitive initiation of referral, and how to work effectively with clients with various psychopathologies. Chapter 8, Cognitive and Behavioral Interventions, includes information on the theoretical basis for behavioral interventions (including the fundamentals of classical conditioning, operant conditioning, and social learning theory), and the theoretical basis of cognitive interventions (including cognitive science research into memory, perception, and attention). The principles of managing problems using cognitive behavioral methods is covered, as are a variety of cognitive and behavioral interventions relevant to physical and manual therapists. These include cognitive restructuring, positive thinking, building self-efficacy, thought stoppage, reframing, systematic desensitization, goal setting, and the use of positive reinforcement. Chapter 9, Relaxation Techniques, outlines clinic-based and home-based relaxation exercises that can serve as useful adjuncts to the physical and manual therapies. The techniques include progressive muscle relaxation, breathing techniques, and autogenic training. For each of these techniques, the rationales for use and sample scripts for practitioners are included. Chapter 10, Imagery, focuses on the application of imagery in illness and injury rehabilitation. Specifically, imagery for healing, anxiety, and rehearsing returning to full activity are discussed, and examples of imagery scripts are included. Chapter 11, Pain and its Management, describes the mechanisms of pain, theoretical explanations of pain and pain behavior, the experience of pain, and assessment of pain in clinical settings. The chapter also includes information on managing pain through cognitive and behavioral therapies. Chapter 12, Terminating the Therapeutic Relationship, addresses the psychological and social factors that come into play when a client–practitioner relationship is drawing to a close. The chapter examines feelings, thoughts, and behaviors of both practitioners and clients, and makes suggestions for effective ways of terminating therapeutic relationships.

Section 3 of the book, Working with Specific Client Populations, incorporates eight chapters covering a variety of common conditions that physical and manual therapists are involved with. Chapter 13 is on Traumatic Brain Injury and Stroke; Chapter 14 addresses Spinal Cord Injury; Chapter 15 looks at Cardiovascular and Respiratory Conditions; Chapter 16 covers Injury from Sport, Exercise, and Physical Activity; Chapter 17 focuses on Arthritides; Chapter 18 provides information on Functional Somatic Syndromes; Chapter 19 covers Personality Disorders; and Chapter 20 considers Terminal Illness. In each of these chapters the areas covered include physical and medical considerations, psychological considerations, psychological interventions, and integrated management approaches.

SUMMARY

This book has been written with the specific purpose of providing user-friendly psychology-based information to those working in the physical and manual therapies. Training and education of healthcare professionals is increasingly dependent on interdisciplinary practice. We believe that the content of this book can assist physical and manual therapists to successfully recognize and incorporate psychological approaches in their management strategies for a range of disorders.

References

Beck A, Rush J, Hollon S et al 1979 Cognitive therapy of depression. Guilford, New York

Chambless D L, Hollon S D 1998 Defining empirically supported therapies. Journal of Consulting and Clinical Psychology 66: 7–18

Frances S R, Andersen M B, Maley P 2000 Physiotherapists' and male professional athletes' views on psychological skills for rehabilitation. Journal of Science and Medicine in Sport 3: 7–29

Goldfried M R, Wolfe B E 1998 Toward a more clinically valid approach to therapy research. Journal of Consulting and Clinical Psychology 66: 143–150

Gordon S, Milios D, Grove J R 1991 Psychological aspects of the recovery process from sport injury: The perspective of sport physiotherapists. Australian Journal of Science and Medicine in Sport 22: 53–60

Graham H 1995 Mental imagery in health care: An introduction to therapeutic practice. Chapman & Hall, London

Ninedek A, Kolt G S 2000 Sport physiotherapists' perceptions of psychological strategies in sport injury rehabilitation. Journal of Sport Rehabilitation 9: 191–206

Shultz J H, Luthe W 1969 Autogenic therapy, Vol 1. Grune & Stratton, New York

Chapter 2

Psychological antecedents to injury and illness

Urban Johnson

INTRODUCTION

Throughout history, the two major causes of early death have been infectious diseases and injury. Epidemiological studies from Sweden (1997) show that injury and intoxication are, after coronary heart diseases, the primary reasons for hospitalization (Socialstyrelsen 2001). Three-fourths of all accidents occur at home or in leisure time, with children, adolescents, and elderly people especially prone to injury. Even though the greatest cost of injury is in human suffering and loss, the economic cost of injury in the United States of America was estimated at more than $US224 billion in 1994. These costs include direct medical care and rehabilitation costs, as well as individual lost wages and national productivity losses (National Center for Injury Prevention and Control 1996). Each year in the US, an estimated 600 000 children are hospitalized for preventable injuries, and almost 16 million children are seen in emergency rooms for their injuries. More than 30 000 children are permanently disabled from injuries each year. The cost of injuries for children is estimated to exceed $US7.5 billion each year (Rodriguez 1990).

Many view injuries as inevitable, random, and not amenable to prevention efforts because they are caused by accidents. Viewing injuries as preventable is possibly the first step in reducing their occurrence. Current convention in the field of injury prevention uses the term "unintentional injury" rather than accident to avoid reinforcing the belief that injuries cannot be prevented. Because many injuries are largely a result of modifiable human behavior, it seems logical that psychologists, who are expert in promoting behavior change, should intervene (Fowler 1990). This chapter provides a review of important issues related to psychosocial antecedents and prevention of injury and illness. An overview of theoretical frameworks related to different kinds of prevention will be described. After that, conceptual models and research are described, specific to the injury prevention literature, including examples of specific injury and illness prevention programs. Factors affecting successful prevention efforts are also discussed. The chapter concludes with recommendations for medical personnel involved with prevention issues.

PSYCHOSOCIAL FACTORS INFLUENCING THE ONSET OF INJURY AND ILLNESS

Even though causes for injury are primarily physical in nature (e.g., faulty biomechanics, low muscle power, cars colliding) or just simply bad luck, psychosocial factors play an important role. Over the last few decades, a growing number of researchers have tried to determine which psychosocial variables influence injury vulnerability and resiliency (resistance to injuries). Researchers have found that individuals who have experienced many recent stressors and who did not have the personal resources and skills to cope with the stressors were most at risk for injuries. A substantial body of research has been directed at identifying mechanisms that might explain why the stress–injury relationship occurs and what interventions will reduce injury risk.

RELATIONSHIP BETWEEN MAJOR LIFE EVENTS STRESS AND ILLNESS OUTCOME

Interest in life event stress evolved initially from the work of Holmes & Rahe (1967). They developed the Social Readjustment Rating Scale (SRRS), a questionnaire that identifies and ranks the magnitude of 40 life change events found in the general adult population. Examples of life events are incidents such as the break-up of a relationship, taking a vacation, and death of a loved one. On the SRRS, each life event is given a numerical weighting based on the presumed degree of adaptation required for the typical individual in the general population. Individuals indicate the frequency of each event's occurrence during a specified period of time. Adding the weighted scores (life change units) for the checked items gives a total life-change score.

Research has supported the relationship of high life event stress to increased illness and even accidents (e.g., Holmes & Rahe 1967, Savery & Wooden 1994).

An example of the link between life stress and illness was provided by Rahe et al (1967). Rahe et al (1967) surveyed over 2000 people regarding their life events and periods of illness they had experienced in the previous 10 years. Those people who reported lower life stress scores for a given year had generally good health the following year. Approximately 50% of those who reported higher life stress scores indicated varying degrees of illness the following year. For those people with life stress scores at the very top end, they experienced varying degrees of illness the following year, and their life stress scores were positively correlated with the number of reported periods of illness. In a prospective study, Rahe & Arthur (1978) found that those who reported low life stress scores experienced less days of illness than those who reported higher life stress scores over the study period. Similar results have appeared in other studies (e.g. Rabkin & Struening 1976). Since these early studies, there have been a large number of research reports substantiating the life events stress–illness relationship.

RELATIONSHIP BETWEEN MINOR LIFE STRESS AND ILLNESS

Daily hassles and uplifts are other forms of stressors that can impact on health. Hassles are characterized as the irritating and often routine demands of life, and can range from minor irritants, frequent annoyances, and low-intensity stressors to chronic difficulties, problems, and pressures (Kanner et al 1981). Common hassles include events such as losing things, traffic problems, minor annoyances from work colleagues, and sleep difficulties. Hassles are often based on unmet expectations that trigger frustration or anger responses. These micro-stressors are cumulative and can be a significant source of stress, especially in the relative absence of compensatory uplifts. Uplifts may counteract hassles. They are pleasant surprises, treats, and events that make people feel good. Typical uplifts include having a good exercise workout, compliments from friends, eating out with a loved one, and completing a difficult task. Compared to major life events, hassles and uplifts are minor stressors. They are less life changing than life events, but do occur repeatedly, and on a daily basis. Hassles and uplifts are highly related to one's appraisals of situations, and can influence the ability to cope with injury and illness.

Research evidence exists for the link between daily hassles and illness. For example, DeLongis et al (1982) showed that scores on the Hassle Scale (Kanner et al 1981) predicted present and future psychological symptoms and somatic illness – sometimes more strongly than life events. The relationship between uplifts and stress, however, is not as clear. Both hassles and life events seem to contribute independently to distress levels and overall functioning. Many life events such as the death of a spouse are difficult, if not impossible, to control or predict. Daily hassles, however, are more easily able to be controlled. Lowering the number of daily hassles holds considerably greater potential for reducing stress and enhancing the quality of life than focusing on trying to reduce major life events. Furthermore, it seems that negative stressors and hassles affect health more strongly than positive life events and uplifts. That is, avoiding stressful situations when possible, or interpreting them more positively is conducive to enhanced levels of health on a psychological and physiological level.

A STRESS-BASED MODEL OF INJURY RISK

One of the most influential stress–injury models aimed at predicting the occurrence of injury was developed by Williams & Andersen 1998 (Figure 2.1). Although the stress–injury model was originally developed for stress and athletic injury, it is generic enough to apply to the wider population. Based on this model, when individuals experience stressful situations, their personality characteristics,

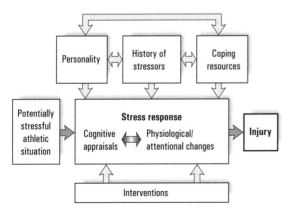

Figure 2.1   The stress and injury model (reproduced by permission from Williams & Andersen 1998, http://www.tandf.co.uk)

history of stressors, and coping resources contribute interactively with, or in isolation to, the stress response. The main idea of the model is that individuals with personality characteristics that tend to exacerbate the stress response, with a history of many stressors, and with few coping resources will be more likely, when placed in a stressful situation, to appraise the situation as stressful, and thus, to exhibit greater physiological activation and attentional disruptions. The muscle tension, distractibility, and perceptual narrowing that occur during the stress response appear to be the mechanisms behind increased injury risk. The center of the model, the stress response, involves a bi-directional relationship between the person's cognitive appraisals of a potentially stressful situation and the physiological and attentional responses to stress. See Chapter 16 for a more detailed account of the stress–injury model.

Personality

An account of the relationship between stress and injury/illness would not be complete without considering personality characteristics. The stress–illness literature identifies many personality variables as moderators in the stress–illness relationship. Some personality characteristics may predispose individuals to perceive fewer situations and events as stressful, or they may predispose individuals to be more susceptible to the effects of stressors such as major life events and daily hassles. Important personality dimensions in relation to the stress–injury model include locus of control, trait anxiety, and achievement motivation.

Locus of control refers to an individual's perception of the extent to which outcomes are within control. For example, a person with a high internal locus of control would perceive that the outcome (injury) is fully within their control. Conversely, someone with a high external locus of control would attribute the outcome (injury) to something outside of their control (e.g., fate or bad luck). In one example of the association between locus of control and injury, Pargman & Lunt (1989) found that injuries were positively correlated with external locus of control in a sample of American football players. More recently, however, Kolt & Kirkby (1996) found no relationship between locus of control and injury in their sample of sub-elite gymnasts, but found that internal locus of control significantly predicted injury in higher-level or elite gymnasts. As there is still a lack of agreement on the link between locus of control and injury in the literature, further research is needed. In relation to illness, it has been shown that people with a higher internal locus of control are more likely to take a more active involvement in their own health (Wallston et al 1983).

Trait anxiety is a behavioral disposition to perceive threatening circumstances, which are objectively not dangerous, and then to respond with disproportionate anxiety. Highly trait-anxious people usually have more state anxiety in highly evaluative situations than people with lower trait anxiety. Researchers using non-specific sport measures have found inconclusive results regarding trait anxiety and the incidence of athletic injury (see Williams & Andersen 1998 for a review). On occasions when researchers used sport-based measurements to assess competitive trait anxiety, athletes who scored high on competitive anxiety had more injuries or more severe injuries (e.g., Lavallee & Flint 1996). In one study, Petrie (1993) found that trait anxiety was positively related to injury rate for football starters but not for non-starters. Furthermore, Petrie (1993) found that competitive trait anxiety moderated the effects of positive life stress such that higher levels of anxiety (when accompanied with positive stress) were associated with more days missed due to injury.

Support also exists for adding mood states to the list of variables that influence injury occurrence. For example, Williams et al (1993) found that athletes who experienced positive states of mind (e.g., keeping relaxed, staying focused) early in the season incurred fewer injuries during their athletic season compared to athletes who had less-positive states of mind. Research also indicates that negative states such as aggression, anger, or dominance relate to injury risk. Van Mechlen et al (1996) determined that more dominant persons (self-reliant) ran a higher risk of sport injury than those who were less dominant, and Thompson & Morris (1994) indicated that high anger directed outwards, but not inward, increased injury risk.

History of stressors

History of stressors includes major life events, daily hassles, and previous injury history. Of these, life event stresses have received the most extensive research. Based on the early work of Holmes & Rahe (1967), Holmes (1970) administered the modified Social Athletic Readjustment Rating Scale (SARRS) to football players at the commencement of a

playing season. He then compared the player's life stress score (life events experienced during the preceding 12 months) to time-loss injury data monitored by athletic trainers throughout the football season. He found that 50% of the athletes who experienced high life stress during the year prior to the football season incurred an athletic injury that required missing at least three days of practice or one game. In comparison, only 9% and 25%, respectively, of athletes with low and moderate levels of life stress experience had equivalent time-loss because of injuries. Holmes (1970) concluded that life stress relates to athletic injuries in much the same ways it does to the occurrence of illness. Since Holmes conducted the first football investigation, at least 35 studies have examined the relationship of life stress to athletic injury (Williams 2001). The vast majority of these studies have found a positive relationship between life stress and injury. The history of stressors portion of the model also includes daily hassles. The stress from many minor daily problems, irritations, or changes may contribute to stress levels and injury risk as much as that encountered from major life event changes. Fawkner et al (1999) found that injured individuals had a significant increase in hassles for the week prior to injury.

Another form of stress is previous injuries. Studies have shown either no relation between previous injury and frequency or severity of injury occurrence (Hanson et al 1992) or a positive correlation between prior injury and subsequent injury (Williams & Andersen 1998).

Coping resources

Coping resources include a wide variety of behaviors and social networks that help the individual deal with the problems, joys, setbacks, and stresses of life. Coping resources may come from the environment (e.g., friends, family) or from personal resources (e.g., social competence, healthy diet). The presence of good coping resources may directly protect the individual against injury, or may attenuate the negative effects of stressors or the effects of personality.

Substantial evidence exists for coping resources either directly affecting injury outcome or moderating the influence life stress has on injury vulnerability. For example, Williams et al (1986) found that the only predictor of injury was the level of coping resources. Hanson et al (1992) continued this line of research and found that coping resources contributed the most in discriminating group differences for both severity and frequency of injuries: the injured people had significantly fewer coping resources than their non-injured counterparts. Social support has also been examined in relation to injury. Some studies have shown that social support directly influences injury risk. That is, those with high levels of social support had a lower incidence of injury, and those with low degrees of social support had more injuries, regardless of life stress (e.g., Hardy et al 1991). Other studies have found that social support moderated the life stress–injury relationship. For instance, Petrie (1992) found that for people with low social support, negative life stress accounted for more variance in injuries than for those with high social support.

In other psychological literature, researchers have examined relationships between different types of antecedents and the onset of psychological illness (e.g., depression). One model that is offered to understand this relationship is the stress and vulnerability model (Wasserman 1999). In relation to Williams & Andersen's (1998) model, the stress and vulnerability model also takes into account genetic and psychosocial inheritance as well as cultural and environmental influences in the onset of psychological illness.

Stressful life events, such as family conflicts, separation, bereavement, somatic illness, and financial problems are common antecedents of psychological illness. The occurrence of stressful life events was investigated among elderly people with potential suicide risk in Sweden, and it was found that somatic illness, family discord, and financial trouble were significant risk factors (Rubenowitz et al 2001). Other risk factors reported in the Rubenowitz et al (2001) study were mental disorder, low level of education, feelings of loneliness, and previous suicides in the family.

PSYCHOSOCIAL FACTORS INFLUENCING HEALTHY AND UNHEALTHY BEHAVIOR

Several theoretical explanations and models capturing various psychosocial antecedents to healthy and unhealthy behaviors have been outlined in the literature. They include attribution theory, explanations around health locus of control, unrealistic optimism, the health belief model, and protection motivation theory. These theories and models are important in order to understand what behaviors could be risk factors for injury and illness development.

ATTRIBUTION THEORY

The origins of attribution theory can be found in the work of Heider (1944), who argued that individuals are motivated to see their social world as predictable and controllable (i.e., a need to understand causality). Since its original formulation, attribution theory has been developed extensively and differentiations have been made between self-attribution (i.e., attributions about one's own behavior) and other attributions (i.e., attributions made about the behavior of others). The dimensions of attributions have been defined as follows:

- Internal versus external (e.g., "my getting sick was due to me not looking after myself" versus "my getting sick was due to that bug going around").
- Stable versus unstable (e.g., "I am always prone to getting sick" versus "I am only sick because of this one incident").
- Global versus specific (e.g., "my getting sick influences other areas of my life" versus "my getting sick only influences this specific aspect of my life").
- Controllable versus uncontrollable (e.g., "my getting sick was controllable by me" versus "my getting sick was uncontrollable by me").

Over recent years, attribution theory has been applied to the study of health and health-related behavior. Herzlich (1973) interviewed 80 people about the general causes of health and illness and found that health was regarded as internal to the individual and illness was seen as something that comes into the body from the external world. King (1982) examined the relationship between attributions for an illness and attendance at a screening clinic for hypertension. The results demonstrated that, if the hypertension was seen as external, but controllable by individuals, then they were more likely to attend the screening clinic.

HEALTH LOCUS OF CONTROL

The internal versus the external dimension of attribution theory has been specifically applied to health in terms of the concept of a health locus of control. Individuals differ as to whether they tend to regard events as controllable by them (an internal locus of control) or uncontrollable by them (an external locus of control). Health locus of control has been shown to be related to whether an individual changes his/her behavior (e.g., gives up smoking). For instance, even if a healthcare practitioner encourages an individual who has a high external locus of control to give up smoking, they are unlikely to comply, as they do not feel responsible for their health.

UNREALISTIC OPTIMISM

Weinstein (1984) suggested that one of the reasons why people continue to practice unhealthy behavior is due to inaccurate perceptions of risk and susceptibility (i.e., their unrealistic optimism). Weinstein (1984) asked participants to examine a list of health problems and to estimate their chances (greater, same, or less) of contracting each of the problems in relation to other people of their age and sex. The results of the study showed that most participants believed that they were less likely to get health problems compared to others. Weinstein (1984) called this phenomenon unrealistic optimism. Weinstein (1987) described four cognitive factors that contribute to unrealistic optimism: (a) a lack of personal experience with the problem, (b) the belief that the problem is preventable by individual action, (c) the belief that if the problem has not yet appeared, it will not appear in the future, and (d) the belief that the problem is infrequent. These factors suggest that the perception of one's own risk is not a rational process.

THE HEALTH BELIEF MODEL

The health belief model, developed by Rosenstock (1966), suggests that behavior is a result of a set of core beliefs. The original core beliefs suggested by Rosenstock (1966) stem from the individual's perceptions of their susceptibility to illness, the severity of illness, the costs involved in carrying out the change in behavior, the health benefits involved in carrying out the behavior, and the cues to action (internal or external).

The health belief model suggests that these core beliefs could be used to predict the likelihood that behavior will occur. Several studies have supported the predictions of the health belief model. Research has shown that dietary compliance, safe sexual practices, having vaccinations, making regular dental visits, and taking part in regular exercise programs are related to the individual's perceptions of susceptibility to related health problems, to their belief that the problem is severe, and to their perception that the benefits of preventive action outweigh the costs (e.g., Becker & Rosenstock 1984).

Other studies, however, have reported conflicting findings. For example, Janz & Becker (1984) found that healthy behavioral intentions were related to low perceived seriousness of health problems. Other studies have suggested an association between perceived low susceptibility to disease and healthy behavior (e.g., Langlie 1977).

PROTECTION MOTIVATION THEORY

The protection motivation theory, developed by Rogers (1985), expanded the health belief model to include additional factors, and suggests that health-related behavior is the product of four components: severity, susceptibility, response effectiveness, and self-efficacy. These components predict behavioral intentions, which are related to behavior. According to protection motivation theory, there are two types of sources of information: environmental (e.g., verbal persuasion, observational learning) and interpersonal (e.g., prior experience). The quality of this information influences the adoption of an "adaptive" coping response (e.g., behavioral intention) or a "maladaptive" coping response (e.g., avoidance).

In one study, Beck & Lund (1981) manipulated dental students' beliefs about tooth decay using persuasive communication. The results showed that the information increased fear, and that perceptions of severity and self-efficacy were related to positive behavioral intentions. The protection motivation theory has been less criticized than the health belief model. Schwarzer (1992), however, criticized the protection motivation model for not explicitly examining behaviors in terms of process and change.

OTHER RESEARCH EXAMPLES

Langius & Björvell (1993) studied coping ability and functional status in a sample of 145 urban-dwelling Swedish people. The researchers used an instrument measuring three aspects of sense of coherence: comprehensibility, manageability, and meaningfulness (Antonovsky 1987). Sense of coherence scores were significantly positively correlated to the overall sickness impact profile scores. That is, people with low sense of coherence scores had poorer health, and those with higher sense of coherence scores had better health. It was also shown that general health was positively correlated to sense of coherence and negatively correlated to dysfunction.

In another study, Steptoe & Wardle (2001a) investigated the relationship between locus of control and health behavior in 4358 female and 2757 male students from 21 different countries in Europe. For five health behaviors, the odds of healthy behavior were more than 40% greater among individuals in the highest versus lowest quartile of internal locus of control. Lack of control was shown to be associated with heightened physiological stress responsivity, poor tolerance of pain, and poor mental health. One of the predictions to emerge from the health locus of control model is that people with a high internal health locus of control will engage in health-promoting activities, whereas the reverse will be true of those with strong beliefs in chance (i.e., high external locus of control).

Jackson et al (2002) conducted a longitudinal study of 198 college students to examine whether pessimistic explanatory style interacts with perceived stress to predict subsequent illness. Their findings confirmed the hypothesis that explanatory style interacts with perceived stress to influence illness risk.

Examining what predicts the onset of illness is important in relation to the development of preventative interventions and strategies. Current thinking points to an interaction among biological, psychological, and situational risk factors. A representative model of these interactive influences is the attribution reformulation of helplessness theory (Peterson & Bossio 2001). According to this theory, stress coupled with pessimistic explanatory styles leads to negative outcomes (including illness) among individuals who are biologically or otherwise at risk. The results from the Jackson et al (2002) study support the prediction of the attribution reformulation of helplessness theory. That is, pessimistic explanatory style interacts with perceived stress to predict subsequent physical illness. Neither perceived stress nor pessimistic attributional style alone predicted subsequent physical illness in the Jackson et al (2002) investigation.

In a subsequent study, Steptoe & Wardle (2001b) investigated health behavior, risk awareness, and emotional well-being in students from Eastern and Western Europe. The results revealed that East European students had less healthy lifestyles than West Europeans according to a composite index of 11 health behaviors. East Europeans were less likely to be aware of the relationship between lifestyle factors and cardiovascular disease risk. In addition, they were more depressed, reported lower social support, and had higher levels of chance and powerful others locus of control.

Health locus of control is a domain-specific control construct that indexes beliefs in different types of means–ends relationship (Skinner 1996). Because it is specific to the domain of health, it may not reflect general perceptions, however, it is particularly relevant to the actions people carry out to maintain health. Analysis of the combined healthy lifestyle index in the Steptoe & Wardle (2001b) study indicated that 47% of East Europeans had healthy lifestyles, compared with 63% of West Europeans. There were striking differences between East and West samples in depressed mood and perceptions of social support.

In a study by Elovainio et al (2001), socioeconomic status, hostility, and health among the Finnish population were investigated. The results showed that men seemed to be more hostile than women, and hostility levels seemed to make men and women vulnerable to different health risks. People with poor economic resources, and who did not feel that they belonged to their family, neighborhood, and/or friends tended to be exceptionally hostile. The results were consistent with the vulnerability model of hostility, which assumes that the health of hostile people is at a greater risk than that of others, at least partly because the coping strategies of hostile persons are less effective in psychosocial stress situations. Hostile women who had experienced many psychosocial risks were at greater risk of a poor state of health than non-hostile women. Hostile men were at greater risk of poor health if they reported that they did not belong to a social network (Elovainio et al 2001).

PRIMARY, SECONDARY, AND TERTIARY ILLNESS AND INJURY PREVENTION

A common way of describing preventive activities is to divide them into primary, secondary, and tertiary prevention. Primary prevention occurs before the onset of a disease or disorder and often involves a population-wide approach. An example is a governmental campaign to increase physical exercise at elementary schools. Secondary prevention involves early intervention with specified risk factors. This could be distribution of smoke detectors to low-income families with young children. Tertiary prevention is prevention in name only (Winett 1995) because it involves improving treatment and restoring function following the initial injury or illness.

PASSIVE VERSUS ACTIVE PREVENTION OF INJURY AND ILLNESS

Another method for categorizing injury prevention is the dichotomization of prevention into active (e.g., wearing a helmet when riding a motorcycle, lights on bicycles when riding, wearing seat belts when driving a car) and passive (e.g., airbags installed on vehicles, noise signals for blind people at crosswalks). The schema of preventive activities is concerned with the extent to which a certain measure requires the active participation of the person in question to have an effect, and the extent to which the measure is built into the environment, having an effect regardless of human activation.

INTERVENTION/PREVENTION METHODS AND RESEARCH TO REDUCE INJURY AND ILLNESS

Several intervention strategies to reduce injury risk have been investigated in both sport and non-sport settings. In relation to sport, Schomer (1990) investigated the effects of associative (monitoring bodily functions and feelings such as heart and breathing rate) versus dissociative thought patterns (distraction and tuning out) on injuries with marathon runners. Schomer (1990) reported an ability to optimize training intensity without increasing injury using associative strategies. The intervention involved shaping associative thought processes over a 5-week training period using audio tapes of attentional strategies. Associative thinking was related to perceptions of increased training effort. Through the use of lightweight recorders worn on the body during training, this study used a simple, yet effective method to shape attentional strategies to produce optimal, injury-free performance.

Davis (1991) used imagery and relaxation with college-level swimmers and football players to reduce injuries. The program was composed of progressive relaxation combined with imagined rehearsal of swimming and football skills and related content during the competitive season. Relaxation instructions usually required 10 minutes and included the guided imagery techniques of Suinn (1982). Davis reported a 52% reduction in swimming injuries and a 33% reduction in football injuries.

Kerr & Gross (1996) conducted a stress-management intervention with 24 elite gymnasts based on Meichenbaum's (1985) stress inoculation training program. The gymnasts were matched into pairs according to sex, age, and performance. One member of each pair was randomly assigned to the intervention group, who received the stress management program. The other member of each pair acted as a control, completing the stress and injury measures, without exposure to the training program. The training consisted of 16 sessions covering skills such as cognitive restructuring, thought control, imagery, and mental rehearsal. The gymnasts were responsible for maintaining training logs that contained homework assignments for the skills in the program. A trend toward significance for reduced injury in the stress management group was reported.

Prevention strategies have also been reported for non-sport injury and illness. Two examples of such studies follow. Each year approximately 2 million people in the US sustain traumatic brain injuries (TBI) and over 10 000 sustain spinal cord injuries (SCI) (Stover et al 1995). In response to the devastating impact of these injuries, more than 200 sites have sponsored the THINK FIRST program. The program is directed towards teenagers and young adults. By using role models who have sustained TBIs or SCIs, the 45–60-minute program stresses "using your mind to protect your body." One of these prevention programs, the Missouri Head and Spinal Cord Injury Prevention Program, has been empirically evaluated. This multicomponent program, based on the health belief model, introduces adolescents to their vulnerability to injury, the injury effects, and educates them about reducing risk and preventing injury. In a follow-up study 3 years after the exposure of the program, students scored significantly higher on measures of knowledge, attitudes, and self-reported safety behavior than students who had never seen the program (Avoli et al 1992). A more rigorous evaluation of the Missouri program used an effective deception method to decrease demand characteristics (Bouman & Frank 1992). It was found (contrary to the hypothesis) that those who viewed the program did not report improved driving habits or increased perceptions of vulnerability to injury. Of note, students at highest risk for injury responded to this educational preventive intervention with the most negative cognitions. This suggests that alternative models that do not rely on traditional educational methods must be considered if high-risk students are going to be influenced.

Psychological distress, including symptoms of depression and anxiety, is an important problem in patients with cardiovascular diseases. Depression has a major impact on mortality, morbidity, and functional recovery in patients with cardiovascular diseases (Hayward 1995). Levels of anxiety in patients after myocardial infarction are also very high. During hospitalization for cardiac events, almost all patients experience significant levels of distress. However, significant levels of anxiety often remain even after the acute crisis resolves. The Taylor et al (1981) study was designed to determine the efficacy of a nurse-case-managed, multifactorial, risk-factor intervention program aimed at reducing distress in patients with myocardial infarction. In the Taylor et al (1981) study, people who were hospitalized for acute myocardial infarction were randomized to receive a nurse-managed, home-based, risk-reduction program or usual care. The program, which began in hospital, included a brief screening for five areas of psychological distress with further evaluation (if indicated), monitoring during the follow-up phone calls, and referral for mental health treatment (if needed). The program included smoking cessation, nutritional counseling, lipid-lowering drug therapy, and exercise training. There was a significant reduction in the psychological distress variables for all patient groups between baseline and 12 months. The program had a significant effect on reducing anxiety in the patient group with frequent episodes of anger, but overall, the treatment and control groups showed equal levels of improvement.

RECOMMENDATIONS FOR HEALTHCARE PRACTITIONERS

Based on the contents of this chapter there are a number of recommendations for healthcare practitioners. First, major life event stress and daily hassles seem to have a direct or indirect effect on injury and illness resiliency and vulnerability. Consequently, it is important to understand the effect of these problems on health outcome. Trying to buffer the effects of life stress or to make the person aware of the relationship is a first major step towards prevention of injury and illness outcome.

The second recommendation is that it is important to recognize the effect that some personality variables seem to have on injury and illness outcome. People with high trait anxiety, external locus of control, pessimistic lifestyles, chronically low

moods, and aggressive behaviors seem to be at greatest risk.

The third point of interest is that coping resources have either a direct effect on illness and injury outcome or seem to moderate the influence life stress has on illness and injury vulnerability. For healthcare practitioners, it is central to be aware that low or restricted amounts of coping resources seem to be related to elevated risks of developing somatic problems. This is especially evident in combination with people who report low levels of social support.

For people with a potentially high risk of becoming ill or injured, some methods and techniques could be used in order to prevent negative outcomes. These include somatic relaxation techniques focusing on breathing and/or progressive muscle relaxation, and general stress management training such as thought control and cognitive restructuring.

SUMMARY

In Western society injuries and coronary heart diseases are some of the leading causes for hospitalization. Although the largest cost for society is in terms of human suffering and loss, the financial cost of such conditions is huge and is steadily increasing. In injury prevention, one of the first steps is to view the injury as preventable. In order to do this it is important to know more about research linking controllable and external factors to the occurrence of injury and illness. Relationships between major life events and illness outcome have been documented. Minor stressors, such as daily hassles have high predictive power for injury and illness risk. A conceptually well-organized framework describing potential psychosocial antecedents leading to injury is described by Williams & Andersen (1998). This model suggests that when a potential stressful situation occurs, the person's personality, history of stressors, and coping resources affect their stress response and injury risk. Even though it is a complicated task to test the whole model, the three interrelated variables have generated substantial support for the utility of the model. Furthermore, the chapter reviewed other models related to predicting healthy and unhealthy behaviors. The role of health beliefs in predicting health-related behaviors has become increasingly salient in injury and illness research. Theories such as attribution theory, health locus of control, unrealistic optimism, health belief models, and protection motivation theory have been adapted to examine beliefs about health and resulting risky behaviors and responses. The models can be used to predict health behaviors and have implications for developing methods to promote change.

A common way of describing preventive activities is to divide them into primary (before the onset of disease), secondary (early intervention) and tertiary prevention (improving treatment following the initial injury). Another method is to classify them as active and passive into the activity level that is required of the individual. Typical psychological intervention methods for reducing injury and illness involve using imagery, stress management (e.g., thought control, somatic relaxation) and cognitive restructuring. Evidence shows that stress management techniques seem to have the potential to buffer stressors influencing injury and illness outcome.

References

Antonovsky A 1987 Unravelling the mystery of health: How people manage stress and stay well. Jossey-Bass, San Francisco

Avolio A E C, Ramsey F L, Neuwelt E A 1992 Evaluation of a program to prevent head and spinal cord injuries: A comparison between middle school and high school. Neurosurgery 31: 557–562

Beck K H, Lund A K 1981 The effects of health threat seriousness and personal efficacy upon intentions and behavior. Journal of Applied Social Psychology 11: 401–415

Becker M H, Rosenstock I M 1984 Compliance with medical advice. In: Steptoe A, Mathews A (eds) Health care and human behavior. Academic Press, London

Bouman D E, Frank R G 1992 Examination of traumatic injury prevention program: Adolescent's reactions and program efficacy. Paper presented at the 100th Annual Convention of the American Psychological Association, Washington, DC

Davis J O 1991 Sport injuries and stress management. An opportunity for research. The Sport Psychologist 5: 175–182

DeLongis A, Coyne J C, Dakof S et al 1982 Relationship of daily hassles, uplifts, and major life events to health status. Health Psychology 1: 119–136

Elovainio M, Kivimäki M, Kortteinen H et al 2001 Socio-economic status, hostility and health. Personality and Individual Differences 31: 303–315

Fawkner H J, McMurray N, Summer J J 1999 Athletic injury and minor life events: A prospective study. Journal of Science and Medicine in Sport 2(2): 117–124

Fowler R D 1990 Psychology: The core discipline. American Psychologist 45: 1–6

Hanson S J, McCullagh P, Tonymon P 1992 The relationship of personality characteristics, life stress, and coping resources to athletic injury. Journal of Sport & Exercise Psychology 14: 262–272

Hardy C J, Richman J M, Rosenfeld L B 1991 The role of social support in the life stress/injury relationship. The Sport Psychologist 5: 128–139

Hayward C 1995 Psychiatric illness and cardiovascular disease risk. Epidemiology Review 17: 129–138

Heider F 1944 Social perception and phenomenal causality. Psychological Review 51: 358–374

Herzlich C 1973 Health and illness. Academic Press, London

Holmes T H 1970 Psychological screening. In: Football injuries: Paper presented at a workshop. Sponsored by Sub-committee on Athletic Injuries, Committee on the Skeletal System, Division of Medical Science, National Research Council, February 1969. Washington, DC: National Academy of Science, p 211–214

Holmes T H, Rahe R J 1967 The Social Readjustment Rating Scale. Journal of Psychosomatic Research 11: 213–218

Jackson B, Sellers R M, Peterson C 2002 Pessimistic explanatory style moderates the effects of stress on physical illness. Personality and Individual Differences 32: 567–573

Janz N K, Becker M H 1984 The health belief model: A decade later. Health Education Quarterly 11: 1–47

Kanner A D, Coyne J C, Schaefer C et al 1981 Comparison of two modes of stress management: Daily hassles and uplifts versus major life events. Journal of Behavioral Medicine 4: 1–39

Kerr G, Gross J 1996 The effects of a stress management program on injuries and stress levels. Journal of Applied Sport Psychology 8: 109–117

King J B 1982 The impact of patient's perceptions of high blood pressure on attendance at screening: An attributional extension of the health belief model. Social Science and Medicine 16: 1079–1092

Kolt G S, Kirkby R J 1996 Injury in Australian female competitive gymnasts: A psychological perspective. Australian Journal of Physiotherapy 42: 121–126

Langius A, Björvell H 1993 Coping ability and functional status in a Swedish population sample. Scandinavian Journal of Caring Science 7: 3–10

Langlie J K 1977 Social network, health beliefs, and preventative health behavior. Journal of Health and Social Behavior 18: 244–260

Lavallee L, Flint F 1996 The relationship of stress, competitive anxiety, mood state, and social support to athletic injury. Journal of Athletic Training 31: 296–299

Meichenbaum D 1985 Stress inoculation training. Pergamon Press, New York

National Center for Injury Prevention and Control 1996 Major causes of unintentional injuries among older persons: An annotated bibliography. Center of Disease Control and Prevention, Atlanta, GA

Pargman D, Lunt S D 1989 The relationship of self-concept and locus of control to the severity of injury in freshman collegiate football players. Sports Medicine, Training and Rehabilitation 1: 201–208

Peterson C, Bossio L M 2001 Optimism and physical well-being. In: Chang E C (ed) Optimism and pessimism: Implication for theory, research, and practice. American Psychological Association, Washington, DC, p 127–145

Petrie T A 1992 Psychosocial antecedents of athletic injury: The effects of life stress and social support on female collegiate gymnasts. Behavioral Medicine 18: 127–138

Petrie T A 1993 Coping skills, competitive trait anxiety, and playing status: Moderating effects of the life stress–injury relationships. Journal of Sport & Exercise Psychology 5: 1–16

Rabkin J G, Struening E L 1976 Life events, stress, and illness. Science 194: 1013–1020

Rahe R, Arthur R J 1978 Life changes and illness studies: Past history and future directions. Journal of Human Stress 4: 3–15

Rahe R, McKean J, Arthur R J 1967 A longitudinal study of life changes and illness patterns. Journal of Psychosomatic Research 10: 355–366

Rodriguez J G 1990 Childhood injuries in the United States: A priority issue. American Journal of Diseases of Children 144: 625–626

Rogers R W 1985 Attitude change and information integration in fear appeals. Psychological Reports 56: 179–182

Rosenstock I M 1966 Why people use health services. Milbank Memorial Fund Quarterly 44: 94–127

Rubenowitz E, Waern M, Wilhelmson K et al 2001 Life events and psychosocial factors in elderly suicides: A case–control study. Psychological Medicine 31(7): 1193–1202

Savery L K, Wooden M 1994 The relative influence of life events and hassles on work-related injuries: Some Australian evidence. Human Relations 47: 283–305

Schomer H H 1990 A cognitive strategy training program for marathon runners: Ten case studies. South African Journal of Research in Sport, Physical Education and Recreation 13: 47–78

Schwartzer R 1992 Self-efficacy in the adoption and maintenance of health behaviors: Theoretical approaches and new model. In: Schwarzer R (ed) Self-efficacy: Thought control of action. Hemisphere, Washington, DC, p 217–243

Skinner E A 1996 A guide to constructs of control. Journal of Personality and Social Psychology 71: 549–570

Socialstyrelsen 2001 Folkhälsorapport. Epidemiologiskt Centrum, Stockholm, Sweden

Steptoe A, Wardle J 2001a Locus of control and health behavior revisited: A multivariate analysis of young adults from 18 countries. British Journal of Psychology 92: 659–672

Steptoe A, Wardle J 2001b Health behavior, risk awareness and emotional well-being in students from Eastern Europe and Western Europe. Social Science & Medicine 53: 1621–1630

Stover S L, DeLisa J A, Whiteneck G M 1995 Spinal cord injury: Clinical outcomes from the model systems. Aspen, Gaithersburg, MD

Suinn R M 1982 Imagery and sport. In: Sheikh A (ed) Imagery, current theory, research and application. John Wiley, New York, p 507–534

Taylor C D, DeBusk R F, Davidson D M et al 1981 Optimal methods for identifying depression following hospitalization for myocardial infarction. Journal of Chronic Disease 34: 1–7

Thompson N J, Morris R D 1994 Predicting injury risks in adolescent football players: The importance of psychological variables. Journal of Pediatric Psychology 19: 415–429

Van Mechlen W, Twisk J, Molendiijk A et al 1996 Subject-related risk factors for sport injuries: A 1-year prospective study in young adults. Medicine and Science in Sports and Exercise 28: 1171–1179

Wallston K A, Smith R A, King J E et al 1983 Expectancies about control over health: Relationship to desire for control of health care. Journal of Personality and Social Psychology 9: 377–385

Wasserman D 1999 Depression en vanlig sjukdom. Natur och Kultur, Stockholm, Sweden

Weinstein N 1984 Why it won't happen to me: Perceptions of risk factors and susceptibility. Health Psychology 3: 431–457

Weinstein N 1987 Unrealistic optimism about illness susceptibility: Conclusions from a community-wide sample. Journal of Behavioral Medicine 10: 481–500

Williams J M (2001) Psychology of injury risk and prevention. In: Singer R N, Hausenblas H A, Janelle C M (eds) Handbook of sport psychology, 2nd edn. John Wiley, New York, p 766–786

Williams J M, Andersen M B 1998 Psychosocial antecedents of sport injury: Review and critique of the stress and injury model. Journal of Applied Sport Psychology 10: 5–25

Williams J M, Haggert J, Tonymon P et al (1986) Life stress and prediction of athletic injuries in volleyball, basketball, and cross-country running. In: Unestähl L-E (ed) Sport psychology in theory and practice. Örebro, Veje, Sweden

Williams J M, Hogan T D, Andersen M B 1993 Positive states of mind and athletic injury risk. Psychosomatic Medicine 55: 468–472

Winett R A 1995 A framework for health promotion and diseases prevention programs. American Psychologist 50: 341–350

Chapter 3

Psychological responses to injury and illness

Diane M. Wiese-Bjornstal

INTRODUCTION

Although people do not always have a choice as to whether or not they require physical or manual therapy to aid in the treatment of an injury or illness, they do have some control over how they psychologically respond to, cope with, and manage the course of the illness/injury and associated therapy. Psychological responses comprise full spectrums of both personal and social responses. Coping involves a broad range of styles, strategies, and mechanisms by which people psychologically adjust to challenging events in their lives. Psychological factors can (a) contribute to the onset of physical illness and injury, (b) contribute to the maintenance of the illness or injury state, and (c) serve as secondary reactions and responses to the onset of injury and illness. This chapter focuses on (b) and (c) as they relate to those seeing physical or manual therapists for treatment. Understanding the broad array of ways in which individuals respond to illness and injury situations, as well as to their prescribed courses of treatment and rehabilitation, will enhance the work of those in the physical and manual therapies by allowing them to accommodate and empathize with those responses that they are unable to change, and to serve as more active agents in enhancing adaptation and changing some of the maladaptive psychological responses of clients.

PSYCHOSOCIAL RESPONSES TO INJURY AND ILLNESS

To provide an overall context, or framework, for understanding the variety of psychological responses to injury and illness, several psychosocial models of response to health events are first described and then integrated into an overarching model of psychological adjustment. Next, some of the most relevant psychological and social components are more fully developed in the context of illness and injury as they relate to the work of physical and manual therapists. Throughout the chapter, suggestions are offered for physical and manual therapists regarding their roles in managing the psychological responses of their clients.

MODELS OF RESPONSE TO INJURY AND ILLNESS

The following brief descriptions of conceptual approaches and models provide snapshot views of the ways in which the individual experience of a medical event might be better understood within the overall context of a person's life. This section concludes with a practical, conceptual model outlining a framework for understanding psychological responses to injury and illness in a way that is relevant for the work of physical and manual therapists.

The biopsychosocial approach

A comprehensive systems approach to understanding health that incorporates the intersection of the biological, psychological, and social components of a person's being (Engel 1977, 1980) provides an overarching context within which to understand psychological responses to medical events. These three components all affect and are affected by a person's health. The biological component includes such elements as genetically inherited characteris-

tics and a person's physiological functioning. The psychological component involves the influential role of mental processes and behavior, such as cognition, emotion, and motivation. The social component encompasses the influences of one's family, community, culture, and society on health. These three major components are a part of a person's health system, which is a dynamic and constantly changing state of affairs. Within the context of this overall approach, it is apparent that in order to understand psychological responses to injury and illness one must also view the broader context of the person's life and their biological capacities and limitations.

Crisis theory

Another model with application toward understanding psychosocial responses to injury and illness is crisis theory (Moos & Shaefer 1984). Developed to explore the context of chronic illness, the theory "deals with the impact of disruptions on established patterns of personal and social functioning" (Brannon & Feist 2000, p 295). In the case of serious, chronic illnesses or injuries that present crisis experiences to be dealt with, not only must people adjust to the symptoms, limitations, and challenges of the illnesses or injuries themselves, but they also must adjust to often radical changes in other areas of their lives. Thus, new coping patterns must be learned to manage the novel crisis experiences.

Psychological responses to the changes imposed by a crisis vary on a continuum ranging from healthy adjustment to unhealthy maladjustment. The intrusiveness of psychological symptoms and their effects on overall health and rehabilitation can vary in frequency, intensity, and duration, which consequently indicate the degree of psychological adjustment difficulty. In turn, the nature and degree of difficulty indicate the type of intervention that would be beneficial.

Cognitive–behavioral models

Behavioral models of psychology suggest that actions or behaviors – both adaptive and maladaptive – are developed and maintained through conditioning and social learning processes. In other words, behaviors are reinforced via the consequences that follow them. Cognitive models focus on the mediating role that thoughts play; within these models cognitive interpretations of the meaning and salience of events affect subsequent behaviors. Recent psychological models have incorporated both the roles of cognitions and behavioral learning principles in understanding affective experiences and overt behaviors. They also reflect the social dimension in that affective and behavioral responses can be learned and interpreted through observations of others (i.e., vicariously) via the principles of social learning (Bandura 1986).

Recent interpretations of social learning/social cognitive theory highlight the importance of perceived control as central to the determination of responses. A perceived capacity to exercise control over destinies is known as human agency (Bandura 2000). In the case of a person's experience during a medical event, for example, agency and control can be reflected in each of the following ways: (a) by self, individual clients serving as active agents in determining their own self-regulation and quality of functioning; (b) by proxy, other individuals such as the therapist serving as agents for the individual client in achieving their best health interests; and (c) by society, socially coordinated and interdependent efforts such as those achieved through healthcare systems exercising collective agency toward achieving the optimal outcomes for individual clients.

STRESS PROCESS MODELS AND COPING THEORY

Stress process models – such as those based on the constructs of Lazarus & Folkman (1984) – present more specific cognitive appraisal-based models that can guide therapists in better understanding, and in turn managing, the psychological adjustments of their clients. Such cognitive-behavior and stress process models have been identified relative to various medical conditions such as lower back pain (Truchon 2001), sport injury (Wiese-Bjornstal et al 1998), and chronic pain (Turk & Okifuji 2002). These models illustrate that the occurrence of a potential stressor, such as a medical event, leads to a dynamic and temporally ongoing process of cognitive appraisals, affecting emotional responses, and leading to behavioral responses and choices.

The writings of Lazarus & Folkman (1984) and the theory of coping and adaptation (Lazarus 1993) suggest that individuals' primary perceptions and appraisals of a situation (perceiving an event as a challenge, a threat, or as harmful) affect secondary or subsequent appraisals of the resources available to meet the situational demands, and the usefulness of various possible coping strategies. In turn, these secondary appraisals lead to behavioral choices

about which coping strategies to employ. For example, by understanding beliefs about the effectiveness of certain coping strategies the therapist might play a role in changing erroneous beliefs (e.g., the belief among many with chronic fatigue syndrome that physical activity avoidance is a useful way to stave off further fatigue, Ax et al 2001) or in offering additional coping strategies for consideration (e.g., suggesting that the client engage in gradually increasing modest physical activity levels during episodes of chronic pain flare-up or chronic fatigue). These approaches may lead to the clients' selection of effective coping strategies that enhance, rather than detract from, their physical and mental recoveries.

A psychosocial model of response to injury and illness

Taking the broad view of seeing the medical event of injury or illness and the corresponding rehabilitation or recovery process as a stressor somewhere along a continuum – be it a minor life event level stressor or a crisis level stressor as illustrated in Figure 3.1 – helps in considering the ways in which pre-existing dispositions, thought patterns, emotional styles, and behavioral tendencies affect adaptation to medical events. Stressors are stimuli, defined as "physically or psychologically challenging events or circumstances" (Sarafino 2002, p 70). Some of the stressors that may face clients appearing for physical or manual therapy include functional impairment, dependency on others, or uncertainty about a prognosis. The consequence of stressors can be strain, defined as "psychological and physiological responses to a stressor" (Sarafino 2002, p 70). The strain that results from these stressors, such as fear, anxiety, or depression, is affected by clients' pre-existing status and dispositions and their interpretation of the meaning of the stressors for their lives. Stressors and strains are part of a process of adjustment in which "a person is an active agent who can influence the impact/strain of a stressor through behavioral, cognitive, and emotional strategies" (Sarafino 2002, p 70, based on Lazarus 1999).

Sequentially, then, clients engage in ongoing cycles of adjustment through which they manage these strains. These cycles involve cognitive appraisals and emotional and behavioral responses, and are reflected in the dynamic model illustrated in Figure 3.2. As they engage in more positive or helpful attempts to cope with strains, they will spiral (Gavin & Taylor 1992) upward toward

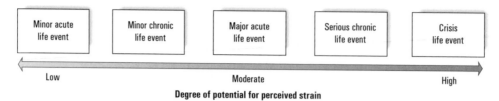

Figure 3.1   Continuum of potential for psychological strain based on the magnitude of the stressor(s)

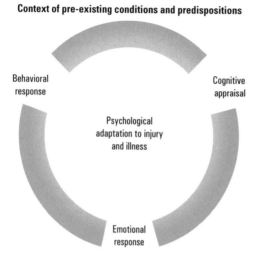

Figure 3.2   Dynamic model of psychological response and adjustment to injury and illness

positive adjustment; with more negative or detrimental approaches toward coping they may spiral downward toward maladjustment. In a manner something like that of a Slinky® toy, they will also likely oscillate over time in both upward and downward cycles (Wiese-Bjornstal, 2003). Temporally, there are immediate reactions to health stressors, which imply unconscious, subconscious, or defensive responses at the time of health events, as well as more long-term process-oriented reactions to health stressors, which imply purposeful and effortful cognitive, emotional, and behavioral responses to ongoing health challenges (see Figure 3.3).

In turn, these factors determine the additional ways in which physical or manual therapists may be of assistance, both within the context of the way they do their own jobs as well as within the context of providing referrals to other health resources as needed for help beyond what would fall within the purview of the therapist's expertise. Such assistance in managing the psychological and social consequences of stressor perceptions benefits clients both

mentally and physically. Research indicates, for example, that because perceptions of greater stressors and strains impair the functioning of the immune system and slow recoveries, physical healing can be improved by reducing stressor perceptions and strain responses (Kiecolt-Glaser et al 2002). Perceptions of stress and strain also impair the cognitive and emotional functioning of clients and delay their ability to psychologically adjust to, and manage, their injury or illness, and negatively affect their quality of life.

In sum, these various models provide the therapist with an understanding of the overall process of responding and adjusting to the stresses and strains of health events. The subsequent discussion provides an overview of the contextual factors also influencing the response choices of clients.

PRE-EXISTING FACTORS INFLUENCING PSYCHOLOGICAL RESPONSE

People enter into a medical event with both personal dispositions and tendencies and social characteristics, which at minimum continue undisrupted through the medical event or which may be exacerbated or magnified in intensity via the experiences of the medical event. The following discussion briefly highlights some of these dispositions, tendencies, and characteristics.

PERSONALITY AND DISPOSITIONAL TENDENCIES

Although recent research indicates that personality can and does evolve over the course of a lifetime, within the window of time encompassing most discrete encounters with a medical event one's basic personality typically remains relatively stable. An understanding of personality and dispositional tendencies helps the therapist better interpret the client's responses to treatment.

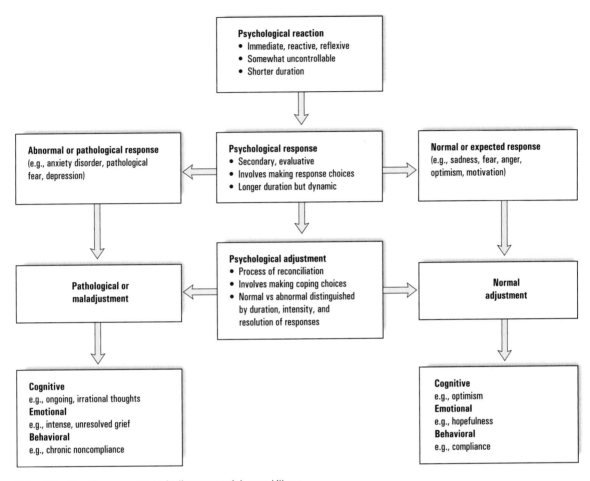

Figure 3.3   Reaction, response, and adjustment to injury and illness

Personality

Individuals bring to a medical event certain unique predisposing personality styles that influence their psychological adaptation to the event (Radnitz et al 2000). These personality styles might be of the kinds that benefit adaptation, or they may be of the sort that leads toward reducing the adaptability or resilience of the client. The consequent effect of these characteristics is also determined by the current condition of the person's overall life in the broader social context. These personality dispositions create the personal context within which later cognitive, emotional, and behavioral responses can be better understood.

Existing psychopathology

A significant number of people seeking physical therapy services have extensive medical histories, including existing psychopathologies such as depression (Boissonnault 1999). These histories and conditions influence their psychological and behavioral management of the presenting medical event. Psychoneuroimmunology studies have demonstrated that existing psychopathologies such as depressive and anxiety disorders can provoke immune system alterations and dysregulations, which in turn affect physical health and healing (Kiecolt-Glaser et al 2002). Existing psychological problems such as anxiety disorders may play a role in the development or exacerbation of chronic pain (Vendrig 2000). Implications for therapists include the importance of becoming familiar with broader medical histories and conditions of clients, having suitable resource and referral networks of mental health professionals in place, and using team approaches to coordinate and manage client care.

Coping dispositional style

Coping involves cognitive, emotional, and behavioral efforts to manage stressful events and the associated psychological strain. Individuals can cope by minimizing, avoiding, tolerating, or accepting the situation. Coping has a trait-like dimension, in that individuals tend to be more easily disposed toward certain preferred strategies and have somewhat consistent dispositional tendencies toward coping strategy choices when coping with a particular type of stressor. The two general dimensions of coping include approach, or monitoring, and avoidance, or blunting. Approach coping occurs via sensory vigilance (having a ruminative focus on the stressor; maintaining attentional and cognitive focus on the source in an attempt to emotionally process the event) and active information seeking (being proactive and problem solving, such as asking questions, talking with other people about the stressor, consulting other information sources) (Bijttebier et al 2001). Avoidance coping occurs by escaping or absenting oneself psychologically or physically from the stressor, or by blunting oneself from having to deal with the stressor head on. Some forms of blunting imply intentional choices and purposeful behavior, such as intentionally distracting oneself from thinking about an injury, whereas others are thought to involve more defensive or unconscious processes, such as denying one's injury (Bijttebier et al 2001).

Anxiety sensitivity

A dispositional tendency to fear the symptoms of anxiety because of a fear of the associated negative consequences of such symptoms has been termed "anxiety sensitivity." These harmful negative anxiety consequences might include anticipated psychological (e.g., inability to concentrate and forgetfulness), social (e.g., humiliation due to flushing of the cheeks), or somatic (e.g., an upset stomach) consequences. Higher anxiety sensitivity plays a role in the fear and avoidance responses of chronic musculoskeletal pain clients, such that they are more likely to experience pain-related fear, negative affect, and avoidance behavior; in addition they report greater use of analgesic medication (Amundson et al 1999).

COGNITIVE-DEVELOPMENTAL LEVEL

Children and adults are different in many ways that relate to their psychological responses to injury and illness, such as their cognitive-developmental level (Wiese-Bjornstal 2003). Children's conceptions of illness and the associated treatments, for example, are not necessarily simpler versions of adult conceptions (Brannon & Feist 2000, Hansdottir & Malcarne 1998, Kalish 1996). Children's early, unpleasant experiences with medical treatment may be cognitively and emotionally generalized to future interactions with the medical system (Dahlquist et al 1986). Younger children may also have misconceptions about their health problems and why things happen. For example, sustaining illness or injury might be viewed as punishment for something they have done, or they might think that having to go to therapy for treatment is a punishment for being bad. Younger persons in general have more immediate, current concerns about their health, such as how they feel right now and whether their activities are impaired. Older persons are concerned with current difficulties but also express greater concern for their future health and lifestyles.

GOAL ORIENTATIONS AND MOTIVES

The reasons or motives that people have for engaging in their life activities can affect their adjustment to health events. For example, people who are highly motivated toward maximum achievement in their professions or who are exclusively focused on specific goals in life might be more traumatized by injuries that impede their progress than those who have more broad-based motives about their work and feel that they would also be happy engaging in alternate forms of employment if necessary. Understanding the goals and motivations of clients might help the therapist better empathize with their responses when injured or ill.

SOCIOCULTURAL FACTORS

In the broader context of people's lives, normative expectations affect both their responses and behavioral choices. For example, in the time-pressed American culture people often show up for work even when ill with something transmittable, almost assuring that whatever it is that they have will be passed along to others. People simply feel that things cannot go on properly without them being there, believe the corporate or work culture in which they are employed demands they be at work regardless of uncontrollable events like illness, or find their life circumstances such that they cannot take time off from their other responsibilities, such as caring for their own families. Within the context of physical activity and sport, for example, the prevailing normative ethic is that in order to be a true athlete, continued participation in exercise sessions or sporting pursuits is necessary even when injured or ill. One who chooses to rest in order to allow recovery is considered undisciplined, undedicated, or weak. This climate may exist in employment situations as well. Conversely, there may be incentives in the work environment that reward people for resting beyond that which might be needed; for example, studies of workmen's compensation situations have found that when factors such as pending litigation and ongoing financial gain without working exist, then the injured person may be likely to return to work more slowly.

SPECIFIC PSYCHOLOGICAL RESPONSES TO INJURY AND ILLNESS

Having highlighted some of the pre-existing conditions and dispositions of clients that influence their responses to injury or illness, the next section contains a description of some of the common cognitive, emotional, and behavioral responses observed in medical illness or injury situations as they might be encountered by a physical or manual therapist (Rusch et al 2002). Figure 3.4 provides an overall example for a chronic pain client of how the complex system of interrelated personal and situational factors might fit together in the context of a medical experience.

COGNITIVE APPRAISAL AND RESPONSES

As discussed earlier, a client's assessment of a stressful situation (cognitive appraisal of the meaning of the situation for personal well-being) results in initial cognitive reactions to a medical event, and secondary cognitive responses to the diagnosis, treatment, and rehabilitation of the medical problem. Perceptions of stress can impair cognitive functioning; the cognitive appraisal in turn affects emotional responses, physiological reactions, and behavioral choices. The general view at present is that cognitions and emotions are closely interwoven, and their separation for purposes of this chapter is somewhat arbitrary, but it is done with the purpose of helping therapists understand the contributions of both.

Identity

Before the occurrence of a medical event, individuals have established identities relative to their roles in such areas as the workplace, home life, parenting or other caretaking responsibilities, and leisure activities such as sport, travel, or music. In addition to disrupting their personal lives, a medical event disrupts identities in other ways, such as by limiting their ability to do their jobs or earn a living, take care of others for whom they feel responsible, or engage in valued leisure activities. Beyond disrupting these important roles, medical events may threaten their very identities, particularly for those who define themselves by the things that they can physically do. When valued things can no longer be done core identities are shaken. This can lead to significant psychological distress in the absence of strong self-perceptions that are not reliant upon the ability to do things, but rather that rely on who one is (i.e., one's personality, character, and spirit) as the basis for identity. The therapist's role might be to reaffirm admired qualities in their clients.

Coping

The coping process involves managing the perceived discrepancy between the demands of a situation and the available personal and social resources. Cognitions play an important role in appraising, responding to, and making choices about how to cope with the situation. Experiential, sociocultural, and gender influences are apparent in the selection of coping styles. The general research findings have been that individuals use a wide variety of coping strategies to manage life events, and methods of coping may differ under short-term versus long-term events. Coping strategies are not inherently adaptive or maladaptive (Lazarus 1993), but their effectiveness varies based on the individual and the situation. Table 3.1 provides a very broad overview of some of the coping strategies that are employed by clients in medical situations. A general indication of the cognitive, emotional, and/or behavioral goal of the strategy is also described.

While reinforcing that there is individual variability in the use and efficacy of these coping strategies, some specific medical research has suggested that there may be desirable or undesirable medical consequences associated with specific strategy use. For example, a strategy of denial, defined as a refusal to believe in or act upon the existence or seriousness of the illness, was associated with greater

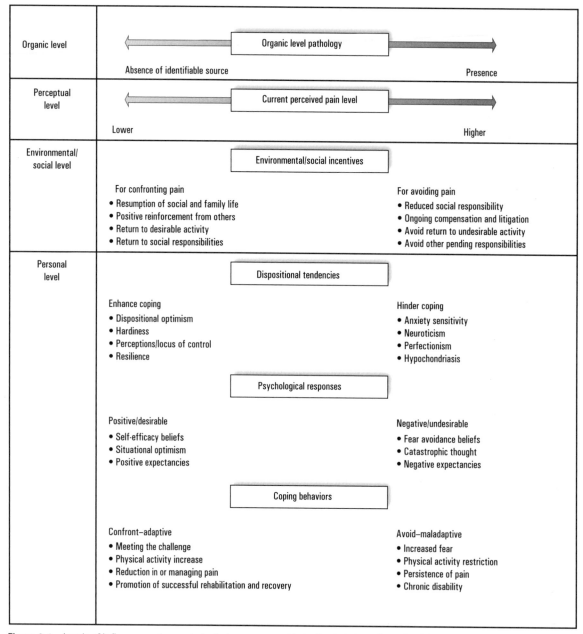

Figure 3.4 Levels of influence on the psychological responses and behavioral choices of people with chronic pain

disruption in social relationships and greater perceived illness burden among clients with chronic fatigue syndrome (Ax et al 2001). Coping strategies have also been found to be related to immunological consequences. In particular, the use of repression, denial, escape-avoidance, and concealment strategies in coping with a medical event have been found to disadvantage immunity (Kiecolt-Glaser et al 2002). Strategies such as positive reappraisal and social support engagement have, in general, been

found to be related to psychological well-being (Ax et al 2001).

One type of dysfunctional pain coping deserves mention at this point relative to its specific occurrence in the types of medical situations seen by physical and manual therapists. Cognitions and the associated emotions involving an "exaggerated negative appraisal of pain sensations" have been labeled "catastrophizing" (Sullivan et al 2000); the interrelated dimensions of which are the tendency toward

Table 3.1   Some common coping strategies in medical situations

Coping strategy	Description	What's the person trying to do?
Comparing with something worse Downward comparison	Compare a stressful medical event with a worse outcome of the accident, with a worse situation when the accident took place, or with a person who is worse off than oneself	Cognitively alter the meaning of the situation to make it seem less stressful or to put it in context
Positive thinking Positive framing Positive reappraisal Comforting self-talk	Focus on real or imagined positive aspects of the problem or focus on positive benefits that might accrue via one's experience of the situation	Cognitively reduce the degree of threat presented by the situation, by viewing situation as a challenge rather than as a threat; construing a stressful encounter in positive terms
Distancing Disengagement Escape-avoidance	Keeping problems at a distance; avoiding immediate response threat	Cognitively using a strategy to avoid the immediacy of the threat; behaviorally distancing oneself
Distracting attention Behavioral distraction Cognitive distraction Social diversion	Divert attention from the problem; keeping busy with other cognitive and behavioral activities	Cognitively and behaviorally distracting oneself in order to minimize and manage negative emotions
Accepting the situation	Trying to make the best of the situation	Cognitively accepting what has happened and seeing what positives might come out of the situation
Seeking social support	Manage emotional and tangible problems by relying on help from others	Cognitively believing that help is available if needed; behaviorally actually requesting and receiving help from others
Maintaining control Sense of control Capacity Relying on personal capacity	Keeping a sense of one's own capacity to manage problems; using tangible strategies for eliminating problems posed by physical limitations Strong belief or efficacy in one's own capacity to manage difficult situations	Cognitively feeling in control by behaviorally doing things for oneself as much as able; behaviorally doing things for oneself by adapting strategies and supplies as needed to accommodate physical limitations Cognitively reinforcing their own mental toughness or control over their responses
Direct tension reduction Pain-relieving actions	Using symptom-directed strategies to moderate distress Taking painkillers, massage or elevation of injured part Distracting attention from pain	Behaviorally relying on substance use Behaviorally or cognitively managing pain
Active processing of the situation in which injury or illness occurred	Trying to find an explanation for why it happened; revisiting the location of the injury occurrence; analyzing the situation	Cognitively put one's mind more at ease about what happened and why it happened (perceived cause)
Unconscious self-deception Ilusion Positive self-assessments	Unrealistic assessments or evaluations of the injury or illness; overly optimistic self-assessments	Cognitively holding beliefs that serve the purpose of maintaining personal well-being and hope
Devices and tricks Concealment Repression	Conscious or subconscious attempts to hide, repress, and trick oneself and others into thinking that there is no problem	Cognitive and emotional self-protection

Continued

Table 3.1 Some common coping strategies in medical situations — cont'd

Coping strategy	Description	What's the person trying to do?
Denial Behavioral avoidance Cognitive avoidance	Refusal to believe in or act upon the existence or seriousness of the illness or injury	Cognitively denying the injury or illness; behaviorally continuing to do everything that one did before as if not injured/ill

Based on information derived from Ax et al 2001, Gustafsson et al 2002, Hadjistavropoulos et al 1999, Hadjistavropoulos et al 1998, Kiecolt-Glaser et al 2002, Sarafino 2002, Smith et al 1990b.

undue focus on pain sensations, magnification of the threat of pain sensations, and a perceived powerlessness to control one's pain intensity. Catastrophizing has been found to be predictive of pain perception and emotional distress (Severeijns et al 2001, Sullivan et al 2000), such as more overt pain behavior, pain-related disability, and use of pain medications (Keefe et al 2001). These overt displays of catastrophizing may be intended as a means by which to communicate emotional need and desire for support from others (Keefe et al 2001).

Cognitive perceptions of the effectiveness of certain coping strategies are related to coping behaviors and choices. The implication, again, is that one area of intervention would be to identify irrational beliefs about the effectiveness of certain techniques. Clients are likely to be more willing to employ coping strategies that they perceive to be effective. As discussed earlier, the effectiveness of different strategies varies based on the person, situation, and medical event, so it advantages therapists to familiarize themselves with a broad range of coping strategies and choices to offer to clients stuck in the rut of relying on their perhaps ineffective dispositional coping tendencies. Coping strategies can be adjusted to the individual client, and result in the client being an active collaborator, which results in greater perceptions of agency or control. Responses to injury/illness are a dynamic process and different coping strategies and efforts are needed at varying points in the temporal process of recovery and rehabilitation.

Optimism/pessimism

Having optimistic views of life, holding positive expectancies, and behaving in positive ways have beneficial implications for both physical and mental health and well-being. Optimism, a tendency toward focusing on the positive features in life, involves using more active coping strategies and asserting more control over difficult circumstances. Physically, an optimistic state is linked to better immune system functioning, faster recoveries from surgery, and less frequent re-hospitalizations following medical procedures (Mahler & Kulik 2000). Optimism and pessimism (defined as a negative bias in perceptions and expectations) should be considered not as functional opposites but as separate constructs. In a study of older coronary bypass surgery clients, for example, it was found that lack of pessimism was more predictive of positive affect, pain, and functional status over time than was optimism (Mahler & Kulik 2000). These authors also implied a dynamic nature to this relationship in finding that the roles of optimism and pessimism may be different at different points during the recovery process.

Unrealistic optimism can potentially be a danger to health. This might occur, for example, when unrealistically optimistic individuals underestimate their chances of suffering negative consequences, and thus, become less concerned about taking actions to prevent them; the thought is "it won't happen to me." For example, an unrealistically optimistic athlete might not believe she is in danger of more permanent injury by continuing to play when mildly injured, and thus, she does not heed recommendations to rest and rehabilitate.

Control

A more dispositional dimension of control related to health events is something termed "health locus of control." The basic loci of control are internal and external. Those with an internal health locus of control have a strong sense of control over health events, a locus that helps them adjust to being injured or ill and promotes their ultimate recovery. Those with an external health locus of control believe they have little control over their health, and as a consequence adopt more pessimistic approaches leading to poorer health habits and more illnesses. In addition, they are less likely to take active steps toward treating illness or injury.

In general, an increased sense of personal control can reduce the strain that results from stressors, in turn leading toward a more positive psychological adjustment. Different types of control relevant to the illness or injury situation include behavioral, cognitive, decisional, and informational (Sarafino 2002). Behavioral control refers to the ability or opportunity to take action, such as the opportunity to engage in gradually increasing levels of physical activity and exercise. Cognitive control refers to the ability to use cognitions to modify stressor effects, such as viewing a rehabilitative situation as a challenge rather than a threat. Decisional control refers to the ability to choose among possible courses of action, such as when the therapist offers some options relative to rehabilitative tasks. Informational control refers to the ability to get knowledge about the stressful event, such as when pamphlets outlining the nature of the injury and the rehabilitative protocols are offered to clients.

The degree of perceived control interacts with situation predictability to affect the basic coping style of the client. A general coping strategy of monitoring is more likely when there is both high controllability and predictability; in general, monitoring would be thought to be a more desirable strategy if prediction and control over processes and outcomes is possible for that unique medical event. The combination of low predictability and controllability is more likely to result in the general coping strategy of blunting (Bijttebier et al 2001). Thus, for example, therapists might be able to help clients gain a better understanding of the expected stages and outcomes of progress with therapy as well as allowing them control over treatment options when possible.

Self-perceptions

Self-perceptions are often affected by illness or injury situations. For example, clients' confidence in their physical abilities may deteriorate as a result of the restrictions and limitations placed on their bodies during rehabilitation. Clients with higher rehabilitative self-efficacy (i.e., confidence in their ability to complete rehabilitative activities) are more likely to adhere to treatment protocols (see Chapter 4), another example of how cognitions can relate to overt behavioral responses. The implication for therapists is to enhance the self-efficacy of clients, such as by adjusting rehabilitation goals to be incremental, challenging, and realistic.

Self-efficacy is also part of a constellation of characteristics comprising what has been termed "resilience." People high in self-efficacy, personal control, and optimism are more likely to view stres-

sors as causing less strain, to exhibit better mental and physical health, and to recover more quickly. In other words, they are more resilient to life's challenges, such as health events. Realizing that there is a dispositional component to resilience that is inherent in the client, it is still possible to structure the therapeutic situation to offer clients opportunities for enhanced perceptions of control, efficacy, and optimism. It is also important for therapists to demonstrate these characteristics in client interactions, such as by displaying a competent, confident, and positive manner that engenders the same in the clients.

Illness cognition/illness attributions

The clients' cognitive assessments about the causes, meaning, and salience of medical events affect their subsequent responses and choices. Thus, their beliefs and expectations about their injury/illness status and their treatments (illness cognitions) affect their emotional and behavioral responses. The accuracy of their attributions for injury or illness causality (illness attributions) is also related to their emotional responses. For example, clients are likely to have more negative beliefs and emotions if they believe that they are in some way to blame for their medical situation. Inaccurate attributions for injury or illness causality also can limit their beliefs about the efficacy of therapeutic treatment, leading to behavioral limitations such as avoidance of treatment.

Faith and religious beliefs

Koenig's (1997) review of over 1000 studies on the relationship between religion and health found that religious involvement can positively affect health by enhancing social support, alleviating stress, and promoting healthy practices. Psychological variables such as perceptions of stress and anxiety delay healing through their immune and neuroendocrine consequences. Psychological interventions lessen the effects of stressors and improve physical recoveries (Kiecolt-Glaser et al 2002). If the intervention of religious faith can aid in the reduction of stress and anxiety, one would expect corresponding physical and mental health benefits. There is also strong evidence that social support can moderate the effects of psychological stress, and one of the primary benefits of religious affiliation and activity is the maintenance of a social support network. The implication for therapists is to recognize that for many clients their religious belief systems affect their cognitive, emotional, and behavioral responses to injury.

EMOTIONAL RESPONSES

Some of the common affective reactions and responses to illness and injury include the more negative emotions of fear, anxiety, sadness, and anger, as well as the more positive emotions of hope, courage, and calmness. These emotional reactions and responses affect physiological functioning as well as behavioral choices. For example, emotional states affect human pain reactivity (Rhudy & Meagher 2000) as well as compliance with physical activity behaviors. In general it has been found that more negative emotions such as pessimism and depression are related to impaired immune functioning, and more positive emotions such as optimism and hopefulness boost immune function. It is also true that some negative emotional responses might be considered as normal and expected following a medical event. Emotional expression, be it the expression of positive or negative emotions, is important in the process of adapting to illness/injury and the associated life changes (Bowman 2001). For example, it seems perfectly reasonable for a person sustaining serious injury in an automobile accident to report some sadness over the incident and anxiety about what is to come. It is important that with time, however, these negative emotions gradually resolve and are replaced by more positive emotions that can more effectively help in the psychological management of the recovery process.

Mood states

Mood state responses to injury often stem directly from cognitions, and change dynamically throughout the injury/illness and recovery process. Some of the most commonly noted mood states postinjury include tension, sadness, and frustration (Smith 1996, Smith et al 1993). Other moods commonly observed include boredom (particularly during long rehabilitative periods), anger, and fatigue (Morrey et al 1999, Smith 1996). Many clients, however, also respond to injury with more positive mood states, such as anticipation, vigor, and relief. Research in the sport injury field has found that mood states fluctuate across the time course from injury through recovery and return to activity, with overall reductions in mood disturbance paralleling perceptions of recovery (Smith et al 1990a, 1993).

Looking only at measures of total mood disturbance over the time course of a medical experience masks the subtleties of individual mood-state changes (Morrey et al 1999, Wiese-Bjornstal 2001). Early in an injury cycle, for example, a client might feel greater sadness, tension, and anger. Over the course of time, the predominant moods may reflect boredom, frustration, and isolation as one feels more able to resume physical activity than actual recovery would allow and as social support sources gradually withdraw. An interesting finding has been that at the time of being given the go ahead to return to activity such as work or sport (Morrey et al 1999), rather than feeling the positive mood states that might be anticipated, many individuals report a return to more negative moods such as apprehension and worry about their ability to perform once again in a valued setting, and avoid re-injury.

Fear and anxiety

Fear is typically used to describe the emotional reaction resulting from an immediate, real, and present threat. Anxiety is thought of as an emotion related to the cognitive anticipation of a future undesired threat. Fear has been found to increase pain thresholds (a stress-induced analgesia) whereas anxiety has been found to decrease them (Rhudy & Meagher 2000). Anxiety has been related to increased pain reports in clinical settings. Clients with high trait anxiety or generalized anxiety demonstrate increased attention to pain (hypervigilance) and greater perceived intensity of pain than do their counterparts with lower anxiety (Rhudy & Meagher 2000).

In considering negative emotional responses, Bowman (2001) suggested that "fear and sadness are discrete emotions associated with specific life events . . . whereas anxiety and depression are a complex combination of emotion and thought" (p 258). He further suggested that anxiety and depression be thought of as psychopathological responses to medical events, and thus abnormal, whereas other negative moods or responses such as fear, sadness, or anger are normal emotions that might be expected when reacting to medical events. The point is that treating all negative emotional and mood state responses as abnormal and in need of psychological intervention is premature, and does not acknowledge the normal feelings that people work through when deciding how to meet unexpected challenges in life. When these normal responses become abnormal and in need of specific interventions is a function of the frequency, intensity, and duration of the emotional experiences.

To illustrate once again how interactive the cycle of cognitions, emotions, and behaviors is, consider the case of chronic pain. As illustrated in Figure 3.5, worry (cognition) and fear (emotion) have been linked to avoidance (behavior) in chronic pain. Another more extreme example would be that of post-traumatic stress disorder. Post-traumatic stress disorder (PTSD) can result as a consequence of an encounter with an extremely severe stressor. The initial reaction to this severe stressor does not dissipate but leads to recurring responses characterized by high arousal (as manifested in difficulty sleeping and concentrating), frequent reliving of the event, and being unresponsive to other people. Recent literature suggests that chronic pain – frequently a result of work-related injuries or motor-vehicle accidents – is often comorbid with PTSD (Sharp & Harvey 2001). This constellation of intrusive cognitions, hyperaroused emotions and physiology, and avoidance behavior provides another example of the cycle of cognitions, emotions, and behaviors in the context of a medical event.

Emotional distress and somatic complaints

Subscales on certain psychological inventories, such as the Minnesota Multiphasic Personality Inventory-2 (MMPI-2), are used as indicators of psychological adjustment. The neurotic triad of subscales on the MMPI is relevant to understanding the psychological responses of clients to medical events (Vendrig 2000). The neurotic triad is reflected in scores on three subscales: hypochondriasis (pre-

occupation with and complaints about physical health), depression (feelings of unhappiness, pessimism, and hopelessness), and hysteria (tendency to cope with problems by using avoidance strategies and developing physical symptoms), again reflecting the cognitive, emotional, and behavioral links.

When in pain due to illness or injury, some clients display elevated neurotic triad scores. The illness attitudes (Hadjistavropoulos & Amundson 1998) and beliefs of clients may also provide evidence of hypochondriasis and somatization, forms of abnormal behavior in which "subjective symptomatology is present in a degree disproportionate to objective signs and pathology" (Currie et al 1999, p 19). These evidences of abnormal illness behavior are often associated with clinically significant levels of depression (Peveler et al 2002) and anxiety. In protracted injury recovery experiences, for example, where negative mood states have frequently been documented, one might expect that these mood states influence health beliefs and behaviors. The presence of multiple somatic complaints can lead to a salient manifestation of emotional distress, which can prolong a pain state via the associated tension and bodily distress (Vendrig 2000).

Kinesiophobia

The term "kinesiophobia" has been used to describe a "fear of physical activity stemming from the belief that it will lead to pain, injury, or reinjury" (Amundson et al 1999). In the case of chronic back pain, for example, it has been found that pain-related fears about physical and work-related activities are more predictive of disability and work loss than are biomedical measures of pain (Amundson et al 1999). Thus, pain beliefs (cognitions), pain fear (emotions), and pain avoidance (behavior) are interrelated.

In addition to specific fears about resuming physical activity, many of those with chronic musculoskeletal pain also fear other situations not necessarily associated with pain such as social activities. They minimize or avoid involvement in social activities, in part in order to avoid any cues that might be associated for them with increased arousal or fear.

Emotional regulation strategies

In order to regulate one's emotions, one must first be able to identify them. The term "emotional approach coping" has been used to describe recognition,

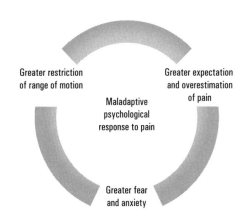

Figure 3.5   Cognitive expectation, anxiety, and avoidance behavior in chronic pain

acknowledgment, and expression of one's feelings (Keefe et al 2001). Greater use of emotional approach coping relates to better health (Stanton et al 1994). Emotional inhibition, failing to experience or express emotions, is associated with poorer health (Keefe et al 2001, Stanton et al 1994). The long-term avoidance of certain thoughts and emotions is associated with poorer psychological adaptation.

The clinical term "alexithymia" has been used to indicate a pattern observed in some clients with difficulty in identifying their own emotional feelings, differentiating emotional feelings from other physical sensations, and communicating emotional feelings to others (Keefe et al 2001). The person exhibiting this pattern typically experiences negative affect, impaired social relationships, and detrimental physiological changes (Keefe et al 2001).

The salient point for therapists is that acknowledging, recognizing, and managing emotions underlies the ability to negate their impact on pain, injury, and illness. Unacknowledged and unexpressed emotions have negative health-related consequences that inhibit rehabilitation and recovery.

Grief

The actual state and/or cognitive perception of having lost something, such as health, can be a stressful event with subsequent emotional responses. This stressful event is often called "bereavement," and is typically thought of relative to the loss of a loved one or other form of interpersonal loss, although in the context of this chapter the loss of health might be considered as an intrapersonal loss. Grief is the term used to reflect emotional reactions and responses to bereavement. Grief is normal and expected when faced with a loss. It can also become abnormal and even pathological, however, when manifested as masked, delayed, or debilitative expressions of grief (Stroebe et al 2000). "Mourning" as a term is used to reflect the behavioral expressions of the emotional grief. Thus, once again we see a cycle of cognitions (sense of loss), emotions (grief), and behaviors (mourning) that characterize a psychological process.

The majority of bereaved individuals exhibit normal grief, that is, they exhibit "moderate disruptions in cognitive, emotional, physical, or interpersonal functioning during the initial months after a loss" (Bonanno & Kaltman 2001, p 709). Concomitant to this process, most individuals also experience some positive thoughts and emotions related to the loss. Although the clinical grief literature does not focus

on intrapersonal losses (losses within oneself such as a loss of identity or status, loss of personal health), many of the characteristics of grief can be present in these losses as well. For example, cognitive disruptions such as confusion and preoccupation, identity disturbance, disrupted futures, and searches for meaning characteristic of grief experiences (Bonanno & Kaltman 2001) can occur among those experiencing personal loss of health. Emotional malaise or dysphoria, characterized by negative emotions such as anger, irritability, hostility, guilt, and sadness as well as other emotions such as yearning or loneliness, is also typical of the process of grieving (Bonanno & Kaltman 2001) and appear within injured or ill populations as well. Somatic manifestations of grief include digestive difficulties, insomnia, and restlessness, and social withdrawal and feelings of isolation associated with grieving can further affect the adjustment process. Positive responses are also characteristic of the grief process, including positive cognitions such as a sense of freedom, positive emotions such as feeling comforted, and positive behaviors such as seeking out and using social support networks.

BEHAVIORAL RESPONSES

Behavioral responses include such overt actions as adherence or compliance to treatment regimens, use of psychological skills (e.g., mental imagery, goal setting, anxiety management), use of social networks, risk-taking behaviors, and the effort and intensity with which the client pursues rehabilitation. Cognitive appraisals and emotional responses of clients will influence their actual behaviors. Clients who adhere to rehabilitation, use psychological skills to manage pain and direct energies, effectively use available social support, reduce risk taking behaviors that inhibit rehabilitation, and pursue rehabilitation goals with optimum effort and intensity are more likely to recover effectively than those who do not engage in these actions (Wiese-Bjornstal et al 1995). Because other chapters in this text specifically explore these behaviors (see Chapters 5 and 16), the following section is brief and intended to serve the purpose of providing examples of behaviors that are influenced by the cognitive and emotional responses of clients to medical events.

Social-support-seeking behavior

Social support comprises the perceived help and caring that individuals receive from others. In general, people with a high degree of social support are healthier and live longer. Social support can have a direct influence in benefiting health regardless of the amount of strain experienced or may serve the function of buffering a person against the negative health effects of high strain (Bianco 2001, Chwalisz & Vaux 2000).

Whether or not clients engage in the behaviors of seeking out and making use of available social support is related to factors such as their personal qualities, their potential providers or sources of social support, and the available forms of support. Personal qualities affecting clients' use of support, for example, might be their introverted/extroverted dispositions, willingness to ask for help, or willingness to let others help them. Potential providers of support may include family members, personal friends, professional colleagues, medical professionals, or mental health professionals. Forms of support are often characterized as emotional/ social, informational, and tangible. Emotional support could best be provided by close friends and family, and involves emotional disclosure as well as social engagement. Informational support, such as providing verbal and written information about the nature of the injury and rehabilitation program worded in a way that clients can understand is a very basic, yet often overlooked and underestimated, form of support. Tangible or material support is routinely provided by therapeutic personnel, such as providing physical therapy and needed medical supplies, or helping to arrange transportation.

Not all social support is perceived positively by the recipient. Social support might be perceived as pressure rather than as support, or may, however well-intentioned, enable the client to avoid challenges that need to be faced. For example, among clients with chronic pain, it has been found that with solicitous and supportive spouses, clients are not only less likely to do things for themselves but also more likely to report greater pain (Chwalisz & Vaux 2000). So, even though social support is used, it does not achieve the ultimate goal of helping clients back to functioning, independent states. Social reinforcement for pain behavior can result in more pain, more disability, and less physical activity.

Emotional disclosure

Engaging in the behavior of disclosing and expressing one's emotions has been found to be helpful in altering negative emotions (Keefe et al 2001). Because of their underlying dispositions and per-

sonalities, some clients are already quite comfortable disclosing their emotional responses to others. Many, however, are not comfortable with such disclosure, whether based on cultural norms, family style, or personal introversion. Helping people engage in the behavior of expressing emotions can help in emotional regulation and pain control (Keefe et al 2001). Writing or talking about emotionally traumatic experiences has been found to result in benefits such as reduced stress perceptions, reduced negative feelings, and improved health (Sarafino 2002). Although the physical or manual therapist would not be the primary target of such emotional disclosure, it would seem helpful to inquire about the client's well-being during a visit.

Adherence behavior

One specific type of behavior essential for successful rehabilitation is adherence behavior, or actually sticking with the treatment and rehabilitation protocol and plan. Multiple factors have been suggested as influencing adherence behavior (Heil 1993), including personal factors (e.g., anxiety, confidence), social factors (e.g., therapy room climate, social support), and physical factors (e.g., pain, recovery progress). Psychological and social factors related to poor adherence might include somatic anxiety, low treatment confidence, low self-motivation, and limited social support. Psychological and social factors predicting successful adherence include client perception of need for particular intervention, expectation for a positive outcome, belief that benefits of rehabilitation outweigh the costs, and a sense of active involvement in treatment (Heil 1993). Thus, in order to achieve optimal adherence to physical and manual therapy, consideration must be given to the psychological and social climate created in the therapy room. For a more detailed account of adherence to rehabilitation see Chapter 4.

Malingering behavior

Another behavioral response consideration involves malingering behavior, or continuing to seek out and remain in the medical setting by presenting with symptoms of discomfort or physical distress when there is no longer an identifiable underlying pathology or need for treatment (Rotella et al 1993). Malingering behavior has been described as a psychological adjustment to negative circumstances, in which there is some sort of incentive to remaining in the medical setting. External incentives might, for example, be the care and attention received in the therapy setting, the alleviation of fear by having someone continue to monitor one's physical recovery, or the avoidance of return to work or responsibility required when healthy. People who appear to malinger may do so as a result of a need for attention or because of fear (Rotella et al 1993); once again, it is apparent that as in the cyclic model, thoughts are affecting emotions and behaviors. Therapists cannot discount out of hand the clients' claims of injury because there may be an as yet undetected underlying physiological cause, but they must also recognize that there are many possible reasons for malingering behavior related to the moderating factors, cognitions, and emotions.

SUMMARY

Physical and manual therapists should recognize that there is much more to treating clients than managing their physical symptoms alone. Both the physical and mental recoveries of clients depend upon the skillful understanding and management of their overall lives, including their internal psychological lives and their external social lives. Each member of the treatment team can contribute toward this goal.

The research data tell us that both the state of clients' personal and social lives and their interpretations of, and responses to, medical events are characterized by a wide variety of thoughts, feelings, and behaviors that have a direct bearing on the success with which they rehabilitate and recover. Thus, the effective physical and manual therapist cannot afford to avoid playing their role – within the boundaries of expertise and ethics – in the psychological management of client responses.

Other chapters in this text are devoted to the elaboration of various intervention strategies, but the general point of this chapter was to clarify how essential it is for physical and manual therapists to recognize the powerful influence that thoughts, emotions, and behaviors have on rehabilitation. The role of therapists encompasses a variety of intervention paths and strategies suggested by our understanding of the psychological responses of clients to injury and illness as illustrated in Figure 3.6. There are some clients for whom the routine practice of effective physical and manual therapy will provide sufficient intervention to enable rehabilitation and recovery, whereas others will require a bit of added assistance from other members of the healthcare team but still will reflect responses within normal or subclinical ranges. For a third subset of clients, the assistance of specialized mental healthcare providers will be helpful in facilitating their psychological adaptations.

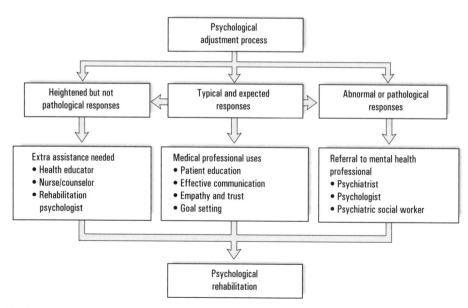

Figure 3.6   Link between psychological response and psychological intervention

References

Amundson G J G, Norton P J, Norton G R 1999 Beyond pain: the role of fear and avoidance in chronicity. Clinical Psychology Review 19: 97–119

Ax S, Gregg V H, Jones D 2001 Coping and illness cognitions: Chronic fatigue syndrome. Clinical Psychology Review 21: 161–182

Bandura A 1986 Social foundations of thought and action: A social cognitive theory. Prentice Hall, Englewood Cliffs, NJ

Bandura A 2000 Social cognitive theory: An agentic perspective. Annual Review of Psychology 52: 1–26

Bianco T 2001 Conceptual considerations for social support research in sport and exercise settings: The case of sport injury. Journal of Sport and Exercise Psychology 23: 85–107

Bijttebier P, Vertommen H, Vander Steene G 2001 Assessment of cognitive coping styles: A closer look at situation-response inventories. Clinical Psychology Review 21: 85–104

Boissonnault W G 1999 Prevalence of comorbid conditions, surgeries, and medication use in a physical therapy outclient population: A multicentered study. Journal of Orthopaedic and Sports Physical Therapy 29: 506–519

Bonanno G A, Kaltman S 2001 The varieties of grief experience. Clinical Psychology Review 21: 705–734

Bowman G S 2001 Emotions and illness. Journal of Advanced Nursing 34: 256–263

Brannon L, Feist J 2000 Health psychology, 4th edn. Wadsworth, Belmont, CA

Chwalisz K, Vaux A 2000 Social support and adjustment to disability. In: Frank R G, Elliott T R (eds) Handbook of rehabilitation psychology. American Psychological Association, Washington DC, p 537–552

Currie A, Potts G, Donovan W et al 1999 Illness behaviour in elite middle and long distance runners. British Journal of Sports Medicine 33: 19–21

Dahlquist L N, Gil K M, Armstrong D et al 1986 Preparing children for medical examinations: The importance of previous medical experience. Health Psychology 5: 249–259

Engel G L 1980 The clinical application of the biopsychosocial model. American Journal of Psychiatry 137: 535–544

Engel G L 1977 The need for a new medical model: A challenge for biomedicine. Science 196: 129–136

Gavin J, Taylor M 1992 Psychosocial recovery from athletic injury: A process model with implications for rehabilitation. Paper presented at the annual meeting of the Association for the Advancement of Applied Sport Psychology, Colorado Springs, CO

Gustafsson M, Persson L O, Amilon A 2002 A qualitative study of coping in the early stage of acute traumatic hand injury. Journal of Clinical Nursing 11: 594–602

Hadjistavropoulos H D, Amundson G J 1998 Factor analytic investigation of the Illness Attitudes Scale in a chronic pain sample. Behaviour Research and Therapy 36: 1185–1195

Hadjistavropoulos H D, Amundson J G, Norton G R 1999 Validation of the Coping With Health, Injuries, and Problems Scale in a chronic pain sample. Clinical Journal of Pain 15: 41–49

Hadjistavropoulos H D, Craig K D, Hadjistavropoulos T 1998 Cognitive and behavioral responses to illness information: The role of health anxiety. Behaviour Research & Therapy 36: 149–164

Hansdottir I, Malcarne V 1998 Concepts of illness in Icelandic children. Journal of Pediatric Psychology 23: 187–195

Heil J 1993 Psychology of sport injury. Human Kinetics, Champaign, IL

Kalish C 1996 Causes and symptoms in preschoolers' conceptions of illness. Child Development 67: 1647–1670

Keefe F J, Lumley M, Anderson T et al 2001 Pain and emotion: New research directions. Journal of Clinical Psychology 57: 587–607

Kiecolt-Glaser J K, McGuire L, Robles T F, Glaser R 2002 Psychoneuroimmunology and psychosomatic medicine: Back to the future. Psychosomatic Medicine 64: 15–28

Koenig H G 1997 Is religion good for your health? Haworth Pastoral Press, Binghamton, NY

Lazarus R S 1999 Stress and emotion: A new synthesis. Springer, New York

Lazarus R S 1993 Coping theory and research: Past, present, and future. Psychosomatic Medicine 55: 234–247

Lazarus R S, Folkman S 1984 Stress, appraisal, and coping. Springer, New York

Mahler H I M, Kulik J A 2000 Optimism, pessimism and recovery from coronary bypass surgery: Prediction of affect, pain and functional status. Psychology, Health and Medicine 5: 347–358

Moos R H, Shaefer J A 1984 The crisis of physical illness: An overview and conceptual analysis. In: Moos R H (ed) Coping with physical illness 2: New perspectives. Plenum Press, New York, p 3–25

Morrey M A, Stuart M J, Smith A M, Wiese-Bjornstal D M 1999 A longitudinal examination of athletes' emotional and cognitive response to anterior cruciate ligament injury. Clinical Journal of Sports Medicine 9: 63–69

Peveler R, Carson A, Rodin G 2002 ABC of psychological medicine: Depression in medical clients. British Medical Journal 325(7356): 149–152

Radnitz C L, Bockian N, Moran A I 2000 Assessment of psychopathology and personality in people with physical disabilities. In: Frank R G, Elliott T R (eds) Handbook of rehabilitation psychology. American Psychological Association, Washington, DC, p 287–309

Rhudy J L, Meagher M W 2000 Fear and anxiety: Divergent effects on human pain thresholds. Pain 84: 65–75

Rotella R J, Ogilvie B C, Perrin D H 1993 The malingering athlete: psychological considerations. In: Pargman D (ed) Psychological bases of sport injuries. Fitness Information Technology, Morgantown, WV, p 85–97

Rusch M R, Gould L J, Dzwierzynski W W et al 2002 Psychological impact of traumatic injuries: What the surgeon can do. Plastic and Reconstructive Surgery 109: 18–24

Sarafino E P 2002 Health psychology, 4th edn. John Wiley, New York

Severeijns R, Vlaeyen J W, van den Hout M A et al 2001 Pain catastrophizing predicts pain intensity, disability, and psychological distress independent of the level of physical impairment. Clinical Journal of Pain 17: 165–172

Sharp T J, Harvey A G 2001 Chronic pain and posttraumatic stress disorder: Mutual maintenance? Clinical Psychology Review 21: 857–877

Smith A M 1996 Psychological impact of injuries in athletes. Sports Medicine 22: 391–405

Smith A M, Scott S G, O'Fallon W M et al 1990a The emotional responses of athletes to injury. Mayo Clinic Proceedings 65: 38–50

Smith A M, Scott S G, Wiese D M 1990b The psychological effects of sports injuries: Coping. Sports Medicine 9: 352–369

Smith A M, Stuart M J, Wiese-Bjornstal D M et al 1993 Competitive athletes: Pre-injury and post-injury mood state and self-esteem. Mayo Clinic Proceedings 68: 939–947

Stanton A L , Danoff-Burg S, Cameron C L et al 1994 Coping through emotional approach: Problems of conceptualization and confounding. Journal of Personality and Social Psychology 66: 350–362

Stroebe M, van Son M, Stroebe W et al 2000 On the classification and diagnosis of pathological grief. Clinical Psychology Review 20: 57–75

Sullivan M J L, Tripp D A, Rodgers W M et al 2000 Catastrophizing and pain perception in sport participants. Journal of Applied Sport Psychology 12: 151–167

Truchon M 2001 Determinants of chronic disability related to low back pain: Towards an integrative biopsychosocial model. Disability and Rehabilitation: An International Multidisciplinary Journal 23: 758–767

Turk D C, Okifuji A 2002 Psychological factors in chronic pain: evolution and revolution. Journal of Consulting and Clinical Psychology 70: 678–690

Vendrig A A 2000 The Minnesota Multiphasic Personality Inventory and chronic pain: A conceptual analysis of a long-standing but complicated relationship. Clinical Psychology Review 20: 533–559

Wiese-Bjornstal D M 2003 From skinned knees and pee wees to menisci and masters: Developmental sport injury psychology. In: Weiss M (ed) Developmental sport and exercise psychology: A lifespan perspective. Fitness Information Technology, Morgantown, WV

Wiese-Bjornstal D M 2001 In the mood. Athletic Therapy Today 6: 38–39

Wiese-Bjornstal D M, Smith A M, LaMott E E 1995 A model of psychologic response to athletic injury and rehabilitation. Athletic Training: Sports Health Care Perspectives 1: 16–30

Wiese-Bjornstal D M, Smith A M, Shaffer S M et al 1998 An integrated model of response to sport injury: Psychological and sociological dynamics. Journal of Applied Sport Psychology 10: 46–69

Chapter **4**

Psychological aspects of rehabilitation

Britton W. Brewer

INTRODUCTION

In the preceding chapters, important roles were ascribed to psychological factors in the occurrence of and responses to the sorts of injuries and illnesses for which practitioners of the physical and manual therapies are likely to be consulted. Psychological factors can also have an impact on key processes and outcomes in the rehabilitation of physical conditions. The purpose of this chapter is to examine three aspects of rehabilitation with prominent psychological components: adherence to rehabilitation, client–practitioner relationships, and psychological readiness to return to pre-injury or pre-illness activity.

ADHERENCE TO REHABILITATION

As defined by Meichenbaum & Turk (1987), adherence is an "active, voluntary collaborative involvement of the patient in a mutually acceptable course of behavior to produce a desired preventative or therapeutic result" (p 20). Although the terms *adherence* and *compliance* are often used interchangeably, adherence is used in this chapter because compliance has the connotation of a more passive role of patients or clients carrying out the requests of healthcare practitioners (Meichenbaum & Turk 1987). Depending on the physical condition when undergoing rehabilitation and the characteristics of the treatment regimen, the specific behaviors constituting adherence in the context of rehabilitation vary widely. Adherence behaviors of relevance to the physical and manual therapies include attending and actively participating in clinic-based rehabilitation appointments, avoiding potentially harmful activities, wearing therapeutic devices (e.g., orthotics), consuming medications as prescribed, and completing home rehabilitation activities (e.g., exercises, therapeutic modalities).

Although adherence would seem to be vital to the success of rehabilitation programs, relatively few intervention studies in the rehabilitation literature have included indices of adherence (Nicholas 1995). In a recent review of adherence to sport injury rehabilitation regimens, Brewer (1999) indicated that adherence rates ranging from 40% to 91% were obtained in six studies that used several different methods to assess adherence. Adherence rates in the general medical literature have varied even more substantially, with a range of 4% to 92% across a wide range of medical conditions and treatment regimens (Meichenbaum & Turk 1987).

MEASUREMENT OF ADHERENCE TO REHABILITATION

Reflecting the diverse array of behavioral requirements of treatment programs in the physical and manual therapies, numerous measures of adherence to rehabilitation have been developed. Some rehabilitation adherence measures pertain to behaviors occurring in clinical settings, whereas other adherence measures address behaviors occurring away from the clinical environment.

Clinic-based measures of adherence to rehabilitation

The simplest and most convenient measure of adherence to the clinic-based portion of rehabilitation programs is attendance at appointments scheduled with rehabilitation practitioners. Typically calculated by dividing the number of rehabilitation sessions attended by the number of rehabilitation sessions scheduled, attendance indices are useful for identifying clients who are having difficulties showing up for clinic appointments. Nevertheless, because clients tend to be present for the vast majority of their scheduled rehabilitation sessions and attendance measures do not provide information about what clients actually do during their clinic appointments, the clinical utility of attendance scores is limited to indicating cases of gross nonadherence to clinic-based rehabilitation activities (Brewer 1999).

The second main measure of clinic-based rehabilitation adherence is practitioner behavioral observations and judgments. Capitalizing on their frequent, personal contact with clients, rehabilitation practitioners can observe, record, and make judgments about the extent to which clients adhere to rehabilitation activities occurring in the clinical setting. Although time- and labor-intensive, observing clients at regular time intervals and recording their behavior can yield a rich account of what clients do during rehabilitation sessions and provide an indication of their level of adherence to the rehabilitation program (Brewer 1999). A prime example of a coding scheme for clinic-based rehabilitation activities is the Sports Medicine Observation Code (SMOC, Crossman & Roch 1991). The SMOC features 13 categories of behaviors that clients may exhibit while attending clinic appointments, including active rehabilitation, waiting, and non-activity.

In clinical settings where implementing a behavioral observation system is impractical, a streamlined alternative method for assessing adherence to clinic-based rehabilitation activities is to have practitioners indicate their judgments of client adherence immediately following each appointment. In such an approach, practitioner judgments are presumably based on their observations of client behavior during the preceding rehabilitation session. The Sport Injury Rehabilitation Adherence Scale (SIRAS; Brewer et al 2000b), which is displayed in Figure 4.1, is an example of a measure of practitioner judgments of clinic-based rehabilitation adherence.

Although the SIRAS was designed to assess adherence to rehabilitation of sport-related orthopedic injuries, the items are sufficiently generic as to be applicable to a wide range of medical conditions and rehabilitation programs. Support has been obtained for the internal consistency, test–retest reliability, interrater reliability, factor structure, and construct validity of the SIRAS (Brewer et al 2000b, 2002, Laubach et al 1996).

Non-clinic-based measures of adherence to rehabilitation

Away from the clinical environment, one of the most common features of rehabilitation programs is home exercises designed to enhance strength, flexibility, and other key rehabilitative attributes. Home exercise completion has traditionally been assessed through self-report methods, most typically by a single retrospective report (Brewer 1999). Retrospective self-reports, however, can be subject to bias, distortion, and inaccuracy (Dunbar-Jacob et

1. Circle the number that best indicates the intensity with which this patient completed the rehabilitation exercises during today's appointment:

   Minimum effort   1   2   3   4   5   Maximum effort

2. During today's appointment, how frequently did this patient follow your instructions and advice?

   Never   1   2   3   4   5   Always

3. How receptive was this patient to changes in the rehabilitation program during today's appointment?

   Very unreceptive   1   2   3   4   5   Very receptive

Figure 4.1   Sport Injury Rehabilitation Adherence Scale (reproduced from Brewer et al 2000b with permission of Churchill Livingstone). *Note*: The Sport Injury Rehabilitation Adherence Scale can also be used with reference to adherence tendencies in general by using the present tense (without reference to "today's appointment")

al 1993, Meichenbaum & Turk 1987). Consequently, daily diaries have been used to decrease the amount of time covered in a given self-observation of home exercise completion and, in the process, boost the accuracy of the account of adherence to home exercises. In addition to the inherently subjective self-report measures, objective means of assessing home exercise completion are available. Examples of objective indices include a motion sensor embedded in an ankle exerciser in the treatment of persons with muscular dystrophy (Belanger & Noel 1990), a portable computer attached to a biofeedback unit in knee rehabilitation (Levitt et al 1995), a battery-powered monitor mounted on an ankle exerciser (Petrosenko et al 1996), an electronic counting device attached to a splint for individuals who have had finger tendon surgery (Dobbe et al 1999), and an accelerometer for persons with fibromyalgia (Schlenk et al 2000). Additional ways of assessing adherence to home exercise regimens involve measuring knowledge of the home rehabilitation program and quality of exercise performance (Friedrich et al 1996, Henry et al 1998, Schoo 2002, Webborn et al 1997). Individuals undergoing rehabilitation provide indirect evidence that they are adhering to rehabilitation outside the clinical setting when they are able to recall the exercises that they are supposed to perform (Webborn et al 1997) or replicate their prescribed exercises correctly (Friedrich et al 1996, Henry et al 1998, Schoo 2002). Remembering what one should do or how one should do it is not the same as actually doing it, so knowledge and cor-

rectness measures are better used to identify non-adherence than to confirm adherence to home rehabilitation regimens. Individuals who cannot recall or correctly perform home exercises are unlikely to have done them consistently.

A variety of measures has been used to assess adherence to aspects of rehabilitation outside of the clinical environment other than home exercises. For example, adherence to medication regimens has been assessed through retrospective and daily self-reports, medication measurements, pharmacy refills, reimbursement records, biochemical and clinical indicators, and, most recently, electronic monitors (Dunbar-Jacob et al 1998), the latter of which are especially desirable because they are unaffected by limitations in memory and motivation. Adherence to recommendations to use therapeutic footwear (e.g., bespoke shoes, orthotics) has been assessed through retrospective self-reports (Donatelli et al 1988, Sawhney et al 1999), a hidden step-counter (Olivier et al 1997), and practitioner observation (Breuer 1994). With respect to recommendations to wear or use therapeutic devices, adherence has been measured by self-report for splint usage (O'Carroll & Hendriks 1989), pain response and analgesic consumption for use of a continuous passive motion (CPM) machine (Laupattarakasem 1988), and self-report and a mechanical timing device for use of an orthopedic brace (Vandal et al 1999). Adherence to a joint protection program among persons with rheumatoid arthritis has been assessed with a measure in which clients' actions while preparing a food and beverage snack are observed and coded (Hammond & Lincoln 1999). Although clinical outcomes have been used as proxies for rehabilitation adherence in some investigations, such an approach to the measurement of adherence is ill-advised because it confounds the processes and products of rehabilitation and yields no information about adherence to the rehabilitation regimen (Brewer 1999, Meichenbaum & Turk 1987). Further, some individuals may adhere perfectly to the rehabilitation program yet show little therapeutic gain. Conversely, other people may show poor adherence but display enhanced clinical outcomes (Dunbar-Jacob et al 1998).

THEORETICAL EXPLANATIONS FOR ADHERENCE TO REHABILITATION

In the general medical literature, literally hundreds of variables have been examined in association with adherence to healthcare regimens (Meichenbaum & Turk 1987). Numerous potential predictors of adherence to rehabilitation have been investigated as well. To facilitate an enhanced understanding of the process by which factors influence rehabilitation adherence, researchers have adapted theoretical models from other areas of psychology to the domain of rehabilitation adherence. Among the theoretical perspectives that have been used to guide research on variables contributing to adherence to rehabilitation are the health belief model/ protection motivation theory, personal investment theory, and cognitive appraisal models.

HEALTH BELIEF MODEL/PROTECTION MOTIVATION THEORY

Developed a half-century ago to help understand why people often fail to take action in ways to prevent adverse health consequences (Rosenstock 1974), the health belief model (HBM) has been applied extensively in investigations of a wide variety of health behaviors, including adherence. According to the model, people are more likely to adhere to medical treatment regimens when they view their physical problem as severe, perceive themselves as susceptible to further negative health effects if they do not adhere to treatment, consider the likelihood of the treatment being effective as high, identify few barriers to adherence, experience few rewards for failing to adhere, and encounter environmental cues supporting the decision to adhere (Clark & Becker 1998). Protection motivation theory (PMT; Prentice-Dunn & Rogers 1986) is essentially an extension of the HBM, adding a self-efficacy component in which people are more likely to adhere to treatment regimens they believe themselves capable of performing.

Research has supported application of the HBM and PMT to rehabilitation adherence. Taylor & May (1996) found that perceived injury severity, perceived susceptibility to adverse health effects without rehabilitation, belief in the efficacy of the treatment protocol, and rehabilitation self-efficacy were positively associated with adherence to sport injury rehabilitation regimens. Similarly, Brewer et al (2003) found that four PMT components (i.e., susceptibility, severity, treatment efficacy, and self-efficacy) accounted for 43% of the variance in four measures of adherence to rehabilitation following knee surgery. As in the Taylor & May study, greater perceived treatment efficacy, self-efficacy, and susceptibility were related to higher levels of adherence. Other studies on adherence to treatments in the physical and manual therapies have documented the relationships with adherence predicted by the HBM and PMT for perceptions of treatment efficacy (Abbott et al 1994, Duda et al 1989, Fong et al 1990, Noyes et al 1983), rehabilitation self-efficacy (Chen et al 1999, Flynn et al 1995, Stenstrom et al 1997), and severity (Fong et al 1990, Sluijs et al 1993).

PERSONAL INVESTMENT THEORY

Maehr & Braskamp (1986) proposed personal investment theory as a cognitive-motivational model in which the subjective meaning of a given behavioral context to an individual is thought to exert a strong influence on behavior in that context. Subjective meaning is defined by constructs (i.e., personal incentives, sense-of-self beliefs, and perceived options) posited to reflect the interaction between personal attributes and characteristics of the situation in which behavior occurs. In the only study to provide an intentional, direct test of personal investment theory in a rehabilitation context, Duda et al (1989) found that variables representing each of the personal investment theory construct categories were significantly correlated with at least one of the three adherence measures administered to a sample of intercollegiate athletes with injuries. Task involvement, a personal incentive variable that pertains to the use of self-referenced standards of competence and success, was positively associated with rehabilitation adherence. Sense-of-self beliefs related to adherence were perceived social support, trait sport-confidence, self-motivation, internal locus of control for rehabilitation, and perceived physical ability (all correlations were positive). Perceived options positively associated with adherence were belief in the efficacy of treatment, knowledge of treatment, plans for future sport participation, and perceived role on the team since becoming injured.

Other studies in which personal investment theory was not explicitly tested have provided additional support for the model. Ego involvement, a personal incentive variable that pertains to using other-referenced (i.e., competitive) standards for evaluating competence and success, has been inversely related to rehabilitation adherence (Lampton et al 1993). Sense-of-self beliefs correlated (positively) with adherence to rehabilitation in investigations other than that of Duda et al (1989) and include: self-motivation (Brewer et al 1999, 2000a, Fields et al 1995, Fisher et al 1988, Noyes et al 1983, Pizzari et al 2002), social support for rehabilitation (Byerly et al 1994, Fisher et al 1988, Pizzari et al 2002), and internal locus of control for rehabilitation (Abbott et al 1994, Chen et al 1999). Perceived option variables showing significant (positive) associations with rehabilitation adherence include belief in the efficacy of treatment (Abbott et al 1994, Fong et al 1990, Noyes et al 1983, Taylor & May 1996) and plans for future return to participation (Shank 1988).

Cognitive appraisal models

With roots in the stress and coping literature (Lazarus & Folkman 1984), cognitive appraisal models are a family of related theoretical perspectives in which cognitions and the emotions that accompany them are ascribed a key role in influencing rehabilitation behavior. The models hold that characteristics of the person and the situation interact in affecting how individuals interpret (or appraise) and respond emotionally and behaviorally to their physical concerns (Wiese-Bjornstal et al 1998). Cognitive appraisal models are dynamic and recursive in that they allow for cognitive, emotional, and behavioral outcomes in rehabilitation to change as a function of fluctuations in personal and situational attributes.

In a recent review of research on adherence to injury rehabilitation programs, Brewer (2001) docu-

mented the utility of using a cognitive appraisal model approach to examine rehabilitation adherence. Brewer presented evidence of correlations of a wide variety of personal, situational, cognitive, and behavioral variables with adherence to sport injury rehabilitation programs. Personal factors linked with adherence included pain tolerance, self-motivation, and toughmindedness. Among the situational factors correlated with adherence were comfort of the clinical environment, convenience of rehabilitation scheduling, and social support for rehabilitation. Cognitive responses associated with adherence included rehabilitation self-efficacy, attribution of recovery to stable and personally controllable factors, and use of goal setting, imagery, and positive self-talk. Brewer also described research demonstrating links between emotional responses (i.e., mood disturbance) and sport injury rehabilitation adherence.

Research findings from other areas of rehabilitation have paralleled those from sport injury rehabilitation. Age (Breuer 1994, Sluijs et al 1993), internal health locus of control (Abbott et al 1996, Chen et al 1999) and surprisingly, the belief that powerful others control one's health (Abbott et al 1996) are among the personal characteristics for which positive associations with adherence have been documented. Level of education (Sluijs et al 1993) is a personal variable that has been negatively correlated with adherence to rehabilitation (for women but not for men). Another personal factor, gender, has also been associated with rehabilitation adherence, with men more likely to attend physiotherapy appointments than women (Armistead 1997).

With regard to situational factors, numerous injury-, illness-, and treatment-related variables have been found to be predictive of rehabilitation adherence. In particular, positive associations with adherence have been reported for perceived seriousness of illness/injury (Fong et al 1990, Sluijs et al 1993), degree of disability, medical prognosis, positive feedback from the physiotherapist (Sluijs et al 1993), level of physical functioning (Lansinger et al 1994), treatment efficacy (Abbott et al 1994, Fong et al 1990), and assistance in completing rehabilitation activities (Abbott et al 1994). Situational factors negatively correlated with rehabilitation adherence include perceived barriers to adherence (Sluijs et al 1993), duration of sick leave (Lansinger et al 1994), pain levels (Lansinger et al 1994, Sawhney at al 1999), and self-presentational (i.e., cosmetic) motives (Breuer 1994).

Although there is only limited research on the hypothesized relations among cognitive responses, emotional responses, and rehabilitation adherence outside of the sport injury domain, the research that has been conducted is supportive of a cognitive appraisal approach. With respect to the proposed relationship between cognitive factors and rehabilitation adherence, self-efficacy (Chen et al 1999) and the expectation of receiving an exercise prescription (Schneiders et al 1998) have been positively associated with adherence in one study each, and health-specific worries have been negatively associated with adherence in two studies (Abbott et al 1996, Fong et al 1990). Sluijs et al (1993) documented an association between an emotional variable and adherence, finding that helplessness was inversely related to adherence across a variety of physical conditions warranting physiotherapy.

Conclusions

Without additional research, it is too early to draw any firm conclusions about the factors that are most critical in affecting adherence to rehabilitation regimens. Nevertheless, based on the studies that have been conducted so far, it can be inferred that adherence is most likely to be maximized when clients:

1. possess personal characteristics that facilitate sticking with a potentially challenging rehabilitation program (e.g., self-motivation, tough-mindedness)
2. experience an environment conducive to adherence (e.g., social support for rehabilitation, comfortable and convenient clinical setting)
3. perceive their medical condition as sufficiently serious to engender concern, but are not overly hampered by pain or emotional distress
4. attribute their health to behaviors within their own control and
5. believe in the efficacy of their rehabilitation programs and are confident in their abilities to complete the programs.

ADHERENCE–OUTCOME RELATIONSHIP

The fundamental assumptions underlying the importance ascribed to adherence by rehabilitation professionals are that the rehabilitation programs they prescribe for their clients are effective and that failing to adhere to the programs has an adverse effect on rehabilitation outcomes. Unfortunately, these assumptions are not always warranted. Very few standard clinical rehabilitation practices have the sort of empirical evidence necessary to label the practices as "effective" (i.e., verified by randomized, controlled clinical trials). Similarly, the consequences of non-adherence on rehabilitation outcomes are not fully understood.

In the general medical literature, positive associations between treatment adherence and treatment outcomes have not been found on a consistent basis (Dunbar-Jacob & Schlenk 1996, Hays et al 1994). In the rehabilitation domain, although five studies did not obtain evidence of a positive adherence–outcome relationship (Cammu & Van Nylen 1995, Friedrich et al 1998, Hahn et al 1993, Linton et al 1996, Noyes et al 1983) and two studies have even reported negative associations between adherence and outcome (Quinn 1996, Shelbourne & Wilckens 1990), there is empirical support for the notion that better adherence is related to better outcomes. As shown in Table 4.1, positive adherence–outcome associations have been documented across a wide variety of medical conditions, interventions, and rehabilitation outcomes.

For some of the studies displayed in Table 4.1, adherence was not predictive of outcomes that were investigated but not listed in the table (e.g., knee symptoms and knee laxity in the Brewer et al 2000a study). Further, the studies presented in the table varied extensively in terms of methodological rigor and the adherence measures used. Thus, the findings on the adherence–outcome relationship in rehabilitation are less uniform than the data in Table 4.1 might suggest.

Interpreting positive adherence–outcome associations is fairly straightforward: recovery is better or faster when adherence to the rehabilitation program is high. Interpreting negative adherence–outcome associations is also straightforward: recovery is worse or slower when adherence to the rehabilitation program is high. Negative associations between adherence and outcome suggest the possibility that the rehabilitation program is ineffective (or perhaps even damaging) and should be modified, as Shelbourne & Wilckens (1990) did after they found that adherence to a conservative postsurgical knee rehabilitation program was inversely related to treatment outcome. Interpretation of non-significant adherence–outcome associations is more complicated. Non-significant findings may accurately reflect the relationship between adherence

Table 4.1   Studies reporting positive associations between rehabilitation adherence and rehabilitation outcome

Study	Medical condition	Intervention	Outcome(s)
Brewer et al (2000a)	Knee (ACL) surgery	Clinic- and home-based activities	Functional performance
Derscheid & Feiring (1987)	Sport injuries	Physiotherapy	Clinical improvement
Di Fabio et al (1995)	Low back pain	Clinic-based exercises	Disability, functional performance
Friedrich et al (1996)	Neck and low back pain	Supervised or home exercise	Pain
Groth et al (1994)	Mallet finger injuries	Clinic and home exercises	Range of motion, joint extension
Hawkins (1989)	Shoulder instability	Activity restriction	Symptoms
Hawkins & Switlyk (1993)	Humerus stress fractures	Supervised postsurgery physiotherapy	Rating scale
Kolt & McEvoy (2003)	Low back pain	Clinic and home exercises	Perceived progress
Meani et al 1986	Pathological apophyseal growth centers	Physiotherapy	Anatomical and functional recovery
O'Reilly et al (1999)	Knee osteoarthritis	Home exercises	Walking, stair-climbing, leg strength
Preisinger et al (1996)	Osteoporosis	Supervised exercise	Bone density, back pain
Quinn & Fallon (2000)	Sport injuries	Physiotherapy	Recovery time
Rejeski et al (1997)	Knee osteoarthritis	Facility- and home-aerobic or resistance exercise program	Disability, pain, functional performance
Rives et al (1992)	Depuytren's disease	Postsurgery splinting	Joint extension
Sawhney et al (1999)	Plantar fasciitis	Orthotics	Pain
Schoo (2002)	Knee/hip osteoarthritis	Home exercises	Hip pain intensity and frequency
Shumway-Cook et al (2000)	Falls	Exercise program	Mobility status, fall risk
Treacy et al (1997)	Knee (ACL) surgery	Exercise program	Knee function, satisfaction, return to activity

and outcome, but they may also be attributable to low statistical power, use of unreliable measures, and, as Cammu & Van Nylen (1995) proposed, reductions in adherence after experiencing treatment gains of sufficient magnitude to elicit perceptions of being "cured." Before abandoning or modifying a seemingly ineffective treatment due to a lack of correspondence between adherence and outcome, further inquiry into the reasons for the low association is needed.

ENHANCEMENT OF ADHERENCE TO REHABILITATION

For tried-and-true rehabilitative interventions that have proven effective in producing desired treatment outcomes, adherence comes at a premium. Assuming a positive adherence–outcome association, it is appropriate to initiate efforts to enhance adherence to the rehabilitation program. Optimally, adherence enhancement interventions should be based on theoretical perspectives and research findings that are directly relevant to the particular form of adherence being addressed.

Educational approaches have predominated in the empirical literature on interventions to enhance adherence to rehabilitation. From a general educational perspective, a meta-analysis of 19 prospective randomized controlled trials of "back school" (i.e., patient education for low back pain) revealed a positive effect on "education/compliance outcomes" (Di Fabio 1995). Other educational interventions have involved alterations in the amount and type of rehabilitation supervision and the ways in which instructional information on rehabilitation regimens is delivered.

Demonstrating the potential importance of supervision to rehabilitation adherence, Bentsen et al (1997) found that 3 months of supervised back strengthening produced better adherence to a home training program than a comparable period of unsupervised back strengthening in a sample of 57-year-old women with low back pain. The characteristics of the practitioners supervising the rehabilitation program may also have an impact on adherence. Helewa et al (1994) reported that clients with rheumatoid arthritis who had physiotherapists with special disease-specific training showed better medication adherence (i.e., salicylates) than those who had physiotherapists with traditional (non-specific) training. Similarly, Hidding et al (1994) found that continued enrollment in supervised group physiotherapy yielded greater adherence to home exercises than unsupervised home rehabilitation exercises in individuals with ankylosing spondylitis who had previously had 9 months of supervised group physiotherapy.

In an example of an instructionally based adherence enhancement intervention, Friedrich et al (1996) reported that persons with neck pain and low back pain displayed better adherence (as measured by quality of exercise performance) when therapeutic exercises were taught by a physiotherapist rather than receiving instruction from a brochure. Several studies have shown that adding various components to traditional instructional methods enhances adherence to home rehabilitation exercises. Added components that have been found effective include an instructional audio tape for women with stress urinary incontinence (Gallo & Staskin 1997), an educational booklet with a credibility-enhancing cue for individuals with low back pain (Jackson 1994), and written and illustrated home exercise instructions

for persons with low back pain (Schneiders et al 1998). Further, in a sample of healthy volunteers, Weeks et al (2002) demonstrated the superiority of a dynamic method (i.e., videotape) over a static method (i.e., still-photograph illustrations) in teaching common rehabilitation exercises. Compared to the static method, instruction with the dynamic method produced greater acquisition and retention of quality of exercise performance and greater motivation to perform exercises in the home environment.

In addition to the mode of instruction, the quantity of home rehabilitation activity assigned to clients may have an effect on adherence. Henry et al (1998) found that among older individuals engaged in home exercises, quality of exercise performance was greater in those randomly assigned to complete two exercises as opposed to eight exercises.

Goal setting is another commonly advocated method of enhancing adherence to rehabilitation. Penpraze & Mutrie (1999) found that setting specific goals produced greater knowledge of the rehabilitation program and time spent doing rehabilitation exercises than setting non-specific goals in a sample of individuals with injuries.

Consistent with the findings of Penpraze & Mutrie, Scherzer et al (2001) reported that for a sample of individuals undergoing rehabilitation following knee surgery, goal setting was positively associated with home exercise completion and practitioner adherence ratings. The data on goal setting in rehabilitation are not unequivocal, however, Bassett & Petrie (1999) found in their study of physiotherapy clients with limb injuries that adherence to home exercises was higher for participants who were given no set goals than for those who received physiotherapist-mandated goals. Among the participants in the Bassett & Petrie investigation who showed clinical improvement, participants who set goals collaboratively with the physiotherapist had greater adherence to home exercises than those who were given physiotherapist-mandated goals. See Chapters 1 and 5 for the importance of the collaborative alliance between the practitioner and the client.

Another approach to enhancing rehabilitation adherence is to combine several potentially beneficial procedures in a multimodal intervention. Friedrich et al (1998) examined the effects of one such intervention on adherence to rehabilitation in persons with low back pain. The intervention focused on increasing motivation to complete the rehabilitation program and consisted of counseling/information, reinforcement of rehabilitation behavior, posting a treatment contract at home, and recording completed exercises in diary. Although no effect on long-term home exercise adherence was found, the intervention produced greater attendance at ten physiotherapy sessions than a control condition. Hammond & Freeman (2001) also assessed the efficacy of a multimodal intervention in a rehabilitation context. For persons with rheumatoid arthritis, a specialized educational intervention consisting of goal setting, contracting, modeling, assigning homework, providing information on motor learning theory, enhancing recall of the rehabilitation program, and facilitating mental practice of treatment procedures produced greater adherence to a joint protection program than standard arthritis education.

Empirical support has been obtained for the potential utility of several other interventions in boosting adherence to rehabilitation. For example, reinforcement of desired rehabilitation behaviors has been associated with elevated levels of adherence to therapeutic exercises for both children with hemophilia (Greenan-Fowler et al 1987) and individuals with severe burns (Hegel et al 1986). Experimental research has shown that adding cryotherapy to a knee rehabilitation program may have a favorable impact on adherence to postsurgical rehabilitation (Lessard et al 1997). Correlational research has indicated that rehabilitation adherence is positively associated with being a member of a self-help group for persons with ankylosing sponylitis (Barlow et al 1993), using positive self-talk for individuals who had knee surgery (Scherzer et al 2001), being referred for physiotherapy by a medical specialist (as opposed to a general practitioner), and having the initial physiotherapy appointments made by telephone instead of by mail (Armistead 1997).

CLIENT–PRACTITIONER RELATIONSHIP

People undergoing rehabilitation do so within a broad social context in which they interact with family members, friends, fellow rehabilitation participants, support staff, physicians, and, especially, rehabilitation practitioners. The nature and quality of the relationships that rehabilitation clients experience with those in their social environment can have important implications for key rehabilitation

processes and outcomes. Given the centrality of rehabilitation practitioners to the planning, implementation, and maintenance of the rehabilitation agenda, the client–practitioner relationship is considered particularly influential (Stenmar & Nordholm 1994).

A defining feature of the client–practitioner relationship is the communication that occurs between clients and their rehabilitation practitioners. One potential indicator of the quality of communication between clients and practitioners is the degree to which client and practitioner perceptions of rehabilitation-related matters converge.

CLIENT–PRACTITIONER COMMUNICATION

In the general medical literature, research on client–practitioner communication has focused on the communication behaviors exhibited by practitioners toward their clients. Such communication has been grouped into the following descriptive categories: competence-related, informational, partnership building, questions, and socioemotional (Hall et al 1988). Characteristics of both clients and practitioners can have an impact on client–practitioner communication. Clients who are anxious, inexperienced with their medical conditions, or unintelligent can have difficulty communicating with their practitioners. Client–practitioner communication can also be hampered when practitioners do not listen to their clients, use jargon and overly technical language, provide overly simplistic explanations, display signs of worry, and stereotype clients in a pejorative manner (Taylor 2003). When client–practitioner communication is problematic, clients may become discouraged from using medical services in the future and have greater difficulty adhering to their rehabilitation regimen (DiMatteo et al 1993, Meichenbaum & Turk 1987, Taylor 2003).

Client–practitioner communication in the realm of rehabilitation, which is addressed in greater detail in Chapter 5, begins with the first appointment (Thornquist 1992) and consists of both verbal and non-verbal interactions. As in encounters between physicians and their patients (Hall et al 1988), socioemotional and informational communication are salient aspects of interactions between rehabilitation clients and practitioners (Hokanson 1994, Owen & Goodge 1981, Talvitie 2000). Non-verbal communication between clients and practitioners can fulfill both socioemotional (e.g., supportive) and informational (e.g., instructional) functions (Perry 1975). Although master physiotherapists tend to focus their verbal and non-verbal communication more effectively than novice physiotherapists (Jensen et al 1992), the interviewing and communication skills of rehabilitation practitioners can be enhanced through training (Ladyshewsky & Gotjamanos 1997, Levin & Riley 1984, Pichert et al 1999).

CLIENT AND PRACTITIONER PERCEPTIONS

Two of the more basic issues that rehabilitation practitioners and their clients may address when communicating about rehabilitation-related matters are the nature of the rehabilitation regimen and the status of their injuries or illnesses. Although it may seem that there should be little disparity in the perceptions of clients and practitioners with regard to these basic issues, research suggests that client–practitioner discrepancies can exist and potentially influence other aspects of rehabilitation. For example, Kahanov & Fairchild (1994) reported significant disagreement between athletes with injuries and their athletic trainers on the extent to which the athletes understood their treatment regimen and were given a written treatment protocol. Other studies with individuals undergoing injury rehabilitation have shown that they underestimate (relative to their physiotherapist's assessment) the amount of time needed to do their home rehabilitation exercises (May & Taylor 1994) and are highly likely to misunderstand at least part of their prescribed rehabilitation regimen (Webborn et al 1997). An investigation of persons with low back pain revealed that incongruence with their chiropractor or rheumatologist in terms of selected aspects of back pain and treatment protocols was associated with a less favorable self-prognosis for the outcome of rehabilitation (Cedraschi et al 1996).

Although client and practitioner perceptions of injury status tend to be positively correlated (Brewer et al 1995a, 1995b, Crossman & Jamieson 1985), indicating a degree of consistency, there is evidence that persons with injuries underestimate how disruptive their injuries will be (Crossman & Jamieson 1985, Crossman et al 1990) and overestimate how serious their injuries are (Crossman & Jamieson 1985). Client–practitioner discrepancies in assessments of injury status have been positively

associated with client pain and emotional distress (Crossman & Jamieson 1985), suggesting that miscommunication between clients and practitioners may have an adverse effect on the rehabilitation experience of clients.

Discrepancies can also occur in assessments of the level of psychological distress experienced by clients. Brewer et al (1995b) reported a lack of correspondence between the behavioral observations made by practitioners at an orthopedic physical therapy clinic and the degree of emotional disturbance indicated by their clients. Such discrepancies do not necessarily represent a breakdown in client–practitioner communication, as clients may consider their emotional states unrelated to their rehabilitation and therefore attempt to conceal them from practitioners. Nevertheless, recognition of client psychological distress is important because emotional difficulties, in addition to being unpleasant to clients, are associated with poorer adherence to rehabilitation (DiMatteo et al 2000) and poorer clinical outcomes (e.g. Brewer et al 2000a, Johnson 1996, 1997).

PSYCHOLOGICAL READINESS TO RETURN

For many individuals, the medical conditions that precipitate their involvement in rehabilitation activities limit or restrict their ability to participate in occupational, social, household, and other valued endeavors. As the conclusion of rehabilitation approaches, it is necessary to ascertain clients' degree of readiness to return to activities from which their involvement had been limited or restricted. Optimally, the return to activity can be phased in gradually, thereby minimizing the degree of readiness required to proceed incrementally from one level of activity to the next. At some point in the process, however, clients may encounter the need to increase their activity levels to an extent that causes apprehension or anxiety. Anxiety-provoking situations such as this reflect the need to consider not only the physical readiness but also the psychological readiness of clients to return to activity.

In the field of vocational rehabilitation, functional capacity evaluations are routinely performed to determine whether clients can safely perform work-related tasks prior to returning to work (Lechner 1998). Similarly, for athletes undergoing rehabilitation, return-to-play guidelines have been established ("The team physician" 2002). Unfortunately, although psychological readiness to return is important to resumption of occupational involvement, little empirical research has been conducted on the topic. Consequently, little is known about what exactly constitutes psychological readiness to return and what rehabilitation practitioners can do to increase the psychological readiness of their clients. The theoretical work of Andersen (2001) suggests that psychological readiness to return can be enhanced by decreasing anxiety associated with activity resumption and reducing psychological risks for recurrence of the medical condition that prompted the need for rehabilitation in the first place.

Anxiety experienced during rehabilitation can signify a reduced level of readiness to return. As Andersen (2001) noted, such anxiety may reflect clients' worries over the possibility of failing to regain 100% of their previous capabilities or of becoming injured or ill once again. The presence of return-related anxiety can be identified through verbal probes (e.g., "What concerns do you have about returning to .... activity?") and observation of behaviors such as bracing and avoidance of certain actions or positions. In the event that potentially debilitating anxiety is observed, it can be addressed through a variety of behavioral (e.g., relaxation, systematic desensitization) and pharmacological means (Andersen 2001).

Another means of enhancing readiness to return is to decrease clients' psychological vulnerability to experiencing future injury or illness. For medical conditions that have psychological stress as an etiological component, stress management interventions can lower clients' stress levels and make them less susceptible to recurrence of their physical problems. In the case of work-related injury, for example, employees can theoretically reduce their risk of re-injury by participating in psychological interventions (e.g., cognitive restructuring, relaxation, imagery) that decrease their stress responsivity (Andersen 2001).

SUMMARY

Psychological factors play an important role in rehabilitation processes and outcomes. Adherence to rehabilitation, which can be measured in a variety of ways depending on the behavioral requirements of the rehabilitation regimen, is a psychological factor that can be enhanced through intervention to improve clinical outcomes. The client–practitioner relationship is a vital part of rehabilitation that involves communication on both informational and socioemotional matters. In concluding the rehabilitation process, practitioners should ensure that their clients are both physically and psychologically ready to return to participation in activities that were medically contraindicated during rehabilitation. By attending to psychological factors in rehabilitation, practitioners can better serve the clients with whom they work.

ACKNOWLEDGMENTS

This chapter was supported in part by grant number R29 AR44484 from the National Institute of Arthritis and Musculoskeletal and Skin Diseases. Its contents are solely the responsibility of the author and do not represent the official views of the National Institute of Arthritis and Musculoskeletal and Skin Diseases.

References

Abbott J, Dodd M, Bilton D, Webb et al 1994 Treatment compliance in adults with cystic fibrosis. Thorax 49: 115–120

Abbott J, Dodd M, Webb AK 1996 Health perceptions and treatment adherence with cystic fibrosis. Thorax 51: 1233–1238

Andersen M B 2001 Returning to action and the prevention of future injury. In: Crossman J (ed) Coping with sports injuries: Psychological strategies for rehabilitation. Oxford University Press, Oxford, p 162–173

Armistead J 1997 An evaluation of initial non-attendance rates for physiotherapy. Physiotherapy 83: 591–596

Barlow J H, Macey S J, Struthers G R 1993 Health locus of control, self-help and treatment adherence in relation to ankylosing spondylitis patients. Patient Education and Counseling 20: 153–166

Bassett S F, Petrie K J 1999 The effect of treatment goals on patient compliance with physiotherapy exercise programmes. Physiotherapy 85: 130–137

Belanger A Y, Noel G 1990 Compliance to and effects of a home strengthening exercise program for adult dystrophic patients: A pilot study. Physiotherapy Canada 43: 24–30

Bentsen H, Lindgarde F, Manthrope R 1997 The effects of dynamic strength back exercise and/or a home training program in 57-year-old women with chronic low back pain. Spine 22: 1494–1500

Breuer U 1994 Diabetic patient's compliance with bespoke footwear after healing of neuropathic foot ulcers. Diabetes & Metabolism 20: 415–419

Brewer B W 1999 Adherence to sport injury rehabilitation regimens. In: Bull S J (ed) Adherence issues in sport and exercise. Wiley, Chichester, UK, p 145–168

Brewer B W 2001 Psychology of sport injury rehabilitation. In: Singer R N, Hausenblas H A, Janelle C M (eds) Handbook of sport psychology, 2nd edn. Wiley, New York, p 787–809

Brewer B W, Linder D E, Phelps C M 1995a Situational correlates of emotional adjustment to athletic injury. Clinical Journal of Sport Medicine 5: 241–245

Brewer B W, Petitpas A J, Van Raalte J L et al 1995b Prevalence of psychological distress among patients at a physical therapy clinic specializing in sports medicine. Sports Medicine, Training and Rehabilitation 6: 138–145

Brewer B W, Daly J M, Van Raalte J L et al 1999 A psychometric evaluation of the Rehabilitation Adherence Questionnaire. Journal of Sport & Exercise Psychology 21: 167–173

Brewer B W, Van Raalte J L, Cornelius A E et al 2000a Psychological factors, rehabilitation adherence, and rehabilitation outcome after anterior cruciate ligament reconstruction. Rehabilitation Psychology 45: 20–37

Brewer B W, Van Raalte J L, Petitpas A J et al 2000b Preliminary psychometric evaluation of a measure of adherence to clinic-based sport injury rehabilitation. Physical Therapy in Sport 1: 68–74

Brewer B W, Avondoglio J B, Cornelius A E et al 2002 Construct validity and interrater agreement of the Sport Injury Rehabilitation Adherence Scale. Journal of Sport Rehabilitation 11: 170–178

Brewer B W, Cornelius A E, Van Raalte J L et al (2003) Protection motivation theory and adherence to sport injury rehabilitation revisited. The Sport Psychologist 17: 95–103

Byerly P N, Worrell T, Gahimer J et al 1994 Rehabilitation compliance in an athletic training environment. Journal of Athletic Training 29: 352–355

Cammu H, Van Nylen M 1995 Pelvic floor muscle exercises: 5 years later. Urology 45: 113–118

Cedraschi C, Robert J, Perrin E et al 1996 The role of congruence between patient and therapist in chronic low back pain patients. Journal of Manipulative and Physiological Therapeutics 19: 244–249

Chen C Y, Neufeld P S, Feely C A et al 1999 Factors influencing compliance with home exercise programs among patients with upper-extremity impairment. American Journal of Occupational Therapy 53: 171–180

Clark N M, Becker M H 1998 Theoretical models and strategies for improving adherence and disease management. In: Shumaker S A, Schron E B, Ockene J K et al (eds) The handbook of health behavior change, 2nd edn. Springer, New York, p 5–32

Crossman J, Jamieson J 1985 Differences in perceptions of seriousness and disrupting effects of athletic injury as viewed by athletes and their trainer. Perceptual and Motor Skills 61: 1131–1134

Crossman J, Roch J 1991 An observation instrument for use in sports medicine clinics. The Journal of the Canadian Athletic Therapists Association April: 10–13

Crossman J, Jamieson J, Hume K M 1990 Perceptions of athletic injuries by athletes, coaches, and medical professionals. Perceptual and Motor Skills 71: 848–850

Derscheid G L, Feiring D C 1987 A statistical analysis to characterize treatment adherence of the 18 diagnoses most seen at a sports medicine clinic. Journal of Orthopaedic and Sports Physical Therapy 9: 40–46

Di Fabio R P 1995 Efficacy of comprehensive rehabilitation programs and back school for patients with low back pain: a meta-analysis. Physical Therapy 75: 865–878

Di Fabio R P, Mackey G, Holte J B 1995 Disability and functional status in patients with low back pain receiving workers' compensation: A descriptive study with implications for the efficacy of physical therapy. Physical Therapy 75: 180–193

DiMatteo M R, Sherbourne C D, Hays R D et al 1993 Physicians' characteristics influence patients' adherence to medical treatment: Results from the Medical Outcomes Study. Health Psychology 12: 93–102

DiMatteo M R, Lepper H S, Croghan T W 2000 Depression is a risk factor for noncompliance with medical treatment. Archives of Internal Medicine 160: 2101–2107

Dobbe J G, van Trommel N E, de Freitas Baptista J E et al 1999 A portable device for finger tendon rehabilitation that provides an isotonic force and records exercise behaviour after finger tendon surgery. Medical and Biological Engineering and Computing 37: 396–399

Donatelli R, Hurlbert C, Conaway D et al 1988 Biomechanical foot orthotics: A retrospective study. The Journal of Orthopaedic and Sports Physical Therapy 10: 205–212

Duda J L, Smart A E, Tappe M K 1989 Predictors of adherence in rehabilitation of athletic injuries: An application of personal investment theory. Journal of Sport & Exercise Psychology 11: 367–381

Dunbar-Jacob J, Schlenk E 1996 Treatment adherence and clinical outcome: Can we make a difference? In: Resnick R J, Rozensky R H (eds) Health psychology through the life span: Practice and research opportunities. American Psychological Association, Washington, DC, p 323–343

Dunbar-Jacob J, Dunning E J, Dwyer K 1993 Compliance research in pediatric and adolescent populations: Two decades of research. In: Krasnegor N A, Epstein L, Johnson S B, Yaffe S J (eds) Developmental aspects of health compliance behavior. Erlbaum, Mahwah, NJ, p 29–51

Dunbar-Jacob J, Sereika S, Rohay J et al 1998 Electronic methods in assessing adherence to medical regimens. In: Krantz D S, Baum A (eds) Technology and methods in behavioral medicine. Erlbaum, Mahwah, NJ, p 95–113

Fields J, Murphey M, Horodyski M et al 1995 Factors associated with adherence to sport injury rehabilitation in college-age recreational athletes. Journal of Sport Rehabilitation 4: 172–180

Fisher A C, Domm M A, Wuest D A 1988 Adherence to sports-injury rehabilitation programs. The Physician and Sportsmedicine 16(7): 47–52

Flynn M F, Lyman R D, Prentice-Dunn S 1995 Protection motivation theory and adherence to medical treatment regimens for muscular dystrophy. Journal of Social and Clinical Psychology 14: 61–75

Fong S L, Dales R E, Tierney M G 1990 Compliance among adults with cystic fibrosis. DICP 24: 689–692

Friedrich M, Cermak T, Maderbacher P 1996 The effects of brochure use versus therpist teaching on patients performing therapeutic exercise and on changes in impairment status. Physical Therapy 76: 1082–1088

Friedrich M, Gittler G, Halberstadt Y et al 1998 Combined exercise and motivation program: Effect on the compliance and level of disability of patients with low back pain: A randomized controlled trial. Archives of Physical Medicine and Rehabilitation 79: 475–487

Gallo M L, Staskin D R 1997 Cues to action: Pelvic floor muscle exercise compliance in women with stress urinary incontinence. Neurourology and Urodynamics 16: 167–177

Greenan-Fowler E, Powell C, Varni J W 1987 Behavioral treatment of adherence to therapeutic exercise by children with hemophilia. Archives of Physical Medicine and Rehabilitation 68: 846–849

Groth G N, Wilder D M, Young V L 1994 The impact of compliance on the rehabilitation of patients with mallet finger injuries. Journal of Hand Therapy 7: 21–24

Hahn I, Milsom I, Fall M et al 1993 Long-term results of pelvic floor training in female stress urinary incontinence. British Journal of Urology 72: 421–427

Hall J A, Roter D L, Katz N R 1988 Meta-analysis of correlates of provider behavior in medical encounters. Medical Care 26: 657–675

Hammond A, Freeman K 2001 One-year outcomes of a randomized controlled trial of an educational–behavioral joint protection programme for people with rheumatoid arthritis. Rheumatology 40: 1044–1051

Hammond A, Lincoln N 1999 Development of the Joint Protection Behaviour Assessment. Arthritis Care and Research 12: 200–207

Hawkins R B 1989 Arthroscopic stapling repair for shoulder instability: A retrospective study of 50 cases. Arthroscopy: The Journal of Arthroscopic and Related Surgery 2: 122–128

Hawkins R J, Switlyk P 1993 Acute prosthetic replacement for stress fractures of the proximal humerus. Clinical Orthopaedics and Related Research 289: 156–160

Hays R D, Kravitz R L, Mazel R M et al 1994 The impact of patient adherence on health outcomes for patients with chronic disease in the Medical Outcomes Study. Journal of Behavioral Medicine 17: 347–360

Hegel M T, Ayllon T, VanderPlate C et al 1986 A behavioral procedure for increasing compliance with self-exercise regimens in severely burn-injured patients. Behaviour Research and Therapy 24: 521–528

Helewa A, Smythe H A, Goldsmith C H 1994 Can specifically trained physiotherapists improve care of patients with rheumatoid arthritis? A randomized health care trial. Journal of Rheumatology 21: 70–79

Henry K D, Rosemond C, Eckert L B 1998 Effect of number of home exercises on compliance and performance in adults over 65 years of age. Physical Therapy 78: 70–277

Hidding A, van der Linden S, Gielen X et al 1994 Continuation of group physical therapy is necessary in ankylosing spondylitis. Arthritis Care and Research 7: 90–96

Hokanson R G 1994 Relationship between sports rehabilitation practitioners' communication style and athletes' adherence to injury rehabilitation. Unpublished master's thesis, Springfield College, Massachusetts, MA

Jackson L D 1994 Maximizing treatment adherence among back-pain patients: An experimental study of the effects of physician-related cues in written medical messages. Health Communication 6: 173–191

Jensen G M, Shepard K F, Gwyer J et al 1992 Attribute dimensions that distinguish master and novice physical therapy clinicians in orthopedic settings. Physical Therapy 72: 711–722

Johnson U 1996 The multiply injured versus the first-time-injured athlete during rehabilitation: A comparison of nonphysical characteristics. Journal of Sport Rehabilitation 5: 293–304

Johnson U 1997 A three-year follow-up of long-term injured competitive athletes: Influence of psychological risk factors on rehabilitation. Journal of Sport Rehabilitation 6: 256–271

Kahanov L, Fairchild P C 1994 Discrepancies in perceptions held by injured athletes and athletic trainers during the initial evaluation. Journal of Athletic Training 29: 70–75

Kolt G S, McEvoy J F 2003 Adherence to rehabilitation in patients with low back pain. Manual Therapy 8: 110–116

Ladyshewsky R, Gotjamanos E 1997 Communication skill development in health professional education: The use of standardized patients in combination with a peer assessment strategy. Journal of Allied Health 26: 177–186

Lampton C C, Lambert M E, Yost R 1993 The effects of psychological factors in sports medicine rehabilitation adherence. Journal of Sports Medicine and Physical Fitness 33: 292–299

Lansinger B, Nordholm L, Sivick T 1994 Characteristics of low back pain patients who do not complete physiotherapeutic treatment. Scandinavian Journal of Caring Science 8: 163–167

Laubach W J, Brewer B W, Van Raalte J L et al 1996 Attributions for recovery and adherence to sport injury rehabilitation. Australian Journal of Science and Medicine in Sport 28: 30–34

Laupattarakasem W 1988 Short term continuous passive motion. The Journal of Bone and Joint Surgery 70: 802–806

Lazarus R S, Folkman S 1984 Stress, appraisal, and coping. Springer-Verlag, New York

Lechner D E 1998 Functional capacity evaluation. In: King P M (ed) Sourcebook of occupational rehabilitation: Plenum series in rehabilitation and health. Plenum, New York, p 209–227

Lessard L A, Scudds R A, Amendola A et al 1997 The efficacy of cryotherapy following arthroscopic knee surgery. Journal of Orthopaedic and Sports Physical Therapy 26: 14–22

Levin M F, Riley E J 1984 Effectiveness of teaching interviewing and communication skills to physiotherapy students. Physiotherapy Canada 36: 190–194

Levitt R, Deisinger J A, Wall J R et al 1995 EMG feedback-assisted postoperative rehabilitation of minor arthroscopic knee surgeries. The Journal of Sports Medicine and Physical Fitness 35: 218–223

Linton S J, Hellsing A, Bergstrom G 1996 Exercise for workers with musculoskeletal pain: Does enhancing compliance decrease pain? Journal of Occupational Rehabilitation 6: 177–190

Maehr M, Braskamp L 1986 The motivation factor: A theory of personal investment. Lexington Books, Lexington, MA

May S, Taylor A H 1994 The development and examination of various measures of patient compliance, for specific use with injured athletes. Journal of Sports Sciences 12: 180–181

Meani E, Migliorini S, Tinti G 1986 La patologia de sovraccarico sportivo dei nuclei di accrescimento apofisari. [The pathology of apophyseal growth centres caused by overstrain during sports]. Italian Journal of Sports Traumatology 8: 29–38

Meichenbaum D, Turk D C 1987 Facilitating treatment adherence. Plenum, New York

Nicholas M K 1995 Compliance: A barrier to occupational rehabilitation? Journal of Occupational Rehabilitation 5: 271–282

Noyes F R, Matthews D S, Mooar P A et al 1983 The symptomatic anterior cruciate-deficient knee. Part II: The results of rehabilitation, activity modification, and counseling on functional disability. Journal of Bone and Joint Surgery 65-A: 163–174.

O'Carroll M, Hendriks O 1989 Factors associated with rheumatoid arthritis patients' compliance with home exercises and splint use. Physiotherapy Practice 5: 115–122

Olivier L C, Neudeck F, Assenmacher S et al 1997 Acceptance of Allgower/Wenzl partial dynamic weight bearing orthosis. Results using a hidden step counting device. Unfallchirurgie 23: 200–204

O'Reilly S C, Muir K R, Doherty M 1999 Effectiveness of home exercise on pain and disability from osteoarthritis of the knee: A randomized controlled trial. Annals of the Rheumatic Diseases 58: 15–19

Owen O G, Goodge P 1981 Physiotherapists talking to patients. Patient Counseling and Health Education 3: 100–102

Penpraze P, Mutrie N 1999 Effectiveness of goal setting in an injury rehabilitation programme for increasing patient understanding and compliance [Abstract]. British Journal of Sports Medicine 33: 60

Perry J F 1975 Nonverbal communication during physical therapy. Physical Therapy 55: 593–600

Petrosenko R D, Vandervoort B M, Chesworth B M et al 1996 Development of a home ankle exerciser. Medical Engineering and Physics 18: 314–319

Pichert J W, Schlundt D G, Boswell E J et al 1999 Improving health professionals' adherence promotion and problem solving skills [Abstract]. Annals of Behavioral Medicine 21(Suppl.): S123

Pizzari T, McBurney H, Taylor N F 2002 Adherence to anterior cruciate ligament reconstruction: A qualitative analysis. Journal of Sport Rehabilitation 11: 90–102

Preisinger E, Alacamlioglu Y, Pils K et al 1996 Exercise therapy for osteoporosis: Results of a randomized controlled trial. British Journal of Sports Medicine 30: 209–212

Prentice-Dunn S, Rogers R W 1986 Protection motivation theory and preventive health: Beyond the health belief model. Health Education Research 1: 153–161

Quinn A M 1996 The psychological factors involved in the recovery of elite athletes from long term injuries. Unpublished doctoral dissertation, University of Melbourne, Australia

Quinn A M, Fallon B J 2000 Predictors of recovery time. Journal of Sport Rehabilitation 9: 62–76

Rejeski W J, Brawley L R, Ettinger W et al 1997 Compliance to exercise therapy in older participants with knee osteoarthritis: Implications for treating disability. Medicine and Science in Sports and Exercise 29: 977–985

Rives K, Gelberman R, Smith B et al 1992 Severe contractures of the proximal interphalangeal joint in Depuytren's disease: Results of a prospective trial of operative correction and dynamic extension splinting. Journal of Hand Surgery 17A: 1153–1159

Rosenstock I M 1974 Historical origins of the health belief model. Health Education Monographs 2: 328–335

Sawhney R, Egidi E, Bukosky J et al 1999 Long-term compliance of patients using functional orthotics for plantar fasciitis [Abstract]. Journal of Orthopaedic and Sports Physical Therapy 29: A–38

Scherzer C B, Brewer B W, Cornelius A E et al 2001 Psychological skills and adherence to rehabilitation after reconstruction of the anterior cruciate ligament. Journal of Sport Rehabilitation 10: 165–172

Schlenk E A, Dunbar-Jacob J, Sereika S et al 2000 Comparability of daily diaries and accelerometers in exercise adherence in fibromyalgia syndrome [Abstract]. Measurement and Evaluation in Physical Education and Exercise Science 4: 133–134

Schneiders A G, Zusman M, Singer K P 1998 Exercise therapy compliance in acute low back pain patients. Manual Therapy 3: 147–152

Schoo A M M 2002 Exercise performance in older people with osteoarthritis: Relationships between exercise adherence, correctness of exercise performance and associated pain. Unpublished doctoral dissertation, La Trobe University, Bundoora, Australia

Shank R H 1988 Academic and athletic factors related to predicting compliance by athletes to treatments. Unpublished doctoral dissertation, University of Virginia, Charlottesville

Shelbourne K D, Wilckens J H 1990 Current concepts in anterior cruciate ligament rehabilitation. Orthopaedic Review 19: 957–964

Shumway-Cook A, Gruber W, Baldwin M et al 1997 The effects of multidimensional exercise on balance, mobility, and fall risk in community-dwelling older adults. Physical Therapy 77: 46–57

Sluijs E M, Kok G J, van der Zee J 1993 Correlates of exercise compliance in physical therapy. Physical Therapy 73: 771–782

Stenmar L, Nordholm L A 1994 Swedish physical therapists' beliefs on what makes therapy work. Physical Therapy 74: 1034–1039

Stenstrom C H, Arge B, Sundbom A 1997 Home exercise and compliance in inflammatory rheumatic diseases – A prospective clinical trial. The Journal of Rheumatology 24: 470–476

Talvitie U 2000 Socio-affective characteristics and properties of extrinsic feedback in physiotherapy. Physiotherapy Research International 5: 173–189

Taylor A H, May S 1996 Threat and coping appraisal as determinants of compliance to sports injury rehabilitation: An application of protection motivation theory. Journal of Sports Sciences 14: 471–482

Taylor S E 2003 Health psychology, 5th edn. McGraw-Hill, New York

The team physician and return-to-play issues: A consensus statement. 2002 Medicine and Science in Sports & Exercise 33: 1212–1214

Thornquist E 1992 Examination and communication: A study of first encounters between patients and physiotherapists. Family Practice 9: 195–202

Treacy S H, Barron O A, Brunet M E et al 1997 Assessing the need for extensive supervised rehabilitation following arthroscopic surgery. American Journal of Orthopedics 26: 25–29

Vandal S, Rivard C H, Bradet R 1999 Measuring the compliance behavior of adolescents wearing orthopedic braces. Issues in Comprehensive Pediatric Nursing 22(2–3): 59–73

Webborn A D J, Carbon R J, Miller B P 1997 Injury rehabilitation programs: "What are we talking about?" Journal of Sport Rehabilitation 6: 54–61

Weeks D L, Brubaker J, Byrt J et al 2002 Videotape instruction versus illustrations for influencing quality of performance, motivation, and confidence to perform simple and complex exercises in healthy subjects. Physiotherapy Theory and Practice 18: 65–73

Wiese-Bjornstal D M, Smith A M, Shaffer S M et al 1998 An integrated model of response to sport injury: Psychological and sociological dimensions. Journal of Applied Sport Psychology 10: 46–69

SECTION **2**

Psychological care in the physical and manual therapies: an integrated approach

SECTION CONTENTS

Chapter 5

Practitioner–client relationships: building working alliances

Al Petitpas, Allen Cornelius

INTRODUCTION

The primary treatment goal for most physical and manual therapists is to assist their clients in the prevention and rehabilitation of injuries. Although much of medical training is focused on the physical aspects of clients' needs, there is considerable evidence that the quality of the working alliance established between medical professionals and their clients is the key predictor of client adherence and positive treatment outcomes (Ray & Wiese-Bjornstal 1999).

Although there are several definitions of the working alliance available in the counseling and medical literature, they all contain a common thread of some type of collaborative relationship between the practitioner and the client in which they work together to help the client manage a specific concern (Osachuk & Cairns 1995). The primary function of a working alliance is to create a climate of trust, and possibly even an emotional bond, in which the client and practitioner come to a clear agreement about treatment goals and the tasks necessary to achieve them (Bordin 1979). Without alliances and agreements, it is doubtful that clients will adhere to the prescribed treatment plan or put forth the effort required to achieve their desired outcomes (Locke & Latham 2002).

In order to be effective in creating working alliances, it is important for physical and manual therapists to define their roles clearly to each of their clients. Research has shown that most clients view medical professionals in a superior or one-up position (Kiesler & Watkins 1989). Many clients place medical professionals in the role of expert and wait for them to take the lead in defining the content and process of their treatment interactions. The initial contacts between practitioners and clients typically set the tone and structure for the working relationship that follows and create a platform for the formation of a collaborative working alliance (Petitpas 1999). To be effective, physical and manual therapists should send a clear message that they are treating people and not just their injuries. For example, medical professionals who approach a new client with statements such as "Are you the knee?"(unfortunately we have heard such questions often in rehabilitation clinics, see Chapter 1), devalue the importance of the client as a partner in the treatment process and jeopardize the development of a collaborative working relationship.

The purpose of this chapter is to provide physical and manual therapists with a general overview of the importance of the working alliance in the rehabilitation and prevention of injuries and a general introduction to some basic techniques for creating positive working relationships with clients. In particular, (a) theory and research supporting the efficacy of the working alliance will be presented, (b) skills and strategies required to enhance client–practitioner relationships will be described, and (c) suggestions for training will be offered.

THEORETICAL AND EMPIRICAL BASIS FOR THE IMPORTANCE OF THE WORKING ALLIANCE

The relationship between clients and their physical or manual therapists is complex. It includes the need for an exchange of information about the condition requiring treatment, the available treatment options, the expected outcomes of treatment, the barriers to adherence and recovery, and other treatment-related information. It may also involve an anxious and uninformed client, a harried therapist, and a healthcare system that may not be supportive. Although some of these factors are beyond the control of physical and manual therapists, it is possible to create a working environment that is based on trust and collaboration even in trying and demanding situations. In this section of the chapter, theoretical and empirical support for the importance of creating a working alliance to help facilitate the process of physical and manual therapy is presented.

MODELS OF CLIENT–PRACTITIONER INTERACTION

Several models describing client–practitioner interaction appear in the literature and provide a basis for understanding how relationships between clients and their physical or manual therapists influence adherence and treatment outcomes. Over the last several decades, there has been a shift from an exclusive adherence to a traditional medical model of client–practitioner interaction to greater acceptance and belief in the efficacy of a collaborative or mutual participation approach. As Parsons (1951) described, healthcare professionals who adhered to the traditional medical model, assumed the role of expert or professional, and interacted with clients who assumed the "sick role." As the experts, healthcare professionals (supposedly) know what is best for their clients and then clients trust without question the knowledge and judgments of the practitioners. This traditional view, however, does not place enough importance on clients' beliefs, skills, emotional states, knowledge, or expectations, and does not enlist clients as participants in their own recovery (Meichenbaum & Turk 1987).

As early as the mid–1950s, researchers began to question the efficacy of the traditional medical model view of client–practitioner interactions for all situations. For example, Szasz & Hollender (1956) suggested that the traditional view might be appropriate for individuals who were unable to act on their own behalf (e.g., infants, comatose adults), but believed that a cooperating or mutual participation mode was more likely to facilitate adherence and encourage clients to help themselves. Empirical support for this belief will be presented later in this section.

The importance of the relationships between practitioners and their clients has been highlighted in two proposed models. In the first, called the process model for client–practitioner collaboration (Jensen & Lorish 1994), a four-component model was developed by examining survey responses from arthritis clients and their practitioners and drawing from related literature, theory, and professional experience. The primary component of this model was the development of a therapeutic relationship, which was viewed as a necessary condition for any subsequent productive work. The other components of the model – mutual inquiry, problem solving, and negotiation – could not be realized without the establishment of a relationship built on rapport, honest dialogue, and disclosure.

Owen & Goodge (1981) described a second model that examined communication between physiotherapists and their clients to determine the types of statements that occur during a physiotherapy session. From these interactions, they identified two distinct types of communication. The first type focused on giving direction and advice, and the second reflected efforts to build a helping relationship. The direction and advice-giving dimension was characterized by asking direct questions, giving advice and directions, and shutting off or ignoring the client's ideas and feelings. The relationship-building component of this model consisted of three types of statements: empathizing statements, constructive feedback, and counseling statements. Empathizing statements showed concern for the client's comfort, an indication of understanding the client's point of view, an acceptance of the client's feelings, a disclosure of the practitioner's feelings, and a willingness to enter a collaborative relationship with the client. Constructive feedback was characterized by giving praise or helpful feedback on performance and progress. Counseling statements included answering clients' questions, building on clients' questions and ideas, encouraging clients to continue, encouraging comparison and description, reflecting statements back to clients, paraphrasing, restating, summarizing, and clarifying what clients said, exploring the meaning of what was said, using silence, and offering observations. The authors concluded that there are at least two types of communication that characterized the client–practitioner interaction. These dimensions likely reflect two aspects of the relationship – one based on the belief that the practitioner has all the knowledge and expertise necessary to help the client and the other based on establishing a relationship within which clients can use this expertise to enhance their recovery processes.

More recently, Szybek et al (2000) applied a psychotherapy model to physiotherapy–client relationships. Their model was based on the multidimensional psychotherapy model of Gelso & Carter (1994), which proposed that any therapeutic relationship is composed of three components: the working alliance, the transference configuration, and the real relationship. This model depicts the working alliance as the fundamental component of the relationship. The working alliance reflects the degree to which the practitioner and client agree on the goals to be pursued and the tasks that need to be undertaken to accomplish those goals. It also includes the emotional bond between the practitioner and client. The working alliance is central to the success of therapy and has been shown to account for up to 45% of the variance in achieving desired outcomes (Horvath & Greenberg 1989). The process of physiotherapy is obviously different from psychotherapy, but the importance of the working relationship should not be overlooked (Szybek et al 2000).

The second component of the model, transference configuration, deals with the concepts of transference and countertransference (Gelso & Carter 1994). Transference occurs when clients transfer their feelings, thoughts, and reactions to significant others in their lives, usually parents, to other parties, often authority figures (e.g., teachers, bosses). These authority figures could include physiotherapists. Countertransference is the parallel process where authority figures, such as physiotherapists, express or transfer their feelings about significant others onto their clients, such as physiotherapy patients. Transference and countertransference can be positive or negative. Positive transference or countertransference occurs when the feelings and thoughts transferred to the other member of the relationship are of a warm and positive nature, and negative transference or countertransference occurs when the feelings and thoughts are of a hostile and negative nature. Either type of transference or countertransference potentially can affect the progress of a therapeutic relationship (see Chapter 6 for an in-depth discussion of transference and countertransference).

The third component of the model, the real relationship, is that part of the relationship that is not influenced by transference or countertransference. If transference and countertransference are examined and dealt with, the relationship can often be deepened and the work between physiotherapists and their clients can be enhanced (Szybek et al 2000, Woltersdorf 1994).

The models discussed above all emphasize the need for physical and manual therapists to establish good working relationships with their clients. There are also philosophical and empirical reasons for the importance of these relationships, and they are discussed in the next section.

THE IMPORTANCE OF THE RELATIONSHIP

The emphasis on establishing a solid working relationship based on effective communication between practitioner and client may reflect a particular philosophical point of view. Physiotherapists who believe that the body and the mind are separate will place less value on the opinions of the patient and rely more heavily on their own expertise concerning the body. The patient would be viewed as a passive recipient of treatment, hence the word "patient" which is derived from "passive." A physiotherapist who believes in a more holistic approach, however, will place more value on the opinions, motivations, and perspectives of the client. The client, in this case, would be seen as a more active participant in treatment, and the need to establish a good working relationship would become more important.

Philosophical motivations notwithstanding, there is empirical support for emphasizing effective communication skills and a strong practitioner–client relationship for physical and manual therapists. In an interview study of clients' perceptions of decision-making in physical therapy, 70% stated that they would like to be more involved in the goal-setting process of their therapies (Payton et al 1998). The authors concluded that a strong emphasis should be placed on relationship-building skills, as there is a strong, positive correlation between healthcare outcomes and the quality of the practitioner–client relationship. Clients do better when they feel they are understood, cared for, and involved in decision-making about their treatments (Ray & Wiese-Bjornstal 1999).

A series of studies investigating the opinions of athletic trainers and physiotherapists about communication and rapport-building skills also supports the need for a good working relationship. Wiese et al (1991) and Larson et al (1996) surveyed athletic trainers in the US and found that a positive communication style, knowledge about goal-setting, knowing how to encourage positive self-thoughts, understanding motivational factors, and knowing how to enhance self-confidence, were important skills. Physiotherapists surveyed in Australia provided similar opinions (Francis et al 2000, Ninedek & Kolt 2000). These surveys support the finding that communication skills on the part of the therapist are viewed as an important element for an effective rehabilitation recovery program, and a number of physiotherapy practitioners and researchers have advocated that the ability to communicate effectively and to establish a sound working relationship are essential skills for physiotherapists (Caney 1983, Croft 1980, Dickson & Maxwell 1985, Wagstaff 1982). These skills may also lead to an environment more facilitative of

rehabilitation and may lead to more positive outcomes (Crossman 1997, Latey 2000, Reynolds 1996).

There is similar evidence for the importance of the practitioner–client relationship from the client perspective. Ford and Gordon (1993) reported that clients described good physiotherapists as those who showed an interest in them, were friendly, empathic, and listened to their concerns. Johnson (1993) reported similar findings in a study in which disabled people described "good" physiotherapists as those individuals who took a more personal approach and "bad" physiotherapists as those who were more impersonal.

The evidence from the broader medical community also highlights the importance of relationship skills. Silverman et al (1998), in their textbook on developing communication skills for physicians, reported support for a positive association between a good practitioner–client relationship and client satisfaction (Bertakis et al 1991, Buller & Buller 1987, Wasserman et al 1984), reduction in client concerns (Wasserman et al 1984), and disclosure of psychosocial problems (Wissow et al 1994). A meta-analysis of 41 studies examining the correlates of client satisfaction found that positive talk and partnership building were positively related to the satisfaction of the client (Hall et al 1988). Silverman et al also described a study by Speigel et al (1989) that examined the effect of a support group on women with metastatic carcinoma of the breast. Over 10 years, women in the support group lived an average of 18 months longer than those in the control group. Silverman et al used the results of this study to highlight the effectiveness of expressing feelings and the power of relationships when dealing with medical issues. There is no reason to believe that an open, honest, and supportive relationship with a healthcare provider, including physical and manual therapists, could not also have powerful therapeutic effects.

The therapeutic relationship, and its possible positive impact, may be especially important for physical and manual therapists due to the unique characteristics of their work (Alexander 1973). Hailstone (1969) stated that because physiotherapists are often viewed as not being directly part of the medical team, clients are more likely to view them as natural allies and accessible outlets for their anxieties and concerns. Pratt (1978) highlighted three additional characteristics of clients' interactions with physical and manual therapists that make these relationships unique. The first characteristic is the amount of time spent with the client. Physiotherapists spend considerably more time with their clients, both during an individual appointment and during the course of treatment, than any other member of the healthcare team. This contact provides more time to establish relationships (Hargeaves 1987), and more in-depth relationships may be needed to make the lengthier appointments comfortable for clients and practitioners. The second characteristic is the physical contact that is typical during physiotherapy sessions. This degree of touching is not usually present in other relationships, except for intimate ones. Within physiotherapy relationships, this personal form of communication can either help the formation of close working relationships, or it can be misinterpreted and lead to confusion, discomfort, and anxiety. The third aspect of physiotherapy relationships is the immediacy of treatment. Treatment is often solution-focused, and results of treatment are often seen and felt quickly, and these two factors can help to build confidence and trust in the physiotherapist. These characteristics give physiotherapists unique opportunities to develop strong and positive working relationships with their clients (Pratt 1978). What are the characteristics of a strong working relationship? The characteristics and components of what is meant by a therapeutic relationship are covered in the next section.

THE THERAPEUTIC RELATIONSHIP

Several physiotherapists (Hamilton-Duckett & Kidd 1985, Pratt 1978) have based their understanding of the therapeutic relationship on the work of Rogers (1967). Rogers believed that practitioners should demonstrate the three facilitative conditions of acceptance, genuineness, and empathy in order to create an environment conducive to growth and positive treatment outcomes.

ACCEPTANCE

Acceptance, sometimes called unconditional positive regard, respect, liking, or prizing, means that therapists accept clients for who they are, regardless of any behaviors, attitudes, or feelings demonstrated by the clients. It simply means "I care" with no strings attached. This attitude on the part of therapists allows clients the freedom to express their

concerns, anxieties, and trepidations without fear of rejection or dismissal.

GENUINENESS

Genuineness, also called congruence, realness, or authenticity, implies that therapists are aware of and honest about their feelings and attitudes. They are comfortable expressing these feelings, when appropriate, and they exhibit consistency in their verbal and non-verbal communications. Being genuine engenders trust in therapists, as clients can sense their honesty. Therapists exhibiting genuineness will not be defensive when challenged, and will express (tactfully) any frustration they feel if clients are not progressing as expected. The honest expression of this frustration will allow therapists and clients to examine the cause of the frustration and work out a solution to the satisfaction of both parties.

EMPATHY

Empathy, also called understanding or attunement, is the ability to enter clients' frames of reference and understand their situations and feelings from their point of view. It is the ability to identify with how clients feel, and to express this understanding, so they believe that their communications have been heard clearly and accurately. Unlike sympathy that contains an element of sorrow, empathy is an impartial but caring understanding of clients' feelings and experiences.

Rogers (1967) believed that these core facilitative conditions were important in a wide variety of situations, from counseling and education to the resolution of social issues. Relationships between physical and manual therapists and their clients are no exceptions (Pratt 1978). The core conditions create relationships based on trust and openness, which in turn encourage the disclosure of concerns and factors that may directly affect the physiotherapeutic process. Although studies that have examined aspects of the three facilitative conditions have yielded some inconsistent results, Patterson's (1984) meta-analysis revealed considerable support for a strong relationship between practitioners' genuineness, empathetic understanding, and acceptance and therapeutic effectiveness.

The core conditions of Rogers (1967) provide physical and manual therapists with specific characteristics that have been shown to promote positive treatment outcomes, but how are these conditions achieved? In the next section, basic relationship building skills, including non-verbal modes of communication, and suggestions for initial client contacts will be examined.

BUILDING THE WORKING ALLIANCE

The working alliance, as described in the previous section, implies a strong command of effective communication skills on the part of the practitioner. The communication of empathy, genuineness, and unconditional positive regard requires an ability not only to deliver information and communicate feelings and attitudes towards clients, but also includes the ability to listen to clients and pay attention to the subtleties of what they are saying. Schwentz (2001) advocated the *look, listen,* and *feel* reminders from CPR training. Physical and manual therapists need to look at their clients' behaviors and body language, listen carefully to what their clients are actually saying, and recognize and respond to their own emotions and use them to better relate to their clients. This recommendation suggests that the communication skills required to respond effectively to clients and to build effective working relationships are more than just listening to what clients say and then verbally responding. Non-verbal behavior, such as facial expressions, gestures, and tone of voice, are also of vital importance in the communication process between therapist and client. This section will begin with an examination of the influence of non-verbal communication on client–practitioner relationships and then continue with an exploration of the attending skills that are used to build rapport and to secure agreement on treatment goals and the tasks necessary to achieve them.

NON-VERBAL COMMUNICATION AND ATTENDING BEHAVIORS

Non-verbal communication involves everything about a person and what they are doing that is not communicated verbally. These behaviors include posture, proximity, touch, body movement, gestures, facial expressions, eye contact, tone of voice, use of time and space, and even physical characteristics such as appearance, gender, and race (Hargreaves 1987, Silverman et al 1998). These attributes and behaviors can be categorized as affiliative or dominant, depending on their intent and how they are interpreted. Affiliative non-verbal messages, also known as attending behaviors, typically create a more personal relationship, and include smiling, friendly tone of voice, eye contact, appropriate touching, and close proximity (Hargreaves 1987). Dominant non-verbal communications are concerned with establishing power and influence, and include speaking loudly and for long periods of time, interrupting, and too much or not enough eye contact (Hargreaves 1987). Non-verbal communication can also be grouped into three categories: kinesics, proxemics, and paralanguage (Martens 1987). Kinesics includes physical appearance, posture, gestures, touching, eye contact, and facial expressions, and is probably what is typically thought of as modes of non-verbal communication. Proxemics involves aspects of personal distance and the environment. These aspects include such factors as how far two people stand from one another when they are interacting and any objects, such as a desk, chair, or table, that could influence communication between individuals. Proxemics in the physical and manual therapies has particular significance in that many treatments involve the invasion of intimate personal space. Paralanguage refers to particular vocal characteristics, such as tone of voice, speed of speaking, and volume. All of these characteristics of the communicators, their appearance, behaviors, and the environment can have a substantial effect on communication between individuals.

Non-verbal communication can be distinguished from verbal communication by several characteristics (Silverman et al 1998). Verbal communication is discrete and has a clear beginning and ending, whereas non-verbal communication is continuous and lasts as long as people are close to one another. Verbal messages are typically transmitted in a single mode, either spoken or written, and non-verbal communication takes place through several modes simultaneously (e.g., facial expression, gestures, posture). Much of non-verbal communication may be at the periphery of conscious awareness, such as fidgeting and eye movement, contrasted to verbal messages, which for the most part are under our direct control. Finally, verbal modes of communication are more suited to conveying ideas, thoughts, instructions, and specific information than are non-verbal channels. Attitudes, emotions, and the quality of interpersonal relationships are more apparent through viewing non-verbal cues than what is actually being said verbally (Silverman et al 1998). Thornquist (1991) observed, in her qualitative analysis of initial sessions of physiotherapy, that caring and feeling was expressed primarily through non-verbal means. Clients communicated how they felt through non-verbal channels and physiotherapists responded to these cues non-verbally.

Research on non-verbal communication

The importance of non-verbal cues in the communication of emotions, attitudes, and relationship information would suggest that these modes of communication are important in establishing a good working relationship. Research has demonstrated that doctors who exhibit positive and relationship-building non-verbal behaviors, such as facing their clients directly, having more eye contact, and more open arm postures are viewed by the clients as more empathic and warm (Harrigan 1985). Client satisfaction has also been related to physicians' non-verbal communication, such as nods, gestures, and interpersonal distance (Weinberger et al 1981); touch, a forward-leaning posture, and eye contact (Larsen & Smith 1981); and physicians' ability to communicate emotion through their facial expressions and tone of voice (DiMatteo et al 1980, 1986). DiMatteo et al also showed that physicians who were able to read clients' non-verbal cues had more satisfied clients, and their clients were more likely to keep their appointments.

Therapist non-verbal behavior

The positive client outcomes related to demonstrating empathy and caring through non-verbal behavior and being sensitive to the non-verbal cues of clients has implications for manual and physical therapists. Hargreaves (1987) reviewed the literature on non-verbal communication and applied the findings specifically to physiotherapy. She emphasized the unique position of physical and manual therapists in regard to the use of touch to communicate non-verbally. Touching can indicate caring, encouragement, and support. This aspect of touching may be particularly important when dealing with amputees, who can be aided in accepting the loss of a limb by therapists who non-verbally (and verbally) communicate care and interest and who accept their clients unconditionally. Hargreaves also advocated smiling, a pleasant facial expression, an open and attentive body posture, affirmative

nodding of the head, and appropriate eye contact as the best means to communicate interest and regard and to create a good working relationship. How the physiotherapist faces the client is also important, as a side-to-side orientation may communicate a more collaborative approach than a face-to-face stance that may be interpreted as more confrontational (Hargreaves 1987).

Therapists need to be aware of the impact of their non-verbal cues and insure that they are transmitting healthy and accepting types of messages. Hargreaves (1987) recommended that the ability to use non-verbal communication requires self-monitoring and feedback from others. Many therapists may not be aware of the non-verbal messages they are sending. Silverman et al (1998) pointed out that conflicting verbal and non-verbal messages often result in confusion and misunderstanding on the part of clients, and when there are mixed messages the non-verbal messages will prevail. For example, therapists who ask clients how their home exercises are going are typically indicating a caring attitude about their clients' therapy programs. Therapists who make notes in their charts and look at their watches while their clients are talking may send a message that they do not care about the importance of home exercise or their clients. Such inattentive behavior on the part of therapists also prohibits them from picking up non-verbal cues from their clients, who may verbally say that things are going fine, but non-verbally exhibit poor eye contact and fidgetiness that could be signs that they are having problems with the home exercise portion of their rehabilitation programs.

Reading clients' non-verbal cues

Interpreting the non-verbal cues of clients must be done with caution (Silverman et al 1998). Poor eye contact, a closed and defensive posture, frowning, and arriving late to therapy sessions obviously are non-verbal cues that transmit a wealth of information, but the precise meaning of these cues needs to be corroborated. The simplest form of corroboration is asking for clarification. An inquiry or comment about clients' non-verbal behavior, such as, "You seem distracted today? Is anything wrong?", not only allows clients to explain and elaborate on anything that may be bothering them, but it also demonstrates an attentiveness that lets clients know that their therapist cares and is paying attention to them as a person and not just treating their illness or condition.

Reading medical charts

An important issue related to non-verbal communication is how the physiotherapist uses case notes or medical charts. It is difficult to maintain good eye contact and appear as though the client is being listened to while reading or writing case notes. Heath (1984) found that consulting client records while trying to listen to a client resulted in clients who

- withheld replies until the eye contact could be maintained
- used gestures to get attention
- paused in mid-sentence to wait for attention.

In addition, physicians who were consulting case notes often missed or forgot information that the client was telling them. Heath concluded that reading or writing in case records while a client is talking actually creates a less efficient session, because information needs to be repeated and reviewed or is missed completely. Heath recommended that healthcare professionals

- should not consult case records until clients have completed their initial statements
- should wait for appropriate moments to consult case records
- clearly indicate to clients when they need to read the case record before shifting their attention away from them.

These procedures will help insure that clients receive the attention that they deserve and that non-verbal signals will not be misinterpreted or send the wrong type of message.

As discussed previously, rapport is most apt to develop when practitioners display acceptance, genuineness, and empathy toward their clients. All three of these characteristics imply a caring toward clients that can only be communicated when both non-verbal and verbal messages are congruent. If physical and manual therapists do not create a caring environment through their non-verbal behaviors, it is doubtful that clients will believe in or adhere to treatment programs.

ATTENDING SKILLS

Although affiliative non-verbal communication sets the stage for the working alliance, effective practitioner–client relationships are not likely to develop unless practitioners are able to build rapport with their clients. The helping professions literature contains a wide variety of models for building rapport (e.g., Corey 2000, Egan 2002, Ivey & Ivey 1999, Kottler 2000), but all of them emphasize the importance of attending to the client's agenda and striving to understand the situation from the client's point-of-view. As discussed previously, the goal is to enlist clients as collaborators in their own rehabilitation or injury prevention process. To accomplish this goal, physical and manual therapists can use a series of skills and techniques that have been shown to facilitate effective communication and empathetic understanding between clients and their healthcare providers. Before examining these skills and techniques, it is important to underscore that empathetic understanding implies that physical and manual therapists not only have the information that they need to make a valid diagnosis or develop a treatment regimen, but also enough information to assess clients' *beliefs* about their injuries, *emotional reactions*, and *expectations*. As described by Meichenbaum & Turk (1987), the three areas that need to be explored are:

1. the personal meanings that clients ascribe to their injuries
2. clients' worries, fears, or concerns about their injuries
3. clients' expectations about treatment and their healthcare providers.

To acquire this information, physical and manual therapists need to ask the right kind of questions, listen attentively, and probe for the messages that may be under the surface of the client's initial responses.

Open and closed questioning

After introducing themselves to their clients, most physical and manual therapists begin their interactions by asking their clients questions. Although this seems quite natural, it is important to recognize that these early exchanges set the tone and the direction for the interactions to follow. Therefore, if the goal is to build rapport and to understand the situation from the client's perspective, then it becomes important to ask questions that allow clients to focus on their agendas. This goal is most likely to be achieved through the use of open questions.

Open questions typically begin with "what," "how," or "why" and may stimulate clients to take the lead and provide more descriptive responses. According to Ivey and Ivey (1999), Egan (2002), and many others, open questions encourage clients to provide more information, elicit examples of particular behaviors, thoughts, and feelings, and empower clients to take a more active role in the diagnosis and treatment process. Each of these factors is important in building empathetic understanding of the clients and their situations. In contrast, closed questions can usually be answered in one or two words and typically reflect the agenda of the practitioner. Closed questions are used to gather specific information, or to refocus or narrow an area of discussion. Nonetheless, extensive or exclusive use of closed questions, particularly during early interactions, can place the practitioner in the power or directing role. When this situation arises, most clients remain passive and wait for practitioners to take the lead and dictate the focus and boundaries of the verbal exchange.

To illustrate the difference between open and closed questioning, consider the following exchange between a healthcare provider (HCP) and a concert violinist (P) who fractured her hand in an accident and is now beginning rehabilitation.

> HCP: Hi, my name is Mary, and I will be your rehab therapist. When did you fracture your hand?
> P: About 6 weeks ago.
> HCP: Has everything gone okay so far?
> P: Yeah, I guess so.
> HCP: When did they remove the Hoffman fixture?
> P: Last Monday.
> HCP: Okay, so you must be ready to get started. Let me take a quick look so I can set you up with a strengthening program.

In this brief example, the practitioner asked a series of closed questions and focused almost exclusively on the injury and not the person. The violinist remained in a passive role allowing the therapist to control the content and direction of the interaction. Although this interaction may seem realistic in light of the time constraints that most physical and manual therapists labor under, it did little to foster empathetic understanding of the client's situation. By substituting open questions in the same scenario, it may be possible to develop a stronger working relationship.

> HCP: How are things going?
> P: Okay, I guess.
> HCP: Sounds like you're not quite sure. What else is going on?

> P: Well, sometimes I worry if I'll ever be able to play again.
> HCP: OK, let's talk about that.

As shown, the use of open questions allowed the client to take the lead and direct the conversation to her fears and worries. If the therapist listens attentively to the client's lead and responds empathetically, it is more likely that the client will perceive the therapist as caring and concerned about them as an individual. The techniques and skills involved in empathetic listening and responding will be discussed in the next section, but there are several other factors to consider before leaving this examination of the use of open and closed questions.

Although the use of open questions has been shown to be beneficial in building strong working relationships, individuals from some cultural groups or those who maintain the expert–"sick client" philosophy may have difficulty with this mode of non-directive interaction. These individuals typically view the healthcare provider as being in a dominant position and may be reluctant to take the lead or voice any concerns. When this situation is the case, it is still important to invite clients' input, while accepting that individuals cannot be forced to take a more active role in their rehabilitation (Petitpas 2000). In addition, it is important to be patient when waiting for a response. Many clients may not respond immediately to open questions during initial interactions because they are having an internal debate over what may be appropriate to disclose. During this delay, it is quite common for therapists to feel a need to ask another question to ensure that the client was clear on the first question. Unfortunately, asking too many or run-on questions can confuse clients or redirect their focus.

There is also consensus that "why" questions should be used sparingly and only after careful consideration. Why questions can put clients on the defensive and can be particularly troublesome to individuals who may be blaming themselves for their own injuries (Petitpas & Danish 1995). Several authors have suggested rephrasing "why" questions to "what" questions in order to lessen the possibility of client defensiveness (e.g., Davis 1998, Silverman et al 1998). For example, instead of asking, "Why don't you keep up with your exercises?", a physical or manual therapist could ask, "What kinds of things are getting in the way of your exercise program?"

Although most researchers agree on the importance of beginning initial interviews with open questions, there is evidence that closed questions or more focused open questions become important as the working alliance develops (Silverman et al 1998). Once physical and manual therapists have created an environment of trust and the client feels understood, targeted open questions or closed questions are often necessary to acquire the specific or detailed information required to make an accurate assessment and treatment plan. This shift from gathering general descriptions of symptoms or experiences as an attempt to understand the specific behaviors or feelings involved in a situation is known as "concreteness" (Sexton & Whiston 1994), and knowing when and how to make this shift without discounting the feelings or experiences of the client is called "pace before you lead." Although the phrase, pace before you lead, may have originated from neuro-linguistic programming (Lankton 1980), it has also been used to describe the technique of matching or attending to clients' present focus before attempting to lead them in new directions (Petitpas 2000). For example, if an injured athlete was angry because she suffered a severe ankle sprain and lost her starting position, it would be important to attend to her immediate feelings rather than try to get her to forget about her playing situation and focus exclusively on her rehabilitation. In this example, failure to attend to the person's immediate concern is likely to have a negative effect on the practitioner–client relationship.

Empathetic listening

Beyond knowing how to use open and closed questions effectively, physical and manual therapists can benefit from learning how to listen empathetically and to acknowledge and validate the responses of their clients. Effective communication is a two-way street. When a person sends a communication, they typically have an *intent* in mind. If the communication, however, has a different *impact* than the person intended, then a communication problem is likely to be present. Therefore, the key to effective communication is clarity in both sending and receiving messages. Unfortunately, many individuals make the mistake of assuming they know what clients are thinking or feeling and miss probing for more explicit information, or they do not acknowledge or validate clients' responses, causing clients to wonder if their communications were understood. Consider the following exchange.

HCP: How is everything going with your exercise program?

P: I don't know. Things are just not right.

HCP: Let me check your range of motion and see how you are doing.

In this example, the practitioner's intent was to gather information about the status of the client's exercise program, and he or she assumed that the client was referring to her physical condition. It is difficult to know what impact this question had on the client. Did the client interpret the question to be an open invitation to talk about "everything" or simply a request for a rehabilitation status report? The client's response of "I don't know," may reflect the client's lack of clarity or something much different. In any case, there may be numerous things that could be bothering the client or getting in the way of her exercise program. In order to prevent such miscommunication, physical and manual therapists should verify their initial perceptions by using listening skills, such as paraphrasing, summarization, and reflection of feelings.

A paraphrase is a response to a client's communication used to ensure that the practitioner has heard what the client said accurately. When paraphrasing, physical and manual therapists encapsulate, rephrase, or repeat back some of the client's communication using inquisitive or tentative language. This strategy serves two primary purposes. First, it shows the client that the practitioner is listening and paying attention to what was said. Second, the use of tentative language (e.g., it appears, it seems) allows the client to clarify or expand on the communication if the practitioner's paraphrase failed to capture the client's intent sufficiently. For example, consider the following exchange.

P: I just don't know whether I can keep pushing myself in rehab.

HCP: It sounds like you have some doubts about whether you can keep it going.

P: Well, I know I can keep it going, but the pain gets to a point where I'm afraid I'm doing more harm than good.

In this exchange, the use of a paraphrase enabled the practitioner to acknowledge not only the client's communication, but to also get a better sense of the client's most pressing concern. As a result, the increased level of understanding between the practitioner and the client may enhance the quality of their working relationship.

A paraphrase is not simply "parroting" back a client's response. A paraphrase should be a sincere attempt to gain clarity and to understand a client's communication empathetically, and it should reflect both the content and the emotion of what was heard. The purpose of a paraphrase is to sharpen understanding rather than just to acknowledge what the client said. Therefore, physical or manual therapists using paraphrases must present congruent caring messages in both their verbal and non-verbal communications.

In many ways, a summarization is quite similar to a paraphrase, except it tries to capture the essence of a longer period of communication. Summarizations are often used to start or end treatment sessions, or to check the accuracy of understanding of clients' facts, emotions, and meanings before moving on to get more depth or on to a new topic. Both paraphrases and summarizations serve not only as perception checks for the practitioner, but they can also assist clients in gaining a better understanding of their own situations through the process of clarifying their statements to the practitioner.

Another basic listening skill is a reflection of feelings. This skill is used when physical or manual therapists sense that there is a lot of emotion connected with a client's injury or recovery process that is not being expressed verbally. When a practitioner suspects that emotions are not being expressed and these emotions may be a barrier to effective treatment, the practitioner, using tentative language, gives the client feedback about what they are observing. In many ways, reflection of feeling serves as a paraphrase, identifying the emotions that a client is communicating through their behaviors. For example, a practitioner, who notices that her client seems tense and does not maintain consistent eye contact, might say something like, "You seem to be a little anxious today." This comment may open the door for a more in-depth analysis of the causes of the anxiety, or lead the client to clarify her non-verbal behaviors as being some frustration or sadness. In any event, the practitioner has reached out to the client and offered some support that may further strengthen the working relationship.

In general, paraphrasing, summarization, and reflection of feelings help practitioners gain a better understanding of clients' perceptions of their injury situations and help to foster rapport. These empathetic listening skills combined with congruent non-verbal messages and the core conditions of acceptance, genuineness, and empathy lay the foundation for the creation of a strong working alliance. Nonetheless, acquisition of effective relationship-building skills requires considerable practice and several training strategies for skill development are explored in the next section.

SUGGESTIONS FOR TRAINING AND SKILL ACQUISITION

Gaining a better understanding of the processes involved in developing rapport and building working alliances is likely to be an on-going learning experience, and one that separates expert practitioners from novices. If physical and manual therapists want to improve their empathetic listening and attending skills, then they need to begin to examine not only *what* they do with their clients, but also *how* they do it. Training and practice are the keys to acquiring what to do, but increased self-awareness and an understanding of the processes involved in the client–practitioner relationship are essential in learning how to do it.

To begin with, most physical and manual therapists throughout the world are governed by certification criteria from their national professional organizations, and most of these criteria include competency in basic listening and counseling skills (Ray & Wiese-Bjornstal 1999). As Ray et al (1999) described, these basic skills do not imply the ability to do psychotherapy, but would include such skills as rapport building, effective communication, education, emotional first aid, and knowing how to make an effective referral. In turn, each of these general skills is dependent on a variety of micro-skills (e.g., paraphrasing, summarization, reflection of feeling) that require considerable practice in order to become an automatic or habitual part of a practitioner's repertoire (Ivey & Ivey 1999). To facilitate this type of practice and skill acquisition, Danish & Hale (1983) have provided a useful model for teaching new skills. They suggest:

1. describe the skill in behavioral terms
2. give a rationale for the skill
3. specify a skill-attainment level
4. demonstrate effective and ineffective uses of the skill

5. provide opportunities to practice the skill with supervision and feedback
6. assign homework to promote generalization of the skill
7. evaluate the skill-attainment level.

Although it may be a relatively easy task to understand these basic skills, using them effectively with a wide variety of clients can be quite challenging. Furthermore, research has shown that healthcare professionals often overestimate their ability to be empathetic. For example, Dockrell (1988) found a large discrepancy between what physiotherapy students reported that they did to build rapport with clients and their actual behaviors, with only seven of 20 participants demonstrating appropriate attending skills. Equally alarming is the finding of Gillium & Barsky (1974) that two-thirds of the healthcare providers in their study believed that adherence problems were caused by clients' personality issues, whereas only 25% of the participants believed that their own behaviors had anything to do with non-compliance. These studies point out that many healthcare providers are unaware of their own behaviors or the effects of their communications on clients. The ability to use basic listening and counseling skills effectively necessitates that physical and manual therapists be willing to look critically at their own behaviors and receive appropriate supervision.

Self-awareness comes from a combination of self-disclosure and feedback (e.g., Meichenbaum & Turk 1987, Sexton & Whiston 1994). Therefore, training programs should afford physical and manual therapists opportunities to share their beliefs and concerns in group and one-on-one supervision activities. Training programs should also contain opportunities for students to get feedback about the advantages and disadvantages of their personal styles in order to identify and help to eliminate any blind spots they may have concerning their self-presentations.

The counseling literature contains a number of training strategies to promote self-understanding and an increased awareness of the processes that take place between practitioners and clients (Petitpas 2000). Several of these strategies may be quite beneficial to physical and manual therapists who want to acquire additional feedback concerning their listening and rapport-building skills. For example, reviewing and receiving feedback on video or audio-taped client interactions allows

practitioners to evaluate their abilities to use facilitative skills and to build rapport with their clients, and also to track the increase in self-awareness of their interpersonal style. In addition, using a training diary would allow individuals to record how their values, thoughts, and emotions play out during their interactions with various clients.

The most effective method of gaining self-knowledge and an understanding of the processes involved in the client–practitioner interactions is through a supervisory or mentoring relationship (Andersen 2000). Practitioners can learn a lot about their interactions with clients by examining their own relationships with their supervisors or mentors. For example, by exploring their own thoughts and feelings concerning their supervisors and supervisory experiences, practitioners can gain insight into process issues (e.g., power differentials, trust) that may parallel what happens in their own client interactions. Even if formal supervisory relationships are not feasible, physical and manual therapists can develop peer-mentoring arrangements that would enable them to share their process concerns with a trusted colleague.

SUMMARY

Client, setting, and practitioner variables have all been shown to influence clients' adherence to treatment regimens. Nonetheless, it is the quality of the client–practitioner relationship that has proven to be the most critical factor (Meichenbaum & Turk 1987). The purpose of this chapter was to examine several aspects of the client–practitioner relationship and to provide physical and manual therapists with suggestions for developing basic listening and counseling skills that would facilitate the development of effective working alliances. The need for these relationship-building skills has become even more important as today's clients are more knowledgeable, demanding, and litigious than ever before.

Although physical and manual therapists cannot control all the variables that influence clients' adherence, this chapter has provided evidence that practitioners who exhibit an accepting, congruent, and empathetic presentation and employ salubrious attending behaviors and skills are in the best position to develop effective working relationships. Nonetheless, creating strong client–practitioner relationships and facilitating treatment adherence is an ongoing process that cannot be learned by reading a book or attending a lecture. Acquiring relationship-building skills necessitates training, extensive practice, continuous feedback, and ongoing supervision. We hope the information and suggestions provided in this chapter will assist physical and manual therapists in developing a client-centered philosophy and acquiring the knowledge and skills necessary to build strong working relationships with all their clients.

References

Alexander D A 1973 Yes, but what about the client? Physiotherapy 59(12): 391–393

Andersen M B 2000 Supervision of athletic trainers' counseling encounters. Athletic Therapy Today 5: 46–47

Bertakis K D, Roter D, Putnam S M 1991 The relationship of physician medical interview style to client satisfaction. Journal of Family Practice 32: 175–181

Bordin E S 1979 The generalizability of the psychoanalytic concept of the working alliance. Psychotherapy: Theory Research and Practice 16: 252–260

Buller M K, Buller D B 1987 Physicians' communication style and client satisfaction. Journal of Health & Social Behavior 28: 375–388

Caney D 1983 Competence, can it be assessed? Newly qualified physiotherapists. Physiotherapy 69(9): 302–304

Corey G 2000 Theory and practice of counseling and psychotherapy, 6th edn. Brooks/Cole, Belmont, CA

Croft J 1980 Interviewing in physical therapy. Physical Therapy 60(8): 1033–1036

Crossman J 1997 Psychological rehabilitation from sports injuries. Sports Medicine 23: 333–339

Danish S J, Hale B 1983 Teaching psychological skills to athletes and coaches. Journal of Physical Education Recreation & Dance 54(8): 11–12, 80–81

Davis C M 1998 Client practitioner interaction: An experiential manual for developing the art of health care, 3rd edn. Slack, Thorofare, NJ

Dickson D A, Maxwell M 1985 The interpersonal dimension of physiotherapy: Implications for training. Physiotherapy 71(7): 306–309

DiMatteo M R, Taranta A, Friedman H S et al 1980 Predicting client satisfaction from physicians' non-verbal communication skill. Medical Care 18: 376–387

DiMatteo M R, Hays R D, Prince L M 1986 Relationship of physicians' non-verbal communication skill to client satisfaction, appointment non-compliance, and physician workload. Health Psychology 5: 581–594

Dockrell S 1988 An investigation of the use of verbal and non-verbal communication skills by final-year physiotherapy students. Physiotherapy 74(2): 52–55

Egan G 2002 The skilled helper: A problem-management approach to helping, 7th edn. Brooks/Cole, Pacific Grove, CA

Ford I W, Gordon S 1993 Social support and athletic injury: The perspective of sports physiotherapists. Australian Journal of Science and Medicine in Sport 25: 17–25

Francis S R, Andersen M B, Maley P 2000 Physiotherapists' and male professional athletes' views on psychological skills for rehabilitation. Journal of Science & Medicine in Sport 3: 17–29

Gelso C J, Carter J A 1994 Components of the psychotherapy relationship: Their interaction and unfolding during treatment. Journal of Counseling Psychology 41: 296–306

Gillium R F, Barsky A J 1974 Diagnosis and management of client non-compliance. Journal of the American Medical Association 228: 1563–1567

Hailstone J D 1969 The importance of the relationship between physiotherapist and client. Physiotherapy 55(6): 230–232

Hall J A, Roter D L, Katz N R 1988 Meta-analysis of correlates of provider behaviour in physicians. Medical Care 26: 657–675

Hamilton-Duckett P, Kidd L 1985 Counselling skills and the physiotherapist. Physiotherapy 71: 179–180

Hargreaves S 1987 The relevance of non-verbal skills in physiotherapy. Physiotherapy 73: 685–688

Harrigan J A 1985 Self-touching as an indicator of underlying affect and language processes. Social Science Medicine 20(11): 1161–1168

Heath C 1984 Participation in the medical consultation: the coordination of verbal and non-verbal behaviour between the doctor and the client. Sociology of Health Illness 6: 311–338

Horvath A O, Greenberg L S 1989 Development and validation of the Working Alliance Inventory. Journal of Counseling Psychology 36: 223–233

Ivey A E, Ivey M B 1999 Intentional interviewing and counseling: Facilitating clients development in a multicultural society. Allyn & Bacon, Boston, MA

Jensen G M, Lorish C D 1994 Promoting client cooperation with exercise programs: Linking research, theory, and practice. Arthritis Care & Research 7: 181–189

Johnson R 1993 "Attitudes don't just hang in the air . . ." Disabled people's perceptions of physiotherapists. Physiotherapy 79: 619–627

Kiesler D J, Watkins L M 1989 Interpersonal complementarity and the therapeutic alliance: a study of relationship in psychotherapy. Psychotherapy 26: 183–194

Kottler J A 2000 Nuts & bolts of helping. Allyn & Bacon, Boston, MA

Lankton S R 1980 Practical magic: A translation of basic neuro-linguistic programming into clinical psychotherapy. Meta, Cupertino, CA

Larsen K M, Smith C K 1981 Assessment of non-verbal communication in the client–physician interview. Journal of Family Practice 12: 481–488

Larson G A, Starkey C, Zaichkowsky L D 1996 Psychological aspects of athletic injuries as perceived by athletic trainers. The Sport Psychologist 10: 37–47

Latey P 2000 Placebo: A study of persuasion and rapport. Journal of Bodywork & Movement Therapy 4: 23–136

Locke E A, Latham G P 2002 Building a practically useful theory of goal setting and task motivation: A 35-year odyssey. American Psychologist 57(9): 705–717

Martens R 1987 Coaches guide to sport psychology. Human Kinetics, Champaign, IL

Meichenbaum D, Turk D C 1987 Facilitating treatment adherence: A practitioner's guidebook. Plenum, New York, NY

Ninedek A, Kolt G S 2000 Sport physiotherapists' perceptions of psychological strategies in sport injury rehabilitation. Journal of Sport Rehabilitation 9: 191–206

Osachuk T A, Cairns S L 1995 Relationship issues. In: Martin D G, Moore A D (eds) First steps in the art of intervention: a guidebook for trainees in the helping professions. Brooks/Cole, Pacific Grove, CA, p 19–43

Owen O G G, Goodge P 1981 Physiotherapists talking to clients. Client Counseling & Health Education 3: 100–102

Parsons T 1951 The social system. Free Press, New York, NY

Patterson C H 1984 Empathy, warmth, and genuineness in psychotherapy: A review of reviews. Psychotherapy 21: 431–438

Payton O D, Nelson C E, St Clair-Hobbs 1998 Physical therapy clients' perceptions of their relationships with health care professionals. Physiotherapy Theory and Practice 14: 211–221

Petitpas A 1999 The client–practitioner interaction and its relationship to adherence and treatment outcomes. In: Bull S (ed) Adherence issues in sport & exercise. Wiley, Chichester, England, p 221–237

Petitpas A J 2000 Managing stress on and off the field: The Littlefoot approach to learned resourcefulness. In: Andersen M (ed) Doing sport psychology. Human Kinetics, Champaign, IL, p 33–43

Petitpas A, Danish S 1995 Caring for injured athletes. In: Murphy S (ed) Sport psychology interventions. Human Kinetics, Champaign, IL, p 255–282

Pratt J W 1978 A psychological view of the physiotherapist's role. Physiotherapy 64(8): 241–242

Ray R, Wiese-Bjornstal D M (eds) 1999 Counseling in sports medicine. Human Kinetics, Champaign, IL

Ray R, Terrell T, Hough D 1999 The role of the sports medicine professional in counseling athletes. In: Ray R, Wiese-Bjornstal D (eds) Counseling in sports medicine. Human Kinetics, Champaign, IL, p 3–20

Reynolds F A 1996 Evaluating the impact of an interprofessional communication course through essay content analysis: Do physiotherapy and occupational therapy students' essays place similar emphasis on responding skills? Journal of Interprofessional Care 10: 285–295

Rogers C 1967 The necessary and sufficient conditions of therapeutic personality change. Journal of Consulting Psychology 21: 95–103

Schwenz S J 2001 Psychology of injury and rehabilitation. Athletic Therapy Today 6: 44

Sexton T L, Whiston S C 1994 The status of the counseling relationship: An empirical review, theoretical implications, and research directions. The Counseling Psychologist 22: 6–78

Silverman J, Kurtz S, Draper J 1998 Skills for communicating with clients. Radcliffe, Abingdon, UK

Speigel D, Bloom K R, Kraemer H C et al 1989 Effect of psychological treatment on survival of clients with metastatic breast cancer. Lancet 2: 888–891

Szasz T S, Hollender M H 1956 A contribution to the philosophy of medicine: The basic models of the doctor–client relationship. Archives of Internal Medicine 97: 585–592

Szybek K, Gard G, Linden J 2000 The physiotherapist–client relationship: Applying a psychotherapy model. Physiotherapy Theory and Practice 16: 181–193

Thornquist E 1991 Body communication is a continuous process. Scandinavian Journal of Primary Health Care 9: 191–196

Wagstaff G F 1982 A small dose of common sense – communication, persuasion and physiotherapy. Physiotherapy 68(10): 327–329

Wasserman R C, Inui T S, Barriatua RD et al 1984 Pediatric clinicians' support for parents makes a difference: An outcome-based analysis of clinician–parent interaction. Pediatrics 6: 1047–1053

Weinberger M, Greene J Y, Mamlin J J 1981 The impact of clinical encounter events on client and physician satisfaction. Social Science Medicine 15E: 239–244

Wiese D M, Weiss M R, Yukelson D P 1991 Sport psychology in the training room: A survey of athletic trainers. The Sport Psychologist 5: 15–24

Wissow L S, Roter D L, Wilson M E H 1994 Pediatrician interview style and mothers' disclosure of psychosocial issues. Pediatrics 93: 289–295

Woltersdorf M A 1994 Transference: Whistling in the dark. PT Magazine of Physical Therapy 2: 60–65

Chapter 6

Transference and countertransference

Mark B. Andersen

INTRODUCTION

This chapter concerns issues of a deeply personal quality that go to the heart of the matter in service delivery for the physical and manual therapies. The core of this chapter involves how we as therapists respond to our clients, both consciously and unconsciously, in the behavioral, cognitive, emotional, and conative (what we desire, what we want) realms, and how they respond to us. The type and depth of those responses will have a profound influence on the quality of the client–practitioner relationships, and even the outcomes of rehabilitation (Giovacchini 1989, Petitpas et al 1999). Because transference and countertransference are such personal topics, I thought that instead of first going through some textbook definitions and theoretical explanations, I would begin with a story of a profound transference–countertransference relationship between a client and her therapist. Then, I will continue with the topic, referring back to the story along the way. I have found that after over 15 years of training future therapists, stories are usually remembered far clearer than theoretical models.

CASE STUDY

Evelyn was a 77-year-old Caucasian woman, of British decent, living in Australia. She was from a financially secure, upper social class family, and had never worried about money. She was active in civic affairs and the arts of the city in which she lived. Those who knew her well would have called her "efficient, solid, demanding, and a bit cool and stand-offish." Her parents' marriage was reserved, and Evelyn could not recall much laughter in the house. Her marriage was not a completely loveless one, but it was not a passionate and affectionate one either. Evelyn married her husband more because it was something that was expected between the two wealthy families in town than because of love. The marriage produced two children, first a daughter, then a son. The daughter followed in the family tradition, and after receiving her graduate degree in business from a prestigious university, moved into the family business. At the time of her mother's rehabilitation, she was essentially running the company. The son, however, rebeled against his family's wealth and the passionless home life, became estranged from the family, and moved to London where he worked as a studio musician along with other odd jobs. He called his mother on her birthday every year, and the conversations would start out pleasant enough, but would deteriorate into "when are you going to grow up?" arguments, leaving both mother and son frustrated, angry, and tearful. Evelyn's husband died 6 years earlier, and except for a housekeeper who was in the house during the daytime, she was alone.

Evelyn was in rehabilitation because of a recent hip replacement operation, and she was also receiving some treatment for rotator cuff tendinosis. She had a cool, aloof, manner within the clinic, and nothing was ever quite good enough for her. The clinic staff she had contact with did not look forward to her visits because of her manner towards them and the other staff.

The physical therapist, Miguel, was a 29-year-old man who immigrated to Australia from Chile with his parents when he was 10 years old. In contrast to Evelyn's family, Miguel's parents actively and daily showed physical affection for each other and for their children. Miguel was the first child, and then three sisters followed. During his 10 years in Chile, his maternal grandmother lived with the family. His maternal grandfather had died when he was 2 years old. Both his parents worked, and so his grandmother did a lot of the keeping of the house and taking care of the children. When Miguel went to his very first day of school, it was his grandmother who accompanied him.

Moving to Australia was difficult for Miguel, but he managed. What was probably the most difficult was leaving his grandmother behind. It was like an Oedipal story one generation removed. His relationship with his grandmother was probably closer than that with his mother. He returned to Chile at the age of 23 after completing his first university degree to visit friends and relatives, and especially his grandmother. She died suddenly of a stroke when Miguel was 27 years old. Miguel was devastated and deeply regretted not being there when she died.

Miguel was attractive looking in the Mediterranean sense, with olive skin and dark hair. He had a smile that made others want to smile, and his laugh was infectious. Clients and staff loved him. Miguel "inherited" Evelyn at the clinic because the therapist who was treating Evelyn moved to another clinic in another city. Evelyn and Miguel did not particularly take to each other well at the first physical therapy session.

THE BEGINNING OF THE RELATIONSHIP

Upon meeting Miguel, the first thing that Evelyn asked was "How old are you?" Miguel told her, and then she began to go on about how he was too young, and she really needed a therapist who was older with more experience, and that she had nothing against him, and that one day he would surely be a fine therapist, but that he just would not do for now. Miguel had been warned about Evelyn and flashed his dazzling smile and said that he was the only therapist available at this time, but that he would try to schedule her future appointments with a "more mature therapist" (his words). She acquiesced and said that they should go ahead with treatment, but that next time she wanted an older therapist. Throughout the treatment session, Evelyn kept saying "Are you sure this is right? I haven't done this exercise before." Miguel would gently respond "This is the next exercise we need to get you doing, don't worry, if you become unsteady, I am here to steady you." While he was working on her shoulder Miguel began to talk to her about how he was fresh out of university, and how she was right that he was young and did not have the experience others had, but that one day he was going to be a dynamite therapist. Miguel knew the art of getting a client on one's side: throw the ego away, agree with them, and tell them they are right. He began telling Evelyn amusing stories from his student days, and she even laughed at a couple of them. Upon completion of treatment, Evelyn said to Miguel "Thank you, and don't forget to check for a new therapist, but if it takes a few weeks to find one, that's OK, you'll do for now." After Evelyn checked out of the clinic, the receptionist came up to Miguel and said "Evelyn just smiled at me! What did you do?" Miguel just winked and said "Damn, I'm good!"

After the second session, Evelyn never mentioned getting a new therapist again. She began to relax more and laugh more at Miguel's stories, and by the fourth session she was beginning to tell stories too, about her childhood and her stuffy parents, but she told them in a way that was amusing and self-mocking. Both Evelyn and Miguel turned out to be gifted storytellers who entertained each other during treatment.

THE EVOLVING RELATIONSHIP

Evelyn and Miguel were getting along quite well when an event occurred that moved their relationship along even further. Miguel was working on Evelyn's shoulder and suddenly he felt something give way, and she let out a yelp of extreme pain. Miguel was frantic. He apologized profusely, put her shoulder in a resting comfortable position, and was about to run for the physician on staff, but did not need to because everyone had heard Evelyn, and the physician was on her way. While the physician was examining Evelyn's shoulder, Miguel was pacing nervously and looking quite anxious. Evelyn looked over at Miguel and said in a mock imperious tone "Oh stop that pacing, and come over here and learn something." Miguel moved to the opposite side of the table from the physician and, with no conscious thought, took Evelyn's hand and held it in both of his until the physician was finished. He was still holding her hand when she said "Do you know how long it has been since a handsome man like you has held my hand?" Miguel blushed and stammered out something like "With a beautiful gal like you, it was probably 10 minutes before your appointment." Evelyn replied, "You flatterer!" Miguel said "That would be me, but you're not bad at it yourself." From that point the quality and depth of their relationship changed.

Evelyn talked a lot about her daughter, but never told stories about her son. As Miguel and Evelyn became closer, stories of hurt and disappointment with her son came out. Miguel's grandmother had always said to him "What is past is past, the important thing is what is happening now, and not letting the past poison today." Miguel knew Evelyn's birthday was coming up soon, and knew a call would

come from London. He translated his grandmother's words for Evelyn by saying "You know Evelyn, you have told me about a lot of past hurt and disappointment with your son, my grandmother always told me that right now is the most important. Maybe when he calls if you can keep it in the 'right now', what is he doing right now? If he is happy right now, be happy with him. If he is sad, be sad with him. Just try and keep it right now. He obviously loves you or he wouldn't call you every year."

On the first appointment after her birthday (the day after), Evelyn came in all cheerful and gave the receptionist half a birthday cake and told her to share it with the staff. Her conversation with her son had been the best one in 20 years, and there was even talk of him coming home for a visit. Evelyn said to Miguel "and I even told him all about you."

LEAVING EACH OTHER

Miguel was down to seeing Evelyn once a fortnight when tragedy struck. Evelyn came in for treatment and said "Miguel, this will be my last day. Remember when I said I was going to the neurologist for that funny stuff in my vision? Well it's bad, it's really bad." Evelyn had an inoperable fast-growing malignancy that had metastasized throughout her brain and into other vital organs. She was given 3 months to live. Miguel and Evelyn held on to each other and cried together.

For the next few weeks Miguel could not sleep, he was anxious, and would think of Evelyn and begin to cry. He lost his appetite, and began to lose weight. He said to his girlfriend. "What is happening to me? She's a patient; we occasionally lose patients. Why am I so upset?" Miguel's crisis resolved considerably when he and Evelyn made a pact that Thursday afternoons were reserved for "Tea with Evelyn," and up until the week she died they kept those afternoon dates. During those times they told more stories to each other, and talked about death and life and living now.

At the wake, Miguel told some hilarious stories about Evelyn that had many of the mourners laughing. Several people came up to him later and said "I never knew that side of Evelyn, thank you!" Evelyn's son came up to him and said "The way she talked about you, I think at the end there you were her best friend, thanks." That night Miguel dreamed of his grandmother, and began to build a deeper understanding of his profound relationship with Evelyn.

THE PROCESS OF TRANSFERRING

The terms "transference" and "countertransference" (Lane 1986, Meyers 1986, Racker 1968) are legacies in clinical and counseling psychology from the work of Freud (Freud 1912, 1915). In the most basic of descriptions, transference stands for a process that occurs in psychotherapy when the client begins to respond (behaviorally, cognitively, emotionally, conatively) to the therapist in ways that resemble patterns of response to significant others in the client's life. For example, if a young man had a turbulent time dealing with an authoritarian father, and rebeled and resisted his father, he may in therapy (especially with an older man) begin to see the therapist as an authority figure and start resisting the therapist's help. The therapist may not be acting in any objective authoritarian way, but the major pattern for relationships with older males for a client like this is one of authority and rebellion. That pattern then gets projected on to the therapist, and in this case, makes for a block in therapy.

The defense mechanism of projection also needs some clarification. The act of projection can present in a variety of forms. One form is where the individual has some ego-dystonic (unacceptable) response to another person (e.g., I hate them), and to defend against that ego-contradictory response, the person projects that response on to the other person (e.g., she hates me). In the case of the male with the authoritarian father above, the process is different, and not so much in service of ego defenses. The young man has a pattern of relationships with older men, the prototype being his relationship with his father. He projects his father and his pattern of responses onto an older man in authority, and then interprets the older man's behavior through the lens of his projections. Another variety of projection involves a fantasized love object. For example, children who have been physically or psychologically abused by a parent may begin to build strong fantasies about the good parent they do not have, but fervently wish they did. They may build up this internal picture of the loving, caring, generous, always-there-for-them parent. This fantasized love object may then later get projected onto a parental-type figure, such as a therapist, teacher, or coach

(see Grant & Crawley 2002). The fantasized good parent projection is often the source of clients falling in love with their therapists.

Freud (1912) believed that transference was essential for therapy to be successful, because transference meant that the person was becoming invested in the process. The transference, whether negative or positive, was also a rich source of information about how clients relate to others in their lives.

Transference processes, however, are not one-way. The name for the similar process whereby the therapist begins to act and respond to clients in similar patterns as he or she has responded to significant others is countertransference (Epstein & Feiner 1983, Gabbard 1995, Greenson 1967, Stein 1986, Strean 1994). For example, a therapist who is older than many of his clients may get big-brother protective feelings about younger clients that stem from their protective feelings for their own siblings.

As transference and countertransference are based on past experiences (not current realities), projections, and fantasies, many in counseling and clinical psychology have misinterpreted these phenomena as something to be avoided. Transference and countertransference are ubiquitous phenomena and are probably a part of most human relationships. Learning how to use them to positive effect is the role of psychologists, teachers, coaches, supervisors, and physical and manual therapists (see Henschen 1991, Mann 1986, Ogilvie 1993, Petitpas et al 1999, Yambor & Connelly 1991). The world of sport offers many examples of transference and countertransference. It is a common experience for athletes to become deeply attached to coaches. Part of that attachment (or love) may have roots in past parental relationships. If an athlete has had loving, healthy, supportive parents, then the probability of responding well to a caring, sensitive coach, and forming a strong bond that helps the athlete perform better in sport, is quite high. In contrast, if an athlete has been psychologically abused by a parent, then that athlete may gravitate to psychologically abusive coaches because that is the model for relationships with powerful others. Psychologically abusive coaches were probably abused by their coaches. Generally, we coach how we were coached, and we parent as we were parented. A happier connection for an abused athlete is to find a coach who represents the fantasized "good parent" they wished they had. With such a coach, the transference can be quite profound.

In the case study presented earlier in this chapter, Evelyn's initial response to Miguel is a good example of immediate negative transference. Evelyn grew up in a family that was reserved, stuffy, and showed little affection. Children crave affection and attention. The hurt that occurs when that affection is not forthcoming can cause children to shut down emotionally and become as cool and stuffy as their parents. As Freud said "the child is father to the man," and he meant that the experiences of the child will shape the adult. Evelyn "knew" from her childhood that to seek affection was to be met with a cold wall. As a result of that lesson, Evelyn developed a pattern of pushing others away before she would want to get close to them in order to not repeat the hurt of her childhood. Evelyn's pushing people away actually confirmed her view of the world as a place where affection was absent. Evelyn pushes away, people leave or respond negatively, Viola! See! the world is a cold place. Her imperious manner was a defense against the hurt of not getting the love she craved as a child.

Fortunately for Evelyn, Miguel had lots of affection and warm models of love in his life. He also had a model of caring for an older woman, his grandmother. If Miguel had responded to Evelyn in a manner that communicated "you're wrong, I am competent, I can handle your case" he would have only helped increase her resistance. Miguel's model for interactions with older women led him to be very respectful, accept her world view, and communicate that he was in agreement with her. Miguel's interactions were probably a mixture of conscious and unconscious processes. He naturally fell into "respect mode." His ability to empathize and take the role of the other helped diffuse Evelyn's basic hostility to the world in general, and to people who would enter her private space specifically. Her interaction with Miguel was something new for Evelyn. She pushed, and he did not run away.

If one reflects on one's clients and how one feels about each of them, that may help to get a feel for transference and countertransference. In an ideal world we should treat and respond to all clients in the same manner, with respect, unconditional positive regard, empathy, and genuineness. But we don't, and why don't we? The answer to that question lies at the heart of transference and countertransference. Below is an example of a therapist and two of his clients.

Freddy is a physical therapist in the US. He has an older brother and a younger sister. His mother is a nurse, and his father is an alcoholic who disappeared from his life when he was 12 years old. All during his childhood Freddy never was sure which father would be home when he got there, the mean drunk, or the regretful sober father. When his father finally left, Freddy's constant background anxiety began to abate. Freddy is heterosexual, but his older brother, who physically defended his mother against his abusive father, is gay. His older brother remains his hero to this day. Freddy has a client, Philip, whom he looks forward to treating every week. They have a great time during these rehabilitation sessions. They laugh a lot and tell stories. Philip is gay, and part of why Freddy and Philip work so well together is that Philip knows Freddy has a gay brother and is sensitive to the gay community and the difficulties gay and lesbian people face. So Philip can be himself and be frank and talk about anything. For Freddy, talking with Philip is like being with his older brother, so he has all those good sibling feelings. Also, Philip flirts with Freddy in a teasing but jovial manner. Despite what heterosexual men often say, many like to know that gay men find them attractive (more on erotic transference later in this chapter). So these two get on well. What is happening is a dance of positive transference and countertransference that is helping the rehabilitation process.

Freddy's other client, Richard, is uncommunicative, surly, and often comes to treatment with bloodshot eyes and smelling of alcohol and marijuana. Freddy dislikes treating him, is also uncommunicative, goes about the treatment methodically, and gets the job done as quickly as possible. So why does Freddy have empathy and unconditional positive regard for Philip, yet for Richard he is almost a robot and hardly human. Many children of alcoholics develop a strong aversion to anything that reflects substance abuse, and often have little tolerance of those who abuse substances. Richard evokes countertransferential responses in Freddy that are tied to both his father's alcoholism, his abuse of his mother and, oddly enough, his being abandoned by his father. There are a jumble of emotions that Richard evokes in Freddy, and in order to handle them Freddy shuts down and goes cold, and gets rid of Richard as fast as possible. Philip is like someone Freddy loves; Richard is like someone who has seriously hurt him.

TRANSFERENCE AND COUNTERTRANSFERENCE IN THE PHYSICAL AND MANUAL THERAPIES

There are few better lessons learned in therapy than the ones that start with the questions: "Which clients do I really like?," "Which clients do I dislike?," "Why do I interact with clients differently?," and "What am I bringing to my interactions with those clients that influences my responses?" Physical and manual therapists have two powerful instruments that they bring to treatment and interactions with clients. They have their clinical knowledge and technique skills, and they have their personalities. This chapter concerns learning about personality and ontogenetic histories in order to understand that second powerful tool of treatment. In the physical and manual therapies, most of the research conducted has to do with descriptions of different syndromes and the effectiveness of different treatments. Rarely is the personality of the therapist discussed, much less the quality of the relationship between the therapist and the client. For a long time, researchers in the fields of clinical and counseling psychology have recognized that when it comes to psychotherapy outcomes, the one variable that is consistently related to outcome is the quality of the relationship between the therapist and the client. What school of psychotherapy one comes from is not nearly as important as the quality of the working relationship. One can use psychodynamic, cognitive-behavioral, or gestalt approaches to psychotherapy, but how the parties get along will have the greatest influence on how much the client improves (see Petitpas et al 1999 for a recent review). Unfortunately, the number of hours physical and manual therapists spend during their training and practice examining their "second instrument" (their personalities) and the quality of their interactions with clients is unknown, but it is most assuredly low. The emphasis on self-reflective practice and examining the self in service does not have the tradition in the physical and manual therapies that it does in clinical psychology. That is a goal of the editors of this book, to increase the emphasis on human interaction in the physical and manual therapies. As one goes through the chapters in this book, it becomes obvious that a core theme of this text is relationships.

Back to the case study of Evelyn and Miguel. The dynamic of what was developing between Miguel and Evelyn should be obvious now. Miguel had an intense passionate relationship with his grandmother, someone he dearly loved, but whom he had to leave, probably with great sorrow. Also, she had died suddenly, and he never got to say goodbye. These events were heartaches in his life that his interactions with Evelyn helped heal. Now, why did the cold Evelyn turn into the warm, caring Evelyn? The first (unconscious) lesson Evelyn learned from her interactions with Miguel was that some people are not cold; some people don't go away emotionally – like her parents, like her son. Evelyn had pushed away a loving son who every year tried to tell his mother that he loved her, yet was pushed away again, and then he, being hurt, pushed back and confirmed Evelyn's world view that those who she wants to love will not love back. One of the patterns we see over and over again in psychotherapy and everyday life is that people often behave in ways that insure that the thing they fear most will happen, does happen. For example, someone desperately wants to be loved, so when he finds someone who shows interest and is affectionate, he throws himself at her with all his might and begins to smother her, insuring that what he fears most, rejection, is bound to happen. That example is only one of the more obvious ones that many people will recognize. Evelyn's case is a bit more subtle and has a long history. Evelyn has a life-long fear of her love being rejected. That fear is so old, and the hurt associated with rejection has turned into a pattern of rejecting first to avoid the investment in love and the subsequent pain of rejection. But along comes Miguel who, despite her best efforts to push him away, stays and keeps caring for her. Miguel shook her world, and did not slam the door on her, but kept it open with a sign saying "human contact here – no rejections." Miguel eventually became the fantasized "good son" that she never had, successful, handsome, responsible, many of the things she believed her real son not to be. No wonder they began to get along so well, willing partners re-enacting an age-old Oedipal drama with no messy father in the way.

The intensity of the mother–son, grandmother–grandson Oedipal connection is illustrated when Miguel unintentionally caused Evelyn a lot of pain and then rushed to hold her hand. Her comment about how long it had been since a handsome man had held her hand has romantic Oedipal overtones, but another message is "it has been a long time since I held my beloved handsome son's hand, and here you are." Miguel was the fantasized "good son" and how Evelyn learned to communicate with Miguel (let her defenses down, open up, and be honest) became a new model for human interaction in general, and interaction with her son in particular, one filled with joy and love, not resentment and regret. She then, at the encouragement of her mentor/son, used her new model of interaction with her real son. And 20 years of resentment, sadness, and estrangement cracked. This change in Evelyn illustrates the transformational power of transference. And what transformed in Miguel? Through Evelyn, Miguel got to fill a gap in his heart. Through her he could see his grandmother, her love, her death, and his being able to say goodbye. Evelyn and Miguel, through their transference and countertransference, helped each other grow and become more whole.

In the case of Evelyn and Miguel, there is an undercurrent of the erotic (hand-holding, flirting, Oedipal desires), but overt erotic transference and countertransferences are not defining features of the relationship. I hesitate to use the words "erotic" or "sexual" in terms of professional relationships or attractions between clients and therapists because those two words often evoke intense responses from professionals. On the one hand, just the thought of erotic involvement with a client brings about a strong aversive reaction and a large denial that it could ever happen. On the "dark" hand, there are too many therapists who exploit their clients sexually and emotionally (Gabbard 1989), and the topic of sex in the physical and manual therapies needs to be more openly discussed.

EROTIC TRANSFERENCE AND COUNTERTRANSFERENCE

I often ask my psychology and other health profession students "If you really wanted to do a great job of seducing someone, how would you go about it? How would you behave?" Some of the suggestions they come up with include:

- I would be a good listener
- I would make sure they knew their health and welfare were important to me
- I would have no agenda but their happiness
- I would pay lots of attention to them
- I would inquire often on how things were going with them
- I would make affectionate, but non-erotic physical contact.

Do any of these seduction strategies sound familiar? Physical and manual therapists probably do all of the above with their clients, and more. From the clients' viewpoints, they have before them someone who is friendly, interested in their welfare, listens to them, wants them to get better, pays attention to them, has no other agenda (like seduction), and touches them in soothing, affectionate, and healing ways. The atmosphere of physical and manual therapy is set up for such processes. It is not a question of why erotic transference would occur, that is obvious. It may be a question of why it doesn't occur more often than it does. On the practitioner side, physical and manual therapists often have clients who look up to them, who rely on them, who think they are wonderful, and who believe they really care. With such attention, why shouldn't a professional begin to respond romantically or erotically. The setting of treatment works to seduce both ways (see Pope et al 1979, 1993).

We all know stories of healthcare professionals and clients falling in love and even becoming partners. This section of the chapter is not a condemnation of erotic transference and countertransference, but rather an examination of why and how it occurs and how physical and manual therapists can handle it when it does (and it will happen). The climate of high quality physical and manual therapy is designed, albeit unintentionally, to seduce. Erotic and romantic attraction is a slippery slope that often starts out quite subtly, and then progresses to become a steeper slope, and if unchecked, becomes a precipice.

The first signs of erotic transference developing in a client may be that the client dresses a bit nicer than usual for appointments. A female client who used to come to treatment in a t-shirt and track pants, may wear a nice blouse. A male client may come to treatment in a dress shirt and tie, or start wearing cologne. Looking good for one's therapist is one sign that the slippery slope has started to rise. Other signs may be when the client starts bringing things to give to the therapist. For example, if the therapist and client have discussed a sport team, the client may bring an article on the team to give to the therapist. Such a gift may be the beginning of an erotic interest, or it may be an "I want you as a friend" interest. Gifts are a sign that the client is looking for something more. An increased interest in the therapist's personal life is also a good sign that something is brewing on the client's part. To stop the pitch of the slippery slope from increasing early in the process (e.g., refuse "innocuous" gifts, avoid talking about oneself somewhat) may actually hurt the working alliance between therapist and client. The therapist may be seen as cold, and the client may withdraw. The slope gets steeper when the client begins to request more of the therapist's time in and out of the treatment session. For example, a client may ask for the therapist's last time slot for the day and then suggest that they go out for coffee afterwards. Saying "Thanks, but I have some paperwork to take care of" may backfire with "That's alright, I'll just wait." How does one meet such requests? No matter how sensitively the matter is handled, someone is going to get hurt. When requests for attention outside treatment occur, that is a good time to bring the slope back down. Physical and manual therapists might want to have some well-rehearsed way to let the client down easy. For example, "Thanks for the offer. You know, I really enjoy being your physical therapist, and working with you has been rewarding for me. I really want to be the best physical therapist I can be for you. If we were to start doing things socially, like coffee or dinner, then it would seem like I wasn't your physical therapist anymore, and I was something else, like one of your friends, and then that would get confusing for me, and maybe interfere with me being your health professional, but I really appreciate the offer. Is it OK with you that we keep our relationship here in the clinic? I really value what we are doing together." Notice, that the therapist here did not hide behind professional ethics by saying "My profession does not allow that." While true, it is a rather cold response to a sensitive situation.

Coffee is innocent enough, isn't it? It would seem so, and I know many healthcare professionals for whom coffee with a client is not an issue. In many cases, it is just that – coffee. But when coffee turns into dinner, then the angle of that slope has just gone up dramatically. So far the erotic attraction has focused on the client's feelings. How may the therapist actually be complicitous in encouraging such feelings? As discussed earlier, we may encourage client attention and interest in how we behave. The countertransference slippery slope starts with the therapist saying "Great, it's Tuesday, Joan will be here today, how nice" and then maybe dressing a bit differently, a bit more attractively, maybe greeting Joan a bit more effusively and complimenting her on how she looks. The slope continues to rise when therapists begin to ask more personal

questions about their clients "So Bob, do you have a girlfriend (or boyfriend)?" When the therapist starts giving gifts to the client (e.g., "Hey, I got some baseball tickets I can't use, would you like them?") the slope jumps several degrees. The dance of erotic transference and countertransference takes two to participate. Some questions for a therapist to ask when clients seem to want to get closer is "What am I contributing to this response?," "How am I encouraging the client?," and "What are my motivations here?"

If the erotic transference and countertransference has reached the point of romantic, sexual involvement, then there is no longer a slope. We now have a vertical cliff. The literature from psychology and medicine has shown that sexual involvement with clients is, in the vast majority of cases, damaging to the client (Bouhoutsos et al 1983, Brown 1988, Butler & Zelen 1977, Gartrell et al 1986). Clients who have had intimate physical relationships with therapists often experience feelings of betrayal, depression, lowered self-esteem, suicidal ideation (and even attempts), anxiety, and a whole host of other distressing symptoms (Bouhoutsos et al 1983, Brown 1988, Butler & Zelen 1977, Gartrell et al 1986). Most helping professions have in their codes of ethics the prohibition against sexual involvement with clients. The prohibition, often in blunt terms resembling "Thou shalt not," is proper and right. The problem is that in the training of many healthcare professionals, physical and manual therapists included, education on how to avoid erotic entanglements, and how to deal with client romantic interest are lacking. This chapter was included in this book to address that lacuna in the background of physical and manual therapists. This chapter, however, is just a start. What is needed in formal education and internship supervision of physical and manual therapists is extended readings and discussions of the topic with students, role playing client erotic overtures to give students some experience in handling sensitive situations that will arise in the future, and encouraging student self-examination in order to understand one's own contributions to the slippery slope.

Some may read this chapter and say "This author is spinning a bunch of Freudian fairy tales, what a bunch of hooey," and I can understand that response. Freud has received a lot of bad press over the last 50 years, and plenty of his ideas are outdated. I often tell my students in psychology "Pick a system (gestalt, cognitive, psychodynamic, behavioral), and learn it well. Learn it inside and out; become an expert, but always remember it's wrong." Each system of psychotherapy, like many systems of manual and physical therapy is a system of metaphors and explanations of illness, injury, and healing. And they are all wrong. I tell my students to find a system that resonates with them and run with it, but always remember that joint mobilization does not work just because it is joint mobilization, ultrasound therapy does not work just because it is ultrasound therapy. All of these systems and metaphors work (or don't work) because they occur in a context of human interaction. I am overstating the point for emphasis. I know there are many forms of treatment that work regardless of who is involved (e.g., a course of antibiotics for bubonic plague). But the readers of this volume are in the business of being right up close and personal with their clients, and the quality of that closeness cannot help but influence outcome. That common feature of the physical and manual therapies, that physical, and often emotional, closeness is what makes the meta-metaphor of transference and countertransference so central to understanding what happens when we touch others on all different levels.

SUMMARY

This chapter began with a long case study of an intimate professional relationship that illustrated the phenomena of transference and countertransference in the physical and manual therapies. The case of Evelyn and Miguel presented an example of how the quality of a working relationship between a therapist and client can transform both their lives. Our ontogenetic histories of relationships with significant others form the bases of how we interact with our clients, and their histories influence how they respond to us. From research in other helping professions, it has been established that the quality of professional relationships is one of the most powerful predictors of treatment outcome.

Transference and countertransference can be found in most human relationships that progress beyond superficial contact, and examples include relationships with teachers, supervisors, coaches, co-workers, and clients. These phenomena can be helpful in the therapeutic process or destructive. One of the most destructive forms of transference and countertransference is when these phenomena move into the erotic realm unchecked. Sexual relationships with clients are almost always damaging for the client, and can lead to depression, feelings of betrayal, and even suicide. What is needed in the physical and manual therapies is more discussions of these topics during training, education, and professional development. Students and practitioners could benefit from learning about these powerful features of treatment, discovering how they contribute to the processes for good or ill, and gaining some skills in handling awkward situations like erotic transference. An appeal is made for a more self-reflective, self-examining ethos in the physical and manual therapies.

References

Bouhoutsos J, Holroyd J, Lerman H et al 1983 Sexual intimacy between psychotherapists and patients. Professional Psychology: Research and Practice 14: 185–196

Brown L S 1988 Harmful effects of post-termination sexual and romantic relationships between therapists and their former clients. Psychotherapy 25: 249–255

Butler S, Zelen S L 1977 Sexual intimacies between therapists and patients. Psychotherapy Research and Practice 14: 139–145

Epstein L, Feiner A H 1983 Countertransference: The therapist's contribution to the therapeutic situation. Jason Aronson, Northvale, NJ

Freud S 1912 The dynamics of transference. In: Strachey J (trans) The standard edition of the complete psychological works of Sigmund Freud, Vol 12. Hogarth Press, London, p 97–108

Freud S 1915 Observations on transference-love: Further recommendations on the technique of psycho-analysis III.

In: Strachey J (trans) The standard edition of the complete psychological works of Sigmund Freud, Vol 12. Hogarth Press, London, p 157–173

Gabbard G O 1989 Sexual exploitation in professional relationships. American Psychiatric Press, Washington, DC

Gabbard G O 1995 Countertransference: The emerging common ground. International Journal of Psychoanalysis 76: 475–485

Gartrell N, Herman J, Olarte S et al 1986 Psychiatrist–patient sexual contact: Results of a national survey I: Prevalence. American Journal of Psychiatry 143: 1126–1131

Giovacchini P L 1989 Countertransference triumphs and catastrophes. Jason Aronson, Northvale, NJ

Grant J, Crawley J 2002 Transference and projection: Mirrors to the self. Open University Press, Philadelphia, PA

Greenson R R (1967) The technique and practice of psychoanalysis, Volume I. International Universities Press, New York

Henschen K 1991 Critical issues involving male consultants and female athletes. The Sport Psychologist 5: 313–321

Lane F M 1986 Transference and countertransference: Definition of terms. In: Meyers H C (ed) Between analyst and patient: New dimensions in countertransference and transference. Analytic Press, Hillsdale, NJ, p 237–256

Mann J 1986 Transference and countertransference in brief psychotherapy In: Meyers H C (ed) Between analyst and patient: New dimensions in countertransference and transference. Analytic Press, Hillsdale, NJ, p 119–129

Meyers H C 1986 Between analyst and patient: New dimensions in countertransference and transference. Analytic Press, Hillsdale, NJ

Ogilvie B C 1993 Transference phenomena in coaching and teaching. In: Serpa S, Alves J, Ferreira V, Paulo-Brito A (eds) Proceedings of the VIII World Congress of the International Society of Sport Psychology. International Society of Sport Psychology, Lisbon, Portugal

Petitpas A J, Giges B, Danish S J 1999 The sport psychologist–athlete relationship: Implications for training. The Sport Psychologist 13: 344–357

Pope K S, Levenson H, Schover L S 1979 Sexual intimacy in psychology training: Results and implication of a national survey. American Psychologist 34: 682–689

Pope K S, Sonne J L, Holroyd J 1993 Sexual feelings in psychotherapy: Explorations for therapists and therapists-in-training. American Psychological Association, Washington, DC

Racker H 1968 Transference and countertransference. Karnac, London

Stein M H 1986 Acting out – transference and countertransference: Technical considerations. In: Meyers H C (ed) Between analyst and patient: New dimensions in countertransference and transference. Analytic Press, Hillsdale, NJ, p 63–75

Strean H 1994 Countertransference. Hawthorn Press, New York

Yambor J, Connelly D 1991 Issues confronting female sport psychology consultants working with male student-athletes. The Sport Psychologist 5: 304–312

Chapter 7

Recognizing psychopathology

Mark B. Andersen

INTRODUCTION

This chapter, along with Chapter 19, is somewhat different from the other chapters in this text. Whereas the other chapters trace the background theory and research into areas such as imagery and relaxation, or cover integrated approaches to the management of a variety of conditions, these two chapters will be more like primers for recognizing different psychopathologies and how they manifest in physical and manual therapy situations. So there will not be references to past research and theories, rather, there will be descriptions of disorders and how people with those disorders may respond to physical and manual therapy. Actually, the literature on psychopathology and the physical and manual therapies is extremely limited. The realm of psychopathology is vast, and covering the theories and research, even in a cursory manner, would be a Herculean task well beyond the scope of this book. This chapter will focus primarily on what is known as Axis I disorders from the Diagnostic and Statistical Manual of Mental Disorders (DSM-IV-TR, 4th edition, text revision) (American Psychiatric Association 2000). Not all the Axis I disorders will be covered, only those that are more likely to appear in common rehabilitation settings. For a list of the classes of disorders on Axis I, see Box 7.1. For those disorders not covered in this chapter, please refer to the DSM-IV-TR (American Psychiatric Association 2000). The chapter will conclude with a case example of a physical therapist working with a client with an eating disorder.

Box 7.1   Diagnostic and Statistical Manual of Mental Disorders: Axis I disorders

Disorders usually first diagnosed in infancy, childhood, or adolescence
Delirium, dementia, and amnestic and other cognitive disorders
Mental disorders due to a general medical condition
Substance-related disorders
Schizophrenia and other psychotic disorders
Mood disorders
Anxiety disorders
Somatoform disorders
Factitious disorders
Dissociative disorders
Sexual and gender identity disorders
Eating disorders
Sleep disorders
Impulse-control disorders not elsewhere classified
Adjustment disorders
Other conditions that may be a focus of clinical attention

WHAT IS PSYCHOPATHOLOGY?

Psychopathology is difficult to define. What is pathological behavior in one setting may be quite normal in a different setting. For example, a woman who hallucinates, claims to talk to the spirit world, goes into trance states, and tells people all about it would be considered at least "odd," if not downright crazy in Dubuque, Iowa, USA. But if this woman was a curandera (medicine woman) in Mexico, then her behavior and her visions would all be well-respected and prized in her community. Culture is only one determinant of whether people get labeled as mentally ill. Other determinants include economics, gender, race, age, and the list goes on. For this chapter, I will take the dominant Western view of mental illness with the caveat that when working cross-culturally, flexibility is needed in determining whether a client has a serious mental condition in need of referral.

Even within a Western view, there are myriad approaches to psychopathology. Psychodynamic paradigms suggest that mental disorders are due to unconscious conflicts, fixations, and childhood experiences. Cognitive psychology viewpoints focus on disorders as the result of irrational thinking. Humanistic theories are concerned, in part, with discrepancies between ideal and real selves. Discussion of these different viewpoints will appear briefly in the sections below when the focus is on a specific disorder. The Axis I disorders that will be covered include anxiety disorders, mood disorders, somatoform/dissociative disorders, adjustment disorders, and eating disorders. In discussions with a wide variety of people working in the physical and manual therapies, it was decided from clinical experience that these were the most common presenting disorders that may appear in physical and manual therapy treatment.

ANXIETY DISORDERS

As the name implies, anxiety disorders have as a defining feature some form of dread, fear, or worry. The anxiety may range from something quite specific (e.g., fear of pain) to a vague free-floating dread with no real target for the discomfort. Several anxiety disorders will be discussed in this chapter. They include panic attacks, social anxiety disorders, obsessive-compulsive disorders, post-traumatic stress disorder, and generalized anxiety disorder.

PANIC ATTACK

Panic attacks can be a feature of any of the anxiety disorders discussed in this section, and so they seem to be a good place to start. Panic attacks are often dramatic periods of time in which the individual experiences any number of physiological and cognitive symptoms. The physiological symptoms reflect intense activation of the sympathetic nervous system and can include tachycardia, hyperventilation, sweating, trembling, nausea, chills, and light-headedness. Cognitive symptoms may be thoughts of losing control and fear of dying. The onset of a panic attack is usually quite sudden, but not in all cases. The attack gains in intensity rapidly and is accompanied often by a strong drive to escape. Attacks may be unexpected and appear to "come out of nowhere," or they may be connected to a situation (e.g., public speaking) or place (e.g., in a physician's waiting room for those with a fear of pain).

Agoraphobia, literally a fear of open spaces (from the Greek "agora" open plaza), is often a feature of panic disorders. The central concern is that one fears being in a situation where a panic attack may occur and escape would be impossible, or difficult, or embarrassing. People with panic disorders with agoraphobia tend to shun those situations (being caught out in the open, so to speak) where they may experience panic. Extreme cases of agoraphobia lead people to become essentially prisoners in their own homes, paralyzed by the thought of going outside and experiencing panic.

In the physical and manual therapies, practitioners may never see a full-blown attack in the clinic, but they have been known to happen under the course of some manual treatment where some stimulus (e.g., massaging a specific body part) or response (e.g., the production of pain) brings about an attack. If such an event were to occur, a physician should be notified immediately. Breathing into a paper bag, despite the jokes made about it, can be quite useful for stemming hyperventilation often associated with panic. What may be more likely is that under the course of treatment, clients may report that they have had panic attacks. A referral at that point would be a salubrious response.

Panic attacks may stem directly from the cause for why the client is in rehabilitation. For example, the client may have experienced severe trauma and has post-traumatic stress disorder (see later in this chapter), a common feature of which is panic attacks. Or there may be some disfigurement associated with why they are in rehabilitation (e.g., significant scars), and they have growing fears of being out in public to the point of agoraphobia and only moving from home to the clinic, avoiding all other social contact.

SOCIAL ANXIETY DISORDERS

Similar to agoraphobia, social anxiety disorder has a central feature of fear of social or performance (e.g., public-speaking) situations. People with this disorder may have fears of evaluation and scrutiny and dread of embarrassing themselves. As a result of these fears, they actively avoid situations where the anxiety will manifest. They recognize that the fear is excessive, and even unwarranted, but are nonetheless incapable of overcoming it.

A specific subset of social anxiety disorder is social physique anxiety, where people are hyperconscious of their bodies and concerned about how others will evaluate them based on their physiques.

Such individuals probably avoid public places where bodies are on display (e.g., public swimming pools and fitness/recreation facilities), and may wear baggy clothing in an attempt to cover up what they believe unsightly to others. In the physical and manual therapies, clients may make comments such as "I hate my body" or "I hate going out in public looking like this." Such disclosures may be signs of social physique anxiety. In the rehabilitation therapies, because people are often attending due to some injury or illness that may have altered the appearance of their body, social physique anxiety is not uncommon. Typical situations where this may be seen is in clients with burns, or following significant motor vehicle accidents.

OBSESSIVE-COMPULSIVE DISORDERS

Individuals with obsessive-compulsive disorders have recurring, repetitive thoughts (obsessions) or behaviors (compulsions) that intrude on daily living in terms of the time they consume, the distress they cause, or the impairment they inflict. Obsessions are cognitive processes that may come in the form of verbal, imaginal, or impulsive intrusions that are contradictory to one's sense of self. For example, one may have recurring thoughts that one is going to hurt someone, and a great deal of anxiety is attached to those thoughts, yet one has no history of violence towards others. Compulsions are the behavioral siblings of obsessions. They are repetitive behaviors aimed at reducing anxiety and often in service of allaying the anxiety brought about by the obsessions. For example, a common obsession is with one's own bodily functions and contamination with "filth." This obsession and anxiety is aroused upon evacuation of the bowel or bladder, and to combat that anxiety, people with obsessive-compulsive disorder may wash their hands (compulsion) for extended periods of time to the point that they damage their skin. People with obsessive-compulsive disorders do recognize that what they are doing and thinking is not normal, but again are powerless to change their thinking and behavior.

Physical and manual therapists may come across those whose compulsions interfere with rehabilitation (e.g., rubbing injured areas excessively, carrying out prescribed exercises excessively). Treatment of obsessive-compulsive disorders is a complex process and will require a referral to a mental health professional. Obsessive-compulsive anxiety disorder is not the same as an obsessive-compulsive personality disorder, and the implications for rehabilitation are quite different (see Chapter 19 for the latter).

POST-TRAUMATIC STRESS DISORDER

Physical and manual therapists will often encounter clients with post-traumatic stress disorder (PTSD) because many people are in rehabilitation because of some extreme traumatic event. In some cases, PTSD develops after someone has experienced a traumatic stressful event that involved a threat to life or functioning, or one has observed such an event happen to another. The response to such an event usually involves feelings of helplessness, intense anxiety, and general extreme distress. War events are only the most obvious examples of experiences that can lead to PTSD. Motor vehicle accidents, natural disasters (e.g., people trapped in earthquake-destroyed buildings), and physical violence (e.g., rape, assault) perpetrated on self or others are other examples where PTSD might develop.

People with PTSD may have ongoing elevated sympathetic nervous system activity, may avoid any activity or place that may be associated with the event, and may have a general blunting of affect, including diminished feelings of intimacy and sexual interest. Often they relive the experience in a variety of ways. They may have recurrent dreams of the event, or they may have waking "flash backs" to the traumatic time. Social interactions may be impaired with feelings of disconnectedness, and the future may seem grim and colorless. PTSD may have a quick onset and last less than 3 months (acute), or may continue for more than 6 months (chronic), or may not become manifest until half a year or so later (delayed onset).

Physical and manual therapists are in the business of helping shattered people get put back together. For people with PTSD in rehabilitation for their injuries, the shattering has occurred on both the physical and the psychological levels. When working with someone who has experienced severe trauma, keeping an eye and ear out for the symptoms of PTSD, asking gentle questions about sleep patterns, social life, and plans for the future may help the physical or manual therapist determine if a consultation with a mental health professional would be a good choice for the client. PTSD can impact on rehabilitation in many ways. For example, the anxiety associated with PTSD could reduce adherence to certain exercises if the client believes that the exercises may reproduce their pain. Further, setting and working towards appropriate rehabilitation goals may also be more difficult in situations of extreme stress.

GENERALIZED ANXIETY DISORDER

We have all encountered individuals with generalized anxiety disorders. These people worry, and are anxious, over a lot of different things, and anxiety seems to be an all-pervasive part of their lives. Often the anxiety is not debilitating, but it is distressing. Common symptoms may include disturbed sleep, irritability, problems staying focused, generalized muscle tension, and fatigue. The worry and distress usually cause some level of impairment in social and vocational situations. For the physical and manual therapist, one of the associated features that may have a large influence on rehabilitation is the generalized muscle tension. Clients with generalized anxiety disorders may have trembling, twitching, and muscle aches and pains. These anxiety symptoms may easily interfere with physical rehabilitation. For example, if a physical or manual therapist is working on mobilizing the joints of the cervical spine, generalized muscle tension around this area can make this more difficult. To address the generalized muscle tension, the physical or manual therapist may want to begin a course of relaxation (see Chapter 9). One is not treating the full disorder, but rather, addressing one of the symptoms that has a direct influence on rehabilitation progress. How successful one would be at combating the generalized muscle tension through teaching relaxation techniques is debatable, but the client may find some relief, both physically and psychologically from learning how to relax. Another symptom of anxiety that can impact on physical and manual therapy rehabilitation is inability to focus. As aspects of rehabilitation require the ability to focus on exercises, body posture, and other therapeutic interventions, someone having difficulties with this task may not progress as rapidly as others.

There are other anxiety disorders (e.g., specific phobias, acute stress disorder, substance-induced anxiety disorder), and the reader can find more information about those in the DSM-IV-TR (American Psychiatric Association 2000). Anxiety is a symptom in a wide variety of disorders, and it will appear again in all of the sections that follow, most notably in the discussion on depression.

MOOD DISORDERS

Mood disorders, at their cores, are disturbances in affect, but they also have obvious manifestations in the cognitive and behavioral realms. The language of mood disorders is firmly planted in the common lexicon, with words like "depressed" and "manic" used to describe a variety of affective states, thought patterns, and behaviors. In this section, the language of mood disorders will be much more specific than what is used in common parlance.

MAJOR DEPRESSIVE DISORDER

Depression is the "common cold" of mental health. The risk of experiencing a major depressive disorder sometime in one's life, depending on demographics, is 5% to 12% for men and 10% to 25% for women (American Psychiatric Association 2000). So the likelihood of physical and manual therapists encountering a client with depression is quite high, especially because many clients are in rehabilitation with conditions that could trigger a major depressive episode, if not a full-blown disorder.

The diagnosis of major depressive episode is complex, involving several levels of determination. It is not the purpose of this chapter to help physical and manual therapists become diagnosticians in the area, but rather to recognize depressive symptoms, respond to them sensitively, consider them in planning rehabilitation programs, and make referrals.

A core feature of a major depressive disorder is the presence of a major depressive episode. An episode is of at least 2 weeks in duration, where the individual experiences depressed mood (e.g., sadness, hopelessness) and loses interest in many, if not all, activities that previously brought pleasure. Accompanying symptoms may include changes in eating (a lot more or a lot less), sleep patterns (hyper- or hyposomnia), weight (gain or loss), along with fatigue, agitation, feelings of worthlessness, suicidal thoughts, and cognitive impairments (e.g., difficulty concentrating).

Major depressive disorders often occur after a severe stressful event such as the death of a loved one or the loss of some aspect of self. This last point is particularly relevant for physical and manual therapists, because some clients with certain conditions (e.g., amputation, spinal cord injury, burns) may have lost a significant aspect of self and be at risk of a major depressive disorder. Individuals with major depressive disorder are at high risk of suicide. Thus, it is imperative that the physical or manual therapist be sensitive to, and alert for, the symptoms of this disorder.

Major depressive episodes or disorders can influence rehabilitation from physical injury or illness in several ways. For example, the loss of interest that accompanies depression can result in poor adherence to rehabilitation activities. Also, difficulty concentrating can affect the learning of rehabilitation exercises. Further, feelings of worthlessness can cause the individual to question why they would want to recover from an injury.

BIPOLAR DISORDER

At the opposite end of the mood spectrum are disorders with manic features. An essential feature of bipolar disorder is the presence of a manic episode (or both manic and depressive episodes). The manic episode must last at least 1 week and is characterized by consistently elevated mood states accompanied by hyposomnia, flights of fancy, grandiosity, and inflated self-esteem. Agitation is also common. People experiencing a bipolar episode may make grand plans, engage in pleasurable activities to excess, and have little regard for personal safety. The individual is often euphoric, but can be irritable, especially if others are "raining on my parade" and trying to bring the person back to reality. Manic episodes in the rehabilitation setting are relatively rare. Bipolar disorders may actually be unipolar with only swings into the manic phase, or they may cover the full spectrum from mania to depressive states. A milder version of bipolar disorder, cyclothymia, may be more common in rehabilitation (see below).

DYSTHYMIC DISORDER

This disorder is relatively common, and we have all met someone who could be described as dysthymic. People with dysthymia have chronically depressed mood, but not to the extent of a major depressive disorder. Their functioning is higher than those with depression, but they experience being sad for more time than not and often have other symptoms related to poor appetite, sleep disturbances, poor self-esteem, and cognitive difficulties (concentration, decision-making). Dysthymia almost seems more like a personality or characterological disorder than a mood disorder because of its long-term chronic course. People with dysthymia will often say "I have just never been a happy person." Diagnosis of dysthymia in adults is made only after a 2-year history of chronic depressed mood.

Many people with dysthymia have in their histories an early loss of a love object such as a parent or sibling, and possibly many of the symptoms of dysthymia (for some) are related to a long-term grief over that loss. Physical and manual therapists will recognize these individuals easily, but treatment requires relatively long-term psychotherapeutic interventions.

CYCLOTHYMIA

People with cyclothymia resemble those with bipolar disorders in that they fluctuate between periods of hypomania and periods of depressed mood. They are on a rollercoaster, but the rollercoaster is not as intense as with bipolar disorders. As in dysthymia, a history of fluctuating positive and negative mood for at least 2 years is necessary for a diagnosis of cyclothymia. Again, as in dysthymia, cyclothymia has a more characterological feel to it than bipolar disorders.

SOMATOFORM DISORDERS

Somatoform disorders are characterized by physical symptoms. These symptoms, at least initially, look like there is some underlying physical medical problem. On closer examination, and often after several medical tests or procedures, no medical or physical explanation can be found for the somatic complaints. These disorders are not malingering, that is, they are not intentional on the part of the client as a means of consciously gaining attention or avoiding responsibilities. The somatoform disorders that will be presented in this chapter include somatization disorder, conversion disorder, and hypochondriasis. Other somatoform disorders are discussed in Chapter 18 under the heading Functional Somatic Syndromes.

SOMATIZATION DISORDER

People with somatization disorder experience repeated somatic problems such as gastrointestinal distress and pain in the head, joints, abdomen, chest, and extremities. Medical attention is sought and medical treatment usually occurs. These clients often baffle medical personnel, and rarely does a year go by where they are free of somatic symptoms. For a diagnosis of somatization disorder there must be at least one sexual or reproductive system problem present at one time, such as irregular menses in women or erectile dysfunction in men. There is also at least one symptom suggesting a neurological condition (weakness in a limb, balance problems, amnesia). People with somatization disorder may enter physical therapy for treatment of problems with joints and limbs that have been diagnosed as a physical disorder. Physical or manual therapy may actually be beneficial and offer some relief for these clients, but the likelihood of other symptoms appearing later is quite high. To emphasize again, these individuals are not "faking it." The pain and the discomfort they experience are quite real.

CONVERSION DISORDER

Conversion disorder is similar to somatization disorder, but it specifically involves neurological symptoms, primarily in motor and sensory pathways. Motor problems include balance impairment, paralysis, and difficulty swallowing. On the sensory side, clients may experience blindness, deafness, numbness or pain upon touch, and hallucinations. A curious feature of conversion disorder is that the symptoms often do not correspond with neuroanatomy. For example, someone may experience a "glove anesthesia" (i.e., no feeling in a hand and forearm up to where a glove would stop), but perfect sensation above that point. There is no neurological damage possible that would produce such symptoms. People with conversion reactions and somatization were in the past labeled "hysterics." Also interesting is that more educated and informed people with this disorder produce more subtle and convincing symptoms. Physical and manual therapists may encounter such clients, especially those who have been referred for treatment on weak limbs. Again, as in somatization disorder, treatment may help, but not for any physical reason.

HYPOCHONDRIASIS

People with hypochondriasis have inordinate fears that they have one or more serious medical conditions. These fears are usually based on negative interpretations of symptoms, that when examined medically reveal that the feared condition is not present, and the worry is misplaced. Even with such information, clients' fears still persist. The anxieties over possibly having some medical disorder cause a significant amount of psychological distress. As with other somatoform disorders, the client is not faking it consciously for attention. The distress is also associated with problems in social and vocational areas. The worry over the feared disease can become a focus for the person's whole life. Individuals with this disorder sometimes undergo repeated medical tests, often at considerable expense. The disorder is often associated with early childhood serious illness, and other mental conditions such as anxiety and depression. The physical and manual therapist may be able to detect hypochondriasis with clients who continually focus conversations on their feared medical conditions, and relate stories about how physicians are not being thorough enough in detecting it.

There are other somatoform disorders and the reader is directed to the DSM-IV-TR (American Psychiatric Association 2000) for further reading. Two sets of disorders, though not really somatoform disorders, are worthy of mention here, and they are factitious disorders and malingering. Factitious disorders involve consciously produced or faked symptoms (either psychological or physical) in the service of assuming a "sick role." Why the person wants to be considered sick is not clear. In the case of malingering, the reason for producing symptoms may be clear, and there is an underlying, and often adaptive, rationale. For example, a person might fake psychological symptoms in order to avoid some hazardous duty in the military. Physical and manual therapists may encounter individuals with these factitious and malingering features. Confrontations with these clients should occur in consultation with other involved medical personnel.

ADJUSTMENT DISORDERS

People with adjustment disorders have recently experienced a significant stressor that in some way taxes their resources to the point where the quality of their lives is diminished. Examples of such stressors could be moving to a new country, major financial setbacks, or a serious injury or illness. Symptoms may include anxiety, sleep disturbance, excessive worry, disruptions in social, vocational, or academic realms, and conduct problems (fighting, reckless driving, excessive consumption of alcohol). Adjustment disorders come in a variety of forms (with anxiety, with depressed mood, with both anxiety and depressed mood, with conduct disturbances, and with all of the above). Many people in treatment with physical and manual therapists have experienced significant stressors that are influencing their lives. For those whose resources are not quite up to filling the demands of the stressor, symptoms of adjustment disorders may appear. These disorders are short lived (usually less than 6 months in duration) and tend to abate in physical and manual therapy as clients get better.

EATING DISORDERS

Of all the psychopathologies discussed in this chapter, eating disorders may be the most difficult to detect and to make referrals for treatment. There is often a considerable amount of shame attached to having an eating disorder, and many people struggling with food and body image keep their problems to themselves. The clandestine quality of these disorders may be more pronounced for males. The DSM IV-TR (American Psychiatric Association 2000) states that 90% of those with bulimia nervosa and anorexia nervosa are female. There is good reason to doubt those numbers, because the prevalence of eating disorders among males is most assuredly underreported. Males may try to hide these disorders because of the stigma of having a "female" disorder. There appears to be a substantially greater prevalence of eating disorders among gay, as opposed to heterosexual, males. It may be that gay men feel less stigma and are more willing to seek help, or it may be that there actually is greater prevalence and incidence of eating disorders in this population. From my own clinical experience in the realm of sport, the prevalence of eating disorders for males is quite high, especially in sports where appearance is important (e.g., diving, figure skating) or where there are weight classes (e.g., rowing, wrestling). Eating disorders can have a variety of etiologies, and in sport the root source of the problem is often the sport environment itself. Coaches can exert huge pressures on athletes to lose weight, and athletes are not natural nutritionists. Many end up resorting to disordered eating in attempts to satisfy the demands of the sport. There is an interesting example of environmental pressure to stay lean in Australian football. In many football players' contracts there are limits set on how high their skinfolds can be, with fines in place if they exceed the limits. In talking with psychologists who work with Australian football teams, it appears that a small, but significant, number of players have serious struggles with weight and eating behaviors. Some eating disorders stem from deep psychodynamic problems that have to do with struggles against a powerful other (often a mother) over control of one's life, and an intense fear for maturing into a sexual being. Such cases are, however, well beyond the scope of this chapter.

Eating disorders are relatively common in industrialized nations where there is a surplus of food, and relatively rare in other parts of the world. Physical and manual therapists working in industrialized nations will surely have clients with eating disorders. Clients who are struggling with weight, body image, and self-esteem may be engaging in behaviors (fasting, bingeing, purging) that will influence the course of rehabilitation. For example, if a client is taking in only a few hundred calories a day, then there are not enough nutrients for proper healing, and the time in rehabilitation may be prolonged. Also for young women with anorexia, who are amenorrheic, osteoporosis may become a problem.

ANOREXIA NERVOSA

The most dramatic aspect of anorexia nervosa is that the individual does not maintain a minimally normal body weight befitting the person's age, gender, and height. People with anorexia nervosa are obsessed and anxious about "getting fat," have issues with self-esteem, and have seriously distorted perceptions of body shape and size. Minimal body weight has been suggested to be 85% of normal on standard growth charts. People with anorexia are easy to spot; they are thin, often painfully so. Not all very thin people are anorexic, and snap judgments should not be made.

There are two subtypes of people with anorexia, restricting and binge-eating/purging types. People who restrict use dieting and fasting in order to lose weight, or maintain a low weight. They may also use excessive exercise as a means of losing weight. People who exercise excessively as part of their regimen are at risk for a variety of musculoskeletal injuries, and if beginning osteoporosis is present, that risk is even higher. These individuals are problematic for physical and manual therapists, because they will often continue to exercise against medical advice and exacerbate their conditions.

People who binge eat and then purge, behaviorally look similar to those with bulimia nervosa, but they have the added feature of low body weight. These individuals may use emetics (pharmaceutical agents to bring on vomiting) or other means to self-induce vomiting, along with using laxatives and diuretics to lose weight. Such behaviors can do serious damage to the gastrointestinal tract, along with damage to teeth as a result of gastric acid often washing over them.

People with anorexia fiercely hold on to distorted images of their bodies and have a great fear of gaining weight. If a physical or manual therapist has a client who is quite thin, there are some things they can do to check if an eating disorder may be the problem. For example, during a treatment visit, the therapist may want to gently comment "You know, while you are in treatment, we might want to talk to a nutritionist to see if we can put a little more weight on you to build up a bit more muscle to help stabilize and strengthen your joints." This comment is put into the context of the weight gain assisting the rehabilitation. If such a comment is met with "Yeah, I just can't keep weight on me, that might be a good idea," then an eating disorder is probably not an issue. If, however, such a comment is met with "No way, I gain weight at the drop of a muffin, and I'll end up fat" then anorexia may be a serious concern.

Other features to look for in underweight clients are evidence of depression (see symptoms above), obsessive-compulsive symptoms, perfectionism, and lack of interest in sex. Many individuals with anorexia also have a diagnosable personality disorder (e.g., borderline, histrionic) (see Chapter 19 for more details). Physical symptoms other than thinness include gastrointestinal distress (e.g., constipation, pain), hypotension, and dry skin. In some cases lanugo (downy hair) may develop on torsos.

A major difficulty for physical and manual therapists is making a referral to an eating disorder specialist for a client with anorexia. Clients with this disorder are often extremely resistant to psychological treatment. If a client complains of some of the physical symptoms, then one step to take would be to refer to a physician who is knowledgeable and sensitive to the problems of eating disorders. It might be easier to get a client to see a physician for physical symptoms first, rather than try to push (and "push" would be how many clients with anorexia would interpret a referral to a psychologist) for psychological treatment. In extreme cases, anorexia is life-threatening, and hospitalization may be necessary to save a life.

BULIMIA NERVOSA

In anorexia nervosa there is an obvious physical symptom that can alert the physical or manual therapist to the potential problem. In bulimia nervosa the symptoms are more subtle than in anorexia. People with bulimia usually do not appear excessively thin, and are often of normal weight or slightly heavier or lighter than normal. The disorder is rare among obese people. The cycle of binge eating and purging is similar to the subtype in anorexia. The bingeing and the purging cycle usually are carried out clandestinely, but in some cases people actually engage in social activities where bingeing and purging are part of the activities. I have had horse-racing jockeys report to me about going to "snarf and barf" parties where the major activity is eating to excess and then vomiting with other jockeys. An episode of binge eating may be triggered by a depressed mood or a stressor, and the bingeing is a sort of stress management technique that helps for a short time. This is then often followed, however, by feelings of self-loathing because of the activity, and purging then follows.

Vomiting is the most common method of purging, but others include use of laxatives, diuretics, and enemas. Those who use these methods are classified as "purging types." There is also another subtype who is nonpurging. Their methods to compensate for bingeing center around periods of fasting or excessive exercise.

Anxiety and depression are often associated with bulimia, as is substance abuse, especially in the form of stimulants to curb hunger. Physical symptoms include dental damage, substantial enlargement of the parotid glands, and lesions or scars on the fingers or hands from contact with teeth when inducing vomiting with the fingers. In severe cases

there can be damage to the esophagus, tears in the stomach and gastrointestinal tract, and with the electrolyte imbalances, cardiac arrhythmias.

People with bulimia would benefit from psychological, nutritional, and medical treatment. As in anorexia, the referral process is a sensitive one. For physical and manual therapists working in clinics with other healthcare professionals, a "team approach" to care is probably the most salubrious option.

OTHER DISORDERS

There are many other disorders on Axis I, including substance abuse, dementias, and schizophrenia. For the complete list of the disorders on Axis I refer to Box 7.1. In the physical and manual therapies, where clients are often experiencing considerable pain, dependency on pain killers may present a concern. Checking in with patients on the use of such medications, and consultation with the attending physician, would be proper client care.

A CASE EXAMPLE

A case study example will now be presented to illustrate the impact that psychopathology can have on the rehabilitation process. This case example demonstrates the dialogue between a physical therapist and a client with intermittent commentary and analysis on that dialogue.

David is a 20-year-old diver at a major Division I (highest level of competition at US universities) school. He has a full scholarship (tuition, books, room and board) to attend the university. He has been referred to the physical therapist in the university sports medicine clinic for treatment of serious tendinosis in both wrists. He is an all-round diver, competing in the one-meter and three-meter springboard events, but his specialty is the ten-meter platform. Diving is especially hard on the wrists, especially with the impact they endure from ten-meter dives. He is 170 cm tall with a slim but muscular build and about 6% body fat. As a result of his injury, he has stopped all diving in the pool and is working on dry land exercises (e.g., trampoline), resistance training that does not involve wrists, and some aerobic training. He is frustrated with his injuries and comes to the physical therapist for his first treatment with somewhat flat emotions. His therapist, Julie, has worked with many divers and swimmers before and is sensitive to the demands of the sport. Their first conversation goes as follows:

> Julie (J): Come on in David, and hop up here (directs him to the treatment plinth). How are you doing today?
>
> David (D): OK, I guess.
>
> J: Hmmm, sounds like you aren't quite sure, having a tough time with those wrists? I got the report from Dr Fawkner.
>
> D: Kind of hard to not be in the pool.
>
> J: Yeah, sort of like that rule, take an unscheduled day off, go backward two days in your training.
>
> D: Exactly, I am going to get so far behind.

A lot has occurred in this brief encounter. Julie right from the beginning has engaged in empathic reflection where she comments on his "I guess" and expresses that she understands the "tough time" he may be going through. She knows the sport well and communicates the training worries that often occur with injuries. She is doing well in establishing rapport as evidenced by David's "Exactly." That one word probably reflects David's thinking that "Cool, here is someone who understands." Finding a health professional that one can relate to is a huge step in the process of a client opening up to talk about their concerns, their injuries, and other aspects of their lives. This brief interchange is a good start in getting David comfortable with working with Julie. Let's continue with Julie and David.

> J: Yeah, getting behind is a worry. What are you doing now that you aren't in the pool?
>
> D: Dryland, weights, mostly trunk and lower body, on the bike too, and getting fat.
>
> J: That's always a concern in diving with weight. Exactly how fat are you getting?
>
> D: (laughing) The way I am going I will end up like the Michelin Man (laughing again).

That David brought up weight so early in the conversation may be because he feels comfortable with Julie, but in the world of diving, athletes always talk about weight and appearance because they are such essential parts of the sport. The truth of the matter is that in diving, if you look good then you get higher points. Divers used to say of Greg Louganis that he got an extra point just for putting on a swimming outfit because he had the perfect diving body. It is not a fair aspect of the sport, but it

is a huge part of competition, so concerns about appearance are always present.

Julie does something interesting here, she empathically reflects but then makes a small joke-inquiry about how fat he thinks he is getting. This tact may reflect her anxiety about once more having to address eating as a problem for a client, and it may be that she is communicating to David that yes, we can talk about weight and not have it be a really difficult topic. David responds well to Julie with his joke about the Michelin Man. People often use humor to compensate for anxiety, and with David's concerns about weight, there is probably plenty of anxiety too. Humor can break the ice, but it is also a way to avoid the topic.

> J: OK, Michelin Man, let's have a look at your wrists, and while we're doing some ultrasound why don't you tell me about your diving list for the ten-meter?
>
> D: OK, cool, my first dive is an inward two and half pike that I usually rip. . . .

Now what has happened here? They were getting to the topic of weight, and then Julie directed him elsewhere to treatment and to his dives. The physical therapist here is really doing a good job. She knows eating and weight are sensitive issues for David, and they have come a long way in feeling comfortable about talking about weight, but Julie does not want to push the issue too fast. So she goes back into further rapport-building by asking David to educate her about his diving. This move helps balance the relationship, so David can feel more like there is equality and give and take on both sides. This balancing will probably help David feel more comfortable about talking over what is really bothering him. We will now move on to their third session together. The session is shortly after lunch. David arrives looking a little haggard, and his eyes are quite bloodshot.

> J: OK, David, you know the drill, hop on up here.
>
> D: OK (Julie notices his eyes).
>
> J: David, I have a question.
>
> D: Yeah, what is it?
>
> J: Have you been crying?
>
> D: No, why?
>
> J: Your eyes are all bloodshot.
>
> D: Really? Must be from getting in the pool for the first time today and doing some partial dives where I go in feet first, all that chlorine. I did that this morning.

Julie knows that "chlorine eyes" do not last a long time and suspects that just after lunch and before this session that David has made himself vomit, which often results in bloodshot eyes. Julie is not about to challenge him at this point.

J: OK, let's get this ultrasound going for now. So how have the last couple of days been?

D: Really screwed, I've gained a kilo in the last week. I told you, Michelin City!

J: Sounds like the weight gain is really bumming you out.

D: I used to have it under control, I used to keep it in check, but with not diving much and not running up the 10 meter for hours on end, I am blowing up.

David is probably referring not only to his weight but also to his bulimia. He most likely had both in control before his injuries disturbed his routine. It is likely that he would binge and purge a couple of times a week and maintain weight. With the injury and lower activity, it has messed up his "control." The bulimia is no longer keeping him on track, but rather it is now a much larger source of anxiety and frustration.

J: Sounds like you are pretty anxious about gaining weight.

D: I gotta be, I gotta look perfect out there.

J: I know, I know, there is so much pressure to look good in your sport. You're out there essentially naked and everyone can see everything.

D: You got that right, it's a nightmare.

Julie is making really strong connections with David because she wants to ask an important question about what he is doing to control his weight. Her empathy and understanding of diving will help David feel more comfortable. It probably also helps that Julie is a woman. It might be more difficult for David to admit to disordered eating to a male physical therapist.

J: So what are you doing to try and keep the weight down?

D: (silent for a while) Well, I am trying to not eat so much, but I get so damn hungry.

J: Are you doing anything more radical than trying to cut down?

D: (looking away) I . . . umm . . . I am doing some other things.

J: Like what? It's OK, this is just between you and me.

D: You won't tell the coach?

J: David, you're my client, not the coach. Whatever we say stays here with you and me.

D: (starting to get tears in his eyes). I have been throwing up a lot, I am so embarrassed . . . I just don't know what to do.

J: It's OK David, and thanks for letting me know. That took some guts (they both have a bit of an anxious laugh at the reference to "guts"). So let's talk a bit about what is happening with you.

D: OK, thanks.

What followed was a long conversation about how David had been engaging in bulimic behavior in a controlled manner for the last 3 years, not enough to do any real damage physically, but always of some concern to him. Lately with his injuries, his bulimic behavior had gotten out of control, and the eating and vomiting were occurring on a daily basis, and he was scared. The example above shows how a sensitive physical or manual therapist can help people talk about their problems and then start the process of referral. Because of the good relationship that was established between Julie and David, David was willing to listen and follow Julie's advice about seeing a nutritionist and a psychologist to help him get back on track. Julie also helped the process along by going with David to both the nutritionist and the psychologist as part of his support team.

Referral is a sensitive issue. People, in general, do not like to hear they have a mental or behavioral problem that requires special treatment. In the above case Julie explained to David that the difficulties he was having were out of her range of expertise, but that she knew of experts she admired and trusted who would be able to help him through these tough times. She also did not just send him away on his own to strangers, but rather remained by his side throughout the whole referral process. Julie's work with David is a good model for physical and manual therapists to have in mind when eating disorders may be present.

SUMMARY

This chapter has covered many of the mental disorders on Axis I of the DSM-IV-TR (American Psychiatric Association 2000). The purpose of the chapter was to describe the disorders in general terms so that physical and manual therapists may recognize the problems easier and earlier. Also included with each disorder were examples of either how the person with the disorder may present in clinical settings, or how the disorder may interfere with the rehabilitation process. The major classes of disorders covered were anxiety disorders, mood disorders, somatoform disorders, adjustment disorders, and eating disorders. Anxiety disorders, in general, are marked by behavioral and cognitive features that are manifestations of some inner dread, and many of the behaviors of people with anxiety disorders are attempts to compensate for that anxiety and dread.

In the area of mood disorders, depression is one of the most common disorders in Western society, and is often called the "common cold" of mental health. Somatoform disorders are particularly difficult to deal with in rehabilitation because there is really no physical underlying problem behind the client's somatic complaints and anxieties. That does not mean that some caring touch will not help. It may help quite a bit, but not for any physical reason.

Many people in rehabilitation have adjustment difficulties, and could benefit from some counseling. Often, however, third party payments for psychological treatment will not be made without a DSM-IV-TR diagnosis. The subtypes of adjustment disorder could probably encompass many "normal" people in rehabilitation.

Eating disorders are extremely complex and often closeted. The chapter ends with a description of the eating disorders of anorexia nervosa and bulimia nervosa, and a case example of a male diver with bulimia nervosa, and how the interactions with a caring physical therapist helped him seek psychological and nutritional help.

Physical and manual therapists should be aware of the signs and symptoms of a variety of psychopathologies so that they can tailor their rehabilitation to suit the needs of the individual. Being aware of such conditions also allows physical and manual therapists to make appropriate referrals to psychologists and other mental health practitioners.

Reference

American Psychiatric Association 2000 Diagnostic and statistical manual of mental disorders, 4th edn (text revision). American Psychiatric Association, Washington, DC

Chapter 8

Cognitive and behavioral interventions

Craig A. White, Esther K. Black

INTRODUCTION

Traditional models of medical illness focused solely on the physical aspects of the person's difficulties, providing surgery, medication, and physical and manual therapies where applicable, in order to maintain the physical health status of the client. In recent years, however, there has been an increasing recognition that psychological factors are also important, not only to the emotional health of the client but that they can also influence the client's physical recovery. Clients who experience physical illness or serious injury are at increased vulnerability in developing psychological problems including depression and/or anxiety (Martin 2001). This contributory factor to the experience of psychosocial morbidity is aside from those whose existing psychological problems are exacerbated by the development of a physical illness. These difficulties can lead to a decrease in resources to deal with the demands of recovery from physical illness and injury.

Although most clients adjust well to the psychosocial aspects of their medical condition, around 20–25% of clients with medical problems experience clinically significant psychological symptoms. Clients often find themselves undertaking a delicate balancing act where they must balance the need to be in control of their lives with the reality that there will be times when it will be more functional for them to surrender control to significant others.

Psychological problems can complicate the management of medical problems. There is a huge variation in the subjective impact of medical conditions of the same objective severity. Two clients may have the same degree of physical disease or damage but yet have markedly different psychological responses to that physical illness. The thoughts that clients have about their illnesses have a significant influence on their emotional reactions to symptoms and on their self-care behavior. Clients with more negative views of their illness are more likely to be depressed and people who view their illnesses as more serious, chronic, and uncontrollable tend to be more passive, report more disability, have poorer social functioning, and more mental health problems (Heijmans 1999). Client perceptions of control over their symptoms and the course of their disease or rehabilitation often relate to mood states such as depression (Affleck et al 1987, Devins et al 1981, Helgeson 1992, Thompson et al 1993). Level of perceived control has been shown to predict recovery from disability (Johnston et al 1999).

Scandlyn (2000) suggested that illness challenges one's views of life as being orderly and having continuity. This challenge can have significant psychological consequences, particularly for clients who have to endure debilitating and demanding treatments. Clients tend to have contact with a greater number of health professionals in what is an increasingly multidisciplinary healthcare system. This contact with numerous professionals involves a need to interact with more people and, for some, increased demands on already limited psychological resources. The move towards care in the community and day care means that clients may spend longer periods of time in non-hospital settings, resulting in some clients feeling unsupported psychologically and therefore contributing to psychological problems.

Many medical problems require a self-management approach to regulate the course and impact of client symptoms and problems. Collaborative relationships must be established with healthcare staff, and clients are often expected to adopt a more active role in managing their problems. Indefinite outcomes and the associated pervasive levels of uncertainty surrounding diagnosis and prognosis can result in psychological problems for some.

A psychological approach that encompasses both the individual client and the system within which their healthcare is managed, needs to be considered. Enright (1997) suggested that a cognitive behavioral approach can assist with both the physical and psychological problems. There is a growing body of research to support this contention. There are an ever-increasing number of psychological disorders for which cognitive behavioral models and therapy

protocols have been developed, many of which have been shown to be effective in research trials. A recent systematic review of the effectiveness of a range of interventions for the treatment and management of chronic fatigue syndrome found cognitive behavior therapy (CBT) and graded exercise therapy to show the most promising results (Whiting et al 2001). Another review compared CBT with other interventions and found that CBT significantly improved physical functioning in adult outpatients with chronic fatigue syndrome as compared with standard medical treatment or relaxation (Price & Couper 1999). Cognitive behavioral approaches have also been shown to be useful in the reduction of long term disability in clients with back pain (Pincus et al 2002). Physical and manual therapists often encounter people with medical problems that occur within the context of problems and disorders (e.g., anxiety or depression) that have been studied from a cognitive behavioral perspective.

Many physical and manual therapy clients will experience problems (or in some cases symptoms of psychological disorders) that can be readily assessed, understood, and managed within a cognitive behavioral framework. Management using a cognitive behavioral approach is implicated at all levels of client care by encouraging the client to be active in the management of their illness, by adopting a self-management approach, and establishing an appropriate collaborative relationship between client and practitioner. There is also a group of people who present with physical health problems that place them at an increased risk of clinically significant psychological/psychiatric disorders that may require CBT. The distinction between a cognitive behavioral approach and CBT will be outlined in greater detail later in the chapter.

CBT has been shown to be effective for depressive disorders (Beck et al 1979, Dobson 1989), panic disorder (Clark et al 1994), generalized anxiety disorder (Butler et al 1991), obsessive compulsive disorder (Salkovskis 1999), post-traumatic stress disorder (Dunmore et al 1999), hypochondriasis (Clark et al 1998, Warwick et al 1996), bulimia nervosa (Hay & Bacaltchuk 1999, Ledanowski et al 1997), schizophrenia (Haddock et al 1998, Jones et al 1999, Tarrier et al 1999), personality disorders (Davidson 2000, Davidson & Tyrer 1996), and bipolar disorders (Scott 1996). Rachman (1998) suggested that the application of psychological approaches to other branches of medicine has been slower than expected when compared with the developments in psychological models and therapies within psychiatry and clinical psychology. CBT has also been applied successfully to the management of medical conditions such as irritable bowel syndrome (Greene & Blanchard 1994), chronic pain (Morley et al 1999,) and cancer (Greer et al 1992). Advances in cognitive behavioral approaches to psychological disorders have not been matched by the application of the model to understanding psychosocial aspects of adjustment to physical illness, injury, and rehabilitation. This application is beginning to emerge (e.g., Salkovskis & Rimes 1997) as therapists start to combine clinical observations with scientific findings (Gelder 1997).

Readers interested in CBT generally are advised to consult comprehensive introductory texts on cognitive therapy such as those by Beck (1995), Leahy (1996), or Blackburn & Twaddle (1996) that provide both introductions and excellent illustrations of cognitive therapy in practice. Readers wishing for a more specific consideration of CBT for medical problems should consult White's (2001) book, *Cognitive behavior therapy for chronic medical problems*.

The application of a cognitive behavioral framework is easier when one considers the theoretical underpinnings of the approach. Psychological approaches to the management of emotional and behavioral dimensions of being physically ill or injured have been, like mainstream applied psychology, significantly influenced by behavioral theories in the 1960s–1980s. Cognitive theories of psychosocial functioning and adjustment began to

appear in the 1980s and have come to dominate mainstream applied psychology over the past 20 years. The basic components of behavioral and cognitive approaches will be outlined in this chapter, and links will then be made with cognitive-behaviorally oriented assessment. Case conceptualization will be covered and some specific examples of how to integrate this into care delivery will be outlined. The ways in which some of these principles can be applied by non-specialist practitioners (i.e., non-specialist in cognitive behavioral therapy) will be addressed in the section on interventions.

THEORETICAL BASIS OF BEHAVIORAL INTERVENTIONS

Behavior therapy emerged in the early 1950s based on assumptions derived from animal learning research carried out earlier in the century by Pavlov (1927) and his colleagues, and an American group of researchers led by Thorndike (1898). Two theories emerged from this work. The first, termed classical conditioning, was based on the work of Pavlov who found that if a bell was rung just prior to feeding dogs, the dogs learned to salivate to the bell ringing rather than to the presentation of food. Pavlov termed the food the unconditioned stimulus, and salivation to food the unconditioned response, as no learning was involved in food resulting in salivation (see Figure 8.1).

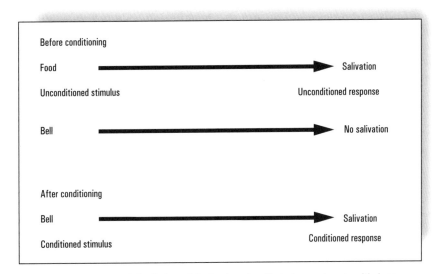

Figure 8.1   The fundamental components of classical conditioning based on Pavlov's experiments with dogs

After repeatedly pairing the bell with the food, the sound of the bell led to salivation, thus the dog had learned to salivate (conditioned response) in response to the bell (conditioned stimulus) rather than in response to food (unconditioned stimulus). Pavlov also showed that if the pairing of the bell with the food stopped, then the conditioned response (salivation to the bell) gradually went away, or was extinguished. Using the same principles, it was discovered that emotions could be conditioned in the same way. For example, Watson & Rayner (1920) presented a small child with a pairing of a loud noise and a rat, and as a result the child came to fear furry animals.

When classical conditioning was first described it was thought that these principles could be used to explain the development of all behavior. It was soon found that classical conditioning was limited, and an alternative conditioning model emerged called operant conditioning. This model was based on the idea that behavior could also be altered due to the consequences of it, as well as what happens prior to or alongside it (classical conditioning). It was found that a behavior followed by pleasant consequences is likely to increase in frequency (positive reinforcement), and conversely, a behavior that is followed by unpleasant consequences is likely to decrease in frequency (punishment). Skinner (1953) went on to describe two further reinforcers that affect the frequency of a behavior. The first was negative reinforcement, where behavior increases when an expected negative event fails to occur because a behavior has helped someone get out of a bad situation. The second was frustrative non-reward, where behavior decreases because an expected reward fails to occur. The use of rewards (positive reinforcement) for desired behavior and the withdrawal of reward (frustrative non-reward) for inappropriate behavior have been used in clinical settings to develop and shape behavior. Operant conditioning principles have also been used successfully in the management of people with pain (Fordyce 1982).

Both of the above models suggest that learning only occurs when an individual has personal experience of an event. Social learning theory, however, suggests that one can also learn through the experiences of others. This learning can occur through vicarious conditioning where someone else is seen receiving a reward or a punishment for a particular behavior, and as a result, the individual watching draws conclusions about the appropriateness or inappropriateness of a behavior. Alternatively this can occur by observational learning, where an individual learns to carry out a behavior after seeing someone else they admire carrying out that behavior even when no reward or punishment occurs. These principles have been used with great success in the treatment of anxiety disorders, overcoming childhood behavioral problems, and working with those with learning disabilities. Little progress was made with depressive or psychotic disorders and the cognitive element of these disorders could not be ignored, thus leading to the development of cognitive theories.

THEORETICAL BASIS OF COGNITIVE INTERVENTIONS

Cognitively based interventions are used to modify patterns of thinking that may be associated with the experience of unhelpful emotions or problem behaviors. It has been shown that a number of the common psychological disorders are associated with characteristic patterns of thinking (see Clark & Fairbairn 1997 for a more detailed account). Anxiety reactions are commonly associated with patterns of thought related to perceived threat or danger, and are associated with related thoughts of an inability to cope. Depressive reactions, on the other hand, are associated with thoughts relating to loss and an inability to cope in the face of seemingly insurmountable problems. People with depressive symptoms traditionally struggle with thoughts relating to low self-esteem, self-blame, personal worth, moral worth, and personal ability. In addition to characteristic thought patterns, psychological problems are often associated with particular changes in attention. Attention and memory tend to operate according to the principle of content specificity – clients will generally pay attention to and recall information that is congruent with their mood. An example of this would be a client who, by virtue of exposure to adversity or loss in their early life, developed negative beliefs regarding loss, failure, and achievement. These beliefs will be activated by events that are thematically congruent with them. An example might be when someone, by virtue of their physical symptoms, is unable to work. This may activate negative beliefs regarding a failure to achieve. A client with a belief about worthlessness is more likely to experience activation of this belief following rejection than someone who has a similar experience but does not have this belief. Belief activation leads to the tendency to process information in a manner that results in experiencing thoughts and images that are associated with predictable emotional, behavioral, and in some cases, physical reactions.

Anxiety and mood disorders are associated with greater levels of self-focused attention (Ingram & Smith 1984, Wells 1985). Contact with medical services often results in clients having to pay greater attention to themselves than they might otherwise. This need for greater self-focused attention can exacerbate pre-existing problems and/or may precipitate problems with an attentional bias that results in an exaggerated self-focus. Clients may display what is known as an attentional bias in that their attention is more likely to be drawn to particular events than others. In the case of anxiety disorders, clients tend to report their attention being specifically drawn to physical stimuli, and have experiences where they are more aware of physiological functioning (see Table 8.1). The focus of an individual's attention has also been shown to be important in that some anxiety problems (particularly those related to social anxiety) are associated with an increase in self-focused attention. This is most commonly seen when clients report being acutely aware of their own thoughts about how they may present to others and increased awareness of the physiological aspects of their response to stressful situations.

Experimental studies have also demonstrated the effects of psychological problems on memory (Kuyken & Brewin 1995). It is well recognized that low mood is associated with a more rapid recall of unhappy memories, a phenomenon that is of particular importance in understanding the ways in which mood can be lowered further by such a recall. The occurrence of visual images is particularly important (McNeil et al 1993). Images have often been shown to be associated with particularly strong emotion. Research in recent years has distinguished particular types of cognition, often important for understanding client experience and planning cognitive interventions accordingly (Greenberger & Padesky 1995). Theoretical work has highlighted the differences between types of thought such as worry or intrusive thoughts. Worries tend to be characterized by repetitive thoughts and images, and are associated with anxiety, preoccupation, and rumination. Intrusive thoughts, on the other hand, are more often short lived, are experienced as involuntary thoughts, and tend to be associated with different consequences (e.g., clients with intrusive thoughts often report the need to avoid thinking about them). People with worrying thoughts are less likely to report this need. In recent times, greater emphasis has been placed on understanding thoughts about thinking itself. In this way, theories have been proposed as to the importance of the ways in which people understand the controllability of their thought processes and/or

Table 8.1 Example of differing impact of problems on thinking, memory, and attentional processes

Problem	Thought	Memory	Attention
Anxiety	I am going to collapse I am having a heart attack	More focused on times when unable to cope; avoided exposure to situations due to fear of fears becoming reality	Drawn to internal and external stimuli that might herald danger or threat With panic problems this will usually be the physical sensations associated with anxious arousal
Depression	I am a failure I am useless	More focused on prior negative life events	Drawn to instances of perceived failure to meet personal standards; instances that are cited as evidence of negative beliefs about self, world and future
Anger	He set out to make things difficult for me They have no regard for how I feel	More focused on times when personal rules have been violated by others (e.g., others should be considerate for how I feel)	Drawn to elements of others' actions that suggest malevolent intent and/or aspects of scenarios that emphasize rule being transgressed

their significance (e.g., "if I keep thinking about the impact of pain on my life then I will go mad").

Examining the ways in which psychological treatments modify the processes and products associated with thinking has led to a greater understanding of the cognitive basis of psychological problems and their treatment. Changing the extent to which someone believes a particular thought, or enabling someone to arrive at an alternative explanation of similar internal or external stimuli, has been shown to be associated with significant changes in emotion. Researchers have made significant headway in understanding the ways in which thoughts influence behavioral responses, particularly in understanding the ways in which such behavioral responses may enforce and maintain dysfunctional thinking.

COGNITIVE BEHAVIORAL ASSESSMENT

Assessment of the client is the starting point of any cognitive behavioral intervention. It aims to identify the specific problems of the client, determine the client's past and present level of functioning, and allows for the formulation and case conceptualization of the individual client's difficulties and concerns. It also helps determine the specific treatment goals and allows for the monitoring of treatment gains and outcome. At the end of the first assessment session the client should begin to feel that it is possible to bring about change. There are a number of methods used to aid the process of assessment. These include self-report questionnaires, diaries, observation, and clinical interview.

Two types of self-report measures are commonly used. The first of these is standardized measures or self-report questionnaires that have been developed to assess a particular problem. Several types of self-report questionnaires have been developed and are readily available for use. Examples of these included the Beck Depression Inventory (Beck et al 1961) and the Beck Anxiety Inventory (Beck et al 1988). This type of inventory can provide information on the symptoms being experienced by the individual and can be used to determine the severity of these symptoms. As these measures are often administered both at initial assessment and throughout treatment, this information can be used to indicate change in severity and type of symptoms, thus providing a reliable outcome measure.

The second type of self-report measures used in cognitive behavioral assessment is diaries. Many of these are available in standard formats aimed at gathering information on a range of topics including frequency of panic attacks, daily pain fluctuation, and weekly activity schedules. Diaries can also be designed to measure the specific problems of the individual, and provide a flexible means of gathering detailed information about the problems experienced. Diaries of this sort can be adapted for use within the physical and manual therapies and can be used throughout treatment both to aid treatment (by using them to encourage and monitor homework tasks) and to measure treatment outcome. An example of a diary can be seen in Figure 8.2.

Observation of the client during assessment can provide useful information relating to their emotional state, and the relevance of particular topics to the client's difficulties. Attention to the client's posture, facial expression, eye contact, and the volume and tone of voice can provide information regarding the emotional and cognitive salience of parts of the assessment and topic areas to the client. It can be useful to note down particular examples of these observations, as the relevance of them may only become apparent later in the assessment process.

Probably the most important component of the cognitive behavioral assessment process is the clinical interview. The next few paragraphs will outline the main components of a clinical interview. At the outset of any cognitive behavioral assessment it is important to establish rapport and begin to encourage a collaborative relationship with the client, ensuring that at every stage of the assessment they have clear understanding of what is happening and why it is happening.

This process begins with ensuring the client has a clear understanding of why they have been referred to see you, and what they expect from the session. This information can be established by asking two straight-forward questions:

- What did Dr X tell you about why you have been referred to me?
- What do you think will happen during today's appointment?

Depending on the answers given to these questions it is then important to fill in any gaps the client may have in relation to these questions by explaining what it is you do, how you can help, and what will happen during the session. This approach is

Please rate your pain intensity on the following scale: 0 (no pain) to 10 (worst pain ever)

Time	Monday	Tuesday	Wednesday	Thursday	Friday	Saturday	Sunday
8 a.m.							
10 a.m.							
12 p.m.							
2 p.m.							
4 p.m.							
6 p.m.							
8 p.m.							
10 p.m.							
12 a.m.							
2 a.m.							
4 a.m.							
6 a.m.							

Figure 8.2   Example of a weekly pain diary

appropriate and applicable across most therapeutic settings, whether that be during the first session of a cognitive behavioral assessment or at an initial physical or manual therapy session. Ensuring the client has a clear understanding of what they can expect from you, and what is expected of them, will help facilitate a good therapeutic relationship with the client, and in the long term, should lead to a better outcome.

The next stage of the clinical assessment is to establish a clear list of what the client feels are their presenting problems. This stage should include a detailed description of the client's thoughts, feelings, and behaviors in relation to each problem they describe. It is important during this process to gain a clear description and understanding of why the client feels each problem they present is a problem for them. This can be done by summarizing the information given by the client and presenting it back to them. This process will help link problems that are related or are the same as a problem described previously, and will also help ensure that the problem list is comprehensive. This formal

process is typical of what psychologists do in assessment. In the physical and manual therapies, such information is usually gathered more informally over the course of treatment through conversation held during clinic visits.

Once a clear and comprehensive problem list has been outlined it is important to assess the cognitive and behavioral factors that contribute to the maintenance of the problem. This involves getting a clear understanding of the situations that trigger, and the factors that maintain, each problem mentioned by the client. It can be useful to think of this part of the assessment using an ABC format; where A stands for antecedents or triggers of the problem; B stands for the behaviors and beliefs attached to the problem; and where C is the emotional and behavioral consequences of the problem (see Figure 8.3). As you will note from the example in Figure 8.3, the client's pain is a clear result of overexertion which has led to some muscle ache. The client, however, assumes the situation is much worse than it is, and their response to cease all physical activity is likely to increase their pain, and therefore their problems.

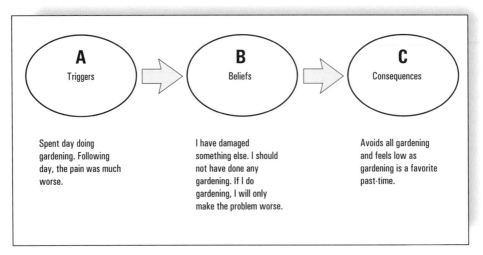

Figure 8.3 Assessment using an ABC format

Some clients struggle to identify the feelings and thoughts associated with their problems, and in these circumstances it can be useful to ask them to describe a recent example of the problem. Using this example, it is then possible to determine the context within which the problem arises, the factors that affect the intensity of the problem, and the consequences of this to the client. Specific details that one hopes to elicit during this period include:

• what makes the problem better or worse
• particular situations within which the problem occurs more frequently or less frequently
• what thoughts and feelings are associated with the problem
• what the consequences of the problem are
• how the client deals with the problem when it occurs.

It is important to note, that the consequences of a client's problems can be positive as well as negative, and that positive consequences will play a significant role in maintaining or reinforcing the problem. How to approach a problem like this is outlined in the sections describing goal setting and activity scheduling.

So far, the assessment should have provided a clear description of the presenting problems and the triggers and consequences associated with each problem. It is then important to gain some insight into the development of the problem, whether the person has experienced similar problems in the past, and how they have coped with these difficulties previously. It can be useful to get some idea of previous family history of psychological problems and how these difficulties were dealt with. This may provide insight into the coping strategies available to the individual.

Throughout the assessment process it is important to determine the client's suitability for a cognitive behavioral style treatment approach. There are several factors that should be considered when determining if a client is suitable for a CBT style approach. These include the client's ability to distinguish between thoughts, feelings, and behavior, the level of motivation of the client, and how easily the client appears to accept a cognitive behavioral explanation of their difficulties. It is not always possible to gather all the necessary information to establish a client's suitability for a CBT style approach during one session, and under these circumstances it may be beneficial to offer a time-limited number of sessions until this decision is made. It is also important to evaluate when onward referral to a CBT specialist is necessary. This decision is based on the severity and complexity of the client's problems and should occur if the client has a significant level of distress or presents with multiple problems.

This section has outlined the main components of cognitive behavioral assessment. It is, however, important to remember that assessment should be ongoing throughout treatment, allowing the therapist to adapt and modify the planned treatment where necessary. The assessment outlined here is a psychological model, but many practitioners in the physical and manual therapies carry out such assessment over the course of treatment, albeit in a less formal way.

COGNITIVE BEHAVIORAL CASE CONCEPTUALIZATION

When client assessment information has been collected, decisions need to be made about the ways in which client problems and their manifestations are related. This information is then used to plan treatment, or in the case of physical and manual therapies, how CBT principles can be incorporated into the physical aspects of care. The process of making links in this way is known as case conceptualization (sometimes known as case formulation). The conceptualization aims to outline how a particular problem/concern or symptom emerged, the way in which it has manifested itself, and how it is being maintained. Box 8.1 contains some examples of questions that may help clarify how an individual's medical condition may be linked to their psychosocial well-being (e.g., general anxiety, social anxiety, post-traumatic stress, depression).

A case conceptualization commonly contains a description of factors that exacerbate the problem, and situations under which it manifests. By having ideas about the ways in which problems are linked, it is possible to begin to suggest strategies to ameliorate or change presenting problems. The construction of a case conceptualization is much easier to do when a detailed assessment of recent problem examples has been carried out. This way, information can be incorporated from this recent example (assuming that the recent example is representative of other times the problem has occurred). A case conceptualization should also aim to outline historical information that might be relevant in understanding the occurrences of problems. Details on previous life experiences (particularly critical incidents) and current life circumstances of clients should all be recorded. Box 8.2 outlines some of the issues that might be relevant in conceptualizing client problems. Box 8.3 provides some examples of the components that sometimes feature in cognitive behavioral case conceptualizations. Critical incidents (see Box 8.3) are usually easy to identify in that they are often the events that are associated with the onset, exacerbation, or recurrence of

psychosocial aspects of client problems. They are usually emotive events, and as such, clients usually find these easy to recall. Critical incidents can be identified by having clients provide information according to a chronological sequence of events.

It is possible to provide some general principles that can be used in conceptualizing client problems. Problems can be divided into emotional, behavioral, cognitive, and physiological components. This way clients can be assisted in gaining a greater appreciation of the ways in which each component influences the others. Clients with anxiety often have conceptualizations that place emphasis on the thoughts that they have about threat, danger, and their inability to cope with these situations. This is usually linked by specifying in detail the ways in which clients try to minimize exposure to anxiety. Commonly, such attempts to minimize exposure are evident in the form of behavioral avoidance, or attempts to avoid thinking about salient issues. Clients are often unaware that their avoidance behavior makes problems worse by denying them the opportunity to discover that the feared outcome does not transpire, and that their coping abilities are usually greater than they estimate. Clients presenting with panic need to have conceptualizations that outline the specific ways in which they misinterpret benign physical sensations into evidence of impending catastrophic mental or physical events. Clients experiencing worry need to understand that there are commonly two types of worry: worries about the nature of their problems, and worries about worry itself. People often become concerned that their worrying will cause secondary physical or psychological problems. Clients can be asked about the things that they do to manage their worries.

INTERVENTIONS

PRINCIPLES OF COGNITIVE BEHAVIORAL MANAGEMENT

Some of the principles that define cognitive behavioral psychotherapy can be useful to clinicians wishing to use cognitive behavioral principles to enable their clients to make changes in their thinking and behavior. These principles should be considered by physical and manual therapists for possible incorporation into their work with clients.

Box 8.1 Questions to guide case formulation

General anxiety–related problems
Does this client's medical condition cause physical sensations that they catastrophically misinterpret?
Has this client been privy to any information recently about people with the same condition experiencing catastrophic or tragic outcomes?
Are any of the client's coping strategies designed to prevent perceived physical catastrophe?
Has the perceived catastrophe occurred in the past? If so, what are the predominant memories of this?
Do any of the client's medications produce physical sensations that could be misinterpreted?
Has this client received instruction in how to cope with the consequences of their medical problems?

Social anxiety problems
Do this person's symptoms worsen when they are in social situations?
How do they think that other people perceive their medical problem?
Are there elements of this person's behavior and appearance that make it apparent to others that they have a problem? If so, might they be exaggerating the extent to which this is the case?
Does their medical management involve them having to pay attention to their physiological functioning? If so, would this have generalized to such an extent that they have an exaggerated self-focus in social situations?
Were they teased or bullied at school because of a medical problem?
Have they heard or witnessed others with similar experiences being embarrassed or humiliated in social situations as a result of their medical problems?
Does their medical problem actually result in them drawing greater attention to themselves than would otherwise be the case?

Post-traumatic stress reactions
Does the content of their re-experiencing symptoms relate to aspects of their medical problems? If so, are these themes reflected in their thoughts about other presenting problems and/or do they contribute to other problems on the problem list?
Does this person have concerns about the significance of their re-experiencing symptoms in the course of their medical problems?
What elements of their premorbid lifestyle have they given up since their diagnosis/treatment, and to what extent is this contributing to them being frozen in time?
Which aspects of the course of their medical problems have been most shocking? Which beliefs might have been shattered to produce this degree of shock?

Depression
What losses has this client experienced with regard to their medical problems?
How much time does this person spend thinking about the negatives of their situation compared with the positives in their life?
Has this client been told that their condition will deteriorate?
Have they experience of witnessing (directly or indirectly) the negative consequences of this or similar illnesses?
Does this client perceive events to be more permanent and uncontrollable than might be the case?

Agenda setting

It may not always be possible to address all of our clients' presenting problems within a single consultation. This, combined with the fact that some presenting problems have no apparent solution, can be overwhelming for clinical staff who may not know where to start. Setting an agenda is a method for maximizing the chance that consultations will make some progress towards solving the presenting problems. This agenda is a vital component of cognitive therapy and can similarly be used to structure the time available to therapists with their clients. If contact with clients is to be repeated over a number of occasions then it may be that a standing item can

Box 8.2 Questions answered by cognitive behavioral conceptualization

What cognitive/behavioral/situational factors make this problem better/worse?

What is the main factor behind changes in symptom severity?

What would need to change in order for this cognitive/behavioral/emotional element to cause less of a problem?

What makes this a problem for this client?

Why should this set of problems have occurred for this person at this time in their lives?

Which problem components are linked?

Which life events are most important in understanding why this is a problem now?

Are there times that this has not been a problem for this client? Why was this? Were there particular cognitive, behavioral and/or emotional factors which explained this?

What have been the most important incidents in influencing this person's beliefs about their illness?

What are this person's beliefs about themselves, their illness, and medical staff and how are these relevant in understanding their adjustment to their medical problems?

How does this client's past psychological history relate to their current experience of chronic medical problems?

Has this person developed a strategy/set of strategies to cope with their problems? If so, how does this relate to their beliefs and the course of their problems?

Box 8.3 Sample components of cognitive behavioral case conceptualization

Early experiences

Physical, sexual or emotional abuse

Neglect

Witnessed negative consequences of relatives' chronic medical problem

Parental anxiety about ill health

Overprotective parental responses to illness

Critical parents or significant adult (e.g., teacher)

Traumatic hospital experiences as a child

Critical incidents

When was diagnosis of chronic medical problem confirmed

Reactions of other people to news of problems

Having to give up work because of difficulties

Actions or memorable statements by medical/health staff

Acute exacerbations in symptoms

Hospital admissions

Media coverage relating to own medical problems

Deterioration in physical health status

Development of a new physical health problem

Change in arrangements for the provision of medical and/or nursing care (e.g., new member of staff)

always be placed on the agenda. This may be a review of a client's progress with aids and adaptations and/or the severity of a commonly occurring symptom such as pain.

Homework

Clients and clinical staff spend only a small proportion of time together. For this reason, it is often useful to ensure that clients address problems outside of clinical contact time. This concept is of course familiar to professionals such as physical therapists and occupational therapists who might provide clients with advice on how to manage between contacts. Clients can be encouraged to keep written information on their progress. Tasks might include inviting clients to write about their thoughts and feelings on their illness and its effects, and their adherence to an intervention. Inviting clients to write about their understanding of their progress and/or the reasons for difficulties can provide information for discussion. The introduction of such homework can promote a self-management approach to their disease.

Collaboration

Cognitive behavioral therapeutic work emphasizes the importance of client and therapist working together on a set of mutually agreed goals. This emphasis is also reflected in the frequent inclusion of invitations to comment on the therapeutic direction, provide feedback, and the general client-centered focus. It should be noted that collaboration need not always be 50:50. Indeed, the initial sessions of contact with a clinician may sometimes be more like 80:20 as the clinicians may wish to provide more of the initial direction while a client gets used to the role of collaboration.

INDICATIONS FOR COGNITIVE BEHAVIORAL THERAPY

It is important at this point to clearly outline the difference between the application of a cognitive behavioral approach to the management of a client's care and the use of CBT with a client. As already mentioned, management using a cognitive behavioral approach is implicated at all levels of client care. Cognitive behavioral therapy, however, only becomes implicated under a specific set of circumstances and with an individual trained as a cognitive behavioral therapist. A client should be considered for cognitive behavioral therapy when they report increased levels of, or experience prolonged durations of, distress respective to their current circumstances. Further indication that an individual may benefit from CBT would include their level of motivation and their ability to link thoughts and feelings. In a situation where these criteria are met, the case should be referred to a cognitive behavioral therapist for psychological case management. It is sometimes possible, however, to have a shared case, where the responsibilities of case management are held by the cognitive behavioral therapist but certain aspects of the treatment plan are carried out by another therapist. This may include carrying out a specific behavioral experiment or encouraging homework tasks.

COGNITIVE BEHAVIORAL MANAGEMENT STRATEGIES

The following section outlines a range of cognitive and behavioral intervention strategies that might be used by therapists to help their clients address particular psychosocial problems.

Reappraisal of historical data

Sometimes clients' difficulties are associated with thoughts that exhibit distortions of prior events. For example, this may occur when clients recall their reactions to the early stages of their rehabilitation, or, as a result of anxiety, their recall of prior events emphasizes distressing elements of their care experiences. Clients can be asked to list the information from the past that they are using to support their particular belief. It is often useful to divide time into manageable chunks (e.g., 5 years). When such thoughts have been listed, clients can then think of alternative ways of viewing this information (sometimes known as reframing the evidence). This is illustrated by someone who listed their early distress following the diagnosis of arthritis as evidence of their weakness but, through discussion, was able to reframe this as a normal response to diagnosis, influenced by a clinic setting that was not attuned to the psychosocial impact of breaking bad news.

Behavioral experiments

When case conceptualizations outline details of how clients' behavior has changed over time, it can be helpful to think about structuring opportunities for clients to try out new behaviors or evaluate the consequences of behaving differently. This technique is most easily appreciated by considering the avoidance behavior that is often seen with anxiety disorders. If clients are asked to articulate their reasons for avoiding particular situations or experiences they will often provide thoughts containing predictions about negative outcomes. An example of this might be someone experiencing feelings of panic who believes that if they were to leave the house alone that they would be overwhelmed by fear and collapse. When clients have an understanding of the self-fulfilling nature of these predictions, they can be encouraged to challenge these predictions. This way, they can begin to gather evidence that their fears of collapsing when alone are the product of anxious thinking and not an actual risk of collapse.

Survey method

Clients often experience beliefs that are characterized by predictions or guesses as to what other people might think. For example, clients with low mood often underestimate the extent to which other people care about them and/or the quality of their relationships. The survey method can be used in this situation to change the thinking of the client. To do this, clients are encouraged to think that their assumptions about how other people think or experience situations might not be as they imagined. In keeping with many interventions strategies, this is presented as a possibility that deserves further scrutiny and, therefore, clients are invited to conduct a survey for the purposes of gathering further information.

Decatastrophizing

Catastrophizing is a characteristic thinking style that is often encountered when talking with clients with anxiety disorders. It is also a frequent component of the thinking style adopted by a subgroup of people with chronic pain problems. The process of decatastrophizing assumes that the person recognizes that their thinking style is reflective of focus upon the worst possible outcome or scenario. When this strategy is being applied it should be done tentatively and sensitively. It could be suggested, in general terms, that their thinking is being colored by this common problem, and it is possible that by considering a range of outcomes (i.e., not automatically the worst one), they will notice a change in the extent to which they are feeling anxious. The following questions can be used to structure this exchange of information: "What is the worst thing that could happen?," "What is the best outcome?," and "Given this, what would be a more realistic outcome?"

Although the technique can be used with people who are actually experiencing negative life events (e.g., someone with an incurable or a progressively deteriorating disease), this should be done only after having considered and practiced the technique (perhaps in role-play with a colleague or supervisor). The reason for this is that the application of this technique can be perceived as in some way minimizing the experience of the client. Consider a client with multiple sclerosis who is experiencing anxiety associated with the thought that they will end up being unable to walk. It would clearly be inappropriate to suggest that this is the reflection of catastrophizing as their thinking is reflective of a possible future outcome. For further information on this approach refer to Moorey (1996).

Using questioning to promote the evaluation of thoughts

If assessment or monitoring of client problems reveals that they experience frequent thoughts along similar lines, they can be taught a simple strategy to alleviate associated distress. Clients are encouraged to note their thoughts during times of elevated distress in a bid to identify commonly occurring thoughts that underlie distress. This approach can be promoted by asking clients to think about the personal significance of an event (e.g., "What did that mean to you when X happened?;" "What does that mean to you about you/the world/your illness/the future?"). When a thought has been identified, clients can use a series of structured questions in a bid to help them consider alternative information. The sorts of questions that can be used to help clients discover less distressing alternative thoughts are outlined in Box 8.4.

Attentional control training

Attentional control training is an intervention that has been shown to be particularly effective for clients who are experiencing a number of psychological difficulties including health anxiety (Papageorgiou & Wells 1998), major depression

---

Box 8.4 Questions that could be used to help clients discover less distressing alternative thoughts

What experiences have you had that show this thought is not completely true all the time?
If you were trying to help someone you love who had a similar thought in this similar situation, what would you tell them?
What would someone who loved you tell you if they knew that you were thinking about your situation in this way?
Do you think about things this way when you are feeling less distressed? If not, how do you think about these things at these times?
Is it possible that you could be underestimating the chances of you being able to do something to lessen your distress?
What is the evidence to support this distressing thought?
Is it a fact?
Might it be the way you are looking at things?
Are you basing your thought on how you feel (as opposed to how things actually are)?

(Papageorgiou & Wells 2000), and social phobia (Wells 2001). This process is based on the modification of self-attention, which is often heightened in these disorders. Attentional control training is designed to reduce the level of self-focus and to modify attentional control. This procedure, that requires the client to practice auditory attentional monitoring on a daily basis, is thought to have its effect by removing the focus from negative beliefs. Further evaluation of the effectiveness of this intervention in other psychological disorders is ongoing.

Goal setting

Goal setting is a fundamental component of a cognitive behavioral approach within a physical health setting. There are a number of reasons why goal setting is so important. Goal setting can help the therapist and client understand each other. As goals are agreed on collaboratively it may become apparent that the therapist has misunderstood the importance of different aspects of the client's problem. Similarly, it may be at this point that the patient realizes they will not be able to work within a cognitive behavioral framework. Goal setting is also important as it places the focus on the future, rather than on the past and its problems. This sends a clear message to the client that change is possible.

Goals should be decided on collaboratively with the patient. This should include identifying goals in a number of areas including employment, social and leisure activities, and household tasks. It is usually easier to identify some long-term goals as clients often report wanting things to return to "normal." It is important in these cases to identify what "normal" is for that individual client, and this will usually lead to the identification of long-term goals. Once a long-term goal has been identified it is usually necessary to break this down into smaller, achievable goals. It is important in any goal setting process that expectations are not placed too high. Clients recovering from mental or physical ill-health cannot expect or be expected to resume their previous level of functioning immediately. Goals such as returning to work or resuming a physical activity may need to be broken down into smaller short-term goals such as increasing social activities or walking round the block at home. It is important that whatever goal is chosen it is achievable for the client so that they will remain motivated to attempt their next goal. A client will quickly become discouraged if repeatedly facing a goal that is unachievable for them in their current physical state. Activity scheduling and graded task assignment (outlined below) are useful tools to facilitate goal setting and achievement.

Activity scheduling

Activity scheduling is used to maximize a client's engagement in mood-elevating activities. The first stage of this task is to ask the client to monitor their current level of activity. This can involve the client completing a chart monitoring their activity levels on an hourly basis. The client is also asked to rate each activity they do on a scale of 0–10 for mastery and pleasure. This process provides an accurate record of the actual levels of activity being achieved by the individual, and can also be used to challenge beliefs that the client may have about their lack of activity and/or lack of enjoyment in activity.

This same schedule can then be used to plan activity in advance. Activity scheduling works on a number of levels. It can be used to increase overall levels of activity, increase the number of pleasurable activities an individual is carrying out, and reduce hour-by-hour decision-making that may hinder an individual carrying out a task.

Graded task assignment

Graded task assignment can be used alongside activity scheduling. If clients repeatedly set themselves tasks that are unachievable given their current mood and level of functioning, their repeated failure will increase their feelings of hopelessness and inadequacy. A graded task assignment requires the client to re-assess each task they wish to perform to determine if their expectations are realistic, and where possible, to break each task down into smaller components. This approach can increase the client's chance of success. In people with anxiety this approach allows them to attempt tasks, which as a whole, would be considered too anxiety provoking.

Activity scheduling, along with graded task assignment, can be particularly useful in clients with pain and other clients who struggle to maintain levels of activity due to mobility problems. Breaking tasks down into smaller components and introducing regular rewards and breaks can make a previously unmanageable task manageable, and as a result, will bring about a sense of achievement and increase overall mood.

Using pie charts

Anxious clients often overestimate the amount of control they have over a particular event or consequence. It is possible to challenge a client's belief that they have a large amount of responsibility or control by asking them to list all possible factors or people who may also play a part in influencing the event. Once this list has been constructed the therapist draws a circle on a piece of paper and asks the client to allocate a section of the circle to each influence on the list. Their own control or responsibility should be allocated at the end. There is usually only a small proportion of the circle left to be allocated to the client's own level of responsibility, thus challenging their exaggerated perceptions of control or responsibility.

Role play and reverse role play

Role play is a useful technique to practice tasks that are going to be carried out as part of homework. They can be used on a number of levels. Firstly, role play can be used as a modeling technique where the client learns an alternative approach or behavior by observing the therapist carry out a task. Secondly, role play can be used as part of a graded exposure program for clients with anxiety, where prior to carrying out a task in a "real life" situation, the task can be practiced in a clinic setting (a less threatening environment). Finally, reverse role play can be carried out where the client plays the therapist or significant other, and the therapist plays the client. This process is similar to modeling, but allows the client to experience the impact the planned intervention will have on the other person.

Imagery modification

The cognitions involved in anxiety and depressive disorders can be images rather than thoughts. These images can be addressed by challenging the meaning of the image using verbal questioning. This process, however, is not always effective, and it can

be useful to use visualization techniques to reduce the distress caused by an image. An example of this can be found in clients with pain who can reduce the distress they are experiencing by visualizing the site and intensity of their pain and then gradually changing the image they have to a less distressing image (see Chapter 11). This process is called guided imagery. Further information about these imagery techniques can be found in Chapter 10.

Continuum method

Many psychological problems or concerns are characterized by rigid styles of thinking or thoughts that are biased toward a particular dimension of experience. In a similar way to decatastrophizing, the continuum method aims to assist the client to consider a wider range of possibilities than they may do ordinarily. Consider a client who reports gaining little pleasure from previously enjoyed activities, or someone who mentions that all of the possible activities that they might engage in are equally difficult. There are also times when clients report experiencing a physical symptom as being present or absent (as opposed to being present to varying degrees/severity at different times). Figure 8.4 illustrates the ways in which continua can be used (in this case to rate pain) to structure discussions with clients about components within their experience of physical symptoms or psychological dimensions.

The technique can be extended when people label themselves using pejorative terms, such as tending to think of oneself as being unable to cope, being worthless, or being helpless. Instead of thinking of experiences in terms of helpless or not helpless, people can be encouraged to think about constructs such as helplessness or worth as occurring along a continuum, taking account of varying

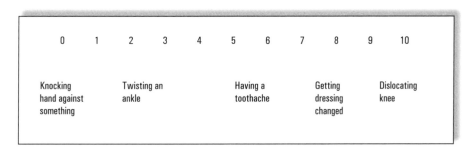

Figure 8.4 Example of the use of a continuum to rate pain. Such continua can be used to structure discussions with clients about components within their experience of physical symptoms or psychological dimensions

degrees of worth. This approach can be communicated by thinking of a scale from 0 to 100.

SUMMARY

Physical illness can result in increased vulnerability to the experience of emotional distress or lead to an exacerbation of existing emotional distress. It is therefore important to use a model of care that considers both physical recovery and emotional recovery following medical problems. Although the cognitive behavioral approach has traditionally been the realm of those with specific training in cognitive behavioral techniques, this chapter outlines how some of the strategies, which fall within the cognitive behavioral framework, can be used by therapists working in other fields. These strategies can be used to ensure there is a collaborative relationship between the practitioner and client, and to encourage the client to take a self-management approach to their illness and rehabilitation. In some cases it may be appropriate to share client care with another clinician with more advanced training in CBT and carry out prescribed cognitive behavioral techniques under their guidance. CBT remains the domain of those with specialist training in this area, and care should be taken to refer clients on where individual CBT is indicated. This chapter outlined the cognitive behavioral approach and how it can be used within the physical and manual therapies. It also provided information on the management of shared cases and set guidelines for appropriate referral to a cognitive behavioral specialist.

References

Affleck G, Tennen H, Pfeiffer C et al 1987 Appraisals of control and predictability in adapting to a chronic disease. Journal of Personality and Social Psychology 53(2): 273–279

Beck J S 1995 Cognitive therapy: Basics and beyond. Guildford Press, New York

Beck A T, Ward C H, Mendelson M et al 1961 An inventory for measuring depression. Archives of General Psychiatry 4: 561–571

Beck A T, Rush A J, Shaw B F et al 1979 Cognitive therapy of depression. Guildford, New York

Beck A T, Epstein N, Brown G et al 1988 An inventory for measuring clinical anxiety: Psychometric properties. Journal of Consulting and Clinical Psychology 56: 893–897

Blackburn I M, Twaddle V 1996 Cognitive therapy in action: A practitioners casebook. Souvenir Press, London

Butler G, Fennell M, Robson P et al 1991 Comparison of behavior therapy and cognitive behavior therapy in the treatment of generalised anxiety disorder. Journal of Consulting and Clinical Psychology 59: 167–175

Clark D M, Salkovskis P M, Gelder M et al 1994 A comparison of cognitive therapy, applied relaxation and imipramine in the treatment of panic disorder. British Journal of Psychiatry 164: 759–769

Clark D M, Fairbairn C G (eds) 1997 Science and practice of cognitive behavior therapy. Oxford University Press, Oxford, UK

Clark D M, Salkovskis P M, Hackmaan A et al 1998 Two psychological treatments for hypochondriasis: A randomised controlled trial. British Journal of Psychiatry 173: 218–225

Davidson K 2000 Cognitive therapy for personality disorders. Butterworth Heinemann, London

Davidson K M, Tyrer P 1996 Cognitive therapy for antisocial and borderline personality disorders: Single case study series. British Journal of Clinical Psychology 35: 413–429

Devins G M, Binik Y M, Hollomby D J et al 1981 Helplessness and depression in end-stage renal disease. Journal of Abnormal Psychology 90(6): 531–545

Dobson K S 1989 A meta-analysis of the efficacy of cognitive therapy for depression. Journal of Consulting and Clinical Psychology 57(3): 414–419

Dunmore E, Clark D M, Ehlers A 1999 Cognitive factors involved in the onset and maintenance of post traumatic stress disorder (PTSD) after physical or sexual assault. Behavior Research and Therapy 37: 809–829

Enright S J 1997 Cognitive behavior therapy – clinical applications. British Medical Journal 314: 1811–1816

Fordyce W E 1982 A behavioral perspective on chronic pain. British Journal of Clinical Psychology 4: 313–320

Gelder M 1997 The scientific foundations of cognitive behavior therapy. In: Clark D M, Fairbairn C G (eds) Science and practice of cognitive behavior therapy. Oxford University Press, Oxford, UK, p 27–46

Greenberger D, Padesky C A 1995 Mind over mood: A cognitive therapy treatment manual for clients. Guilford, New York

Greene B, Blanchard E B 1994 Cognitive therapy for irritable bowel syndrome. Journal of Consulting and Clinical Psychology 62(3): 576–582

Greer S, Moorey S, Baruch J D et al 1992 Adjuvant psychological therapy for clients with cancer: A prospective randomised trial. British Medical Journal 304: 675–680

Haddock G, Tarrier N, Spaulding W et al 1998 Individual cognitive behavior therapy in the treatment of hallucinations and delusions: A review. Clinical Psychology Review 18: 821–838

Hay P J, Bacaltchuk J 1999 Psychotherapy for bulimia and binging. Cochrane Database of Systematic Reviews, 4

Heijmans M 1999 The role of clients' illness representations in coping and functioning with Addison's disease. British Journal of Health Psychology 4: 137–149

Helgeson V S 1992 Moderators of the relation between perceived control and adjustment to chronic illness. Journal of Personality and Social Psychology 63(4): 656–666

Ingram R E, Smith T W 1984 Depression and internal versus external focus of attention. Cognitive Therapy and Research 8: 139–152

Johnston M, Morrison V, MacWalter R et al 1999 Perceived control, coping and recovery from disability following stroke. Psychology and Health 14: 181–192

Jones C, Cormac I, Mota J et al 1999 Cognitive behavior therapy for schizophrenia. Cochrane Database of Systematic Reviews, 4

Kuyken W, Brewin C R 1995 Autobiographical memory functioning in depression and reports of early abuse. Journal of Abnormal Psychology 104: 585–591

Leahy R 1996 Cognitive therapy: Basic principles and applications: Jason Aronson, New Jersey

Ledanowski L M, Gebing T A, Anthony J L et al 1997 Meta-analysis of cognitive behavioral treatment studies for bulimia. Clinical Psychology Review 17: 703–718

McNeil D W, Vrana Scott R, Melamed B G et al 1993 Emotional imagery in simple and social phobia: Fear versus anxiety. Journal of Abnormal Psychology. 102(2): 212–225

Martin F 2001 Co-morbidity of depression with physical illnesses: A review of the literature. Mental Health Care 4(12): 405–408

Moorey S 1996 When bad things happen to rational people: Cognitive therapy in adverse circumstances. In: Salkovskis P (ed) Frontiers of cognitive therapy. Guilford Press, New York, p 450–469

Morley S, Eccleston C, Williams A 1999 Systematic review and meta analysis of randomised controlled trials of cognitive behavior therapy and behavior therapy for chronic pain in adults, excluding headache. Pain 80: 1–13

Papageorgiou C, Wells A 1998 Effects of attention training on hypochondriasis: A brief case series. Psychological Medicine 28: 193–200

Papageorgiou C, Wells A 2000 Treatment of recurrent major depression with attention training. Cognitive & Behavioral Practice 7(4): 407–413

Pavlov I P 1927 Conditioned reflexes (Anrep G V, trans.). Oxford University Press, London

Pincus T, Vlaeyen J W, Kendall N A et al 2002 Cognitive behavioral therapy and psychosocial factors in low back pain: Directions for the future. Spine 27(5): 133–138

Price J R, Couper J 1999 Cognitive behavior therapy for chronic fatigue syndrome in adults. Cochrane Database of Systematic Reviews, 4

Rachman S 1998 Progress toward a cognitive clinical psychology. Journal of Psychosomatic Research 45(5): 387–389

Salkovskis P M 1999 Understanding and treating obsessive-compulsive disorder. Behaviour Research and Therapy 37 (Suppl. 1): S29–S52

Salkovskis P M, Rimes K A 1997 Predictive genetic testing: Psychological factors. Journal of Psychosomatic Research 43: 477–487

Scandlyn J 2000 When AIDS became a chronic disease. Western Journal of Medicine 172: 130–133

Scott J 1996 The role of cognitive behavioral therapy in bipolar disorders. Behavioral and Cognitive Psychotherapy 24(3): 195–208

Skinner B F 1953 Science and human behavior. MacMillan, New York

Tarrier N, Yusupoff L, Kinney C et al 1999 Randomised controlled trial of intensive cognitive behaviour therapy for clients with schizophrenia. British Medical Journal 317: 303–307

Thompson S C, Sobolew-Shubin A, Galbraith M E 1993 Maintaining perceptions of control: Finding perceived control in low-control circumstances. Journal of Personality and Social Psychology 64(2): 293–304

Thorndike E L 1898 Animal intelligence: An experimental study of the associative processes in animals. Psychological Monographs 2 (8)

Warwick H M C, Clark D M, Cobb A M 1996 A controlled trial of cognitive-behavioural treatment of hypochondriasis. British Journal of Psychiatry 169: 189–195

Watson J B, Rayner P 1920 Conditioned emotional reactions. Journal of Experimental Psychology 3: 1–14

Wells A 1985 Relationship between private self consciousness and anxiety scores in threatening situations. Psychological Reports 57: 1063–1066

Wells A 2001 The maintenance and treatment of social phobia: A cognitive approach. Tidsskrift for Norsk Psykologforening 38(8): 717–724

White C A 2001 Cognitive behavior therapy for chronic medical problems. Wiley, Chichester, UK

Whiting P, Bagnall A M, Sowden A J et al 2001 Interventions for the treatment and management of chronic fatigue syndrome: A systematic review. Journal of the American Medical Association 286(11): 1360–1368

Chapter 9

Relaxation techniques

Rosemary A. Payne

INTRODUCTION

In rehabilitation, relaxation techniques can be used for coping with pain, managing the stress of recovery, establishing better sleep patterns, and handling everyday hassles. Thus, they can play a useful role following injury and illness. They are also useful as health promotion strategies in the context of challenging experiences such as competitive sport, artistic performance, and other life-events where they can ameliorate stress responses and help to protect the individual against stress-related disease. It can be seen that relaxation techniques have wide applications in health and illness.

Some relaxation techniques make a direct approach to physical organs such as the musculature where their effect extends to promoting healing by relieving muscle tension around the injured part and improving the blood supply. Other techniques target thoughts where they can suggest more adaptive ways of viewing events. But whether somatic or cognitive in style (and there are elements of both in most techniques), relaxation techniques tend to have a global effect on the individual.

As relaxation therapy has always featured in some form in physical therapy training, the physical therapy clinic becomes an appropriate setting for such work with clients (Potter & Grove 1999).

EFFECTIVENESS OF RELAXATION TECHNIQUES

It is important to establish the effectiveness of relaxation techniques. A review of the area (Kerr 2000) found evidence that relaxation training is an effective component of treatment in a wide range of disorders. Both clinicians and researchers view it as a useful adjunct to a variety of medical treatments, and reviews testify to its potential in reducing both physiological and psychological indicators of stress. However, not all the research in this area is methodologically sound, so it is not possible at this stage to draw firm conclusions. Many researchers have approached the topic of relaxation by testing the effectiveness of particular techniques in the context of specific conditions.

For example, relaxation in conjunction with guided imagery has been shown to elevate mood levels in competitive athletes recovering from long-term injury (Johnson 2000). As well, relaxation with imagery was found to result in a significant reduction in pain and re-injury anxiety following reconstructive surgery to the anterior cruciate ligament (Cupal & Brewer 2001). Clients with postoperative pain have also benefited from relaxation. In the study by Good et al (2001), pain was significantly relieved by relaxation techniques administered with and without music in the first 2 days following surgery. Other conditions that have benefited from relaxation training include mild hypertension (Yung et al 2001) and anxiety related to cardiac rehabilitation (Wilk & Turkoski 2001).

Some studies have compared one technique with another. For example, Salt & Kerr (1997) compared the effectiveness of progressive relaxation with Mitchell's physiological approach, and Öst & Breitholtz (2000) compared applied relaxation with cognitive therapy. In neither of these studies, however, was it found that one method was more effective than the other, but all were found to be effective.

Given that relaxation training appears to perform a useful role, the next question concerns the choice of technique. Some relaxation techniques are physically oriented (e.g., progressive relaxation and breathing awareness) whereas others are cognitively oriented (e.g., autogenic training and meditation). None of these techniques fall neatly into any particular category, because there are both somatic and cognitive elements in most techniques. However, in relation to technique selection, one might first consider the presenting symptoms: should a physical disorder be matched with a predominantly physical relaxation technique? Is a painful joint more likely to respond to a muscular approach than to a psychological one? These questions are not easy to answer, as a painful joint does not simply involve physical symptoms but can also involve psychological factors such as worry.

Another factor to be considered when deciding on the most appropriate technique is the preference of individual clients (Fanning 1988, Lichstein 1988). Techniques that appeal to a given client are more likely to gain their cooperation and will result in more effective therapy. Some clients like to have different techniques combined in a single session, and this approach has been shown to be more effective than using single techniques (Davis et al 1988, Poppen 1988).

PREPARING THE CLIENT FOR RELAXATION

As part of the assessment phase of client management, therapists need to give the client space to talk. From this, it will be possible to get some idea of the client's feelings with regard to the injury or disorder and help to steer the treatment in a satisfying way for the client. With a sensitive practitioner, client fears and aspirations may be expressed, giving the therapist a framework for the relaxation training. It needs to be borne in mind, however, that the client has come expecting physical therapy and may resent the imputation of stress if such an idea is presented before a certain level of confidence and rapport has been established. When this point has been reached, an explanation of the physiology of stress can be introduced. For example:

Healing can be influenced by your general health which includes good diet, adequate sleep, and low stress. Injury of any description, however, can create varying levels of stress and this can interfere with recovery. If you are under stress the body's healing mechanisms cannot work properly because body energy goes into maintaining a state of high alert. To get the most out of treatment we need to relax that state of alert. A calm mind can promote recovery. (*If the client begins to nod in agreement, the therapist can continue in the following manner.*) I can see that you understand. Would you like me to show you how it is possible to minimize or prevent some of that stress?

Most techniques are best performed in a supine position but a reclining chair can be used as an alternative. The tone is conversational at this stage. As the therapist approaches the induction passage, the tone of the delivery changes and the volume and pace are gradually reduced. Bernstein & Borkovec (1973) suggested that a smooth and quiet (but not purposely hypnotic) tone is appropriate. The words should be spoken slowly with lengthy pauses (indicated in the text by ellipsis points). Tone of voice should also convey the mood of the particular instruction, distinguishing between the tension phase and the relaxation phase.

Formal termination of the relaxation exercise allows the client's blood pressure, which tends to fall during relaxation (Benson 1976), to normalize. A sample script might run as follows.

I am going to bring this relaxation session to an end . . . in your own time, I'd like you gradually to become aware of the room . . . put out your hand and feel the floor/chair underneath you . . . open your eyes . . . bend and stretch your limbs a few times . . . make a fist with both hands . . . and regain the feeling that you are alert and ready to carry on with your day.

Debriefing after a relaxation induction is a central element of the whole process. The therapist introduces it with remarks such as: "I'm very interested to know your reaction to that. Can you describe its effect on you?," and "Did you feel noticeably more relaxed?" Encouraging feedback in this way, the therapist might also ask whether the client found the explanation confusing. Did they understand what the therapist meant when he/she described body parts, and which body parts were easier or more difficult to relax? Asking questions about what worked, what did not work, and what needs more emphasis can influence the approach taken during the next session.

Group relaxation work necessitates longer discussion than individual work because clients often share their experiences. Many difficulties may be revealed, and discussion is encouraged by the practitioner who acts as facilitator. If the discussion dries up it can be revived by the strategy of circular questions (Powell & Enright 1990), which entails drawing one participant into conversation with another. For example, "Jenny, you've done muscle relaxation before. Would you like to tell Peter how you found it?"

The importance of home practice should also be emphasized. Relaxation training is a skill, which means that competence is directly related to the amount of time spent on it. To encourage the client to practice, timeslots can be carefully selected to fit in with the client's daily routine. Practice sheets and tapes can be given out and clients asked to keep a record of the time they spend practicing relaxation (as they do with other aspects of home rehabilitation in the physical and manual therapies) and how they feel before and afterwards (see Figure 9.1). Ideally, the practice period should be related to any home physical therapy exercises they have been asked to carry out in order to create an integrated experience of treatment. If the session was successful, plans can be discussed for the further development of the technique. In the event that the session was not positive, the therapist might consider an alternative approach.

Clients often release their feelings during this debriefing period. The relaxation experience may have tapped into feelings related to past trauma, and painful experiences may be voiced for the first time. Emotional reactions however, are not necessarily confined to the client. Sometimes the shared disclosures can touch feelings in the therapist (see Chapter 6). At other times the therapist can become emotionally fatigued in a condition known as vicarious traumatization or burn-out when the capacity to feel compassion becomes temporarily exhausted. Effective supervision provides the support needed to help the therapist understand these experiences and to deal with them if they occur. Therapists also need to recognize the point when the client's distress is too deep for them to handle effectively and to seek professional assistance.

To assist in assessing the effectiveness of relaxation techniques during rehabilitation, measurement can be carried out at the beginning and end of a course of treatment. Both physiological (heart rate, respiration rate, blood pressure, range of motion, electromyographic recordings) and psychological self-rating scales for anxiety and pain can be used. While the course of relaxation is in progress, simple measures such as heart rate and self-rating can be used before and after each session. Not only do such measurements assist the physical therapist in determining the effectiveness of the intervention, but they also help clients see the relative benefits they are gaining.

Physical and manual therapists are well placed to incorporate relaxation in the rehabilitation process. They are, however, working in a sensitive area and using powerful tools. It is therefore essential for them, as with any aspect of treatment, to have some form of structured training in the correct use of the technique.

Date	Time	Type of relaxation	Relaxation level before 0–10	Relaxation level after 0–10	Comments on relaxation today

Figure 9.1 Form for recording relaxation training homework

RELAXATION TECHNIQUES

This chapter will focus on three relaxation techniques: progressive relaxation training, breathing, and autogenic training. Many other methods exist including Benson's Relaxation Response (Benson 1976, see Chapter 11), the Mitchell method (Mitchell 1987), biofeedback, and exercise. For further details and reviews of other relaxation techniques see Payne (2000) and Kerr (2000).

PROGRESSIVE RELAXATION TRAINING

History and development

Progressive relaxation training (PRT) was developed by two American psychologists (Bernstein & Borkovec 1973) as a modified version of progressive muscle relaxation, previously devised by the physiologist Jacobson (1938).

In the course of his work on muscle activity Jacobson had observed that a relaxed musculature was associated with a reduction in the mental activities of thinking, memory, emotion, and imagery. Such a finding, Jacobson suggested, could have application in the treatment of anxiety and stress-induced conditions. Developing this notion, he devised a technique for inducing the skeletal muscles to relax. It involved a system of tensing and releasing applied to the major muscle groups, a technique called progressive muscle relaxation. The purpose of the tensing and releasing was to teach the client how to recognize tension and how to release it. Both isotonic and isometric forms of muscle activity were used, but as the client became more skilled, the tension component was gradually reduced until it was eliminated altogether. In this progressive manner, the client learned the skill of muscle relaxation.

The tensing component was used solely as a means of teaching the client to recognize tension in a muscle. Once this was learned, Jacobson considered there was no further use for it. He claimed that further tensing procedures were not only unnecessary, but also obstructive to relaxation, because the muscle tension that had built up during the contracting phase would, to some extent, persist when the muscle was called upon to relax (Lehrer 1982, Lehrer et al 1988, Lucic et al 1991).

Bernstein & Borkovec (1973) suggested, however, that the tensing component held intrinsic value; it was a fundamental element in the production of the relaxed state and the stronger the contraction, the more effective would be the relaxation that followed it. Lehrer et al (1988) tested this hypothesis but no clear result emerged. These researchers considered it was unlikely that the release of a strong muscle contraction would produce an automatic decrease in muscle tension. This view was supported by Lucic et al (1991) who demonstrated that tensing muscle groups prior to relaxation was physiologically detrimental to the relaxation process. The matter remains unresolved.

Another feature of the method was the use of suggestion. Bernstein & Borkovec (1973) used suggestion to augment the effect of the tensing, although they insisted it should be of an indirect nature. "Notice how your arm is feeling more relaxed" is an example of indirect suggestion, as opposed to the more commanding "Now your arm is limp," which is a more direct suggestion. Direct suggestion, employed in some versions of hypnosis, would not be appropriate here. Whereas Bernstein & Borkovec (1973) looked upon suggestion as a useful means of enhancing the overall effect, Jacobson (1938) was totally opposed to its use in any form, believing that it interfered with the acquisition of the skill.

Perhaps the most marked difference between the two approaches is the amount of time needed to acquire the skill. Jacobson's course entailed a total of at least 40 sessions, which was a major drawback for the client in terms of both commitment and financial burden. If the system were to have wide appeal it would have to be reduced. PRT can be learned in as few as 8–12 sessions and is achievable by reducing the number of muscle groups worked and by covering them all in a single learning session. Jacobson, by contrast, often devoted a whole session to just one or two muscle groups.

Description of the procedure

PRT consists of a sequential tensing and releasing of the major muscle groups (Box 9.1), allowing 5–7 seconds for the tensing period and 30–40 seconds for the releasing period. Later in the course, when the client is able to generate relaxed responses, the routine can be presented in a summarized form where both arms are worked together, both legs together, face and head items combined, and torso movements combined.

A more advanced stage involves the tensing component being dropped, leaving only the release component. This advance stage is referred to as "relaxation through recall." The client recalls the

---

Box 9.1 Order for working muscle groups in Bernstein & Borkovec's (1973) progressive relaxation training

Make a fist with the dominant arm
Press the dominant elbow down into the floor or into the arm of the chair
Work the non-dominant arm in the same way
Raise the eyebrows
Screw up the eyes and wrinkle the forehead
Clench the teeth and pull back the corners of the mouth
Press the head back while keeping the chin in
Draw the shoulders back
Tighten the abdominal muscles
Tense the thigh of the dominant leg
Plantarflex the dominant foot
Dorsiflex the dominant foot
Work the non-dominant leg in the same way

---

sensations that accompanied the release component in the full format, and reproduces a similar level of relaxation. Relaxation through recall is a form of passive muscular relaxation.

Further developments of PRT include conditioned relaxation, sometimes referred to as cue-controlled, and differential relaxation, where the aim is to reduce the tension in the working muscles to a level where it is just consistent with task performance, and to eliminate any unnecessary muscle activity that may accompany it.

Rationale for use

In relaxing the skeletal musculature, PRT is believed to exert a calming effect on the whole organism via the neuromuscular network. The effect is psychological as well as physiological. A critical review by Kerr (2000) indicated that muscular techniques based on progressive relaxation have repeatedly been associated with reductions in stress indicators, both physiological and psychological. Studies have shown decreases in blood pressure, heart rate, respiratory rate, electromyographic activity, depression, and anxiety. These results suggest that progressive relaxation and its derivatives have the potential to promote health (Kerr 2000).

As a component of treatment, muscular relaxation has been found to be effective in a wide range of disorders (Carlson & Hoyle 1993). In their review of abbreviated PRT techniques, these researchers noted that the largest effects were found in studies investigating the effect of relaxation on tinnitus, migraine, and tension headache.

When progressive relaxation has been compared with other stress-reducing approaches, it often appears equally effective. For example, Salt & Kerr (1997) compared progressive relaxation with the Mitchell method in 24 normotensive participants. Whereas significant reductions in heart rate, respiratory rate, and blood pressure were found in both methods, the study did not show any significant difference in effectiveness between them. Similarly, Crist & Rickard (1993) found no difference in outcome between muscular and imaginal relaxation in 100 healthy students, although significant training effects were found. Öst & Breitholtz (2000) also found applied relaxation (a form of progressive relaxation) and cognitive therapy equally effective in 33 people experiencing generalized anxiety. Some studies have identified differences in effects between methods. For example, Yung et al (2001) found that muscular relaxation was more effective than cognitive imagery for lowering blood pressure in people with mild hypertension. Canter et al (1975) found muscular relaxation to be less effective than biofeedback in 28 participants with symptoms of anxiety.

The picture is far from clear but, as all reviewers have suggested, much of the research had questionable methodological rigor. In spite of this, Carlson & Hoyle (1993) concluded that the evidence is strong enough to support the continued use of these methods in the clinical setting. They suggested that such approaches are more effective when performed on an individual basis than in a group, and when recipients are provided with training tapes. Improvement in stress-relief is strongly associated with the amount of practice carried out.

Practical example of integration into care

Although progressive relaxation has cognitive elements, it can be seen as a predominantly physical approach. Because some researchers in the past have recommended a physical approach for a physical disorder (Davidson & Schwartz 1976, Lehrer 1996, Yung et al 2001), it has been suggested that muscular relaxation would make a useful contribution to a program of rehabilitation to relieve stress following athletic injury (Cupal & Brewer 2001, Johnson 2000, Potter & Grove 1999, White

1998). Such stress could arise from a variety of sources: pain on movement, doubts about recovery, or fear of re-injury when play is resumed. Additional to the stress-relieving effects, are the physiological benefits of releasing tension in the muscles leading to an improved blood supply.

An example of introducing relaxation to clients follows in the script below.

> Relaxation has physical and psychological aspects. On the one hand, we feel an absence of bodily tension, and on the other, we begin to feel less anxious about things. It is a state that we can promote either by addressing the muscles and releasing their tension, or by quietening the thoughts in the head. Relaxing the muscles is particularly helpful after injury because it can promote the blood supply to the injured part, and blood has healing properties. Knowing this will give you a feeling of being more in control of your recovery. Progressive relaxation training is a system of relaxation that addresses the muscles. It consists of specified contractions followed by their release in muscle groups throughout the body. It is believed that the firmer the contractions, the more total will be the release which follows, in a sequence resembling the action of a pendulum swinging high on both sides. While we are going through this exercise, you will be asked to pay particular attention to the feelings in the working muscles to help you recognize the state of tension. You will also be asked to notice the sensations associated with relaxation so that you can reproduce that state. All this applies to the healthy parts of the body. When we come to the injured part itself I want you to be very gentle, working only as far as you can without pain. There are 16 muscle groups to work through and the program takes 30 or 40 minutes to complete. I'll first demonstrate the actions and will give you a chance to try them out.

After demonstrating the actions, the therapist asks if the client has any questions, and once all the questions are answered, the practitioner asks the client to adopt a lying or reclining posture, before beginning the relaxation exercise. A sample script follows.

> Let's begin now. We'll work through all the 16 actions. I'll announce each muscle group as we come to it but I don't want you to carry out the tensing instruction until I give you the cue word "Now." The cue word for

letting go is "Relax." When you hear this word I would like you to release the tension immediately and completely. You may find it easier to focus your attention if you close your eyes. I'm going to ask you to draw your right hand into a tight fist . . . Now . . . clench the fingers . . . pull hard . . . and as you do so, feel the sensation of tension throughout your hand and forearm . . . and . . . Relax . . . let it go . . . let it go completely . . . feel the fingers losing their tension as they uncurl . . . feel the tension flowing out . . . and continuing to flow out . . . notice the changing sensations as the hand and forearm return to their inactive state . . . as they come to rest . . . getting more and more relaxed . . . and . . . when you feel they have lost all their tension, compare in your mind the two sensations of tension and release.

This routine is repeated once and followed by a full minute of extended relaxation to give the muscle plenty of time to release its tension. Using this kind of format, the remaining muscle groups are worked through bringing this first session to a close. After the termination of the relaxation exercise, a short debrief is useful.

The therapist would want to know if the clients felt more relaxed now. What sensations did they have in their muscles? Could they now recognize the feeling of tension? In particular, what sensations did they have in the injured part? Do they feel they are beginning to understand the technique of muscle relaxation? Did the therapist pace things well for the client? Should the therapist spend more time on certain muscle groups? Would three or four repetitions be better? The answers to these questions will guide the therapist in planning the next lesson.

At some point the therapist will feel the clients are ready to move on to relaxation through recall (described above). A further introductory passage, such as that below, will lead them in.

Your earlier sessions will have made you highly sensitive to the feelings which accompany changes in the muscles. You are now aware of the presence of tension – you are able to recognize it and release it, and so, you are ready to be introduced to the next stage in which we leave out the tensing part. We'll work on the summarized schedule as we work through these groups. I'll ask you to look for any signs of residual tension and then, to let it go by recalling the sensations associated with its release. The injured limb can take full part in this exercise.

The therapist then presents the technique to the clients:

With your eyes closed, please focus your attention on the muscles of your arms and hands. Are you aware of any tension in them? If so, try and locate it . . . notice what it feels like . . . then, recalling the feelings you have previously experienced when releasing tension in these muscles, relax it away . . . continue to release it . . . recalling previous sensations . . . relaxing further and further . . . feel the tension flowing out . . . go on until you are totally free of it . . . feeling deeply relaxed . . . and when you have reached this point, indicate with a lifted finger.

Relaxation is induced in this manner for 35–40 seconds before moving on to the leg muscle groups and then to the head and torso groups.

BREATHING AND RELAXATION

History and development

Breathing routines have a long history in the East where they feature in approaches such as yoga. In the West, they tend to appear as one component of a wider relaxation program. Breathing relaxation techniques include slow breathing, deep breathing, diaphragmatic breathing, breathing meditation, and breathing with imagery. Some of the reasons for its general appeal are that breathing routines can be discreetly carried out, which makes them available in a stressful situation itself. Breathing techniques are also easy to learn, and offer an alternative to those who find other approaches difficult.

Description of the procedure

Breathing in the context of relaxation is often referred to as breathing awareness. This simply means that attention is centered on the respiratory pattern. A gentle, responsive approach is adopted rather than one that commands and disrupts. The form may vary, but in general it consists of a series of breathing procedures that begin with explorations of thoracic and abdominal movement, leading to a variety of routines for inducing relaxation. These approaches focus on slow diaphragmatic breathing.

When performing breathing for relaxation a few points should be considered. For example, inhalation should lead smoothly into exhalation. Breathing should be seen in terms of "letting the air in" rather than "taking a breath," and wherever possible, breathing should take place through the nose rather than the mouth because the nasal passages are able to warm and filter the air before it reaches the lungs. This way of breathing features in a large number of breathing routines. Some techniques use inhalation through the nose and exhalation through the mouth. It should be remembered that artificially deep breaths, when repeated in quick succession, could lead to hyperventilation.

Rationale for use

A direct link exists between respiration and the system that controls physiological arousal. Stimulation of the sympathetic branch leads to breaths that tend to be fast and staccato-like, whereas stimulation of the parasympathetic branch is associated with slow breathing (Keable 1989). A resting individual displays a slow breathing rate, and because the oxygen requirement is low, breathing tends also to be rather shallow. The individual may occasionally take a deep breath and find it profoundly relaxing, but the natural tendency is for such a breath to be followed by the original pattern of slow and fairly shallow respiration. This connection between slow breathing and parasympathetic dominance has created a perception that slow breathing has stress-relieving properties and has led to its adoption as a relaxation technique (Sudsuang et al 1991, Wallace & Benson 1972). The mechanism is, however, unclear. Lum (1983) proposed that slow breathing had a corrective effect on an abnormal pattern of breathing, whereas Garssen et al (1992) suggested that it may reduce stress for other reasons such as distraction.

Diaphragmatic (otherwise known as abdominal) breathing is also associated with parasympathetic dominance and the resting state. This kind of breathing emphasizes the downward expansion of the chest cavity, causing the abdomen to swell slightly.

As slow diaphragmatic breathing is traditionally offered as part of a broader relaxation strategy, it is difficult to estimate its intrinsic effectiveness. So what evidence is there for the effectiveness of breathing routines?

One of the few published works on the topic is the comparison study of Bell & Saltikov (2000). These researchers compared the effectiveness of the Mitchell method (including diaphragmatic breathing) with diaphragmatic breathing alone in 45 normal male participants. Using heart rate as an outcome measure, significant reductions were found in both experimental groups relative to the control condition of lying in a supine position. However, no significant difference in effectiveness was found between the two groups themselves. In other words, diaphragmatic breathing appears to be an effective relaxation technique on its own and is rendered no more effective by being presented in conjunction with the Mitchell method. In their analysis, Bell & Saltikov (2000) suggested that physiological benefits of the Mitchell method may be largely due to the component of diaphragmatic breathing, and that the technique of Mitchell may be only as effective as diaphragmatic breathing alone. However, there is currently so little work available on this topic that firm conclusions cannot be drawn.

Practical example of integration into care

Slow diaphragmatic breathing has a place in the relaxation programs presented in most conditions because of its relation to the parasympathetic arm of the autonomic nervous system. A situation to which it is particularly suited is the surgical setting. Miller & Perry (1990), investigating 29 patients after cardiac surgery, demonstrated significant decreases in physiological responses and pain reports following training in breathing routines. In a review of complementary therapies, Petry (2000) reported the benefits of relaxation strategies in the relief of pre- and postoperative distress. Such interventions may also reduce the need for pain-relieving medication.

Breathing awareness is often presented to the client pre-operatively. An example of a script for presurgery use follows.

> Surgery can be a stressful time so perhaps you'd like me to show you a few relaxation techniques to help you cope with it. These are breathing routines that, besides relaxing you, will help your body deal with the effects of the anesthetic. They are easy to learn and involve the kind of breathing which is gentle and slow, and characteristic of a body at rest. But as a first step, I'd like to ask you to explore the different ways in which the chest can expand. Place your hands flat over your lower ribs ... feel the sideways expansion taking place as the air enters ... take your time ... feel also the recoil as air flows out ... Next, place one hand over your solar plexus (the soft part between your ribs and your navel) and the other hand over the chest, just below the collar bone, and notice the movements under your hands as the air enters and leaves ... spend a few moments focusing on this

idea ... don't be in a hurry ... and when you are ready (for those who are seated), I'd like you to try something else. Would you now lean forwards with your forearms resting on your thighs. With movement in the front of your chest now restricted, you may have the sensation of expansion taking place in the back of your chest ... give yourself time ... So relaxed breathing is slow and gentle. But it is also "diaphragmatic," which means it is focused on a downward expansion. I'd just like to remind you what happens during the breathing process. The lungs, as you know, lie inside the chest cavity, which is bounded by the ribs. Situated beneath the lungs is the diaphragm, a sheet of muscle whose edges are attached to the lower ribs creating a floor to the chest. In the resting state it is dome-shaped. Contraction of the diaphragm flattens the dome, thereby lengthening the chest and sucking in air. Relaxation of the muscle causes it to reassume its dome shape, which helps to push the air out. But the diaphragm also forms the roof of the abdomen and as such, its movements affect the position of the internal organs: as the contracting diaphragm presses down on the organs, it causes the abdomen to swell slightly. Similarly, as the relaxing diaphragm releases its pressure on the organs, the abdomen sinks back again.

Clients may wish to ask questions or seek clarification at this point. When these matters have been settled, they transfer from a seated to a lying position (if possible) and the therapist proceeds with the breathing relaxation exercise.

Please make yourself as comfortable as possible ... release your shoulders ... and spend a few moments quietly resting ... you might like to run through a sequence of pleasant imagery ... then, as your body relaxes turn your attention to your breathing ... lay one hand lightly over the upper part of your abdomen ... focus your attention on this area ... After a few minutes notice what is happening under your hand ... you will have discovered that your hand moves ... Let's just run through that in the form of an exercise ... it begins with a breath out ... a naturally occurring breath out ... notice a sinking of the area under your hand ... Next, allow air to flow into the lungs, noticing the slight swelling which takes place under your hand ... then, as the air is expelled, notice the same area sinking back again ... allow the breathing to take place naturally ... We'll just try that again ... and this time, as the air flows in, I'd like you to think "down" ...

this helps to make the abdominal movement a natural one ... continue breathing in this way, taking care to maintain your normal breathing rhythm ... If, however, you feel the urge to have one deep breath, do so, but don't repeat it ... just let your breathing return to its gentle resting rhythm ... and now ... I'll run through it again with you.

In the ensuing debriefing session clients may be asked to describe their reactions to the breathing approach and to share their views. Do they feel calmer? Perhaps a client reports no benefit, in which case time is spent exploring the reason. The client is reminded that relaxation is a skill, that it takes time to learn, and not to expect too much the first time; home practice is essential. Other clients, perhaps awaiting abdominal surgery, may wonder how they are going to carry out diaphragmatic breathing postsurgery. The therapist will need to reassure them that the procedure will be introduced gradually and that they will not be asked to do anything that is painful or uncomfortable.

Hyperventilation needs to be discussed, and the clients should be warned of its dangers. The symptoms are wide-ranging but palpitations, dizzy spells, chest pain, tachycardia, paresthesia, and the inability to take a satisfying breath are common (Gardner & Bass 1989, Innocenti 2002). Breath-holding and slow shallow breathing will usually correct it.

On the first postoperative occasion, the diaphragmatic breathing routine can, if necessary, be modified to allow for postsurgical difficulties. An example follows.

Settle down as comfortably as you can ... and close your eyes ... feel your body getting heavier as the tension ebbs away ... let your mind gradually become calm by using some pleasant imagery ... Now bring your attention to focus on your breathing ... be aware of the movements which occur without trying to change them ... just observe them in the knowledge that your body takes full care of your breathing ... let your breathing continue on its own ... flowing gently and smoothly ... perhaps you can feel the rate getting slower ... this is because your resting body doesn't need so much oxygen as when you are active ... Your heart rate also is lowered, and your blood pressure falls, as a state of quiet settles on you ... Allow yourself to enjoy the feeling of tranquillity ... let your mind continue to focus on your breathing for a few minutes longer.

This relaxation exercise is probably enough for the first postoperative attempt. A short debriefing session could follow if the client were up to it. For subsequent sessions other gentle routines may be presented. Below are three brief and gentle breathing techniques.

Breathing with cue words

In this exercise the individual picks a word such as "relax," "calm," or "healing" and begins silently to recite it on each breath out. Following many repetitions, an association is built up between the word and the relaxed state, whereby the word alone becomes capable of inducing relaxation. The word has thus become a cue. The stronger the association, the greater the power of the cue word. A script follows.

> Spend a few moments quietly resting with your eyes closed ... signal to me when you feel settled by raising your right index finger ... there's no hurry ... And ... now ... if you are ready, turn your attention to your breathing ... tune into its rhythm ... letting it proceed at its own pace ... Do not be tempted to alter it ... and just before you release the next breath, think the word "relax."

The practitioner leads with the instruction "relax" for five breaths, and then asks the client to continue for a further five breaths. After a few minutes of rest, the full sequence is repeated (Öst 1987). Twenty pairings a day of the cue word with exhalation are recommended to build up the skill.

The path of the breath

Another brief breathing technique involves following the path of a breath in the mind. An example of an appropriate script of this technique follows.

> Follow the path of the breath in your mind, taking care not to change its pace or its rhythm. Imagine the air flowing in through your nostrils, along your nasal passages, down your windpipe and into your lungs ... then, gently and smoothly turning, it is carried out along the same route ... turning again as the air is drawn back in ... Notice the feel of the air ... cool as it enters, and warm as it leaves ... and as a state of quiet settles on all your body systems, imagine the healing process taking place ... See it helped by your relaxation ... Continue on your own for a few minutes.

In this exercise, imagery has been used to help induce relaxation.

"Out tension, in peace"

Following is a script for another short breathing exercise.

> Listen to your breathing without altering its pattern ... imagine your tensions being breathed out ... imagine them being carried away, a little at a time, with each breath out ... and now, imagine that every time you inhale, you are breathing in relaxation and healing ... a little at a time with each breath ... building up a mental state of relaxation ... breathe out tension ... breathe in relaxation ... gently breathing ... feeling relaxation flowing through your mind and your body ... always keeping your breathing natural.

As can be seen from the breathing-based relaxation exercises above, many of them could be incorporated into physical therapy management as an adjunct to other physical therapy methods.

AUTOGENIC TRAINING

History and development

Autogenic training (AT) is an approach derived from self-hypnosis. It dates from the 1930s, when Johannes Schultz, a psychiatrist at the Berlin Neurobiological Institute, noticed that some patients were using images of heaviness and warmth to create a light trance. As they seemed to be benefiting in terms of their mental health, Schultz encouraged them, and set about organizing his discoveries to create a formal program of treatment.

Description of the procedure

AT is a gentle technique in which a resting individual recites simple phrases. These phrases are based on six themes: heaviness in the arms and legs, warmth in the arms and legs, calm and regular heartbeat, gentle breathing, warm solar plexus, and cool forehead. Other requirements are an absence of bright light and loud noise, a mental connection with the bodypart to which the phrase refers, and an attitude of passive concentration. This form of concentration is a state of mind that is non-striving, relaxed, and unconcerned with the end product. The technique involves not forcing any change, but just letting the exercise work (Achterberg 1985). Rosa (1976) described it as an "allowing" rather than a "doing."

Each phrase is recited by the instructor and repeated three times or more mentally or vocally by the learner to emphasize its effect. When the exercise has been worked through in this manner, a cancellation procedure is carried out as a safeguard against deep trance states. It consists of fist-clenching, brisk arm and leg stretches, and one deep breath. The whole schedule is then repeated, three times. This relaxation pattern largely follows the work of Kermani (1990).

It is a central principle of AT that the client is in control. Although the practitioner presents the method, it is the client who carries it out. The phrases are thus styled in the first person for the client to repeat. Schultz & Luthe (1969) worked slowly through the schedule, taking 6 months to complete the instruction, but more recent versions are presented in short periods of time (Kanji & Ernst 2000).

Rationale for use

Schultz & Luthe found that the recited phrases, following many repetitions, created a light hypnotic trance. They proposed that this trance allowed the body's intrinsic powers of healing to become more available (Schultz & Luthe 1969, Shone 1984). A Freudian interpretation would see the recited phrases as lowering the mental defenses enough to allow communication with the interior, where ideas can be given access and unconsciously internalized.

In their review of the area, Kanji & Ernst (2000) suggested that AT does reduce stress and anxiety. Medium to large clinical effects have been found after treatment with AT, and these tend to be stable at follow-up and to exceed placebo effects (Stetter & Kupper 2002). The meta-analysis of Stetter & Kupper (2002) showed that benefit has been found from AT in psychological disorders such as anxiety, mild to medium depression, and functional sleep disorders. Positive effects of AT have also been observed in psychosomatic disorders such as tension headache, migraine, essential hypertension, coronary heart disease, asthma, Raynaud's disease, and certain kinds of pain (Stetter & Kupper 2002).

The effectiveness of AT compares with that of other relaxation techniques (Stetter & Kupper 2002). One study (Takaishi 2000), however, comparing AT with progressive relaxation, found AT significantly superior in terms of lowered EMG arousal levels and effects on symptoms. AT was also judged easier to carry out by patients with anxiety disorders. In other words, an approach that involves passive listening (e.g., AT) may be perceived to be easier than one that demands more active concentration (e.g., PRT).

Results of effectiveness studies should be viewed with caution as methodological quality of the individual studies varies widely (Stetter & Kupper 2002). However, AT does appear to have much to offer as a relaxation technique in conditions associated with stress, either as a preventive measure, or as an adjunct to conventional treatment (Broms 1999). AT also has the advantage of being available to individuals with conditions where movement is painful such as arthritis, and conditions where certain movements are not possible because of paralysis.

Practical example of integration into care

Anxiety exists as a secondary feature in the experience of most disease and injury. It can also occur in primary forms. In either case, the physical or manual therapist might be looking for a way of reducing it. Kanji & Ernst (2000) suggested that AT might be useful in such situations. Faced with a client, or a group of clients, who are anxious, the therapist would first introduce them to the method with an introductory talk, as follows.

Autogenic training is a method that has been shown to calm the mind. It is believed to provide individuals with access to the deeper parts of the mind where ideas are more readily accepted and where they are able to introduce changes they may wish to make, for example, to become more relaxed. The method consists of short phrases describing sensations of heaviness and warmth in the limbs. I'll read the phrases out, and as I do, I'd like you to focus your attention on each in turn, repeating the phrase silently to yourself several times. Your repetitions will tend to create a feeling of relaxation, which makes you more receptive to the suggestions you make to yourself. In this sense it resembles self-hypnosis. I would like you to feel passive and casual about it. Please don't try to force any response to occur. The sensations of heaviness and warmth must be allowed to arise on their own. You may find that your private thoughts intrude. Do not attempt to fight them. Just let them pass through, then gently bring your attention back to the phrases – allowing them to work on you in their own way.

The relaxation process consists of a series of lessons, each one preceded by a winding-down passage in which you'll be asked to scan your body to release any tension.

The clients will now take up the position they have chosen for the procedure or the one that has been assigned to them.

With your eyes closed I'd like you to spend a few moments quietly resting. To help you unwind I'm going to lead you round the body, helping you to make contact with each part of it in turn and checking that it feels relaxed. Begin by bringing your attention to your feet . . . are they relaxed? . . . then, slowly working up through the legs . . . the abdomen . . . chest . . . shoulders . . . traveling down the arms . . . slowly . . . to reach the fingertips . . . now, moving to the lower spine . . . is that relaxed? . . . rising gradually up to the shoulder blades . . . and into the neck, the scalp . . . over the crown of the head . . . into the forehead . . . and down through the face . . . to the jaw . . . focus on it for a moment . . . feel that every part of your body is relaxed. Begin with the dominant arm.

My right arm is heavy.

I am relaxed.

Following the repetitions, this concludes the first lesson. When clients are again seated a debriefing session begins in which they are encouraged to describe their reactions. Do they feel less anxious as a result? Do they feel that AT will be a useful way of calming their thoughts? If, for example, a client had difficulty in evoking a state of heaviness the therapist could suggest images of lead; and a sense of warmth could be heightened by images of warm water and sunshine (Rosa 1976). Clients are reassured that it can take time to master the technique. The training continues through a series of lessons with the following self-statements:

- my right arm is heavy (left, both)
- my right leg is heavy (left, both)
- my arms and legs are heavy
- my right arm is warm (left, both)
- my right leg is warm (left, both)
- my arms and legs are warm
- my arms and legs are heavy and warm
- I believe in myself
- my heartbeat is calm and regular
- my breathing is calm
- I believe in myself
- my solar plexus is warm
- my forehead is cool
- I believe in myself
- I am at peace.

When using AT, the practitioner might suggest including affirmations. These are phrases, some of which express changes that clients may wish to make in their behavior, and others contain confirmations of their positive attributes or encouragement to carry out tasks they have set themselves. The affirmations should be short, simple, positive, in the first person, and in the present tense. In the case of the client with anxiety, an appropriate affirmation might be "I believe in myself" but clients themselves should decide on the one best suited to them and incorporate it in the schedule.

Other exercises known as "advanced" belong to an area described as therapy rather than training, and are beyond the scope of this chapter.

CONTRAINDICATIONS AND PRECAUTIONS FOR RELAXATION TECHNIQUES

The literature has shown that there are several contraindications for relaxation techniques. It can be tempting to attribute greater power to a therapy than is warranted. Relaxation techniques are not panaceas and therapists should know how to separate the need for relaxation from the need for medical attention. Relaxation training is not a substitute for medical treatment and any organic disorder, whether diagnosed or suspected, should be appropriately addressed.

Deep relaxation states may occasionally lead to out-of-body experiences. As a safeguard against this happening, grounding strategies can be carried out when terminating the treatment.

Benson warned against inducing deep relaxation immediately following a meal because of competing demands on the vascular system (Benson 1976, Bricklin 1990). A further caveat relates to the terminating procedure, which should be conducted slowly. This gives the body organs a chance to adapt to normal waking life and protects the client from the ill-effects of sudden rising.

These contraindications and precautions apply to all approaches. With regard to specific methods there are additional caveats. In the case of PRT, sustained muscle contractions can raise the blood pressure, so "release-only" may, on some occasions, be preferable to tensing procedures (Madders 1982). "Release-only" techniques are useful for people who cramp easily and for women in labor, where tensing strategies can interfere with uterine contractions (Polden & Mantle 1990, Priest & Schott 1991).

Breathing exercises carry a risk of hyperventilation, but it can be prevented by ensuring that any deep respirations are adequately spaced. It should be remembered that the routines presented here are designed for relaxation, not cardiorespiratory therapy, so that in the case of clients receiving cardiorespiratory physical therapy treatment, it will be necessary to consult with the relevant healthcare professional.

The AT phrases may occasionally cause distress, but this response can be mitigated by changing the messages from "heavy and warm" to "light and cool." Alternatively, the lesson can be stopped. Rosa (1976) drew attention to the inadvisability of using the "abdominal warmth" phrase in people with any kind of abdominal inflammation. Although care should be taken in the selection of techniques, the relaxation techniques described here suit most people.

SUMMARY

Relaxation training consists of a variety of techniques that provide a means of coping with stress. The techniques may be somatic or cognitive.

Somatic techniques are directed towards body parts such as the breathing system or the muscles, and the cognitive techniques are directed towards mental concerns such as thoughts and feelings. Many techniques contain both cognitive and somatic elements, giving them a psychophysiological quality.

Three techniques were described in this chapter. Two are predominantly somatic, PRT and breathing, and the other is predominantly cognitive, AT. For each technique, information is presented on its history and development; there is a description of the procedure, a rationale for use, and a practical example of its application.

It is important to prepare the client adequately for relaxation as well as debriefing after the exercise. Debriefing is a necessary part of the procedure as it enables the client to leave the clinic feeling satisfied with the time spent, having fully comprehended the reason for attending. Debriefing also helps the therapist modify future sessions. Home practice should be seen as an essential part of relaxation training, carried out on a daily basis to reinforce the learning.

Relaxation training can have a powerful effect on the individual, and its techniques can be easily integrated into physical and manual therapy care.

References

Achterberg J 1985 Imagery in healing: Shamism and modern medicine. New Science Library, Boston

Bell J A, Saltikov J B 2000 Mitchell's relaxation technique: Is it effective? Physiotherapy 86(9): 473–478

Benson H 1976 The relaxation response. Collins, London

Bernstein D A, Borkovec T D 1973 Progressive relaxation training: A manual for the helping professions. Research Press, Champaign, IL

Bricklin M 1990 Meditation: The healing silence. In: Bricklin M (ed) Positive living and health. Rodale Press, Emmaus, PA

Broms C 1999 Free from stress by autogenic therapy: Relaxation technique yielding peace of mind and self-insight. Läkartidningen 96(6): 588–592

Canter A, Kondo C Y, Knott J R 1975 A comparison of EMG feedback and progressive muscle relaxation training in anxiety neurosis. British Journal of Psychiatry 127: 470–477

Carlson C R, Hoyle R H 1993 Efficacy of abbreviated progressive muscle relaxation training: A quantitative review of behavioral medicine research. Journal of Consulting and Clinical Psychology 61(6): 1059–1067

Crist D A, Rickard H C 1993 A "fair" comparison of progressive and imaginal relaxation. Perceptual and Motor Skills 76: 691–700

Cupal D D, Brewer B W 2001 Effects of relaxation and guided imagery on knee strength, reinjury anxiety and pain following anterior cruciate ligament reconstruction. Rehabilitation Psychology 46(1): 28–43

Davidson R J, Schwartz G E 1976 The psychobiology of relaxation and related states: A multiprocess theory. In: Mostofsky D I (ed) Behavior control and modification of physiological activity. Prentice-Hall, Englewood Cliffs, NJ

Davis M, Eshelman E, McKay M 1988 The relaxation and stress reduction workbook, 3rd edn. New Harbinger, Oakland, CA

Fanning P 1988 Visualization for change. New Harbinger, Oakland, CA

Gardner W N, Bass C 1989 Hyperventilation in clinical practice. British Journal of Hospital Medicine 41: 73–81

Garssen B, De Ruiter C, Van Dyke R 1992 Breathing retraining: A rational placebo? Clinical Psychology Review 12: 141–153

Good M, Stanton-Hicks M, Grass J A et al 2001 Relaxation and music to reduce post-surgical pain. Journal of Advanced Nursing 33(2): 208–215

Innocenti D M 2002 Hyperventilation. In: Pryor J A, Prasad S A (eds) Physiotherapy for respiratory and cardiac problems: Adults and paediatrics, 3rd edn. Churchill Livingstone, Edinburgh, p 563–581

Jacobson E 1938 Progressive relaxation, 2nd edn. University of Chicago Press, Chicago

Johnson U 2000 Short-term physiological intervention: A study of longterm injured competitive athletes. Journal of Sport Rehabilitation 9(3): 207–218

Kanji N, Ernst E 2000 Autogenic training for stress and anxiety: A systematic review. Complementary Therapies in Medicine 8(2): 106–110

Keable D 1989 The management of anxiety: A manual for therapists. Churchill Livingstone, Edinburgh

Kermani K S 1990 Autogenic training: The effective holistic way to better health. Souvenir Press, London

Kerr K M 2000 Relaxation techniques: A critical review. Critical Reviews in Physical and Rehabilitation Medicine 12: 51–89

Lehrer P M 1982 How to relax and how not to relax: A re-evaluation of the work of Edmund Jacobson-1. Behavior Research and Therapy 20: 417–428

Lehrer P M 1996 Varieties of relaxation methods and their unique effects. International Journal of Stress Management 3: 1–15

Lehrer P M, Batey D M, Woolfolk R L et al 1988 The effect of repeated tense–release sequences on EMG and self-report of muscle tension: An evaluation of Jacobsonian and post-Jacobsonian assumptions about progressive relaxation. Psychophysiology 25: 562–567

Lichstein K L 1988 Clinical relaxation strategies. John Wiley, New York

Lucic K S, Steffen J J, Harrigan J A et al 1991 Progressive relaxation training: Muscle contractions before relaxation? Behavior Therapy 22: 249–256

Lum L C 1983 Physiological considerations in the treatment of hyperventilation syndromes. Journal of Drug Research 8: 1867–1872

Madders J 1982 Stress and relaxation: Self-help ways to cope with stress and relieve nervous tension, ulcers, insomnia, migraine and high blood pressure, 3rd edn. Martin Dunitz, London

Miller K M, Perry P A 1990 Relaxation technique and post-operative pain in patients undergoing cardiac surgery. Heart and Lung 19(2): 136–146

Mitchell L 1987 Simple relaxation: The Mitchell method for easing tension, 2nd edn. John Murray, London

Öst L G 1987 Applied relaxation: Description of a coping technique and review of controlled studies. Behavior Research and Therapy 25: 397–407

Öst L G, Breitholtz E 2000 Applied relaxation versus cognitive therapy in the treatment of generalized anxiety disorder. Behavior Research and Therapy 38(8): 777–790

Payne R A 2000 Relaxation techniques: A practical handbook for the health care professional. Churchill Livingstone, Edinburgh

Petry J J 2000 Surgery and complementary therapies: A review. Alternative Therapy in Health and Medicine 6(5): 64–76

Polden M, Mantle J 1990 Physiotherapy in obstetrics and gynecology. Butterworth-Heinemann, Oxford, UK

Poppen R 1988 Behavioral relaxation training and assessment. Pergamon, Oxford, UK

Potter M, Grove J R 1999 Mental skills training during rehabilitation: Case studies of injured athletes. New Zealand Journal of Physiotherapy 27(2): 24–31

Powell T J, Enright S J 1990 Anxiety and stress management. Routledge, London

Priest J, Schott J 1991 Leading antenatal classes: A practical guide. Butterworth-Heinemann, Oxford

Rosa K R 1976 Autogenic training. Victor Gollancz, London

Salt V L, Kerr K M 1997 Mitchell's simple physiological relaxation and Jacobson's progressive relaxation techniques: A comparison. Physiotherapy 83(4): 200–207

Schultz J H, Luthe W 1969 Autogenic methods. Grune & Stratton, New York

Shone R 1984 Creative visualization. Thorsons, Wellingborough, UK

Stetter F, Kupper S 2002 Autogenic training: A meta-analysis of clinical outcome studies. Applied Psychophysiology and Biofeedback 27(1): 45–98

Sudsuang R, Chentanez V, Veluvan K 1991 Effect of Buddhist meditation on serum cortisol and total protein levels, blood pressure, pulse rate, lung volume and reaction time. Physiology and Behavior 50: 543–548

Takaishi N 2000 A comparative study of autogenic training and progressive relaxation as methods for teaching clients to relax. Sleep and Hypnosis 2(3): 132–137

Wallace R K, Benson H 1972 The physiology of meditation. Scientific American 266: 85–92

White J 1998 Alternative sports medicine. The Physician and Sportsmedicine 26(6): 92–105

Wilk C, Turkoski B 2001 Progressive muscle relaxation in cardiac rehabilitation: A pilot study. Rehabilitation Nursing 26(6): 238–243

Yung P, French P, Leung B 2001 Relaxation training as complementary therapy for mild hypertension control and the implications of evidence-based medicine. Complementary Medicine in Nursing and Midwifery 1(2): 59–65

Chapter 10

Imagery

Helen Graham

INTRODUCTION

In this chapter, the history of imaginative medicine is briefly outlined, together with contemporary understanding of the psychophysiology of imagery, and its applications in medical diagnosis, treatment, and rehabilitation. It includes examples of rehabilitation scripts that illustrate each of these applications, and discusses various aspects of working with imagery. This chapter also is a bit different from others in this book, in that it devotes a good deal of time and words to the history of imagery. I take this approach for a couple of reasons. First, I am a firm believer in "knowing where one comes from," and second, the evidence for the usefulness of imagery in medicine has roots more firmly established in history, anthropology, and psychoanalysis than it does in positivist scientific traditions.

THE HISTORY OF IMAGINATIVE MEDICINE

THE ANCIENT ORIGINS OF MEDICINE

The imagination has always played a key role in medicine. Folk medicine throughout the world is based on vivid imagery, and the oldest and most widely used system of healing in the world, shamanism, has been described as the "medicine of the imagination" (Achterberg 1985). Shamanic healing works on the body by creating powerful images that alter the expectancies people have regarding their health, and this imaginal process, it seems, brings about physiological effects. So too, Achterberg (1985) claims, do shrines (e.g., Lourdes, miracle cures, unproven remedies, and placebos work to produce change through imaginal processes).

Although the imagination has been used throughout the history of medicine, whether explicitly as a means to manipulate cure, or implicitly in every interaction between the medical practitioner and the client, its role in health and illness has largely been ignored or overlooked in orthodox Western medicine. It is only relatively recently that the psychological functions and physiological effects of imagery have been determined and applied in conventional healing.

In the ancient world, the soul was viewed as the essence of man and imagination the expression of it. Images – the products of the imagination – revealed the nature, powers, and potentials of the human soul or essence. Images could be used diagnostically to reveal how an individual's true nature was being thwarted, or therapeutically to give expression to the soul and bring its powers and potentials to fruition.

The art of interpreting and manipulating the imagination fell to shamans, and their many-faceted roles included healing the sick, divining the future, and, most importantly, restoring the soul to those who had lost sight of, or contact with it, which was understood to be the fundamental cause of all ills. Throughout the world these shamanistic principles underpinned medicine, which was closely linked with magic, and the origins of many systems of healing can be traced back to this source. This origin is evident in Eastern systems such as traditional Chinese medicine and Ayurveda, traditional Indian medicine, and also in the West, which inherited its medicine from traditions established in ancient Egypt and Greece.

Like the ancient Egyptians, the ancient Greeks used dream images in diagnosis and treatment. The interpretation of dream images was of the greatest importance in healing because all illness was seen fundamentally as sickness of the soul, and images were the expression of that illness. Many cures were attributed to the practice known as "incubatio" in which diagnosis and treatment took place just prior to sleep, when what are now referred to as hypnogogic images occur.

MEDICINE IN THE RENAISSANCE

Jumping ahead to the 16th century, the essayist Montaigne reflected medical wisdom in his essay "On the Imagination" in which he highlighted the ways in which imagination contributed to the onset and development of illness, and also to cure. With the development of science during the 17th century and its application to medicine, the role of the imagination in illness and its treatment became progressively overshadowed by medical orthodoxy, and by the 19th century it was all but lost.

THE INFLUENCE OF MESMERISM

Within folk medicine, however, the imagination still flourished throughout the 18th century as was highlighted by the phenomenon widely known as Mesmerism, after its pioneer, Franz Anton Mesmer. In France, at that time, thousand of cures were attributed to this practice, which is now recognized as the forerunner of hypnotherapy. Mesmer's treatment was so popular with the poor, who were unable to afford orthodox medical treatments, that it threatened to undermine the medical profession, and a commission by the French Government was set up to investigate Mesmer's claims under the chairmanship of Sir Benjamin Franklin, American Ambassador to France.

Mesmer attributed the effectiveness of his treatment to "animal magnetism" but when magnetometers failed to detect any magnetic effects, the Commission ruled in 1785 that there was no substance to Mesmer's claims and that the cures attributed to Mesmerism were achieved solely by the imagination. The implication of this finding was neither recognized nor explored. Rather, imagination was dismissed as roundly by the medical orthodoxy as Mesmerism.

Mesmer retreated into obscurity, but his practices continued to be used to good effect, albeit under the name of hypnosis, and proved to be of great interest to both physicians and psychologists. Hypnosis was used widely as an anesthetic and analgesic throughout the 18th and 19th centuries until the introduction of ether and chloroform, which were easier and quicker to administer. Many operations were conducted using hypnosis as the sole anesthetic and many remarkable cures effected, which made it hard to deny that imagination had an influence on perception and sensation. It was Sigmund Freud, however, who irrevocably achieved a rapprochement between medicine and psychology.

IMAGINATION, THE UNCONSCIOUS MIND, AND PSYCHOTHERAPY

Freud recognized the implications of hypnosis for examining unconscious mental processes. He initially applied hypnosis to his explorations, he soon gave up the practice, but not its content – images – in revealing the dynamics of the unconscious. Instead he used other imaginative methods such as word association and dream interpretation as ways of accessing unconscious processes, describing dreams as the "royal road to the unconscious." In this way, Freud pioneered modern psychotherapy. His practices, and the principles they embodied, were those used throughout history by practitioners of imaginative medicine.

IMAGINATIVE MEDICINE IN THE TWENTIETH CENTURY

In the field of psychotherapy, imaginative techniques flourished during the 20th century. They were, however, all but extinct in the field of physical medicine. They might have remained so, were it not for the oncologist Carl Simonton and psychotherapist Stephanie Simonton, who in the 1970s, saw the potential of the imagination in the treatment of cancer. Fundamentally, Simonton and Simonton, along with their collaborators, drew together insights derived from different fields of research and applied them in a novel approach to cancer. This approach involved clients systematically imagining their cancer being successfully overcome by their body's immune system.

Of 159 clients with a diagnosis of medically incurable malignancy, and treated by Simonton over a 4-year period in the 1970s, none of which were expected to live more than a year, 22.2% were reported as having made a full recovery (Simonton et al 1978). The disease regressed in a further 17% of clients and stabilized in 27%. Further tumor growth was reported in 31% of the clients but the average survival time increased. Those who eventually succumbed to the malignancy were reported as having higher than usual levels of activity, and achieved a significant improvement in their quality of life.

These results suggest that by changing fundamental beliefs and expectancies about their malignancies through imaginative methods clients could bring about significant changes in their physical condition. Following their publication, imaginative methods were enthusiastically promoted and widely adopted in the USA and Europe. Effectively, therefore, the Simontons' therapeutic use of imagery brought about the second major rapprochement between mind and body since that of Mesmer. In themselves, however, neither of these developments, individually or jointly, would have been particularly influential because the medical establishment has been as much inclined to dismiss the Simontons' claims as those of Mesmer, and on a similar basis (i.e., lack of proof, inadequately controlled clinical trials). Developments and discoveries in cognitive psychology and in neuroscience towards the end of the 20th century, however, began to suggest ways in which images could achieve their physiological and psychological effects. These came together within the interdisciplinary field of psychoneuroimmunology, and this new area represents the third major rapprochement between mind and body.

CONTEMPORARY UNDERSTANDING OF IMAGINATIVE MEDICINE

IMAGINATIVE THINKING

As a means of non-verbal representation or thinking, mental images complement thinking in words and increase mental capacity and flexibility, facilitating problem-solving, decision-making, and creativity. Furthermore, because images convey simultaneously and instantaneously much more complex information than verbal thought (which is linear and sequential) images can be much more efficient.

Within Western culture, which emphasizes linguistic skills, there is a tendency to represent issues verbally, and because images are also often fleeting, they are frequently overlooked. As a result, individuals are to a great extent unaware of the role of imaginative processes in their ordinary cognitive functioning.

Certainly psychological research on imagery during the 20th century shed light on the workings of the unconscious. Most of the research focused exclusively on visual imagery, and demonstrated that it and visual perception are functionally equivalent. That is, imagining something is neuropsychologically nearly equivalent to actually seeing it. The precise neurophysiological and neuropsychological mechanisms are still far from understood, and images generate similar, albeit not necessarily identical, response states as do actual perceptual stimuli. Contemporary research supports the ancient view of a link between imagination and physiology, and prompted the awareness that through imagery one might be able to control physiological functions formerly thought to be automatic or involuntary.

THE PHYSIOLOGICAL EFFECTS OF IMAGERY

The physiological effects of intense imagery were first examined in the 1920s when the Russian psychologist Luria demonstrated that the pneumonist Sheresheveskii could increase his heart rate by imagining himself running, and alter the size of his pupils and his cochlear reflex by imagining sights and sounds. It was later established that subtle tensions of small muscles accompany imagery, and that motor neurons are activated when particular body movements are imagined (Jacobsen 1929).

Later studies indicated that images can elicit changes in salivation (Barber et al 1964), blood sugar levels, gastrointestinal activity, and blister formation (Barber 1978). It was also established that intense sexual and phobic imagery is accompanied by dramatic physiological changes (Kazdin & Wilcoxin 1975, Laws & Rubin 1969, Marks & Huson 1973, Marks et al 1971, Marzillier et al 1979, Smith & Over 1987, Stock & Greer 1982). Changes in heart rate, galvanic skin response, respiration, and eye movement are associated with negative images; and images of sadness, happiness, anger, and fear can be differentiated by cardiovascular changes (Schwartz et al 1981). Unpublished research (Schneider et al 1988) also suggested that aspects of immune functioning could be influenced by mental images. More recently, the effects of imagery on various physiological functions, notably heart rate, blood pressure, blood flow, electrodermal activity, and immune response have been confirmed.

BODY–MIND COMMUNICATION

Attempts to explain the mechanisms by which psychological factors or states influence physiological functioning are the focus of the interdisciplinary field of psychoneuroimmunology. Research in this field has established that thought and emotion produce molecules known as peptides that have receptors throughout the entire body. Peptide chains within the body can effectively be considered as streams of thought, and greater understanding of the biochemistry of these processes leads to the conclusion that thinking or consciousness occurs throughout the body. This means that the body is effectively the subconscious mind. This awareness has prompted a new way of thinking about the human being as a field of information where thought and emotion travel instantaneously everywhere.

It would seem that the key to understanding the function of images lies in their role as transformers and transducers of information. They facilitate the translation of both verbal and non-verbal outputs and "communication." Images can be regarded as building a bridge between the physical (physiological) and the psychological allowing information to cross those domains, and vice versa. Physiological information may therefore be perceived in symbolic form as images that can provide important clues to functioning and be used as a tool for accessing ordinarily unconscious, or hidden, psychological and emotional processes. Physiological effects can also be induced by the psychological and emotional information conveyed by images.

PSYCHOLOGICAL AND PHYSIOLOGICAL FUNCTIONS OF MENTAL IMAGERY

It is clear from research into mental imagery since the early 20th century, that mental imagery has a number of important psychological and physiological functions.

● It promotes mental absorption and a shift in the time sense enabling relaxation of attitudes, beliefs, preoccupations, and expectations.

- It provides an alternative mode for representation of issues, also a means of accessing information relevant to unconscious processes.
- It makes it possible to influence in a conscious way normally unconscious psychological and emotional processes.
- Mental images relate to physiological states, and may precede or follow physiological changes, indicating both a causative and reactive role.
- Imagery may influence the voluntary or peripheral nervous system, and autonomic functions, and therefore has both direct and indirect effects on the body. These effects are not only on the musculoskeletal system, but also the involuntary nervous system and the immune system, and are in turn affected by these reactions.

Greater understanding of these functions has led to the application of mental imagery in many diverse fields.

CONTEMPORARY APPLICATIONS OF MENTAL IMAGERY

Increasingly, mental imagery is being used to promote decision-making and problem-solving skills, and stimulate creative thinking in various contexts, such as business organization and management. It is also exploited in the commercial field, in product development, advertising, marketing, and market research and public relations. By way of mental imagery, possibilities can be explored in the imagination without taking the time, making the effort, or running the risk of carrying out those operations in physical reality. It is therefore used in many fields involving planning, design, and research. By going through the motions of an intended action imaginally, flaws in planning or performance can be identified and avoided. Mental rehearsal of an activity is widely used to develop strategy, overcome performance anxiety and self-doubt, cope with problems, and raise the level of performance (e.g., for actors, dancers, musicians, sports persons). Because positive mental imagery is inherently absorbing and therefore relaxing, it is used as an aid to stress management and coping skills in industry, business and commerce, and in assertiveness training. The tension-reducing features of imagery are applied in classroom control and management, to assist learning at all levels of education, and to help students cope with potentially stressful situations such as examinations. Imagery is also used by social workers and educational psychologists to encourage the discussion of issues that may be difficult for individuals, especially children, to articulate – issues such as abuse, anxieties, bullying, emotional and physical pain, and phobias. Using imagery to give insight into the normally hidden realm of children's experiences – their fears, needs, wishes, and preoccupations – enables their emotional and psychological development to be monitored more sensitively. Imagery has long been used to uncover and explore unconscious processes within psychotherapy. It is a feature of many therapeutic approaches including psychoanalysis, Jungian analysis, Gestalt therapy, behavior therapy, aversion therapy, and arts and drama therapies. Imagery is used to enhance feelings of control and coping skills in various situations such as promoting awareness and reducing fear of usually avoided situations, and to rehearse alternative strategies for dealing with them. Imagery is also a source of detail about past experiences and can provide access to significant memories of childhood before language became predominant. It can promote a richer experience of a range of emotions, bypass defenses and resistances, and open up new avenues for exploration when therapy reaches an impasse (see Graham [1995] for a thorough review of these uses).

HEALTH IMPLICATIONS OF IMAGERY

Clearly, imagery has numerous implications for health. By promoting relaxation, both mental and physical, it can reduce stress and its effects, and help ameliorate and steady body functions. Imagery can also provide new perspectives on, and insights into, emotional and psychological factors relevant to health and illness, and clues to emotional and physical functions that are of value in treatment. It may be used to influence these processes consciously in support of treatment or prevention of disease, and the management of symptoms including pain. Accordingly, imagery is now widely used in healthcare and related professions where its benefits are increasingly being recognized and supported by research.

Although the use of imagery has been validated on clients with chronic pain, severe orthopedic trauma, rheumatoid arthritis, cancer, diabetes, burn injury, alcoholism and stress disorders, and in childbirth (Achterberg & Lawlis 1978), direct systematic research on the therapeutic outcome of imaginative methods in relation to various specific ailments is limited, and so it is considered here broadly in relation to three areas of application: diagnosis, treatment, and rehabilitation.

IMAGERY IN MEDICAL DIAGNOSIS

The Simontons recognized two important factors in the etiology of cancer: the effect of stress in depressing the immune system, and the influence of a person's beliefs and emotional states. They observed that clients with cancer typically responded to problems and stresses with a deep sense of hopelessness or "giving up," and this emotional response, they believed, triggers a set of physiological responses that suppress the body's natural defenses and make it susceptible to producing abnormal cells. Simonton and Matthews-Simonton (1975) argued that the first step in getting well is to understand how psychological factors have contributed to illness and to find ways of influencing them in support of treatment. They recognized that in helping promote and enhance relaxation, imagery has an important role in decreasing tension and effecting positive physiological changes, including improved immune function. Imagery is also a means whereby clients can confront their fears, and feelings of hopelessness and helplessness, and gain a sense of control and a change in attitude. It also allows them to communicate with the unconscious, where beliefs antithetical to health may be hidden, yielding valuable insights into their condition.

The Simonton method

Simonton & Matthews-Simonton (1975) developed a method in which clients were taught a simple form of relaxation, imagining a pleasant place and holding it in consciousness. They were then asked to imagine their illness in any way that it appeared to them, and to imagine the form of treatment they were receiving. They found that the clients' images of their cancer or pain provided invaluable information regarding their beliefs, attitudes, fears, and expectations. Those clients who succeeded in overcoming their cancer usually employed imagery with certain features: the cancer cells were represented as weak, confused, and susceptible to breakdown, and the treatment as strong and powerful. The body's immune system was imagined as an aggressive army of white blood cells, eager to do battle with invading organisms and destroy them. Dead cancer cells were imagined as being removed from the body normally and naturally, leaving it clear of cancer and healthy. Simonton & Matthews-Simonton (1975) identified images matching these features as essentially positive and advocated their use by clients attempting to overcome cancer.

CRITERIA FOR ASSESSING IMAGERY

Achterberg & Lawlis (1978) drew up a list of tentative criteria for assessing the images of cancer clients. They observed that representation of cancer cells as ants, or eggs in an incubator, is essentially negative, suggesting the likely proliferation of the disease. They argued that it is especially important in treating malignancy that the most powerful images relate to the person's own natural defense system, rather than to the disease or treatment. They proposed that the individual should be encouraged to imagine the white blood cells of the body at least as vividly as the malignant cells, but as more numerous and powerful. The individual must also achieve powerful images of the latter being removed from the body. In addition, treatment should be imagined as a friend or ally, and clients were encouraged to personalize it in any way that seemed appropriate. This approach, they suggested, helps to reduce the aversive side effects of treatment.

Simonton & Matthews-Simonton (1975) recognized that imagery involves a highly personal symbolic language, and that the emotional meaning of any one symbol will vary greatly from one person to another. Thus, one person's image of strength and power may signify weakness to another. Given such variation, they emphasized the importance of exploring personal imagery with an individual rather than imposing meaning on it. The meaning of this personal imagery may not be readily apparent to the individual, and so in order to translate its inherent beliefs and expectations, and discover its meaning, it may be necessary for the person to "try on" the image. Simonton & Matthews-Simonton (1975) therefore advocated free drawing and other means of exploring imagery as valuable methods for facilitating discussion and understanding.

Similar methods have been used to good effect by the psychiatrist Kubler-Ross (1977) in helping people express and confront their fears about death, dying, and bereavement. These methods may involve a person imagining journeying through his or her body in order to gain insight into physical problems and attitudes, taking an imaginary inventory of the body, imagining communication between the two hemispheres of the brain, engaging in imaginary dialogue with individual internal parts of oneself, dying in one's imagination, and exorcising pain.

IMAGERY AND TREATMENT

In the Simonton method, after clients had imagined their illness and the treatment they were receiving, they were instructed to imagine their cancer being destroyed and disposed of by their body's immune system and their bodies free of disease and healthy. They were also encouraged to imagine pain in the same way rather than trying to suppress it, and to rehearse this process three times daily for periods of at least 20 minutes. They found that while those who succeeded in overcoming cancer generally had, or achieved, imagery that matched their criteria, in many cases it did not necessarily contain all the elements at the outset. Thus, while in some instances the insights clients derived from imagining the state of their bodies was sufficient to promote images embodying positive changes, in many cases, they needed assistance in creating images embodying a positive expectancy. This process, termed guided imagery or creative imagination, is often used in psychotherapy, where a person's representation of issues is too limited to enable coping in a given area, or where a therapist wishes to challenge existing representations.

Abundant anecdotal evidence appears to confirm the Simontons' claim that this method is effective in the treatment of cancer as an adjunct to orthodox medical treatment. Support for their claims also comes from a number of studies. Improved cancer outcomes related to the uses of imagery have since been reported (Borysenko 1987) and a number of studies have confirmed that imagery has numerous effects, including cancer regression (Fiore 1974, Meares 1981). Imagery has also been found to provide cancer clients with significant relief from pain, nausea, vomiting, anticipatory emesis, and anxiety (Bradley & McCanne 1981, Donovan 1980), and to be effective in reducing the aversiveness of cancer chemotherapy (Lyles et al 1982).

Current thinking, however, is that the early applications of imaginative approaches to cancer, focused as they were on an initial client group of servicemen in the US Air Force, placed too much emphasis on anger, attacking, and killing, and assumed that most clients would be comfortable with these notions. Subsequently this proved not to be the case. Many people object to the idea of attacking and killing anything, including an invading disease organism, and may reject it, either consciously or unconsciously. Left to summon their own images, they may devise equally effective but gentler ways of dealing with their disease.

There are other reasons why gentler images may be more appropriate. Although the immune system is commonly viewed as the body's defense system, designed to seek out and destroy harmful and alien substances, such as bacteria and viruses, it is now recognized as functioning with more subtlety than this metaphor suggests. In the light of evidence (Taylor 1990) suggesting that the immune system operates cooperatively and collaboratively to support the integrity of the body and its optimal relationship to its environment rather than combatively, this battlefield terminology has to be re-appraised. From this perspective, disease can more appropriately be viewed as disharmony or lack of coherence rather than an unnatural entity or state that needs to be fought.

Nevertheless, the importance of "fighting" imagery is still promoted in treatment by those who consider it important that anger is released. This is partly because people are generally more powerful when angry than when passive, and can mobilize this strength in support of healing (Manning 1989), and also because research has linked inability to express anger with cancer. Significantly better outcomes have been noted for clients who can express their anger compared with those who cannot. Moreover, it appears that cancer may be caused by failure of cell death, rather than cell proliferation per se.

Although it is preferable to work with a person's spontaneous imagery where possible, recognition of the effectiveness of guided imagery as an adjunct to conventional treatment has led to its proliferation in healthcare settings. An increasing number of contemporary practitioners in the USA use imagery in both diagnosis and treatment, and to relieve the pain and anxiety associated with medical conditions. In Britain, psychological approaches involving imagery have been introduced into a number of orthodox cancer treatment programs, most notably at Hammersmith Hospital, London, where, following studies of the use of such methods at the Bristol Cancer Help Centre, physicians have come around to the view that these methods work and are perfectly compatible with traditional methods of treatment. Generally, however, the medical profession has been slow in implementing psychological approaches in general, and imaginative approaches in particular, or conducting controlled trials of their effectiveness. Research concerning imaginative interventions is still very limited and further controlled clinical trials are needed. Meanwhile, popular enthusiasm for imaginative approaches to treatment has created a demand for appropriate source material, and guided imagery scripts directed towards personal growth, psychological transformation, positive mental health, spiritual development, stress management, self-healing and self-help, pain control, and symptom alleviation have been compiled and published for a general audience.

IMAGERY AND REHABILITATION

One of the applications of imagery and rehabilitation is in sport for recovery from injury or heavy training. Physically, greater blood flow to an injured area and warmth in the locality of damaged tissue promotes recovery. It has been shown that imagining increased blood flow and warmth can lead to measurable increases in temperature in areas as specific as a finger (Blakeslee 1980). These principles are already well established and supported by research in the field of autogenic training (Schultz & Luthe 1969).

Sometimes imagery is facilitated by flotation in an enclosed tank of salt-water solution dense enough to support the body. Flotation not only induces relaxation conducive to imagery by reducing sensory stimulation and distractions but also removes much of the effect of gravity allowing more rapid healing, and helps relax the muscles, enhancing their recovery. Studies have suggested that restricted environmental stimulation therapy (REST) can facilitate a whole range of positive physical, behavioral, and psychological changes (McAleney et al 1990, Suedfield et al 1993, Wagaman et al 1991).

Imagery can also be used in training, whether in sport, dance, or on the job, in the absence of ordinary practice. The first studies to suggest a physiological relationship between imagery and motor skills were carried out in the 1930s (Jacobsen 1930, 1931). They demonstrated that changes in muscle activity occur while people imagine performing a physical task, and that these are the same muscles used during actual physical performance. It has been proposed that the electrical stimulation of the muscles and central/peripheral nervous system that occurs when performing intense imagery is similar to that which occurs during physical movement. The apparent difference between imagery and actual physical performance is the amplitude of the electrical stimulation of muscles. Proponents of this theory, known as "muscle memory," claim that imagery strengthens the muscle memories by causing the muscles to fire in the correct sequence similar to actual physical activity (Vealey & Walter 1993).

A different kind of explanation offered to explain imagery enhancement of physical skills, the symbolic learning theory, is supported by a number of studies (e.g., Sackett 1934, 1935). This theory proposes that imagery symbolizes in the brain the movements needed to perform skills and hence facilitates performance. As such, images act as a mental blueprint and their rehearsal strengthens the blueprint enabling skills to become automatic. Imagery rehearsal of physical activities (e.g., job activities, leisure activities, activities of daily living) may be added to rehabilitation programs to help clients return to past levels of functioning.

Imagery and stroke injury

Currently, many of the performance and recovery benefits of imagery are confined within the field of sport psychology, although clearly they have wider application within the broad field of recovery from a wide range of medical conditions including orthopedic trauma and a variety of neurological conditions. A promising area of application currently being investigated is in relation to rehabilitation following stroke (Dirske van Schalkwyk et al, unpublished work 2002). Preliminary investigations have suggested that people who have had strokes commonly experience high levels of disempowerment and despair, along with the feeling that many areas of their rehabilitation are out of their control. Working with imagery can help these clients gain a sense of empowerment and control, and may be effective in aiding recovery.

A key finding of this research, however, is that therapists often unwittingly use negative imagery in therapy, referring, for example, to clients' paralyzed limbs as their "bad" legs or arms, and so reinforce negative expectations the clients might have about their condition and recovery. Negative programming of this kind is by no means confined to physical and manual therapists; it is common throughout orthodox medicine. Typically, healthcare professionals prime clients to experience pain by telling them "this may sting a little" before administering injections or taking blood, and midwives routinely focus on the pains of childbirth rather than the pleasures. This lack of awareness of the power of the imagination in matters of health and illness is only one of many potential pitfalls to be overcome if imaginative methods are to be more widely and effectively implemented in practice. Other problems in working with imagery are considered below.

USING IMAGERY IN PRACTICE

It is important to reiterate that, wherever possible, it is preferable to work with a person's spontaneous imagery because this will reveal information regarding attitudes, beliefs, preconceptions, and anxieties. It may also provide clues to possible solutions to a specific problem. In some cases, the insights derived may be sufficient to promote effective strategies and solutions, but more usually clients have to be guided or directed in order to produce and understand images, and modify them in such a way as to embody positive expectancies.

Exercising the imagination

A fundamental problem when introducing imaginative methods is that many people consider themselves to be unimaginative. They do not realize that imagery is an everyday activity engaged in by everyone except a small number of people with certain kinds of brain damage. Part of the problem is that many people do not readily appreciate what an image is, and the explanation – that it is a sensory experience in the absence of sensory stimulation – may not enlighten them greatly. It is easier to ask them to imagine themselves in a certain place, such as a beach, and to imagine the sea, sky, and shoreline and other aspects of the situation.

Most people will have little or no difficulty doing so, but what they imagine will differ. Some individuals will "see" the entire scene. Others will hear the sounds of the sea and seagulls. Others will smell the air, or taste the salt spray on their lips, and some

will feel the breeze, the sand under their feet, or the water. These are important differences, because they tend to reveal the sensory modality that dominates for an individual. Although everyone produces visual, auditory, olfactory, gustatory, kinaesthetic, and somatic images, most people tend to favor one type over the others. Broadly speaking, people can be categorized as predominantly visual, auditory, or kinaesthetic types, meaning that visual images, sound, or body sensations are most salient for them.

Because psychological research on mental imagery has almost exclusively focused on the production of visual images – it is generally assumed that all people are equally capable of visualizing. Hence, guided imagery scripts tend to be based on this premise. However, a script that focuses exclusively on visual images will be sub-optimal for many people who will find it difficult or unappealing. It is preferable to use imagery scripts that are directed towards all the senses and encourage subjects to imagine sights, sounds, smells, and other sensations. It is best to do an imagery assessment and find out what are the strongest image modalities and work with those first.

Performance anxiety

Being relaxed is the key to successful imagery. It is often claimed that it is necessary to be deeply relaxed in order to produce imagery, and various relaxation techniques are invariably recommended as a prelude. Ordinarily, however, deep relaxation is not necessary, although it may be helpful if clients are very tense, anxious, or mentally overactive. Such states can inhibit the imagination.

Anxiety about imagery often reflects a general anxiety about performance, achievement, success, failure, or evaluation – concerns that create tensions in a person's life and limit experience. "Trying" to produce images is counterproductive as it involves effort and creates tensions that inhibit imagery. Rather, images should be "allowed" to emerge spontaneously and sufficient time needs to be set aside for this to occur.

Regular practice

Although imagery does not involve extensive effort, it does require discipline. The more regularly it is practiced the more likely it is to produce results. If imagery is used as an aid to relaxation, self-awareness, personal or spiritual development, problem solving, or creative thinking, 20–30 minutes daily is normally enough. If it is used in the treatment of illness, pain management, symptom alleviation, rehabilitation, or skilled performance, several periods each day are preferable but 20 minutes is sufficient for each exercise period.

Preparing for imagery

Feeling at ease about imagery is more important than the context in which it is done. It is advisable to practice imagery when sitting in a position where the back, trunk, and legs are supported, feet set apart and firmly on the ground, and no parts of the body crossed or twisted. Prone postures are not usually recommended as they encourage sleep. Closing the eyes may help production of images but is not essential. Clothing should be loose and spectacles removed.

Once comfortable, the person can be encouraged to turn their attention inward by gradually withdrawing it from the wider situation. This inwardness can be achieved through attention to breathing, or focusing upon parts of the body and allowing them to become heavier.

Initial difficulties

With practice, external stimuli are easily screened out and so the setting in which imagery takes place is largely irrelevant, but some people become distracted regardless of context or personal comfort. But in the beginning, external distractions such as voices and traffic noises may interfere. Mind wandering is often a problem for people who embark on imagery. It is usually a sign that the person is trying to maintain self-control. Some people will find their mind wanders around, turning again and again to certain issues and not progressing beyond them.

To allow the imagination free rein, the rational mind needs to be allowed to release its grip and let go of thoughts, anxieties, concerns, and preoccupations that dominate everyday thinking. Fear of losing control, even temporarily, may be a source of anxiety for some individuals.

Some people may feel anxious if they believe that by relaxing they are losing conscious control. If anything, consciousness or awareness is enhanced during imagery and self-control increases. Letting go of the constraints normally imposed by rational conscious thoughts enables not only awareness of the physical, physiological, emotional, and psychological processes ordinarily beyond conscious control, but also allows them to be influenced directly, which is how imagery achieves its effects.

Some people, especially those with strong fundamental religious bents, fear that by looking inwards into ordinarily hidden aspects of themselves they will encounter evil and terrible features and lose their souls. Experiencing images that emerge from and reveal aspects of this ordinarily hidden realm may be emotionally painful, unpalatable, or unpleasant, and strongly resisted. If examined, this resistance invariably reveals negative beliefs and expectancies about the self that prevents the person achieving successful outcomes, and thus, imagery and relaxation may be contraindicated.

Anxieties and fears may effectively prevent some individuals producing any images. On the other hand, there are people who have little or no difficulty producing images but try to control unexpected or unacceptable images by censoring or directing them. This defeats the whole point of imaginative exercises.

In addition to mind-wandering, pre-occupations with aches, pains, minor irritations, noise, and draughts are other ways in which engaging in imagery is typically avoided. Such avoidance often conceals resistance to confronting the self. Identifying these tendencies may promote awareness of the resistance that needs to be overcome if imagery is to be used effectively.

Imagery may challenge beliefs or compromise self-image in significant ways, with the result that many people who begin imagery do not continue with it even when they derive benefits from it. Some women might feel guilty about taking time for themselves and worry that others might consider them self-indulgent if they do so. Men may also feel guilty about "taking it easy" when they have work to do, a living to earn, and other goals to achieve. Self-imposed imperatives such as these often generate stress, illness, and dysfunctional behavior. Even if individuals give themselves permission to relax, these imperatives may prevent them doing so effectively.

People are often unaware that they are reluctant to look at themselves and so deny that they are resisting self-awareness. Examining the reasons people give for not being able to do imagery often exposes their avoidance strategies and the underlying beliefs and fears. Encouraging them to become aware of what is stopping them generating images allows them to observe this process. In this way they may discover the rules of conduct they impose on themselves and the anxiety and problems they generate. Also, by uncovering fears and anxieties they may discover other areas of life they influence and inhibit. Hence, it is important that a therapist does not simply accept this difficulty but helps the person to examine and understand the underlying factors. Once again, as in many other places in this book, the reasons for resistance may have roots way beyond the understanding of the physical and manual therapist, and would be better addressed by another healthcare professional (e.g., a psychologist).

This difficulty may be more marked when guided imagery is used to achieve specific outcomes. Simonton et al (1978) found that some of the cancer clients he treated were unable or unwilling to engage in imagery because they believed that to imagine their cancer shrinking when they had been told it was growing constitutes lying. Imagery, therefore, compromised their view of themselves as honest. It is important to realize that guided imagery is not a method of self-deception and that what is being imagined is the desired outcome rather than what is happening at the time. The belief that they are deluding themselves by imagining their bodies eliminating a cancer may conceal a strong fear of the disease and doubt about the body's ability to overcome it. Images people have difficulty creating or accepting, and wish to change need to be examined, along with the reasons for the difficulty.

Recording images

Keeping a record (an imagery log book) helps to cultivate a disciplined approach to self-examination and a record of this kind is particularly important if images are being used in the treatment of illness, in rehabilitation, or to improve skilled performance where certain kinds of outcome are desired. In such cases, it is advisable to establish that the images used are suitable to the task in hand.

Interpreting images

One of the most widespread misconceptions about working with images is that they have universal meanings known to experts who can interpret them. This mistaken view owes much to authoritative interpretations of dream and fantasy images. It is perpetuated in books on dreams and other imagery. Although imagery may have certain universal features, it represents nonetheless an individual's unique symbolic language or representational system that he or she can learn to translate and

understand. Two individuals may produce the same image, but it may have quite different meanings for each of them. Interpretation of a person's imagery by others, however "expert," will reveal details of their symbolism rather than that of the person who produced it, and may be highly misleading.

Exploration of a person's imagery can be assisted by carefully examining the context of the images and other available clues, their components, similar kinds of images, the associations they evoke, the memories they stir, and the responses they produce. In this way, a person can become expert in his or her own symbolism. Those people working with others in this enterprise should ensure that the personal meaning of symbols is not lost in their translation of them, and that they do not impose their personal meanings on the images. Although the interpretation of images may be beyond the realm of physical and manual therapist skills, these sections are presented here to illustrate some of the pitfalls and the depths that can happen when imagery is explored. A common occurrence in the physical and manual therapies is that during some soft-tissue massage or other manipulation, the client suddenly reports an intense visual image, or the images from an important memory emerge.

Understanding images

The meaning of imagery will not always be immediately obvious and individuals may need help to understand it. Without help they may be left puzzled, confused, alarmed and, in some instances, distressed by images and the powerful feelings that sometimes accompany them. If "untranslated" images are rehearsed without comprehension of their full meaning the resulting outcome may be far from what is intended or desired, especially if the images are distressful.

Similarly, limiting and negative thoughts can reduce the likelihood of positive outcomes and effects from imagery. For example, the healing "force" mobilized by one man in an attempt to prevent the spread of a rapidly advancing cancer consisted of two men blocking off a flooded underground railway tunnel with a portable cement-mixer, a bucket, and two spades. Inappropriate imagery, such as this, is unlikely to be effective.

Brain-storming

Working with imagery is like puzzling over a vast jigsaw and trying to establish the connections between its many features. This is achieved primarily by identifying the links between elements. Simple word association may be effective, but any tendency to generate lists of words should be avoided. It is preferable to "brain-storm" by writing or drawing the image and its component features in the center of a large piece of paper or blackboard. To this can then be added the words and pictures the creator associates with it. Each associated item can be "mapped" by placing each one as it emerges close to the word or picture that triggered it until no further associations can be made or the available space is used up. Drawings, paintings, various kinds of artwork, and color can be included. In this way thousands of items can be produced, each linked to the others. Connections between items can be made by joining them up. This process results in a plan that represents a mental map far more rich and varied than the linear pattern of associations lists typically produce.

These maps can be used not only to help amplify and elaborate images, but also to generate ideas, plan essays and projects, and stimulate creative thinking of all kinds. Nevertheless, as most people have not been educated and trained to organize their thoughts in lists and flow diagrams, clients may need a good deal of practice before they feel comfortable with this procedure and can use it effectively.

Other ways of working with imagery

Images can be worked on in many other ways. Imaginary scenes may be dramatized using cartoon figures, puppets, dolls, toys, other persons, or by acting out or talking through each of the "parts," themes, or characters of the fantasy. These techniques are particularly useful when working with children in rehabilitation.

The meaning of certain images may become clear as a result of other activities, in sudden flashbacks or images, flashes of insight, which in some cases may be dramatic. Whereas "flashes" usually bring about a sudden transformation of consciousness, understanding, or awareness, images may recur without any increased insight or understanding. These should not be dismissed or ignored but carefully noted. Usually resolution will occur quite spontaneously, but other people, whether therapists or friends, can have a valuable role in helping understanding. They can encourage exploration of feelings and responses to images and the associations they have. They can

also amplify responses to images by expressing the associations and responses these images elicit in them, point to similar symbols in mythology and esoteric traditions, and suggest possible meanings. Nevertheless they should never interpret images for the person.

GUIDED IMAGERY SCRIPT

Two guided imagery scripts are presented below: one dealing with light breathing, and the other, a healing imagery script.

BREATHING LIGHTLY

Here is an example of how one might talk a client through an imagery session (see also Chapter 9).

Find somewhere you can sit comfortably, and having done so simply be aware of how your body is located in relation to its surroundings. Be aware of your feelings in this situation. How do you feel? Do you feel comfortable and ready to begin? Do you feel silly or guilty about taking time to do this exercise? Having identified how you feel, close your eyes or focus them on a fixed point or object within your line of vision, such as a mark on a wall, ceiling, or floor. Then gradually withdraw your attention from your surroundings and bring it to the boundary between your body and the surfaces your body is touching. As you do so, notice whether the contact is comfortable or uncomfortable, and adjust your position so as to maximize comfort. When you are positioned as comfortably as possible, bring your attention to the tip of your nose. Imagine that you are breathing colored light, which may or may not be scented, in through your nose. This enters your body and is drawn upwards and over the crown of your head, then down the back of your neck and the length of your backbone, filling your head and body with light. At the base of your spine the colored light curls upwards, and as you breathe out, it is drawn upwards, forcing a dark dense fog of tension towards and out of your mouth, leaving your body feeling light and clear. Continue breathing in this way for several minutes.

This imagery script has numerous applications. In itself, breathing through the nose slows and deepens breathing and produces greater relaxation.

Imagining breathing in color, which involves visualization, is for most people absorbing and promotes relaxation more easily. The imagery being guided also has kinaesthetic and olfactory components, and the script itself is verbal, so it is appropriate for many people with different dominant image modalities.

The brief induction focuses specifically on areas that may be problematic for individuals and that may prevent them from engaging in the exercise and/or producing images. Through debriefing the breathing imagery exercise with the client, it is possible to identify areas in the body where the light cannot pass, or does so only with difficulty. When examined more closely, these areas are usually those in which a person experiences tension, and often symptoms such as pain, discomfort, and other difficulties. Hence, the exercise has a diagnostic function.

By encouraging a person to breathe more deeply and thereby push light through areas where it appears to be blocked, tension can be relieved, together with attendant pain, discomfort, and other symptoms. This process deepens relaxation and counteracts stress and its effects, and hence has broad treatment applications.

In addition to relieving and reducing stress, repeating or rehearsing this exercise can improve flexibility and function in areas affected by chronic tension. By relieving muscle tension it also releases energy and can improve feelings of well-being. The exercise may also increase blood flow to areas where this is restricted, and may be used to good effect in conditions such as sport injury, stroke, and paralysis as part of rehabilitation programs.

HEALING IMAGERY SCRIPT

Here is an example of a script that one might use with a client undergoing rehabilitation for a hamstring strain. It is often a good idea to have an anatomy text handy to show the client the structure of the muscle, or other organs involved, the neural pathways, and the blood flow patterns. Using such a text may help the client produce more vivid images.

Please get yourself into a comfortable position and take a couple of nice deep breaths. Go ahead and close your eyes and feel yourself becoming more and more relaxed, letting yourself go, as you continue to breathe in an easy and comfortable manner. First we are going to send a slow wave of relaxation from the top of your head down to your toes. Imagine this wave of relaxation starting to cross your forehead leaving the muscles behind a bit more relaxed than they were, and the wave moves down across your nose and upper cheeks, down across your lips, and into your jaw. The relaxing wave continues into your neck and spreads down into your shoulders, through your upper arms, then into your lower arms, and the wave moves into your hands pushing the tension out of your fingertips and away from your body. The wave now continues down your chest and upper back, through your stomach and lower back, across your hips and down into your thighs. Feel the wave of relaxation leaving loose muscles behind it as it moves across your knees, into your calves and shins, across your ankles, down into your feet, pushing that last tension out of your toes and away from your body. Now continue to breathe comfortably while you very keenly focus on your hamstring and see and feel the fresh warm blood flowing into your injury. Your hamstring is getting warmer and more relaxed as you see the bright red blood bringing nutrients to the injury and helping lay down new healthy tissue. You can actually see and feel each pulse of new blood, see the muscle fibers beginning to grow and reconnect, and see the dark venous blood taking away the damaged tissue. Watch the process as the muscle is repaired. You are helping by warming the area and sending a healing flow of blood and nutrients, while removing the damaged fibers. Your hamstring is getting stronger every day as you help it heal. Watch the healing process now for several more minutes.

Such an exercise, like many others in this book, needs a solid debriefing to determine what modifications should be made so that the client feels they are getting the most out of it. As rehabilitation progresses, the healing imagery can move into other areas such as exercising the damaged muscle and seeing it contract and relax and grow even stronger.

SUMMARY

Ancient systems of healing are based on the premise that all illness results from sickness of the soul, and that the soul expresses itself through the imagination. Hence, the processes of the imagination or imagery reveal the sources of disease and can be used to treat it. Imaginative medicine survived in secret oral traditions and informed medical practice throughout the Middle Ages and until the 18th century. The spiritual aspects of ancient medicine were obscured with the advent of scientific medicine from the 17th century onwards. While the role of the soul in health and illness was no longer considered, the influence of the mind on the body, and specifically the role of the imagination, was highlighted by Mesmerism in the 18th century. During the 20th century, the imagination was reintroduced into orthodox Western medicine when imagery was used in the diagnosis and treatment of cancer. During the 20th century, understanding of the cognitive and physiological functions of imagery was revealed through research in cognitive psychology and the interdisciplinary field of psychoneuroimmunology.

Imagery has been applied in diverse fields and has been recognized as having many applications in the field of health, notably in diagnosis, treatment, and rehabilitation. Powerful images spontaneously emerge in the physical and manual therapies and practitioners need to have some skills for helping clients understand their images. Practitioners can also purposefully use imagery to help the rehabilitation process. The chapter concludes with two practical examples (and scripts) for physical and manual therapists of the use of imagery in the rehabilitation setting.

References

Achterberg J 1985 Imagery in healing: Shamanism and modern medicine. Routledge, London

Achterberg J, Lawlis G F 1978 Imagery and cancer. Institute for Personality and Testing, Chicago

Barber T X 1978 Hypnosis, suggestions and psychosomatic phenomena: A new look from the standpoint of recent experimental studies. American Journal of Clinical Hypnosis 21: 13–27

Barber T X, Chauncey H H, Winer R A 1964 Effects of hypnotic and non-hypnotic suggestion on parotid gland responses to gustatory stimuli. Psychosomatic Medicine 26: 374–380

Blakeslee T R 1980 The right brain. Anchor, New York

Borysenko M 1987 Area review: Psychoneuroimmunology. Annals of Behavioral Medicine 9: 3–10

Bradley B, McCanne T 1981 Autonomic responses to stress: The effects of progressive relaxation, the relaxation response and the expectancy of relief. Biofeedback and Self Regulation 6: 235–251

Donovan M 1980 Relaxation with guided imagery: A useful technique. Cancer Nursing 3: 27–32

Fiore N 1974 Fighting cancer: One patient's perspective. New England Journal of Medicine 300(6): 284–289

Graham H 1995 Mental imagery in health care: An introduction to therapeutic practice. Chapman & Hall, London

Jacobsen E 1929 Electrical measurement of neuromuscular states during mental activity e.g. imagination. American Journal of Physiology 91: 597–608

Jacobsen E 1930 Electrical measurement of neuromuscular states during mental activities. American Journal of Physiology 94: 24–34

Jacobsen E 1931 Electrical measurement of neuromuscular states during mental activities. American Journal of Physiology 96: 115–121

Kazdin A E, Wilcoxin L A 1975 Systematic desensitisation and non-specific treatment effects: A methodological evaluation. Psychological Bulletin 83(5): 729–758

Kubler-Ross E 1977 On death and dying. Tavistock, London

Laws D R, Rubin H B 1969 Instructional control of an autonomic response. Journal of Applied Behavioral Analysis 2: 93–99

Lyles J N, Burish T G, Krozely M G et al 1982 Efficacy of relaxation training and guided imagery in reducing the aversiveness of cancer chemotherapy. Journal of Consulting Clinical Psychology 50(4): 509–524

McAleney P J, Barabasz A, Baraabasz M 1990 Effects of flotation restricted environmental stimulation on intercollegiate tennis performance. Perceptual and Motor Skills 71: 1023–1028

Manning M 1989 Matthew Manning's guide to self-healing. Thorsons, Northants

Marks I, Huson J 1973 Physiological aspects of neutral and phobic imagery: Further observations. British Journal of Psychiatry 1222: 567–572

Marks I, Marset P, Boulougouris J et al 1971 Physiological accompaniments of neutral and phobic imagery. Psychological Medicine 1: 299–307

Marzillier J J, Carroll D, Newland J R 1979 Self-report and physiological changes accompanying repeated imagining of a phobic scene. Behaviour Research and Therapy 17: 71–77

Meares A 1981 Regression or recurrence of carcinoma of the breast at mastectomy site associated with intensive meditation. Australian Family Physician 2(2): 181–218

Sackett R S 1934 The influences of symbolic rehearsal upon the retention of a maze habit. Journal of General Psychology 10: 376–395

Sackett R S 1935 The relationship between amount of symbolic rehearsal and retention of a maze habit. Journal of General Psychology 13: 113–128

Schneider J et al 1988 Psychological factors influencing immune system function in normal subjects: A summary of research findings and implications for the use of guided imagery. Paper presented at the 10th Annual Conference of the American Association for the Study of Mental

Imagery, New Haven, CT. Cited in Sheikh A A, Kunzendorf R G, Sheikh K S 1989 Healing images: from ancient wisdom to modern science. In Sheikh A A, Sheikh K S (eds) Eastern and Western Approaches to Healing: Ancient Wisdom and Modern Knowledge. Wiley, New York, p 470–515

Schultz J H, Luthe W 1969 Autogenic training (Vol. 1). Grune & Stratton, New York

Schwartz G E, Weinberger D A, Singer J A 1981 Cardiovascular differentiation of happiness, sadness, anger and fear following imagery and exercise. Psychosomatic Medicine 43: 344–364

Simonton O C, Matthews-Simonton S 1975 Belief systems and management of the emotional aspects of malignancy. Journal of Transpersonal Psychology 82: 29–47

Simonton O C, Matthews-Simonton S, Creighton J L 1978 Getting well again: A step-by-step self-healing guide to overcoming cancer for clients and their families. Bantam, New York

Smith D, Over R D 1987 Fantasy-induced sexual behaviour habituate? Behavior Research and Therapy 25: 477–485

Stock W E, Greer J H 1982 A study of fantasy-based sexual arousal in women. Archives of Sexual Behavior 11: 33–47

Suedfield P, Collier D, Hartnett B 1993 Enhancing perceptual-motor accuracy through flotation REST. The Sport Psychologist 7: 151–159

Taylor R 1990 The immune system: Guardian of our chemical identity. Caduceus Winter: 26–30

Vealey R E, Walter S M 1993 Imagery training for performance enhancement and personal development. In: Williams J M (ed) Applied sport psychology: Personal growth to peak performance, 2nd edn. Mayfield, Mountain View, CA, p 200–224

Wagaman J D, Barabasz A, Barabasz M 1991 Flotation REST and imagery in the improvement of collegiate basketball performance. Perceptual and Motor Skills 79: 119–122

Chapter **11**

Pain and its management

Gregory S. Kolt

INTRODUCTION

Pain is a symptom of a variety of conditions treated and managed by physical and manual therapists. These conditions include injuries, as well as illnesses and diseases, many of which are covered in separate chapters of this book. In some circumstances, pain can also be associated with the usual components of treatment and rehabilitation administered by physical and manual therapists.

Pain can be debilitating and act as an obstacle to effective rehabilitation and recovery from illness and injury. Given that pain is still poorly understood, physical and manual therapists tend to spend too little time educating patients about pain. In particular, healthcare practitioners should increase their focus during rehabilitation on discussing with patients the large number of ways pain can affect them, and how they can manage it within the confines of their rehabilitation programs. Pain, and the psychological and physiological responses it evokes, if not adequately addressed, can greatly inhibit progress during rehabilitation.

People experience and interpret pain in a variety of ways. The way pain is communicated differs greatly from individual to individual, and is associated with factors such as gender, culture, age, social norms regarding acceptable pain behavior, and the type of the underlying injury, illness, or disease. Measuring and quantifying pain can be difficult, and at best, it can be relatively scaled, qualified, or described. The difficulty in quantifying pain makes working with individuals who are experiencing such symptoms challenging. It is important, however, to have an adequate understanding of the psychological and biological mechanisms of the pain process, and their interrelationships.

Healthcare practitioners working in the physical and manual therapies play an important role in assisting people with managing and coping with pain. For many clients, pain has become persistent, and influences many areas (and in some cases, all areas) of their everyday lives. Such pain can have a significant impact on functions including basic activities of daily living, occupations, personal relationships, and general quality of life. Having a thorough knowledge of the biopsychology of pain, theoretical explanations of pain, pain behavior, and pain management strategies is, therefore, essential for physical and manual therapists in designing effective interventions that integrate with other aspects of their management programs.

This chapter will provide physical and manual therapists with a background on the mechanisms of pain, theoretical explanations of pain, assessment methods for pain, and a range of pain management strategies. It is not, however, the aim of this chapter to provide a detailed and complex discussion of the neurophysiological aspects of pain, or describe particular approaches for managing pain in individual pathologies. The information presented will focus on general principles of pain and pain management that can be adapted and applied to a large number of conditions that physical and manual therapists encounter. A more detailed discussion on pain for healthcare practitioners can be found in Strong et al (2002b) and Monga & Grabois (2002).

DEFINITIONS AND MECHANISMS OF PAIN

There are several definitions of pain that have been used both clinically and in research. The most common definition used in the physical and manual therapies, and for most areas of health practice, has been that adopted by the International Association for the Study of Pain. That is, pain is an unpleasant sensory and emotional experience associated with actual or potential tissue damage, or described in terms of such damage (Merskey & Bogduk 1994). This definition is widely accepted for research and clinical purposes because it incorporates both psychological and physical experiences of pain. This definition also suggests that pain can be an indication of potential damage to tissue, without damage actually having taken place. The Merskey & Bogduk (1994) definition will be used to describe the phenomenon of pain throughout this chapter.

Melzack & Casey (1968) identified three interacting dimensions relevant to pain: sensory-discriminative, cognitive-evaluative, and motivational-affective. In their discussion, Melzack & Casey (1968) described the sensory-discriminative dimension as the ability to analyze the pain location, quality, and behavior. The cognitive-evaluative dimension relates to the individual's ability to perceive and evaluate the pain, and interpret it in light of previous pain experiences and knowledge about pain. The motivational-affective dimension refers to the emotional responses of an individual experiencing pain, and how these influence the response to the pain.

Several neuroanatomical structures are important in the recognition and transmission of pain. In particular, the nociceptors and spinal cord warrant discussion in the context of this chapter.

NOCICEPTORS

The nociceptive system of the nervous network is responsible for the sensation, transmission, and perception of pain. Nociceptors respond to stimuli that damage tissue, or those that have the potential to damage tissues, and are present in a variety of body tissues including skin, muscle, joint capsules, bone, blood vessels, peripheral nerve sheaths, meninges, and viscera (Galea 2002).

According to Heil & Fine (1999), the process of nociception involves four components: transduction, transmission, modulation, and perception. Transduction refers to the translation of noxious stimuli into electrical activity at the sensory nerve endings. During transmission, the transduced electrical impulses are propagated throughout the sensory nervous system. During the third stage, modulation, the nociceptive transmission is modified by a number of neural influences, including central, cortical, and peripheral sensory inputs. The fourth process, perception, describes the cognitive-emotional experience of pain from the resultant transduction, transmission, and modulation (Heil & Fine 1999).

The nociceptors usually have a threshold of excitation that is too high to be stimulated by normal innocuous stimuli. Their main function is to monitor the body for noxious stimuli (Charman 1994). Activation of the nociceptors, and subsequent input of nociceptive impulses into the central nervous system (CNS), ensures rapid, aversive, and non-conscious reflex responses to noxious stimuli. Noxious stimuli are carried predominantly by small-diameter thinly myelinated alpha-delta (A-δ) fibers and unmyelinated C fibers. The A-δ fibers conduct activity at 5–30 meters/second and carry well-localized sensations of sharp pricking pain. Conversely, the small-diameter unmyelinated C fibers conduct diffuse pain sensations (e.g., dull, not well localized, aching, and persistent) at a slower velocity (0.5–2 meters/second) (Torebjörk & Ochoa 1980).

There are three main types of nociceptors: unimodal, bimodal, and polymodal (Charman 1994). Unimodal nociceptors (predominantly A-δ fibers) are mechanosensitive or thermosensitive, and respond to sharp mechanical pressure or tissue temperatures of 45°C or more, respectively. The bimodal nociceptors (mainly A-δ mechano-heat receptors) also respond to mechanical and thermal stimulation, or a combination of both (Campbell & Meyer 1986). The majority of receptors, however, are polymodal (predominantly C fibers). These nociceptors respond to strong mechanical stimuli, as well as noxious thermal stimuli and chemical stimulation. These three types of nociceptors are found at the cutaneous (skin) and deeper levels (e.g., joint structures) (Charman 1994).

Joint nociceptors are located in several joint structures including ligaments, bone, periosteum, joint capsule, and the surrounding blood vessels. Such receptors include those that respond to high levels of pressure and extreme joint movement, and those that react to high levels of pressure but not to joint movement. Inflammation within a joint (e.g., with various forms of rheumatoid arthritis, see Chapter 17) activates all joint nociceptors (Galea 2002). The skeletal muscle nociceptors respond to a variety of mechanical (pressure, muscle stretch, or muscle contraction), thermal, and chemical stimuli. The visceral nociceptors respond to stimuli such as inflammation, tension, and ischemia (Galea 2002).

SPINAL CORD

In the spinal cord, the unmyelinated C fibers unite to form a single nerve fiber that enters the peripheral nerve sheath before reaching the dorsal root ganglion. The A-δ fibers travel as individual myelinated fibers to the dorsal root ganglion. When both of these fiber types enter the dorsal root of the spinal cord they separate; the myelinated fibers form the dorsomedial bundle and the unmyelinated fibers form the anterolateral bundle of the spinal cord (Figure 11.1) (Fitzgerald 1989).

In the spinal cord, the anterolateral ascending system carries information related to pain and temperature, as well as some tactile information (the dorsal column–medial lemniscal system carries most of the tactile information). The anterolateral system comprises the spinothalamic tract, the spinoreticular tract, and the spinomesencephalic tract. There are a number of ascending nociceptive pathways or tracts in the spinal cord that transmit pain sensations to the brain (Smith 1976). In particular, the lateral and anterior spinothalamic tracts receive axons that have crossed into the gray commissure and transport the impulses to the thalamus, the point at which they terminate (Mehler 1962). The spinothalamic tract relays information related to sharp, discriminatory, and spatial pain stimuli, predominantly of A-δ origin. Several more diffuse ascending pathways carry multisynaptic unmyelinated and thinly myelinated fibers (Charman 1994).

THEORETICAL PERSPECTIVES AND EXPLANATIONS OF PAIN

To implement effective pain management strategies, an understanding of the theoretical perspectives of pain is important. Two widely accepted and used theoretical conceptualizations of pain are the gate control theory of pain (Melzack 1986, Melzack & Wall 1965) and the parallel processing model of pain distress (Leventhal & Everhart 1979).

GATE CONTROL THEORY OF PAIN

The gate control theory of pain explains pain from a neurophysiological perspective, and conceptually, has been described as the most comprehensive and relevant of all pain theories for understanding the cognitive aspects of pain (Weisenberg 1999). The

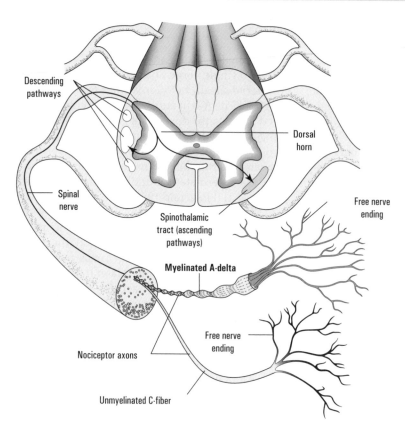

Figure 11.1 The spinal cord and peripheral nociceptors: pain transmission fibers from the periphery enter the central nervous system via the dorsal root and synapse within the dorsal horns of the spinal cord (reproduced with permission from Heil 1993)

predominant assumption in the gate control theory is that the substantia gelatinosa of the dorsal horns of the spinal cord contains a neural mechanism that acts as a pain gate (Melzack 1973, 1990, Melzack & Wall 1965). This gate can increase or decrease (i.e., control) the flow of nerve impulses from the peripheral nerves of the CNS by using the reciprocal activity of the large diameter A-β, the small diameter A-δ and the C fibers. The influence from the cortex, via the descending pyramidal and extrapyramidal tracts, can also contribute to the control of nerve impulses. When the amount of information that passes through the gate exceeds a critical level, the neural mechanisms responsible for the pain experience and control are activated. The A-β fibers can close the gate by depolarizing the intermedullary afferent terminals. This reduced effectiveness of the excitatory synapses decreases the perception of pain (Figure 11.2)

Melzack & Casey (1968) expanded the gate control theory of pain by suggesting different systems for the motivational, affective, and cognitive aspects of the pain experience. In these modifications, the sensory-discriminative information of pain (e.g., location, intensity, duration) is processed by the neospinothalamic projection, and the unpleasant affect and aversive (motivational) drive results from activation of the reticular and limbic areas. The neocortical area of the brain (higher center) can influence the sensory-discriminative and motivational-affective systems after evaluating past pain experience. The modified version of this theory is shown in Figure 11.3.

PARALLEL PROCESSING MODEL OF PAIN DISTRESS

The parallel processing model of pain distress focuses on the psychosocial influences that affect the pain experience. The model is based on the premise that pain is processed along two pathways: informational or emotional (Leventhal & Everhart 1979). The informational pathway deals with information including the location, the cause, and the sensory characteristics of pain. The emotional pathway is responsible for particular emotional responses to pain (e.g., avoidance, distress, fear) and a generalized

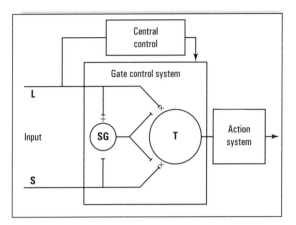

Figure 11.2 Schematic representation of the gate control theory of pain mechanisms: L = large diameter fibers; S = small diameter fibers; + = excitation; – = inhibition. The fibers project to the substantia gelatinosa (SG) and first central transmission (T) cells. The inhibitory effect exerted by the SG on the afferent fiber terminals is increased by activity in L fibers and decreased by activity in S fibers. The central control trigger is represented by a line running from the large fiber system to the central control mechanisms; these mechanisms, in turn, project back to the gate control system. The T cells project to the entry cells of the action system (reproduced with permission from Melzack R, Wall P D 1965 Pain mechanisms: A new theory. Science 150: 971–979. Copyright (1965) American Association for the Advancement of Science)

state of arousal. Individuals, through their historical experiences of pain, develop schemata comprising both informational and emotional components of painful events. When subsequent episodes of pain occur, the experience of that pain will be influenced by aspects of the particular pain schemata that are activated (Taylor & Taylor 1998). According to Leventhal & Everhart (1979), the main function of these schemata in the way pain is processed is in the selection of what people attend to when experiencing pain. Their research suggests that when people focus on informational elements of pain, they experience less pain than when they focus on its emotional aspects. This information has important clinical implications for pain management techniques. It could be that implementing approaches that distract people from emotional aspects of pain reduces the perception of that painful stimulus.

OTHER COMPONENTS IN EXPLAINING PAIN

The definition of pain being used throughout this chapter (Merskey & Bogduk 1994) highlights both the physiological and psychological aspects of the pain. Cognitive appraisals, beliefs, and attitudes can

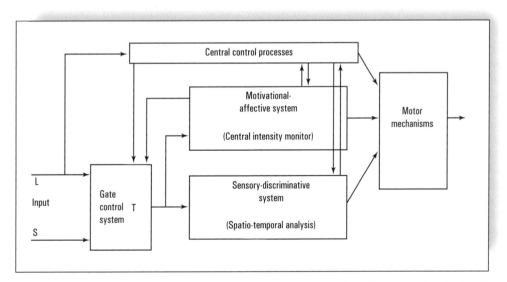

Figure 11.3 Conceptual model of the sensory, motivational and central determinants of pain. The output of the T cells of the gate-control system projects to the sensory-discriminative system (via neospinothalamic fibers) and the motivational-affective system (via the paramedial ascending system). The central control trigger is represented by a line running from the large fiber system to central control processes; these, in turn, project back to the gate-control system, and to the sensory-discriminative and motivation-affective systems. All three interact with one another, and project to the motor system (reproduced from Melzack R, Casey K L 1968 Sensory, motivational, and central control determinants of pain: A new conceptual model. In: Kenshalo R (ed) The skin senses. Courtesy of Charles C Thomas, Publisher, Ltd., Springfield, IL)

influence pain perception, and ultimately, the ways in which people cope with pain. For example, in some situations chronic pain can exist without any clearly defined underlying pathology. It is possible in such cases, that an individual will believe that underlying tissue damage is the cause, and reduce activity levels to avoid further damage to that tissue. This reduced physical activity may have a negative influence on the rehabilitation process.

Other psychological processes, such as stress, can also influence pain. Chapman & Gavrin (1999) suggested that long-term or persistent pain can promote a stress response producing neuroendocrine dysregulation, impaired mental and physical performance, fatigue, and dysphoria. Such stress can also lead to sleep difficulties and postural adaptations. These responses from stress can contribute to further pain in a cyclical manner.

Several environmental factors can also influence pain. These include secondary gains, family, and culture. Although there is a widely held belief that financial compensation (a particular type of secondary gain) can influence the pain experience, the evidence is not strong. Rohling et al (1995) reported, from a meta-analysis of 32 studies, that compensation status accounted for only a small proportion (6%) of the pain experience. Families can also exert a strong influence over the pain experience. For example, Unruh & Campbell (1999) reported that children model pain behavior from their parents. Further, Sternbach (1986) reported that adults were more likely to have a variety of musculoskeletal pain if their parents had severe pain at some point in their lives. Another factor that can influence pain is culture. Cross-cultural differences exist in many aspects of illness prevalence and healthcare usage (Main & Parker 2000). Although a large number of studies conducted on cultural differences in response to pain (e.g., back pain) exist (see Main & Parker 2000), little research has been carried out on cultural influences on the perception or experience of pain (Bates et al 1993). Bernstein & Pachter (1993) suggested that practitioners should be familiar with the health beliefs and practices common to cultural groups they work with, and accommodate such cultural issues within acceptable medical practice.

CONDITIONING OF PAIN BEHAVIORS

Pain behaviors can be conditioned in several ways. In basic psychological terms, respondent conditioning is defined as a learned association between a neutral stimulus and a reflexive response as a result of frequent co-occurrences. For example, when a person with osteoarthritis of the knee experiences an increase in nociceptive input they may grimace and adopt an antalgic posture. It may be that, for an individual, walking does not normally produce pain, but if that individual expects intense pain as they weight bear in walking they may emit learned responses such as limping, grimacing, and protecting the joint. In this case, the pain behavior that was previously produced only by actual pain in the knee is now being produced by walking.

Environment factors can also influence pain behavior. For example, if a person with lumbar spine pain receives sympathetic attention when they indicate signs of pain, a particular pattern of behavior is more likely to develop. In this case of operant conditioning, the pain behavior is not only a result of the nociceptive input, but is also a behavior that is being operantly maintained.

EXPERIENCE OF PAIN

DESCRIPTIONS OF PAIN

Melzack & Dennis (1980) suggested that, temporally, three different forms of pain can be distinguished, and that each of these is associated with distinct affective states (Craig 1994). These forms of pain are phasic, acute, and chronic. In addition, Crue (1983) described subacute pain and recurrent acute pain. Pain is not always an immediate consequence of injury or illness, and a large proportion of people report that pain emerges some time after the injury itself (Wall 1979).

Phasic pain

Phasic pain is of very short duration and suggests that injury has had an immediate impact (Craig 1994). Phasic pain often involves reactions such as reflexive withdrawal from the stimulus, non-verbal and expressive behaviors that are recognizable as pain to onlookers, and protective movements (Craig et al 1992). This initial reaction to the stimulus is subject to modulation dependent on the biological, physical, and social context in which it occurs.

Acute pain

Acute pain is caused by tissue damage and comprises a phasic state as well as a continued tonic state that persists until healing takes place (Craig 1994). Such pain is usually self-limited. That is, when the condition that produces the pain resolves (including blocking of the input by analgesic agents), the pain will be eliminated. Acute pain is most often associated with a well-defined cause (Elton 1995). Elton (1995) suggested that from a biochemical perspective, acute pain is similar to an anxiety state, in that excessive sympathetic nervous system activity occurs, and feelings of anxiety and fear develop. Weisenberg (1999) reported that the contradictory findings of the relationship between pain and anxiety may be accounted for by inconsistencies in definitions of pain between studies, a variable response bias due to people's willingness to complain of pain when anxious, and the moderating role that attention has on both pain and anxiety (Crombez et al 1998). Another complex factor that healthcare practitioners face when dealing with pain is that of causality. What needs to be considered with each individual is whether pain levels are leading to anxiety, whether high levels of anxiety are influencing pain, or whether both of these directional relationships are occurring. Physical and manual therapists should recognize that anxiety can be linked to both acute and chronic pain.

Chronic pain

A distinguishing factor in chronic pain is that the tonic component that begins after the phasic component is over can persist long after actual healing of the injury or illness. Chronic pain can be summarized as constant, persisting long after the initial injury, and comprising physical, social, and psychological components. A variety of definitions of chronic pain have been reported. For example, the American Medical Association (1988) described chronic pain as a syndrome in which pain has persisted beyond the normal time of healing, while the IASP (1986) has referred to chronic pain as one that is constant or recurring in nature, and that has endured for longer than 3 months. Despite the variety of definitions reported in the literature, chronic pain involves a prolonged time course, with an increasing likelihood of anxiety, depression, and social dysfunction as pain continues (Craig 1994). It is these psychosocial aspects of pain that physical and manual therapists should be giving more attention to, and integrating into their treatment and rehabilitation programs.

Healthcare practitioners often face the difficulty of deciding when acute pain becomes chronic. This distinction is often required for third-party insurers or compensation bodies, and is increasingly being required for medico-legal purposes. Equally as important, is the ability to make this distinction for the purpose of adopting effective approaches to helping people manage their pain. Although the term "chronic pain" suggests a temporal difference to acute pain, other features are important in distinguishing the two. Loeser (1996) reported that acute pain can lead to dorsal horn CNS changes that last longer than the nociceptive input from the periphery. The affective responses to perceived noxious stimuli may be related to individual genetics, mood, interpretation of the meaning of pain, and past pain experiences (Shipton 1999). Although it is difficult to clearly delineate acute from chronic, Thienhaus & Cole (1998) suggested that a telling sign that a pain problem is chronic is a letter of referral from one health practitioner to another that starts with an apology.

A particular aspect of chronic pain that is of relevance to physical and manual therapists is depressed mood or even clinical depression. Symptoms of depression in people with chronic pain range from minor (e.g., "feeling down") to a major depressive episode. Symptoms such as depressed mood, difficulties in concentration, appetite changes, sleep disturbances, and loss of interest in usual activities are common with chronic pain (Sullivan et al 1995). Despite the large number of attempts that have been made to explain the causal relationship between depression and pain, no definitive model is evident. Biomedical theories, psychodynamic theories, and theories based on past experiences have all been suggested. For example, Eich et al (1990) suggested that pain increases unpleasant affect, and through this pathway, promotes access to memories and thoughts of previous unpleasant events. The negative cognitions generated intensify the negative affect and perpetuate pain. Biomedical theories have suggested that depression and pain share common biological systems (Magni 1987). From a psychodynamic perspective, patients with chronic pain and those who are depressed both have an inability to modulate or express intense unacceptable feelings (Beutler et al 1986).

Subacute pain

Subacute pain refers to pain that is evident regularly but not on a constant basis (e.g., daily pain over several weeks) (Crue 1983). From the perspective of etiology and nociceptive mechanisms, subacute pain is similar to acute pain. According to Thienhaus & Cole (1998), once subacute pain has been present for greater than 6 months, the likelihood of complete relief is small. They also advocate that subacute pain responds better to the types of management approaches used for chronic pain rather than those used in acute pain.

Recurrent acute pain

Recurrent acute pain has been defined as the acute exacerbation of peripheral tissue pathology resulting from an underlying chronic pathology (e.g., headache, degenerative disk disease) (Crue 1983). Recurrent acute pain refers to discrete acute episodes that return over time. Whereas a good example of subacute pain would be daily pain for several weeks, several time-limited pain episodes over months or years could be described as recurrent acute pain (Thienhaus & Cole 1998).

The predominant reason for distinguishing between the various types of pain described above is to allow the practitioner to implement the management approach best suited to the quality and quantity of pain.

CLASSIFICATION OF PAIN

Classifying pain is complex, mostly due to the subjective nature of pain and the variety of physical and psychological presentations that are possible. Without an accepted and commonly used method of classifying pain, communication between practitioners is made difficult and open to misinterpretation. The IASP (1986) developed a pain classification system that has been of particular use for both research and clinical purposes. This system classifies pain by topography, organ system, and underlying pathology. More specifically, a five-axis coding scheme is used to describe various elements of pain.

- Axis I indicates the region of the pain (e.g., lumbar spine, upper limbs).
- Axis II indicates the organ system involved (e.g., nervous system, musculoskeletal system and connective tissue).
- Axis III indicates the temporal characteristics and pattern of occurrence of the pain (e.g., single episode of limited duration, continuous or nearly continuous and non-fluctuating).

- Axis IV pertains to the patient's statement of pain intensity and duration since onset (e.g., mild with a duration of 1 month or less; medium with a duration of 1 month or less).
- Axis V indicates the presumed etiology (e.g., inflammatory, trauma, burns, operation).

Axes III and IV are further divided into ten detailed gradations of severity (assigned numerical codes), easily allowing pretreatment to posttreatment comparisons.

By using the IASP classification for chronic pain, the physical and manual therapist can record important information on the definition, anatomical location, main features, associated symptoms, laboratory findings, usual course, and potential complications for the majority of pain problems. The system also summarizes information on the physical and social disabilities, pathology, diagnostic criteria, and differential diagnoses for chronic pain conditions. Despite the IASP system providing rich information, it is currently not in wide use (Thienhaus & Cole 1998). As the IASP system is based on inclusion rather than exclusion criteria, it probably has further potential to be used more widely. After all, pain syndromes are diagnosed by signs and symptoms that are present, as opposed to those that are not present. Further information on the IASP pain classification system can be found in the original source (IASP 1986).

PAIN THRESHOLDS AND TOLERANCE

Pain threshold has generally been defined as the point at which a person first reports pain. This point of pain is usually related to the way in which people experience pain. More specifically, however, Melzack & Wall (1996) reported several threshold points to pain, and suggested that distinguishing between them for clinical purposes is essential. The thresholds to pain are sensation threshold, pain perception threshold (lower threshold), pain perception threshold, pain tolerance (upper threshold), and encouraged pain tolerance (see Box 11.1).

Research has repeatedly shown that the majority of people (with normal central and peripheral nervous systems) have a uniform sensation threshold to recognize different stimuli (Charman 1994, Large et al 2002). That is, as stimulus intensity increases, the majority of people will indicate that they initially perceive sensation at a common baseline level. It is

---

> **Box 11.1 Definitions of the various thresholds to pain (Melzack & Wall 1996)**
>
> **Sensation threshold (or lower threshold)**
> The lowest stimulus value at which a sensation is reported
>
> **Pain perception threshold**
> The lowest stimulus at which a person reports that the stimulation feels painful
>
> **Pain tolerance (upper threshold)**
> The lowest stimulus level at which a person withdraws from the painful stimulus
>
> **Encouraged pain tolerance**
> The level at which the person withdraws from the stimulus after encouragement to tolerate higher levels of stimulation

the pain perception and pain tolerance thresholds that differ between people (Charman 1994, Large et al 2002). These can vary with mood and motivation, and across and within individuals.

There are a number of factors such as attention, depression, anxiety, past experiences with pain, age, coping skills, and social reinforcement that can influence an individual's perception of and tolerance to pain (Feuerstein & Beattie 1995, Harsha 1998, McCaffery & Pasero 1999, Melzack & Wall 1996). Despite some research indicating that increasing age is related to decreased tolerance to a variety of potentially painful stimuli (e.g., Jensen et al 1992), Harkins et al (1994) reviewed the literature and suggested that age does not significantly influence the sensory-discriminative dimension of pain experience in healthy older people. They do point out, however, that older people with health problems may experience pain in different ways than their younger counterparts.

Anxiety is another factor suggested to be related to pain. For example, Choinière et al (1989) found that in patients with burns, the more anxious they were, the more pain they reported. Further, support for the relationship between anxiety and pain comes from Cipher & Fernandez's (1997) work with chronic pain. Harsha (1998) has also reported that depression lowers pain tolerance, thereby increasing pain perception. This is important clinically when one considers that the experience of pain over

a prolonged period of time can manifest in depression, which in turn can lower pain tolerance, setting up a pain–depression cycle.

A particular population that physical and manual therapists often work with is athletes and those who participate in sport and physical activity (see Chapter 16). Some evidence exists that athletes have higher levels of pain tolerance than non-athletes (Tajet-Foxell & Rose 1995), and that differences in pain tolerance exist between participants in different sports (Egan 1988). Two general explanations for higher pain thresholds in athletes than non-athletes have been suggested. First, the exposure of athletes to physical training and increased fitness results in higher levels of circulating endogenous opioids, a factor in reducing pain perception. The second explanation relates to psychological factors. Athletes, as part of their training and performance, explore boundaries in relation to extreme physical activity and pain experience, giving a perception of control over the pain–physical activity interface (Tajet-Foxell & Rose 1995).

Given the variety of factors that can potentially influence pain, practitioners should be acutely aware of how to implement interventions that respect individual differences in pain tolerance, and work around those differences to target both the pathology itself, and the individual's interpretation of the painful event.

ASSESSMENT OF PAIN

The assessment of pain is something that is not often performed well in the physical and manual therapies. McCaffery & Pasero (1999) have suggested that the failure of practitioners to ask their patients about their pain is probably one of the more common causes of unrelieved pain. Research has shown that when healthcare practitioners do not assess pain or obtain pain ratings from their patients they are more likely to underestimate pain, particularly when it is in the moderate to severe range (Larue et al 1997, Zalon 1993). A common misconception regarding pain is that the best judge of pain existence and severity is the healthcare practitioner. As individuals experience pain in different ways, assessment of pain is central to understanding pain from the patient's perspective, and to show treatment effectiveness.

The literature contains a variety of pain assessment methods, and it is up to the healthcare practitioner to establish the most relevant method for a given case. Making pain tangible through the use of assessment tools ensures that pain is understood as important information that can facilitate rehabilitation (Taylor & Taylor 1998).

Physical and manual therapists predominantly use patients' subjective interpretations of their pain to gauge or measure changes brought about by intervention and rehabilitation programs (McDowell & Newell 1996). For a pain assessment method to be suitable, the method used must have clinical utility, be valid, reliable, and responsive (Sim & Arnell 1993, Strong et al 2002a). By clinical utility, I mean that the pain assessment method must be suitable for both the client and the clinical environment in which it is being used. Often, this approach means that it should be relatively quick to administer and provide information that is useful to the practitioner in deciding the most relevant form of intervention. Validity refers to the ability of an instrument to measure what it purports to measure, thereby allowing meaningful information to be gained from the data. Reliability relates to the extent to which an instrument yields the same measurement on repeated uses, either by different practitioners (interobserver reliability) or by the same practitioner (intra-observer reliability). Responsiveness refers to the capability of detecting relatively small but clinically important gradations of change.

TYPES OF PAIN MEASURES

There are three types of pain measures: self-report measures, observational measures, and physiological measures. Self-report measures are most often used in clinical settings because they fit with the definition of pain as a subjective phenomenon. These measures include pain scales, pain questionnaires, pain drawings, and pain diaries, and are all completed by the patient themselves, and thus, have limited use in certain populations (e.g., young children, people with impaired communication skills).

Observational measures involve direct observation of a patient's behavior and activity performance by a healthcare practitioner or someone else known to the patient. Although such measures take considerable time, they do relate to functional status of the individual and can provide important information to the practitioner regarding suitability of certain rehabilitation approaches. Observational

approaches have been shown to be more accurate for acute pain conditions. In chronic pain, many behaviors have become habitual and may not represent dysfunction directly resulting from the painful stimuli.

Physiological measures include heart rate, pulse, blood pressure, and muscle tension. Although such measures are useful, their clinical utility for physical and manual therapists is somewhat limited, and there are a variety of other factors than can influence such measures.

In this section I will focus predominantly on self-report measures of pain because they are used most commonly in clinical settings.

MEASUREMENT OF PAIN

A variety of measurements can be used to assess the degree and quality of pain during rehabilitation. Some examples include numerical rating scales (NRS), verbal rating scales (VRS), pain drawings (Ransford et al 1976), visual analogue scales (VAS; Huskisson 1983), the McGill Pain Questionnaire (MPQ; Melzack 1975), and the Short-form McGill Pain Questionnaire (SF-MPQ; Melzack 1987). A large number of scales can also be used to measure responses to pain and the impact of pain. It is not the intent of this chapter to review each of these measures in detail, but some of the more commonly used tools and their applications in the clinical environment will be highlighted.

Rating scales

VRSs are some of the more commonly used and extensively reviewed measures of pain (Bolton & Wilkinson 1998, Sim & Waterfield 1997). VRSs usually consist of a series of verbal descriptors of pain ordered from least to most intense (e.g., no pain, mild, moderate, severe) (Jensen & Karoly 1991). These scales are scored by allocating a value of zero to the least intense descriptor, a value of 1 to the next intense descriptor word, and so forth (Figure 11.4). Despite their ease of use, however, VRSs lack responsiveness (Sim & Waterfield 1997).

NRSs are commonly used and comprise a series of numbers (e.g., 0 to 10 or 0 to 100) anchored by words such as "no pain" and "extreme pain." Patients choose the number that best reflects their intensity of pain (Figure 11.5). Although these scales are simple, clear, and efficient, and therefore easy to use in clinical settings, they lack validity, as they

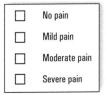

Figure 11.4   A verbal rating scale. The patient is instructed to mark the verbal description that best represents their pain

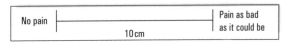

Figure 11.6   A horizontal visual analogue scale for pain intensity

represent only a single pain element (e.g., intensity) (Smith 1999). Adequate reliability has been demonstrated for both VRSs and NRSs (Melzack & Katz 1999), and Strong et al (1991) found that practitioners preferred the use of NRSs (along with VASs) over several other measures, when assessing patients with chronic pain. Responses given on measures like the VRS and NRS do not reflect the complexity of the pain experience as well as multidimensional pain measures might. McCaffery & Pasero (1999) have provided translations of NRSs in a variety of languages that can be reproduced for use in clinical practice. The languages include Chinese, French, German, Greek, Hebrew, Italian, Pakistani, Russian, and Vietnamese, among others.

The VAS most commonly takes the form of a 10 cm horizontal or vertical line that is anchored at each end with terms representing the minimum score (e.g., "no pain") and the maximum score (e.g., "worst ever pain") (Figure 11.6). Patients can rate their pain by placing a vertical mark on the 10-cm line that corresponds to the level of pain intensity they are experiencing. The VAS is scored by measuring the distance in millimeters between this mark and the left-hand end of the scale (in the case of a horizontal VAS). Strong et al (2002a) suggested that the horizontal scale is preferred in clinical practice. Although the reliability of the VAS has been shown to be high when repeatedly used on the same individual (Bowsher 1994, Collins et al 1997), it measures only a single aspect of pain (e.g., intensity) (Sim & Waterfield 1997). The responsiveness

of VASs is high due to the ability to mark a large number of points to reflect pain intensity.

VASs are commonly used due to their brevity of administration and scoring, minimal intrusiveness, and simplicity (Melzack & Katz 1999, Price et al 1983). VASs can also be used to measure other aspects of pain. For example, patients could be asked to rate the unpleasantness of the pain experience by using a VAS with anchors of "not bad at all" to "the most unpleasant feeling imaginable" (Price et al 1987).

Pain drawings

Pain drawings are a simple method by which patients can indicate on an outline drawing of the body (front and back) the location and type of pain they are experiencing (e.g., dull, sharp, aching). Although researchers have developed scoring systems based on the total body area in pain (e.g., Margolis et al 1986, 1988) they have not been widely used or investigated. Despite poor reliability, pain drawings do provide useful information on location and distribution of pain that can be used during rehabilitation sessions.

McGill Pain Questionnaire

The MPQ (Melzack 1975) is a multidimensional measure that includes a numerical intensity scale, a pain drawing, and a set of descriptor words. The MPQ is probably one of the most widely used measures of pain, and can provide valuable information on the sensory, affective, and evaluative dimensions of the pain experience. It has been shown to readily discriminate among different pain problems (Reading 1984). The MPQ (Figure 11.7) contains 20 groups of adjectives (ranging from two to six adjectives in each group) divided into four dimensions: sensory, affective, evaluative, and miscellaneous. Patients are instructed to choose one word in each category to describe their present pain. Quantitative scores (pain rating indices) can be obtained for each of the four dimensions, as well as an overall or total pain score. The MPQ also contains a pain drawing to record spatial distribution of the pain and words that describe the temporal

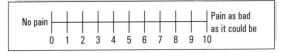

Figure 11.5   A numerical rating scale. The patient is instructed to mark the numbered vertical line as appropriate

McGill Pain Questionnaire

Patient's name _____ Date _____ Time _____ am/pm

PRI: S _____ A _____ E _____ M _____ PRI(T) _____ PPI _____
(1–10)   (11–15)   (16)   (17–20)   (1–20)

1 FLICKERING QUIVERING PULSING THROBBING BEATING POUNDING	11 TIRING EXHAUSTING
	12 SICKENING SUFFOCATING
2 JUMPING FLASHING SHOOTING	13 FEARFUL FRIGHTFUL TERRIFYING
3 PRICKING BORING DRILLING STABBING LANCINATING	14 PUNISHING GRUELLING CRUEL VICIOUS KILLING
4 SHARP CUTTING LACERATING	15 WRETCHED BLINDING
5 PINCHING PRESSING GNAWING CRAMPING CRUSHING	16 ANNOYING TROUBLESOME MISERABLE INTENSE UNBEARABLE
6 TUGGING PULLING WRENCHING	17 SPREADING RADIATING PENETRATING PIERCING
7 HOT BURNING SCALDING SEARING	18 TIGHT NUMB DRAWING SQUEEZING TEARING
8 TINGLING ITCHY SMARTING STINGING	19 COOL COLD FREEZING
9 DULL SORE HURTING ACHING HEAVY	20 NAGGING NAUSEATING AGONIZING DREADFUL TORTURING
10 TENDER TAUT RASPING SPLITTING	**PPI** 0 NO PAIN 1 MILD 2 DISCOMFORTING 3 DISTRESSING 4 HORRIBLE 5 EXCRUCIATING

BRIEF MOMENTARY TRANSIENT	RHYTHMIC PERIODIC INTERMITTENT	CONTINUOUS STEADY CONSTANT

E = EXTERNAL

I = INTERNAL

COMMENTS:

Figure 11.7 McGill Pain Questionnaire. The descriptors fall into four major groups: sensory, 1–10; affective, 11–15; evaluative, 16; and miscellaneous, 17–20. The rank value for each descriptor is based on its position in the word set. The sum of the rank values is the pain rating index (PRI). The present pain intensity (PPI) is based on a scale of 0–5 (reprinted from Pain, 1, Melzack R, The McGill Pain Questionnaire: Major properties and scoring methods, p 227–299, Copyright (1975), with permission of International Society for the Study of Pain)

properties of the pain. The MPQ also includes a present pain intensity (PPI) scale that measures the pain intensity at the time of completion of the questionnaire.

The MPQ is a widely used tool in both research and clinical settings and has been translated into several languages. It has good clinical utility in identifying the many qualitative features of a person's pain. The reliability and validity of the MPQ are well established (see Melzack & Katz 1999). In relation to clinical utility, the MPQ usually takes up to 10 minutes to administer (Melzack 1987). Hence, many people have sought a shortened version for more regular use.

Short-form McGill Pain Questionnaire

The SF-MPQ (Melzack 1987) (Figure 11.8) incorporates elements of the MPQ but allows for a quick and simple gathering of pain data. The SF-MPQ has three components: a descriptive component, the PPI, and a VAS. The descriptive component contains 15 descriptors (11 sensory and four affective) that patients rate on an intensity scale (0 = none, 1 = mild, 2 = moderate, and 3 = severe). The PPI is the same as that used in the MPQ (see above), and the VAS is anchored by the terms "no pain" and "worst possible pain." The PPI and VAS are included to provide indices of overall pain intensity. The SF-MPQ has been shown to be highly correlated with the sensory, affective, and total pain rating indice scores of the MPQ (Melzack 1987), and is highly sensitive to clinical changes brought about by various therapies (Melzack & Katz 1999). High content validity has also been demonstrated for the SF-MPQ (Melzack & Katz 1992). Using a VAS in this questionnaire has been shown to enhance the test–retest reliability beyond that of the MPQ (Bowsher 1994).

Measuring responses to pain

An individual's response to pain depends on several factors including psychological states and traits, previous experience with pain, and cultural practices. Therefore, when evaluating pain it is often necessary to assess attitudes to pain, coping strategies, pain beliefs, and pain self-efficacy. Although this chapter does not contain a review of a large number of questionnaires that can assess components of pain responses, Strong et al (2002a) summarized many measures (Table 11.1). Readers can source further details on each questionnaire from the original references.

MANAGEMENT OF PAIN

Management of most forms of pain is complex and usually comprises several forms of therapy or interventions being used concurrently. Often, combinations of physical and manual therapies, pharmacological treatment, and cognitive behavioral interventions are used. Given that each pain experience can be influenced by a variety of factors, it is important to focus more broadly than just the presenting signs and symptoms. Consideration of the impact of pain on the individual and all aspects of their lives is integral to successful rehabilitation and pain management.

This section will outline some guiding principles of approaches to managing pain. Specific chapters of this book cover particular psychological approaches that can be used for pain management and readers will be referred to those chapters where appropriate. Readers are also referred to Weiner (1998a, 1998b) for a more detailed account of pain management.

PHYSICAL AND MANUAL REHABILITATION THERAPIES

Although it is not the intent of this chapter to cover specific physical and manual therapy techniques that can be used to manage pain, it is important to note that the amount of time spent on such interventions allows the integration of more psychological approaches into overall management strategies. Many patients who consult physical and manual therapists do so because of a pain complaint. For example, rarely does a patient present complaining of poor gait biomechanics, but rather, they will present with knee and back pain that, upon assessment, is linked to poor biomechanical sequencing of their gait. The physical therapist will probably attend to both the presenting pain, and the underlying cause of that pain, as well as the broader impact that the pain can have on their lives.

The typical modalities that physical and manual therapists use in managing pain include electrophysical agents (e.g., transcutaneous electrical nerve stimulation, a variety of thermal agents, several electrical modalities), manual techniques (e.g., joint mobilization and manipulation, soft tissue massage), exercise, and interventions that change movement patterns thought to provoke pain (for a general review of these approaches to

Short-form McGill Pain Questionnaire
Ronald Melzack

Patient's name _____ Date _____

	NONE	MILD	MODERATE	SEVERE
THROBBING	0) ____	1) ____	2) ____	3) ____
SHOOTING	0) ____	1) ____	2) ____	3) ____
STABBING	0) ____	1) ____	2) ____	3) ____
SHARP	0) ____	1) ____	2) ____	3) ____
CRAMPING	0) ____	1) ____	2) ____	3) ____
GNAWING	0) ____	1) ____	2) ____	3) ____
HOT-BURNING	0) ____	1) ____	2) ____	3) ____
ACHING	0) ____	1) ____	2) ____	3) ____
HEAVY	0) ____	1) ____	2) ____	3) ____
TENDER	0) ____	1) ____	2) ____	3) ____
SPLITTING	0) ____	1) ____	2) ____	3) ____
TIRING-EXHAUSTING	0) ____	1) ____	2) ____	3) ____
SICKENING	0) ____	1) ____	2) ____	3) ____
FEARFUL	0) ____	1) ____	2) ____	3) ____
PUNISHING-CRUEL	0) ____	1) ____	2) ____	3) ____

No pain |————————————————————| Worst possible pain

PPI
0   NO PAIN   ____
1   MILD   ____
2   DISCOMFORTING   ____
3   DISTRESSING   ____
4   HORRIBLE   ____
5   EXCRUCIATING   ____

Figure 11.8   The Short-form McGill Pain Questionnaire. Descriptors 1–11 represent the sensory dimension of pain experience and 12–15 represent the affective dimension. Each descriptor is ranked on an intensity scale of 0 = none, 1 = mild, 2 = moderate, 3 = severe. The present pain intensity (PPI) of the standard long-form McGill Pain Quesionnaire and the visual analogue scale are also included to provide overall pain intensity scores (reprinted from Pain, 30, Melzack R, The Short-form McGill Pain Questionnaire, p 191–197, Copyright (1987), with permission of International Society for the Study of Pain)

Table 11.1 Commonly used evaluations for pain responses (adapted from Strong et al 2002a with permission from Churchill Livingstone)

Assessment	Style	Psychometric status	Utility
Fear-avoidance beliefs questionnaire (Waddell et al 1993)	Self-report 16 items on a single page	Only the initial study so far, however this showed good reliability, and a relatively stable 2-factor structure	To measure fear-avoidance beliefs about work and physical activity, specifically for patients with low back pain
Movement and pain predictions scale (MAPPS) (Council et al 1988)	Ten items on a 10-point rating scale with sequential drawings of particular movements	Correlations between 7 of the self-efficacy responses and actual movements	Assesses self-efficacy expectations, pain response expectancies and the reason for not completing the movement
Survey of Pain Attitudes – Revised (SOPA-R) (Jensen & Karoly 1991)	Self-report (57 items) 5-point Likert scale	Internal consistency, discriminant validity, construct validity, and factor structure are all adequate	Assesses seven beliefs which may affect long-term adjustment to chronic pain Is of most value for chronic low back pain
The Guage (Gage et al 1994)	Self-report 27 items on a 1–10-point Likert scale	Has shown good internal consistency and test–retest reliability Convergent validity supported	Assesses the person's confidence in their ability to do a range of basic activities at home, without help
Illness Behaviour Questionnaire (Pilowsky & Spence 1983)			Seven scales to assess abnormal illness behavior in chronic pain and other conditions where the patient's response may appear discrepant to the physical pathology. This is widely used
Coping Strategies Questionnaire (Robinson et al 1997)	Self-report		To determine the use of cognitive and behavioral coping strategies used to deal with pain This is widely used
Pain Beliefs and Perceptions Inventory (Williams & Thorn 1989)	Self-report Has 16 items	Some debate about whether it has 3 or 4 valid subscales	This tool has some usage, but not as broadly as the SOPA-R
Pain Self-Efficacy Questionnaire (PSEQ) (Nicholas 1994)	Self-report on a 10-item questionnaire, using a 7-point scale	Internal consistency and test-retest reliability acceptable Support for construct and concurrent validity	Developed specifically for chronic pain To rate confidence in performing activities despite pain

pain management see Weiner (1998a, 1998b)). What is important in relation to these approaches, is that psychological techniques can be taught and used with patients while these more physical techniques are being used. For example, if a patient is receiving some form of heat or electrical treatment, time would be well spent on relaxation techniques to reduce pain or imagery to distract the person from painful stimuli.

Manual therapy techniques (e.g., joint mobilization and soft tissue massage) are often used by healthcare practitioners. Some of these techniques, despite best intentions of practitioners, are uncomfortable or even painful when being administered.

This pain can potentially cause reflex muscle contraction that contributes to further pain from the techniques. It stands to reason, that cognitive skills such as relaxation, imagery, and dissociation could be used to reduce the pain during these facets of rehabilitation.

Exercise is commonly used in the physical and manual therapies and plays an important role in the management of long-term or chronic pain (Carabelli et al 1998). Aside from the evidence available for the physical benefits of exercise in patients with pain (e.g., muscle strength, muscle endurance, flexibility, changes in body composition), exercise is important in improving several psychological aspects of pain. For example, Bahrke & Morgan (1978) suggested that exercise distracts people from stressful stimuli (e.g., pain). Another suggestion indicates that people assess their self-efficacy in physical activities by using levels of fatigue, fitness, and pain. Therefore, as fitness increases through exercise, feelings of pain and fatigue will reduce, and self-efficacy should be increased resulting in a further desire to continue exercise (Petruzzello et al 1991).

Another important area of pain management is the use of pharmacological agents. To improve the effectiveness of this form of therapy, patients need to be adherent to medication regimes. Chapter 4 outlines the various psychological factors that can influence adherence to health and rehabilitation procedures, many of which can be applied to the use of pharmacological therapy. These include self-efficacy and self-motivation, and should be considered by healthcare practitioners when establishing the most comprehensive approach to pain management.

COGNITIVE BEHAVIORAL THERAPIES

Physical and manual therapists (in addition to many other healthcare practitioners) are becoming increasingly aware of psychosocial factors that influence injury and illness, and are enhancing their management skills by adding a psychological dimension (see Chapter 1). Due to their work, physical and manual therapists are in ideal situations to provide some form of basic psychological assistance to aid the rehabilitation process (Kolt 2000, Ninedek & Kolt 2000). Given that pain, and particularly chronic pain, has psychosocial elements, knowledge of managing pain from a cognitive behavioral perspective may be useful. I am not suggesting that

physical and manual therapists perform the work of psychologists, because such factors would clearly be crossing professional and ethical boundaries. Rather, physical and manual therapists should be integrating basic cognitive behavioral skills into their approaches to treatment and rehabilitation, and be able to recognize more significant issues that need to be referred to a psychologist for management.

Psychological approaches to pain management focus predominantly around cognitive behavioral techniques (CBTs) (see Chapter 8). CBTs are techniques that address patients' cognitions (thought processes) and behaviors. Techniques often used include those aimed at reducing pain, those that change a patient's focus on their pain, and those that teach people how to cope with pain. I strongly emphasize the education of patients about their pain and injury or illness. As physical and manual therapists, that is something we do well, but should be further enhanced using cognitive behavioral principles.

Turk & Okifuji (1999) suggested that the cognitive behavioral approach to pain management is based around the following five assumptions.

1. People are active processors of information and not passive reactors.
2. Thoughts can influence mood, affect physiological processes, can serve as an impetus for behavior, and can have a variety of social consequences. The converse can also occur: that is, mood, physiological changes, environmental factors, and behavior can influence cognitive processes.
3. Behavior is reciprocally determined by both the individual, and environmental factors.
4. Individuals have the ability to learn more adaptive ways of thinking, feeling, and behaving.
5. Individuals should be active and collaborative in changing their maladaptive thoughts, feelings, and behaviors.

There are a number of common features in different psychological approaches used in managing pain (Turk & Holzman 1986). The features are:

- encouraging the patient to reconceptualize their pain
- instilling optimism
- individualizing the treatment to the patient and their needs
- encouraging the patient to play an active role (and take some responsibility) in the treatment

- encouraging patients to actively participate in the intervention
- encouraging self-efficacy in the patient
- having the patient acknowledge their successes in the rehabilitation.

These are all approaches that physical and manual therapists are taught and that can be integrated with the other more physical techniques that they use in practice.

A brief summary of some CBTs and other psychological techniques that can be useful in the management of pain follows. More detailed information on the use of these techniques can be found in Chapter 8 (Cognitive and behavioral interventions), Chapter 9 (Relaxation techniques), and Chapter 10 (Imagery). As suggested above, the management of pain usually works best with several forms of therapy being used concurrently.

Pain reconceptualization

Reconceptualizing pain from being vague, undifferentiated, and overwhelming to being addressable, manageable, and controlled is an important feature of cognitive behavioral approaches. Education of the patient on the basis and causes of pain, and the treatment and rehabilitation program is an important part of reconceptualization. Reconceptualization encourages a change in perception of pain (from one that is predominantly sensory) to a more broader view with cognitive, affective, and socio-environmental factors considered as contributors to the experience of pain (Turk & Okifuji 1999). This approach can provide patients with better control over aspects of their lives, even if the pain itself is not eradicated.

Relaxation

A large number of relaxation techniques have been reported in the literature (see Chapter 9). One approach is to use relaxation techniques that target muscular relaxation (e.g., progressive relaxation, Jacobson 1938). This is based on the premise that pain can elicit muscle tension, that in turn, restricts blood flow and further increases pain (Cousins & Phillips 1985). Progressive relaxation involves systematically relaxing major skeletal muscle groups by firstly recognizing the muscle tension that is present (by contracting the muscles), and then by relaxing that muscle group. As the individual becomes more familiar with the technique, they can simply relax muscle groups from whatever condition it is in at rest, rather than having to contract

muscle groups first. This point is important given the divided opinion on the value of muscle contraction before relaxation (Lucic et al 1991, O'Bannon et al 1987, Payne 2000). When working with people with pain, it is important to monitor that the level of muscle contraction used in the exercise does not aggravate symptoms of pain (both at the time of the exercise and later).

Benson's relaxation response (Benson 1975) is another commonly used technique. This technique is based on the suggestion that there are four common elements underlying the elicitation of a relaxation response: a quiet environment, which allows for the reduction of external distractions; adopting a comfortable position to reduce undue muscular tension; having an object to dwell on, such as the repetition of a word; and adopting a passive attitude that includes emptying all other thoughts from the mind, and allowing distracting thoughts that do return to pass by while returning to a highly focused state. The relaxation response involves a focus on breathing, repetition of a word in time with breathing, and in more recent adaptations, imagery that focuses on an object that moves in time with the person's breathing (Kolt & McConville 2000). Wallace et al (1971) suggested that the relaxation response works by reducing the sympathetic nervous system activity that can accentuate pain. Aspects of this relaxation technique can act as distractions, drawing focus away from the pain and onto the more pleasant feeling of relaxation. The technique also provides a greater sense of control over pain and a reduction in the negative emotions associated with the pain and injury (Taylor & Taylor 1998).

For a more detailed account of similar relaxation techniques refer to Chapter 9 and Payne (2000).

Imagery

A variety of types of imagery have been used in healthcare (see Chapter 10), and specifically in pain management. Imagery of pleasant situations, guided by either a practitioner or by the patient, is an internal dissociative strategy that has been shown to be effective in reducing pain in medical and sport settings (Whitmarsh & Alderman 1993). Imagery generally involves a patient imagining themselves in a relaxing environment (i.e., one that has a relaxing meaning to that person), and focusing on how it feels to be in that environment. This form of imagery encourages the distracting of the patient from pain. A number of types of imagery have also been developed and used for pain management (Ievleva & Orlick 1999) where patients imagine the pain being washed away or see "cool" colors soothing and reducing any inflammation and pain that may be present. Ievleva & Orlick (1999) presented some examples including imagining cool blue colors running through the painful area, imagining the pain exiting the body, and imagining a cold ice pack over the painful area. For a more detailed account of imagery techniques refer to Chapter 10.

Association and dissociation

Association involves having patients focus their attention on their pain. As strange as this sounds (given the variety of distraction methods used in pain management), Taylor & Taylor (1998) suggested that such techniques allow patients to use their pain to learn the extent to which they can push themselves in rehabilitation. Heil (1993) suggested that association methods can increase perceptions of control over pain, heighten body awareness, and encourage a sense of emotional detachment. This emotional detachment can, in turn, act to separate the sensory aspects of pain from its physical presentation.

Dissociative strategies have also been recommended in pain management. Such strategies involve directing a patient's attention away from the pain to make it more manageable (Fisher 1999). A variety of distraction methods can be used including exercise, relaxation techniques, or listening to music. Fisher (1999) suggested that dissociation strategies are more effective for increasing pain threshold than are associative strategies. An obvious clinical implication of this strategy is to prepare patients for painful aspects of treatment.

Self-efficacy

Improving self-efficacy is another method commonly used in pain management. Self-efficacy refers to the conviction that one has about being able to successfully execute the behavior required to produce a certain outcome (Bandura 1977). For example, for a person with pain from osteoarthritis of the knee, self-efficacy would relate to their belief that they can do something about the pain. The encouragement of higher levels of self-efficacy by the physical and manual therapist should be an underlying aspect of all communications with patients during treatment and rehabilitation.

SUMMARY

Managing pain is complex. Pain is a subjective experience, and two people with the same presenting injury or illness could experience and report pain in vastly different ways. An understanding of the mechanisms of pain and how pain can influence rehabilitation and other areas of people's lives is integral to effective rehabilitation. The pain management techniques outlined in this chapter have their place in the clinic and at home. The strong message in the extensive pain management literature is that to be effective, pain management should combine both physical and psychosocial techniques.

References

American Medical Association 1988 Guides to the evaluation of permanent impairment, 3rd edn. American Medical Association, Washington, DC

Bahrke M S, Morgan W P 1978 Anxiety reduction following exercise and meditation. Cognitive Therapy and Research 2: 323–333

Bandura A 1977 Self-efficacy: Toward a unifying theory of behavioral change. Psychological Review 84: 191–215

Bates M S, Edwards W T, Anderson K O 1993 Ethnocultural influences on variation in chronic pain perception. Pain 52: 101–112

Benson H 1975 The relaxation response. William Morrow, New York

Bernstein B A, Pachter L M 1993 Cultural considerations in children's pain. In: Schechter N L, Berde C B, Yaster M (eds) Pain in infants, children and adolescents. Williams & Wilkins, Baltimore, MD, p 113–122

Beutler L E, Engel D, Oro-Beutler M E, Daldrup R, Meredith K 1986 Inability to express intense affect: A common link between depression and pain. Journal of Consulting and Clinical Psychology 54: 652–759

Bolton J E, Wilkinson R A 1998 Responsiveness of pain scales: A comparison of three pain intensity measures in chiropractic patients. Journal of Manipulative and Physiological Therapeutics 21: 1–7

Bowsher D 1994 Acute and chronic pain and assessment. In: Wells P E, Frampton V, Bowsher D (eds) Pain management by physiotherapy, 2nd edn. Butterworth-Heinemann, Oxford, p 39–43

Campbell J N, Meyer R A 1986 Primary afferents and hyperalgesia. In Yaksh T L (ed) Spinal afferent processing. Plenum Press, New York, p 59–81

Carabelli R A, Pertes S M, Koob K, Ames P F 1998 The role of exercise in the management of chronic pain. In: Weiner R S (ed) Pain management. A practical guide for clinicians (Vol 2), 5th edn. St. Lucie Press, Boca Baton, FL, p 549–562

Chapman C R, Gavrin J 1999 Suffering: The contributions of persistent pain. The Lancet 353: 2233–2237

Charman R A 1994 Pain and nociception: Mechanisms and modulation in sensory context. In: Boyling J D, Palastanga N (eds) Grieve's modern manual therapy, 2nd edn. Churchill Livingstone, Edinburgh, p 253–270

Choinière M, Melzack R Rondeau J et al 1989 The pain of burns: Characteristics and correlates. Journal of Trauma 29: 1531–1539

Cipher D J, Fernandez E 1997 Expectancy variables predicting tolerance and avoidance of pain in chronic pain patients. Behaviour Research and Therapy 35: 437–444

Collins S L, Moore R A, McQuay H J 1997 The visual analogue pain intensity scale: What is moderate pain in millimetres? Pain 72: 95–97

Cousins M J, Phillips G D 1985 Acute pain management. Clinics in Critical Care Medicine 8: 82–117

Council J R, Ahern D K, Follick M J et al 1988 Expectancies and functional impairment in chronic low back pain. Pain 33: 323–331

Craig K D 1994 Emotional aspects of pain. In: Wall P D, Melzack R (eds) Textbook of pain, 3rd edn. Churchill Livingstone, Edinburgh, p 261–274

Craig K D, Prkachin K M, Grunan R V E 1992 The facial expression of pain. In: Turk D C, Melzack R (eds) Handbook of pain assessment. Guilford Press, New York, p 257–276

Crombez G, Eccleston C, Baeyens F, Eelen P 1998 When somatic information threatens, catastrophic thinking enhances attentional interference. Pain 75: 187–198

Crue B L 1983 The neurophysiology and taxonomy of pain. In: Brena S F, Chapman S L (eds) Management of patients with chronic pain. Spectrum, New York, p 21–31

Egan S 1988 Acute pain tolerance amongst athletes. Physiotherapy in Sport 11(2): 11–13

Eich E, Rachman S, Lopatka C 1990 Affect, pain, and autobiographic memory. Journal of Abnormal Psychology 99: 174–178

Elton D 1995 Injury and pain. In Zuluaga M, Briggs C, Carlisle J et al (eds) Sports physiotherapy. Applied science and practice. Churchill Livingstone, Edinburgh, p 77–91

Feuerstein M, Beattie P 1995 Biobehavioural factors affecting pain and disability in low back pain: Mechanisms and assessment. Physical Therapy 75: 267–280

Fisher A C 1999 Counseling for improved rehabilitation adherence. In: Ray R, Wiese-Bjornstal D M (eds) Counseling in sport medicine. Human Kinetics, Champaign, IL, p 275–292

Fitzgerald M 1989 The course and termination of primary afferent fibres. In: Wall P D, Melzack R (eds) Textbook of pain, 2nd edn. Churchill Livingstone, Edinburgh, p 46–62

Gage M, Noh S, Polatajko H J 1994 Measuring perceived self-efficacy in occupational therapy. American Journal of Occupational Therapy 48: 783–790

Galea M P 2002 Neuroanatomy of the nociceptive system. In: Strong J, Unruh A M, Wright A, Baxter G D (eds) Pain. A textbook for therapists. Churchill Livingstone, Edinburgh, p 13–41

Harkins S W, Price D D, Bush F M et al 1994 Geriatric pain. In: Wall P D, Melzack R (eds) Textbook of pain, 3rd edn. Churchill Livingstone, Edinburgh, p 769–784

Harsha W 1998 Understanding and treating low back pain. In: Weiner R S (ed) Pain management. A practical guide for clinicians (Vol 1), 5th edn. St. Lucie Press, Boca Raton, FL, p 231–238

Heil J 1993 Psychology of sport injury. Human Kinetics, Champaign, IL

Heil J, Fine P G 1999 Pain in sport: A biopsychological perspective. In: Pargman D (ed) Psychological bases of sport injuries, 2nd edn. Fitness Information Technology, Morgantown, WV, p 13–28

Huskisson E C 1983 Visual analogue scales. In: Melzack R (ed) Pain measurement and assessment. Raven, New York, p 33–37

Ievleva L, Orlick T 1999 Mental paths to enhanced recovery from a sports injury. In Pargman D (ed) Psychological bases of sport injuries, 2nd edn. Fitness Information Technology, Morgantown, WV, p 199–220

International Association for the Study of Pain 1986 Classification of chronic pain: Descriptions of chronic pain syndromes and definitions of pain terms. Pain 27: S1–S225

Jacobson E 1938 Progressive relaxation. University of Chicago Press, Chicago

Jensen M P, Karoly P 1991 Control beliefs, coping efforts, and adjustments to chronic pain. Journal of Consulting and Clinical Psychology 59: 431–438

Jensen R, Rasmussen, B K, Pederson B et al 1992 Cephalic muscle tenderness and pressure pain threshold in a general population. Pain 48: 197–203

Kolt G S 2000 Doing sport psychology with injured athletes. In: Andersen M B (ed) Doing sport psychology. Human Kinetics, Champaign, IL, p 223–236

Kolt G S, McConville L C 2000 The effects of a Feldenkrais Awareness Through Movement program on state anxiety. Journal of Bodywork and Movement Therapies 4: 216–220

Large R G, New F, Strong J et al 2002 Chronic pain and psychiatric problems. In: Strong J, Unruh A M, Wright A, Baxter G D (eds) Pain. A textbook for therapists. Churchill Livingstone, Edinburgh, p 425–442

Larue F, Fontaine A, Colleau S M 1997 Underestimation and undertreatment of pain in HIV disease: A multicentre study. British Medical Journal 3144: 23–28

Leventhal H, Everhart D 1979 Emotion, pain and physical illness. In: Izard C E (ed) Emotions in personality and psychopathology. Plenum, New York

Loeser J D 1996 Pain: Concepts and management. 150 years on – a selection of papers presented at the 11th World Congress of Anaesthesiologists. Bridge, Rosebery, Australia

Lucic K S, Steffen J J, Harrigan J A, Stuebing R C 1991 Progressive relaxation training: Muscle contraction before relaxation? Behavior Therapy 22: 249–256

McCaffery M, Pasero C 1999 Assessment: Underlying complexities, misconceptions, and practical tools. In: McCaffery M, Pasera C (eds) Pain. Clinical manual, St. Louis, MO, Mosby, p 35–102

McDowell I, Newell C 1996 Measuring health: A guide to rating scales and questionnaires, 2nd edn. Oxford University Press, New York

Magni G 1987 On the relationship between chronic pain and depression when there is no organic lesion. Pain 31: 1–21

Main C J, Parker H 2000 Social and cultural influences on pain and disability. In: Main C J, Spanswick C C (eds) Pain management. An interdisciplinary approach. Churchill Livingstone, Edinburgh, p 43–61

Margolis R B, Tait R C, Krause S J 1986 A rating system for use with patient pain drawings. Pain 24: 57–65

Margolis R B, Chibnall J T, Tait R C 1988 Test-retest reliability of the pain drawing instrument. Pain 33: 49–51

Mehler W R 1962 The anatomy of the so-called 'pain tract' in man: An analysis of the course and distribution of the ascending fibres of the fasciculus anterolateralis. In French J D, Porter R W (eds) Basic research in paraplegia. Thomas, Springfield, IL

Melzack R 1973 The puzzle of pain. Penguin, Harmondsworth, UK

Melzack R 1975 The McGill Pain Questionnaire: Major properties and scoring methods. Pain 1: 227–299

Melzack R 1986 Neurophysiological foundations of pain. In: Sternbach R A (ed) The psychology of pain. Raven, New York

Melzack R 1987 The Short-form McGill Pain Questionnaire. Pain 30: 191–197

Melzack R 1990 The tragedy of needless pain. Scientific American 262: 19–25

Melzack R, Casey K L 1968 Sensory, motivational, and central control determinants of pain: A new conceptual model. In: Kenshalo R (ed) The skin senses. Thomas, Springfield, IL, p 423–443

Melzack R, Dennis S G 1980 Phylogenic evolution of pain expression in animals. In: Kosterlitz H W, Terenius L Y (eds) Pain and society. Verlag Chemie, Weinheim

Melzack R, Katz J 1992 The McGill Pain Questionnaire: Appraisal and current status. In: Turk D C, Melzack R (eds) Handbook of pain assessment. Guilford Press, New York, p 152–168

Melzack R, Katz J 1999 Pain measurement in persons with pain. In: Wall P D, Melzack R (eds) Textbook of pain, 4th edn. Churchill Livingstone, Edinburgh, p 409–420

Melzack R, Katz J 2001 The McGill Pain Questionnaire: Appraisal and current status. In Turk D C, Melzack R (eds) The handbook of pain assessment, 2nd edn. Guilford Press, New York, p 35–52

Melzack R, Wall P D 1965 Pain mechanisms: A new theory. Science 150: 971–979

Melzack R, Wall P D 1996 The challenge of pain, 2nd edn. Penguin, London

Merskey H, Bogduk N 1994 Classification of chronic pain. Definitions of chronic pain syndromes and definition of chronic pain, 2nd edn. International Association for the Study of Pain, Seattle, WA

Monga T N, Grabois M (eds) 2002 Pain management in rehabilitation. Demos Medical, New York

Nicholas M 1994 Pain Self-Efficacy Questionnaire (PSEQ): Preliminary report. Unpublished paper, University of Sydney Pain Management and Research Centre, Sydney, Australia

Ninedek A, Kolt G S 2000 Sports physiotherapists' perceptions of psychological strategies in sport injury rehabilitation. Journal of Sport Rehabilitation 9: 191–206

O'Bannon R M, Rickard H C, Runcie D 1987 Progressive relaxation as a function of procedural variations and anxiety level. International Journal of Psychophysiology 5: 207–214

Payne R A 2000 Relaxation techniques. A practical handbook for the health care professional, 2nd edn. Churchill Livingstone, Edinburgh

Petruzzello S J, Landers D M, Hatfield B D, Kubitz K A, Salazar W 1991 A meta-analysis of the anxiety reducing effects of acute and chronic exercise – outcomes and mechanisms. Sports Medicine 11: 143–182

Pilowsky I, Spence N D 1983 Manual for the Illness Behaviour Questionnaire, 2nd edn. University of Adelaide, Department of Psychiatry, Adelaide, Australia

Price D D, McGrath P A, Rafii A, Buckingham B 1983 The validation of visual analogue scales as ratio scale measures for chronic and experimental pain. Pain 17: 45–56

Price D D, Harkins S W, Baker C 1987 Sensory-affective relationships among different types of clinical and experimental pain. Pain 28: 297–307

Ransford A O, Cairns D, Mooney V 1976 The pain drawing as an aid to the psychologic evaluation of patients with low-back pain. Spine 1: 127–134

Reading A E 1984 Testing pain mechanisms in persons with pain. In: Wall P D, Melzack R (eds) Textbook of pain. Churchill Livingstone, Edinburgh, p 195–204

Robinson M E, Riley J L, Myers C D et al 1997 The Coping Strategies Questionnaire: A large sample, item level factor analysis. Clinical Journal of Pain 13: 43–49

Rohling M L, Binder L M, Langhinrischsen-Rohling J 1995 Money matters: A meta-analytic review of the association between financial compensation and the experience and treatment of chronic pain. Health Psychology 14: 537–547

Shipton E A 1999 Pain. Acute and chronic, 2nd edn. Arnold, London

Sim J, Arnell P 1993 Measurement and validity in physical therapy research. Physical Therapy 73: 102–115

Sim J, Waterfield J 1997 Validity, reliability and responsiveness in the assessment of pain. Physiotherapy Theory and Practice 13: 23–37

Smith A 1999 The effects of the Feldenkrais Method on pain and anxiety in people experiencing low back pain. Bachelor of Physiotherapy (Honours) thesis, La Trobe University, Melbourne, Australia

Smith M C 1976 Retrograde cell changes in human spinal cord after anterolateral cordotomies: Location and identification after different periods of survival. Advances in Pain Research and Therapy 1: 91–98

Sternbach R A 1986 Survey of pain in the United States: The Nuprin Pain Report. Clinical Journal of Pain 2: 49–53

Strong J, Ashton R, Chant D 1991 Pain intensity measurement in chronic low back pain. Clinical Journal of Pain 7: 209–218

Strong J, Sturgess J, Unruh A M et al 2002a Pain assessment and measurement. In: Strong J, Unruh A M, Wright A, Baxter G D (eds) Pain. A textbook for therapists. Churchill Livingstone, Edinburgh, p 123–147

Strong J, Unruh A M, Wright A et al (eds) 2002b Pain. A textbook for therapists. Churchill Livingstone, Edinburgh

Sullivan M J L, Bishop S R, Pivak J 1995 The pain catastrophizing scale: Development and validation. Psychological Assessment 7: 524–532

Tajet-Foxell B, Rose F D 1995 Pain and pain tolerance in professional ballet dancers. British Journal of Sports Medicine 29: 31–34

Taylor J, Taylor S 1998 Pain education and management in the rehabilitation from sports injury. The Sport Psychologist 12: 68–88

Thienhaus L, Cole B E 1998 The classification of pain. In: Weiner R S (ed) Pain management. A practical guide for clinicians (Vol 1), 5th edn. St. Lucie Press, Boca Raton, FL, p 19–26

Torebjörk H E, Ochoa J L 1980 Specific sensations evoked by activity in single identified sensory units in man. Acta Physiologica Scandinavica 110: 445–447

Turk D C, Holzman A D 1986 Commonalities among psychological approaches in the treatment of chronic pain: Specifying the meta-constructs. In: Holzman A D, Turk D (eds) Pain management: A handbook of psychological treatment approaches. Pergamon Press, New York, p 257–267

Turk D C, Okifuji A 1999 A cognitive-behavioural approach to pain management. In Wall P D, Melzack R (eds) Textbook of pain, 4th edn. Churchill Livingstone, London, p 1431–1444

Unruh A M, Campbell M A 1999 Gender variation in children's pain experiences. In: McGrath P J, Finley G A (eds) Chronic and recurrent pain in children and adolescents. IASP Press, Seattle, WA, p 191–241

Waddell G, Newton M, Henserson I et al 1993 A fear avoidance beliefs questionnaire (FABQ) and the role of fear-avoidance in chronic low back pain and disability. Pain 52: 157–168

Wall P D 1979 On the relation of injury to pain. Pain 6: 253–264

Wallace R K, Benson J, Wilson A F 1971 A wakeful hypometabolic physiologic state. American Journal of Physiology 221: 795–799

Weiner R S (ed) 1998a Pain management; A practical guide for clinicians (Vol 1), 5th edn. St. Lucie Press, Boca Raton, FL

Weiner R S (ed) 1998b Pain management; A practical guide for clinicians (Vol 2), 5th edn. St. Lucie Press, Boca Raton, FL

Weisenberg M 1999 Cognitive aspects of pain. In: Wall P D, Melzack R (eds) Textbook of pain, 4th edn. Churchill Livingstone, London, p 345–358

Whitmarsh B G, Alderman R B 1993 Role of psychological skills training in increasing athletic pain tolerance. The Sport Psychologist 7: 388–399

Williams D A, Thorn B E 1989 An empirical assessment of pain beliefs. Pain 59: 71–78

Zalon M L 1993 Nurses' assessment of postoperative patients' pain. Pain 54: 329–334

Chapter 12

Terminating the therapeutic relationship

Lynda M. Mainwaring

INTRODUCTION

Saying goodbye is not a moment, it's a process. It's an echo down canyon walls and into the depths of caves, magically vibrating the air for years to come and coming back to us in waves, often when we least expect it.

(Chance 1987, p 21)

The ultimate goal of therapy is to restore individuals to autonomous functioning. Termination of treatment, the gateway to autonomous functioning, is a critical, yet often neglected, phase in therapy (Kramer 1990, Weddington & Cavenar 1979). It involves the process of ending a relationship, the breaking of a bond between a client and therapist in which intimate details of the client's physical and psychological functioning may have been shared. Care and attention is warranted when ending therapeutic relationships that have fostered any degree of attachment. The management of termination is especially important if therapy has been long term, involved elements of psychological counseling, or if the client has difficulty ending relationships. This chapter focuses upon the end or "termination phase" of treatment in the physical therapies, describes the process of structuring a good ending, and provides guidelines for navigating the complex web of feelings that can emerge in termination for both client and therapist. The overall aim of the chapter is to describe best practices for terminating therapeutic relationships (e.g., between physical therapist and client) in the most salubrious manner. In this chapter, the term therapy refers to the wide variety of physical therapies covered in this book.

TREATMENT AND DISCHARGE PLANNING (THE PROCESS)

The process of any therapy involves a beginning, middle, and end phase. Well before treatment ends, therapists or treatment teams establish plans for discharging clients from care. These are thoughtful exercises that integrate physical, psychological, and social considerations for future management of cases. The therapist focuses upon planning the details of discharging the client, bringing treatment into the termination phase, and working toward the final session that terminates treatment. Once plans are outlined, they are discussed with clients for their input. This facilitates client participation in treatment/discharge and ensures that therapeutic relationships do not end abruptly. The transition from the middle phase of treatment to the termination phase prepares the client for the end of treatment and the end of a partnership. During the termination phase a client comes face to face with the reality that the supportive relationship developed through consultation will end soon. Figure 12.1 identifies the process of therapy with an emphasis on the process of termination, which will be described in the sections to follow.

TREATMENT GOALS AND EXPECTATIONS: THE BEGINNING OF A GOOD ENDING

A good ending to therapy starts with a good beginning. The foundation upon which the entire therapy process and the gateway to autonomous functioning are built is the beginning of treatment. From the outset, clear goals and expectations need to be established. Once the initial intake has identified the presenting problem, the treatment team or treating therapist, prepares a treatment plan and discusses it with the client. Treatment goals are most effective when established in conjunction with the client (Bassett & Petrie 1999, Cott & Finch 1990, Gilbourne & Taylor 1998, Wiese & Weiss 1987). Open communication about the goals and process of therapy provides direction and helps to create a trusting relationship. Not only does this help build rapport, but removes the uncertainty associated with the initiation of therapy by informing the client of the anticipated course and direction of treatment. Uncertainty can be distressing for clients and the more informed they are about the injury or illness, the course of treatment, and the expected outcome,

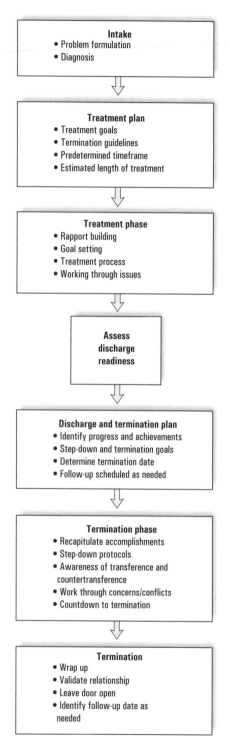

Figure 12.1 Components of the termination process in therapy

the better they can learn to adjust and cope with their current circumstances. Unambiguous goals provide benchmarks for progress, the pinnacle of which is termination. Clear goals create positive expectations about goal attainment. Information about what to expect from treatment and its estimated time course sets the stage for future discussions about bringing treatment to an end. Negative endings typically start prior to the termination phase of therapy; they do not suddenly occur but originate in the early or mid-phase of therapy (Kramer 1990).

DISCHARGE PLANNING

Discharge planning is initiated once the therapist, client, or treatment team decides that the client is approaching termination – the time that regular treatment sessions are no longer needed. Typically, treatment goals are within reach, or the client is clearly not benefiting from treatment such that an alternate form of treatment or termination is appropriate. Often, clients recognize that it is time to modify the treatment schedule, and they themselves raise the topic with their therapists. Regardless of who broaches this topic first, client input into discharge planning is an important part of a successful termination. In a multidisciplinary setting, the treatment team meets and discusses the client's progress or future management needs. A plan is outlined and discussed with the client by the person responsible for the case. Independent practitioners would assess the client's status, progress, and future needs to determine the course of the discharge plan, which is then discussed with the client. Clients involved in lengthy rehabilitation programs have usually established therapeutic and supportive relationships with their therapists. Often therapists provide psychological support and are recognized by their clients as critical social support providers during rehabilitation (Mainwaring 1999, Udry 1996). It is important, especially for long-term cases, to gradually adjust the treatment schedule so that an abrupt ending is avoided. Gradual tapering of treatment sessions serves an important psychological step-down function in the termination process.

Step–down goals

An integral component of the discharge plan and the termination phase is the timeline that explicates target goals, dates, and a tapered schedule of treatment. This information provides both the client

and the therapist with clear directions of the course of treatment and a firm but flexible end date. Setting target dates for reducing and ending treatment provides clients with additional markers for success. For example, a specified date, along with an observable increase in range of motion (ROM), resumption of activities of daily living (ADLs), less time in treatment, and increased time for independent functioning helps the move toward termination in a positive manner. Figure 12.2 presents an example of a termination goals worksheet that a therapist and client can prepare together. Such worksheets offer therapists an opportunity to chart target goals, dates, criteria, and potential concerns. The timeline provides the client with hope about moving forward, reaching a new level in the recovery process, and gaining resumption of normal ADLs. The identification of a termination date makes the upcoming ending "more real" (Firestein 2001) and may stimulate affective reactions such as grief, sorrow, dependency, and insecurity that can lead to treatment relapse (Firestein 2001, Teyber 2000). The therapist must always be alert to new emerging problems, an exacerbation of symptoms, or a regression of progress. Step-down goals establish a gradual progression towards the end of treatment that provides an opportunity for the client to feel comfortable with ending the therapeutic relationship. This tapering may also include adjustments to treatment protocols or interactions. The client may spend time working independently on specific tasks in the clinic and applying a particular modality on their own. This behavior helps promote client confidence and independent execution of rehabilitation exercises that assist with the progression toward termination. Tapering and modifying goals allow therapists to assess client reactions to the upcoming termination.

Discharge and termination goals

The discharge plan confirms or modifies the outcome goals mutually agreed upon in the treatment plan at the commencement of therapy. The goals may be physical, psychological, social, or any combination thereof. These goals address the desired outcome, the number of scheduled visits prior to the last treatment session, the nature of follow-up visits, maintenance exercises, and routines to be followed after discharge. In keeping with the recommendations from the goal setting literature (see Chapter 8), goals for the termination phase of treatment should also be specific, measurable, attainable, realistic, time-targeted, evaluated, and recorded

Date initiated:	April 15th
Client:	D.M. – Elite athlete
Therapist:	J.J.
Physical diagnosis:	ACL tear
Surgery date:	February 15th (reconstruction)

Goals/concerns	Target date	Criteria	Concerns
Discuss termination (client concerned)	April 15th	• Full range of motion • 8/10 strength	• Pain • Nightmares
Reduce appointments (3–4 sessions/week)	April 20th	• Full range of motion • Good strength • Adherence to gym exercises	
(2 sessions/week)	June 30th	• Sufficient motivation to comply with home and gym exercise protocol	
Modify treatment • Increase independence • Increase home exercises • Consult psychologist • Provide relaxation tape	May 1st	• Assess fear of re-injury • Motivation and adherence	• Fear • Hesitation with dynamic movements
Strength assessment	May 15th	• 8/10 muscle tone/mass • 8/10 thigh circumference	• Watch over-exertion • Hesitation
Pivot and stop	June 15th	• Strength and mobility	
Return to full activity (resume contact sports)	July 1st	• Strength and function • No nightmares	
Termination	July 15th	• Full function and strength • Full pivot and stop • 8/10 confidence	
Follow-up (3-month if warranted)	Sept 30th		

Figure 12.2 Example of a terminations goals worksheet

(SMARTER), to be the most effective. Both short-term and long-term outcome goals can be established as well as process-oriented goals. For example, a client who has undergone anterior cruciate ligament reconstruction may be told that increased strength, as measured by muscle tone and number of completed front lunges, is necessary prior to reducing rehabilitation sessions (termination phase outcome goal), and that full stopping, starting, and pivoting capabilities are necessary before rehabilitation is over (termination goal). The therapist can also set process-oriented goals such as suggesting that the client focus on the movement quality of flexion and extension exercises, or that visual or kinesthetic imagery is added to the exercise protocol. Communication of such information provides the client with direction, assists in estimating his or her progress, and offers clear information on when termination of treatment, and thus recovery, is likely to occur. As with all goals, there needs to be sufficient flexibility to accommodate individual variation in progress.

Setting termination goals can create both anxiety and hopeful anticipation. End of rehabilitation, for some, means the resumption of normal ADLs. Adhering to therapy can be an intrusive and frustrating event that clients are only too happy to end. Many look toward the end of therapy with great anticipation and relief. For others, raising the prospect of termination can evoke myriad negative emotions. In moving treatment into the termination phase, the therapist needs to be aware that the client's physical and psychological readiness for discharge may be at conflict. When discussing termination goals, it is a good idea to observe and record a client's response. Like treatment goals, discharge and termination goals should be clear and obtainable. In order to set obtainable termination goals that address both the physical and psychosocial domains of functioning, therapists need to be aware of the kinds of psychological events that warrant special attention and have the knowledge to address them. For example, if a client is intensely self-conscious of a disfigurement from a severe burn injury, the therapist will want to make a referral to a psychologist or psychiatrist prior to termination. Alternatively, in consultation with a psychologist, the therapist can proceed in one of two ways:

- set step-down goals that incorporate a systematic desensitization program to alleviate the cosmetic, or social anxiety prior to discharge, or

- conclude that this particular client would benefit from having her feelings validated and then provide her with practical strategies to manage the feelings along with any adaptive devices that she may need.

WHEN SHOULD THE RELATIONSHIP BE TERMINATED?

"Try as we may to find the optimal moment for termination, there is always something arbitrary about every ending" (Bergmann 1988, p 137). There is never a perfect recipe for termination of any therapeutic relationship. Whether explicit or implicit, therapists usually have their own guidelines to help them decide when to terminate treatment. For treatment that involves strictly short-term physical or manual therapy, therapists are guided by the interplay of their professional training and experience, and the client's response to treatment. Nevertheless, the treatment is conducted within the context of an interpersonal relationship and requires attention to psychosocial issues. Many professional therapy associations such as the American Physical Therapy Association explicitly state that the psychological well-being of clients falls within the purview of physical therapy (American Physical Therapy Association 1995). For psychologically focused therapy, or manual therapy where psychological support is an integral component, therapists are best guided by client-centered therapeutic objectives that are based on mutual agreement and involve more than the restoration of anatomical structure and function.

The therapist's training and experience informs decisions about the course of treatment and what needs to be accomplished. Therapists' objectives for treatment and termination may be quite different from those of their clients. Consequently, the therapist and the client need to work together in a mutually respectful way to gain a consensus of treatment direction and goals. In the event that clients believe that the therapist's objectives for termination are unreasonable, or not in line with their own, they probably will not agree or comply with the plan. Therefore, it is important to understand the client's perspective on treatment and work toward a mutually manageable schedule for ending therapy favorably.

The client may have specific objectives for therapy depending on the nature of the presenting problem and the client's history of injury and treatment. In such cases, treatment and termination goals need to be negotiated by reference to the client's perspective (not necessarily in agreement with their perspective, but in consideration of it). If the client's needs are ignored, adherence to treatment will be affected no matter how scientific and evidenced-based the treatment plan is. Termination may then be unsettled for both the client and the therapist.

Termination criteria

It is difficult for therapists to establish strict termination criteria for ending therapy because of the large number of variables that need to be considered. All clients and their respective circumstances differ so that the criteria for terminating therapy with one client naturally differ to those from another. Even so, there are some commonalities across therapists and clients with respect to decisions about ending treatment. Kramer (1990) examined therapist and client criteria for termination in psychotherapy. He identified similar criteria for termination used by therapists and clients. Over 50% of therapists reported using "global improvement" as a termination indicator; that is, they judged their clients to be "doing much better," "greatly improved in all areas," or "handling life well" (p 50). The second most frequently used criteria by therapists were "specific intrapsychic or internal improvement factors . . . and specific external or observable improvement factors" (Kramer 1990, p 50). These relate to factors such as improved self-esteem or resolution of internal conflict, and the resumption of work or ability to engage in a healthy relationship. Other criteria included the assessment of the cost/benefit ratio: the therapist or the client independently assessed whether the resources (time, effort, and money) spent on therapy were beneficial. Interestingly, only a small percentage of therapists identified a reduction in the presenting problem as instrumental in terminating decisions.

Client decisions about termination have been reported to focus primarily on global improvement factors (e.g., feeling better) that were sometimes gauged by "specific external or internal factors" (Kramer 1990). The other main criterion was some form of cost/benefit analysis: would treatment continue to make a difference, and can I afford it relative to my financial resources or the emotional investment? A few clients registered dissatisfaction with treatment or the therapist, and a few stated

financial cost alone (regardless of a cost/benefit analysis) motivated them to end psychotherapy.

In order for both the therapist and the client to proceed with a clear picture of how the therapy progresses and ends, objective, clear, realistic, and mutually agreed upon termination criteria should be established at the beginning of treatment (Kramer 1990). Once in the termination phase, "the single most important guideline for negotiating a successful termination is to unambiguously acknowledge the reality of the ending" (Teyber 2000, p 297). Experienced practitioners usually gauge readiness to end therapy by reference to criteria in one or more of four general categories: symptom relief, intuition, improved physical and behavioral functioning, or improved psychological functioning.

Symptom relief Therapists, especially those who work within a therapeutic framework that is structured, short-term, and goal-oriented, may decide to terminate the therapeutic relationship based on resolution of symptoms. Therapists may observe, or clients may communicate, that their symptoms have resolved, reduced, or are more manageable. For longer-term therapy that addresses more involved psychological issues, several authors in the psychoanalytic literature agree that symptom relief can be a clear sign that termination is approaching (Epstein 1980, Siporin 1975).

Generally, new symptoms do not arise in the termination phase. However, an exacerbation of symptoms can occur in cases in which there are underlying conflicts about leaving therapy. For example, if a client recognizes that ending treatment means losing insurance benefits and returning to a job that he dislikes or in which he was injured, he may experience a recurrence of psychological symptoms (e.g., elevated anxiety) he experienced at postinjury and during the early phase of treatment. Therapists should not automatically presume that this is a case of malingering. In traumatic injuries, there is often anxiety about returning to the site where the injury occurred or to surroundings that have similar sights, sounds, or odors to the accident site. Similarly, the anniversary of the trauma usually evokes symptom exacerbation or resurgence. For traumatic injuries, discharge plans need to address the timing of termination and the context to which the client is returning. Symptom exacerbation can also be triggered by dependency and separation anxiety that are related to unresolved conflicts about losing a relationship (see Chapter 6 for a discussion of transference reactions). In such a case, therapists may have to proceed slowly and deliberately with the termination process and be mindful of clients' potential threats of self-harm. This is especially true for certain personalities (see later section in this chapter on Strategic planning for terminations with vulnerable individuals).

Practitioner intuition   Most experienced therapists have developed an array of cues, signs, judgments, and evidence-based information that gives them knowledge of when therapy is approaching termination. Often this is a tacit knowledge that translates into what may be called intuition: practitioner intuition is often used when terminating therapy (Kramer 1990). These intuitions about the psychological readiness of a client to end therapy are difficult to explicate into a set of objective criteria, but nevertheless may play a key role in decisions about termination (Firestein 2001, Kramer 1990, Levenson 1976). The therapist has a sense, or impression, that therapy is progressing toward dissolution and in the upcoming sessions endeavors to test this postulate by looking for cues and signs of readiness to end treatment. For neophyte therapists, not knowing when to end treatment can be unsettling, and can feel like trying to find an unfamiliar object in the dark. However, experience, a reflective attitude toward the process of therapy, and good supervision will shed light on the appropriate timing for initiating the discharge and termination phase.

Improved physical and behavioral functioning   In physical and manual therapy, the primary objective is to restore physical functioning, and so, observable and measurable signs of such improvement are indicators that therapy will be ending soon. With the increased emphasis on client-centered, holistic treatment, however, the psychosocial realm of functioning cannot be ignored. Some clients may progress through treatment without any need for psychosocial issues to be addressed, and thus, termination can be guided by physical rehabilitation protocol guidelines for a particular condition. Others will benefit from a therapeutic relationship that integrates psychosocial goals with the physical outcome goals. Assessing readiness for termination involves more than identifying physical markers for recovery. Client behaviors can be clear markers for psychosocial progress in that behaviors are observable and measurable. For example, a client is making small, yet slower than expected gains in muscle strength following reconstructive hand surgery; the therapist notices that the client has recently begun to interact with other clients, smiles

more readily when asked how he is feeling, and has rejoined a social activity club one night a week. These signs are indicators that the client is starting to feel more at ease with himself and others, as well as the observed optimism about his future and readiness to return to work options. His slow physical progress was influenced by his initial psychological state, and the behavioral indicators are signs that the client's psychological state is improving, and gains in physical functioning, and perhaps strength, will follow.

Improved psychological functioning   When clients feel better about themselves, can cope with stressful situations more effectively, or show and experience improved intrapsychic or internal improvements (e.g., improved self-esteem, reduced anxiety), along with the necessary physical improvements, they are ready to move into the termination phase. Clients such as that described in the section above may be showing improved emotional functioning and increased energy levels such that home exercises will most likely be carried out. Physical and manual therapists know that they can move clients into the next phase of treatment when reports of change or functioning across sources converge and are consistent:

1. clients themselves report feeling better
2. therapist observations reveal improved behavioral and psychosocial functioning such that the client can withstand daily hassles and cope better than at the beginning of treatment
3. indirect or direct reports from clients' significant others about observed positive changes in behavior.

Caution is necessary when using improved psychological functioning as a guideline for termination. First, physical and manual therapists should not be making or communicating a psychiatric diagnosis. If a psychiatric diagnosis has been made by a psychologist or psychiatrist, physical or manual therapy may be provided in light of that information, but does not necessarily continue until the psychiatric condition is resolved. The psychiatric disorder may remain despite improved psychological functioning. Second, as clients experience increased psychological functioning, it is important not to confuse treatment goals with larger life goals or therapist goals. For example, trying to help a client overcome longstanding lifestyle difficulties such as alcoholism should not be one of the therapist's goals for treatment. Within the limits of physical and manual therapy, and psychotherapy itself for that matter, realistic goals commensurate with client goals, need to be established. If a therapist believes that a particular client needs to change what amounts to a personality characteristic, then the therapist needs to assess whether this goal is realistic, reasonable, and within the therapist's professional competence, and contained in the contract of therapy. Furthermore, in such a case the therapist needs to assess his or her own issues of countertransference (refer to Chapter 6). When therapists' criteria for termination become detached from the clients', ending therapy can present great difficulties for the client and the therapist.

FOLLOW-UP

Follow-up sessions are determined during the termination phase and are planned according to individual needs. Some clients may require a 3-, 4-, 6-, or 12-month follow-up depending on the nature of the issues to be addressed. In some cases, follow-up may not be necessary or manageable. For example, no follow-up is necessary if there are no concerns with the client's psychological and physical functioning during the termination phase or during the last session. For complex or long-term cases, however, follow-up sessions may provide comfort and reassurance to clients who have difficulty with ending relationships or for those who would benefit from further assistance that may be deemed necessary at follow-up. Regardless of whether a formal follow-up session is scheduled or not, it is usually prudent to let clients know that they can contact you in the future should they have concerns.

TERMINATION

The last session of therapy is typically a blend of positive feelings and sadness about the end of a working relationship for both client and therapist. All the treatment goals have been accomplished and the last session is the concrete step to autonomous functioning; it provides the opportunity to recapitulate what has been accomplished, what remains to be addressed, and it allows an interchange of feelings about the relationship coming to a close. Any difficulties anticipated with termination have already been addressed, but may

need revisiting as the parties exchange goodbyes. It is appropriate for therapists to express feelings about the relationship ending because this self-disclosure validates clients' feelings related to the bond that has been established between the two. Termination issues and affective reactions such as grief and sorrow may extend beyond the last session for the client (Firestein 2001). Depending on the length and intensity of treatment, and the coping style of the client, the grief reaction will vary. The last session may be the end of personal contact between the therapist and client, but it is not the end of the therapist's professional responsibilities toward their clients. The same ethical, practical, and legal standards apply to former clients as current ones even though the file has been closed. Once the file has been closed, it is securely archived for the period of time as required by law. This time may vary among jurisdictions.

TERMINATING THE RELATIONSHIP

A trusting and respectful practitioner–client relationship is the most important quality of the therapeutic enterprise. Within this relationship the client moves towards the ultimate goal of therapy, which is termination and autonomous functioning. To accomplish this goal the client and the therapist need to be in psychological contact whereby empathy, tolerance, respect, and honesty are expressed by the therapist. The success of effective psychotherapy, for example, greatly depends on the strength and integrity of the client–therapist relationship (see Chapter 5). The greater the compliance with treatment, the better the functional outcome (Di Fabio et al 1995). Many client-centered psychotherapists follow the tradition of Carl Rogers who believed that the essence of therapeutic change is the relationship itself (Kramer 1990). Similarly, there is ample evidence that the medical practitioner–patient relationship is instrumental in patient compliance and satisfaction (Ross & Duff 1982) and clients adhere better to services that satisfy emotional needs rather than medical needs (Eisenberg et al 1993). In any context, having established an intimate working relationship, the practitioner is responsible for ensuring the relationship ends salubriously. Figure 12.3 provides a checklist of issues to address in the termination phase that will facilitate an optimal termination for the client regardless of who initiates it.

Termination objective	Status
1. Discuss the ending of therapy in advance	☑
2. Set a specific date to end treatment	☑
3. Review treatment goals and progress	☑
4. Express therapist's feelings of pleasure with client's progress and interactions	☑
5. Invite client to discuss feelings about termination	☑
6. Invite client to express feelings about therapist related to termination	☑
7. Identify therapist's own defensive or countertransference reactions	☑
8. Validate client's feelings and experience especially about loss or previous difficulties with relationship endings	☑
9. Watch for relapse or exacerbation of symptoms	☑
10. Watch for anniversary of trauma or termination triggered conflicts	☑
11. Discuss the meaning of the relationship for the therapist	☑
12. Periodically reinforce the timeframe remaining in treatment	☑
13. Examine termination themes of abandonment, betrayal, resentment, anger, rejection, grief, loss, and responsibility for self	☑
14. Distinguish between client goals and therapist goals	☑
15. Maintain empathy	☑
16. Be mindful of and observe termination cues	☑
17. Respect and encourage the client's autonomy	☑
18. Accept the limitations (what can be changed and what cannot)	☑
19. Avoid encouraging the cultivation of a different kind of relationship after termination	☑
20. Say goodbye and leave the door open for follow-up if necessary	☑

Figure 12.3   Termination phase checklist

CONSENSUAL TERMINATION: BILATERAL NATURAL ENDINGS

A natural ending to treatment emerges when the therapist and client agree that the client's work, as identified in the treatment plan, is complete. Goals have been attained, activities have been resumed or modified, or the predetermined timeframe has run its course. Regardless, there is a mutual sense that it is time to terminate the client–therapist relationship. Often, therapists are at the stage of wondering what the next step should be when the client begins questioning or hinting about termination. In essence, for natural endings, both client and therapist sense, at about the same time, that the ending of therapy is close (Kramer 1978). In such cases, short-term termination phases of about 2 weeks are appropriate (Teyber 2000). In natural endings, the therapist must give the client permission to leave, review treatment achievements, set a definite date for therapy to end, and probe the client's reactions about ending treatment. Even in natural endings, conflicts may be triggered by the anticipation of ending this important relationship. A primary goal in natural endings is to affirm the clients' potentially mixed feelings about ending the relationship. That is, the therapist can praise the client's achievements and progress made toward independence and autonomous functioning, but acknowledge the importance of the relationship and the sadness likely associated with ending the relationship. It is also important for the client to know that the therapist will be available should the client need assistance in the future.

CLIENT-INITIATED TERMINATION: UNILATERAL UNNATURAL ENDINGS

Unilateral client-initiated endings to treatment can be termed "unnatural" and precipitated by different reasons: a perceived lack of progress; frustration with the treatment, therapist conflict, time commitment for therapy; beliefs that sufficient recovery has been made and a return to normal activity is a priority; or external demands are creating such stress that the client needs to address them (e.g., financial concerns). The therapist may have an idea that treatment is not progressing smoothly, but is often caught off guard and will want to evaluate his or her own countertransference reactions to the client's announcement that treatment is over. There is a

greater likelihood of negative transference or countertransference reactions to occur in unnatural endings. If therapeutic work remains to be done, therapists need to assess their motivation for this opinion and invite clients to discuss their reasons for wanting to terminate treatment prematurely. If clients could harm themselves by not continuing, therapists should provide their opinion and document that they have done so (see later section in this chapter on Professional responsibility relating to the termination of the therapeutic relationship). The therapist can offer to continue, or find alternative avenues for treatment if the client is dissatisfied with the therapist. Once the topic of termination is mentioned, however, clients have usually made up their minds to end treatment if they have not quit already; forcing them to stay is not productive, nor in line with codes of ethics. For example, the code of ethics for the British Association of Occupational Therapists specifically states that the autonomy and choice of the client must be respected (College of Occupational Therapists 2000). Nevertheless, it is always a good idea to indicate that clients can return if they so wish.

THERAPIST-INITIATED TERMINATION

Endings initiated by the therapist may arise in the following four instances:

1. the therapeutic objectives have been reached and termination is imminent
2. the student therapist has graduated or finished her term
3. the therapist becomes impaired for intrapersonal, interpersonal, grief, or medical reasons
4. a referral to another professional is required in order to address certain therapeutic issues beyond the therapist's competence.

In all but the first instance, which will depend on the client's perspective, termination is imposed by external circumstances and leads to an unnatural ending. Therapy may be in different phases when unnatural termination looms; some clients may have already made substantial therapeutic gains whereas others may have only begun to scratch the surface of the problem. Regardless, adequate provision for continuity of care/referral is indicated. If not handled sensitively, this unnatural ending of one relationship may negatively influence those to follow, or dissuade clients from trusting a therapist again. It is critical that the therapist and client work through the complex issues arising from any unnatural or externally imposed ending. Clients need time to work through their feelings of anger, frustration, abandonment, disappointment, betrayal, and loss associated with interrupted therapy and relationship endings. Sufficient advance notice of the termination date is always necessary so that client concerns, frustrations, defenses, and transference distortions can be addressed adequately. The success of moving through this phase depends on "therapists' ability to remain nondefensive and tolerate clients' protests – rather than feel guilty, become defensive, and make ineffective attempts to talk clients out of their feelings" (Teyber 2000, p 300). In the case of student therapists, the limits of their own availability, and level of responsibility and contact information of their supervisor should be established from the outset of therapy and emphasized again during the termination phase. Following the checklist in Figure 12.3 enables therapists to assist clients through the feelings that may be experienced during the termination process. It may not be easy for the therapist to take the time to work through these issues when his own life stressors are overwhelming and perhaps the reason for the unilateral termination, albeit, working through these issues with the client is necessary and the therapist's responsibility.

As mentioned previously, there is greater likelihood of client transference reactions and therapist countertransference reactions occurring in unnatural endings, especially when they are therapist initiated (Kirk-Sanchez & Roach 2001, Kramer 1990). For example, the unexpected ending could bring back difficult memories and feelings for either the client, the therapist, or both, about an important relationship that ended abruptly. That previous experience may not have allowed the necessary preparation for ending relationships to evolve such as coming to terms with why the relationship is dissolving. If such transference reactions are evoked, it is critical for therapists to help clients navigate through these painful feelings, and it is their professional responsibility to do so. Manual and physical therapists need to exercise judgment about how they can facilitate an optimal ending that is within their realm of competence and is appropriate to the situation. It is important to always be mindful of the numerous and complex issues that can arise in the process of terminating therapy, especially prematurely.

FUNDER-INITIATED TERMINATION

With increased third party payer involvement (e.g., clinic, hospital, insurer, employer), the potential for interrupted service because of payment withholding is heightened. Here, professionals must be clear about their professional obligations, and insure that the client understands the nature of the engagement and the limits of confidentiality. Once a treatment plan has been approved by a third party insurer, for example, funds are usually forwarded to the service provider; however, there are many cases in which treatment is not approved beyond a set number of sessions. To avoid an interruption of service for the client, or payment for the therapist, the practitioner needs to present a written rationale for continued treatment well before the treatment time has elapsed. Should there be a delay or withdrawal of continued funding, the therapist needs to discuss the situation with the client in order to establish a course of action: this may involve an appeal to the funding source for continued financing of treatment based on client need, seeking alternative funding or arranging payment with the client, initiating a referral or termination of treatment based on appropriateness, or continuing treatment on a pro bono basis. The involvement of insurance agencies or worker's compensation boards introduces another layer of potential stress and conflict for the client, especially if the client has financial concerns or the agency is creating barriers to continued treatment by withholding funds. Often, clients will find comfort in discussing these stressors with their therapists.

PROFESSIONAL RESPONSIBILITIES RELATING TO THE TERMINATION OF THE THERAPEUTIC RELATIONSHIP

CONFIDENTIALITY AND REGULATORY OBLIGATIONS

The starting point of the professional's obligation to maintain confidentiality over the confidences reposed in the therapist by the client or discovered in a therapeutic setting is simple – nothing is to be disclosed.

There are three exceptions to the general rule:

1. disclosure may be made to a third party with the consent of the client

2. disclosure may be made when warranted to avoid death or grievous bodily harm to the client or third party at risk of the client
3. disclosure must be made when compelled by law.

Consent to disclosure may be either expressed or implied. The expressed consent for disclosure is usually given with written authority of the client. If the healthcare professional has doubts concerning whether the consent of the client is informed, they should make no disclosure until that doubt is resolved.

The client may be under a practical compulsion to consent to the disclosure of confidential information by the practitioner to a third party. The third party may be an insurer or funding agency with the right to know, arising either under a contract with the client or by operation of law. The professional may be concerned with determining whether the degree of compulsion effectively spoils or lessens the consent of the client. The professional may also be concerned in determining whether the disclosure may be made without harm to the client. That situation may require the professional to engage in a balancing of interests: if more harm would befall the client in not making than in making disclosure, then the professional may elect not to disclose when a client has been "forced" to consent. Great care is required here, because by not honoring the direction of the client to disclose, the professional runs the risk of being exposed to a legal suit initiated by the client or facing disciplinary complaint.

Consent to disclosure may be implied, where, for example, the professional has been engaged by a third party (e.g., an insurer) to assess the insured. By submitting to the assessment in such circumstances, it is implied that the professional may communicate the assessment to the insurer. Here, however, the concern is with the underlying therapeutic relationship. Yet, implied consent arises because the funding depends on disclosure. Unless an implied consent to disclosure is plain from the circumstances, the healthcare practitioner should insist on the expressed written consent of the client.

Disclosure without the consent of the client may be warranted and so, legally permissible. Where a client is at risk of death or grievous bodily harm, the professional is warranted in making limited disclosure to the competent authority to obviate the risk. Such instances include the potential for suicide or when the client is unconscious or unable to communicate.

Similarly, where a third party is at risk of death or grievous bodily harm at the hands of the client, the practitioner is warranted (and indeed may be under a civil as well as ethical duty to warn) in making limited disclosure to the third party or the competent authority to avoid the harm.

Disclosure without the consent of the client may be compelled by statute, court order, or lawful investigative demand. In those cases, the protection of the interests of the client generally lies with the courts and the due process of law. Even here, however, the practitioner may be required to exercise his or her professional judgment having regard to the best interests of the client. For example, the professional or manual therapist may be called upon to testify and make disclosure carrying the risk of harm to the client. The practitioner may be both legally and ethically duty bound to raise objection before the court to answering questions that could bring psychological harm to the client. It is open for the court to exercise its discretion and not cite the practitioner for contempt for a failure to answer where the potential harm to the client vastly outweighs the benefits to be served by the disclosure.

The duty of confidentiality, although it springs from the professional relationship, survives its termination. It also survives the death of the client. In some areas, there is a belief that the executor, administrator, or other legal personal representative of the former client has the lawful authority to consent to wholesale disclosure of confidential information by the professional. There is reason to doubt that, particularly where that office is related to the administration of an estate or property. Even where the client has been committed to the care of a guardian, the test for disclosure should be by reference to what is warranted rather than by reference to consent. In such cases, any consent of the client is wholly illusory.

Again, obligations of confidentiality survive termination of therapeutic relationships. Even though the relationship has ended, the therapist or service provider has ethical and legal obligations related to client information. Often in the course of the termination phase, questions arise about the clients' records. For example, in hospital settings clients may want to know how they can access their files for insurance, litigation, or medical purposes. Clients may also want to know how to access information if their current therapist is no longer in that setting or if they initiate therapy with another service provider. Typically, in a hospital or clinic setting, laws and policies are in place for file storage and access. For independent practitioners, file retention, storage and accessibility need to comply with professional ethics, standards, and local laws. The therapist must maintain appropriate confidentiality in storing, accessing, transferring, and disposing of records.

CONTRACTUAL OBLIGATIONS

From the outset, the terms of agreement with the client or third party need to be established. The nature of the relationship with each party, the probable use of information or reports, and the limits of confidentiality all need to be addressed. This tactic keeps all parties adequately informed and precludes difficulties at termination. All relevant parties are informed that termination is approaching or has occurred. Any letters, contracts, terms of agreement, treatment plans, and their acknowledgments or approval, should be kept in the client file. If any difficulties arise at termination from a third party, or litigation is initiated post-termination, the client's file houses important documentation.

It would be a mistake to equate the termination of the therapeutic relationship with the discharge of the underlying professional services contract. The professional services contract, both by reference to the expressed as well as implied terms, may subsist well beyond the termination of the therapeutic relationship. There may be on-going obligations relating to a host of matters of which records retention and access, and provision for payment are but limited examples. There may be a host of other contractual matters that survive the termination of the supply of professional services.

It is often the case that the individual being treated is neither the retaining nor paying party, and it would not be strictly correct to characterize that person as the "client" in those circumstances. In other settings, the client is the retaining party and looks to the insurer, employer, or other funding agency for reimbursement of the professional service fees incurred. In those cases, the professional service provider looks to the client for payment in the event of any controversy with the funding agency. In other settings (e.g., National Health schemes), the client may be the retaining party, and the prevailing statutory regime requires the practitioner to look to a designated funding agency for the payment of professional fees without the possibility of recourse against the patient in the event of non-payment. In this case, the concern is with the contractual obligations relating to the termination of the therapeutic relationship. The contract may make express provision for services to be performed over a fixed period or number of sessions without regard to therapeutic result. The contract may be open-ended, in which case, ordinarily, the professional services cannot be terminated by the practitioner without reasonable prior notice of termination. What is reasonable varies with the facts of the particular case and the terms of the specific contract in question.

It seems to be generally accepted as an implied term of all contracts that each party is required to perform in good faith. A serious failure to do so may justify the other in treating the contract as terminated by the breach of the defaulting party. In some cases, the conduct may be so egregious that there is no reasonable doubt that one party has stepped entirely outside of the contract and the acceptance of termination is warranted. In other cases, it may be the culmination of a series of events warranting termination. In those cases, however, determining when a culminating event occurred may be very difficult.

Eventually all contracts come to an end whether by performance, breach, or an agreement to end (what common-law lawyers refer to as "accord and satisfaction"). Recognizing from the beginning that there will be an end, practitioners should make explicit provision for termination of the therapeutic relationship upon the happening of stated events or the achievement of objectively ascertainable results. Admittedly, this may be the counsel of perfection that cannot be safely realized in all cases, and particularly, when the client is unable to bring those matters within his or her mental grasp at the time of contracting. Ethical and legal norms will determine when those contractual provisions may be safely relied on by the practitioner in terminating the therapeutic relationship.

Legal obligations

Legal issues related to termination of therapeutic relationships concern professional malpractice: the failure of the professional to exercise the requisite degree of skill, care, judgment, and diligence measured by professional community standards, resulting in compensable physical (including psychological) harm to the patient. The potential for liability springs from the existence of the professional relationship. The termination of professional services does not by necessity terminate the professional relationship. Indeed, the abrupt or inept termination of professional services may amount to malpractice.

FIDUCIARY OBLIGATIONS

The practitioner–client relationship is unique, sanctioned by law, and involves a special trust between client and practitioner. The client and society repose trust in, and reliance on, the practitioner to do what is best for the client. The practitioner is obligated to protect the relationship and maintain appropriate professional boundaries. The nature of the relationship is such that the client is vulnerable to an exploitive relationship with, and the improper influences of, the therapist or former therapist, if therapy has terminated. If the therapist is impaired, as discussed previously, he or she may not act in the client's best interest and may actually harm the client. For example, the therapist may decide that referrals are down this month and scheduling termination for clients will be postponed. Such a decision clearly involves countertransference issues in that the therapist's needs interfere with what is best for the client. Another more obvious example is in the case where a sexual relationship between client and therapist is initiated shortly after termination. This transgression is a blatant abuse of client trust and contravenes most, if not all, professional standards of practice. Even though treatment has ended, the professional relationship, which is imbued with power imbalances, leaves the client vulnerable. Rules for professional conduct and ethical guidelines for practitioners are developed by reference to the inherent power imbalance in practitioner–client relations and emphasize the need for respecting the fiduciary obligations.

ETHICAL OBLIGATIONS

Rangell (1980) suggested that there are two possible errors that psychoanalysts can make when encountering clients accidentally post termination:

1. they may maintain an analytic attitude at inappropriate times and places
2. they conduct themselves with "premature and excessive" displays of intimacy that may precipitate anxiety or difficulty for the client.

Following termination, it is critical for the therapists to maintain their ethical obligations especially as they relate to avoiding dual or multiple relationships with clients. Kagel & Giebelhausen (1994) suggested that dual relationships are those where a boundary violation has, or may occur. When a therapist engages in a different type of relationship, or second role, with a client so that the client is now also the therapist's business associate, friend, student, or romantic partner, there has been a boundary violation that will probably change the nature of the therapeutic relationship and render the client vulnerable. The client is vulnerable because the professionals' ability to be objective or effective in performing their functions as therapists, may be impaired.

Ethical codes vary with respect to the length of time that is required to elapse between the termination of a therapeutic relationship and the beginning of an intimate relationship, between therapist and client. Many major professional associations stipulate that sexual contact less than 2 years after termination of a professional relationship is unethical. Others, however, maintain that a sexual relationship before or after termination is never ethical.

STRATEGIC PLANNING FOR TERMINATION WITH VULNERABLE INDIVIDUALS

Many individuals treated for physical conditions bring psychological experiences or characteristics to treatment that may put them at risk for a tumultuous termination. Individuals with personality disorders or those with histories of early, intense, repeated, or prolonged psychic trauma are especially challenging to treat; special attention is always warranted when it comes to ending treatment with such cases. When the safety of the therapeutic relationship is in question for these clients, many may feel abandoned and rejected again.

Ideally, with psychological trauma (such that can come from motor vehicle accidents, traumatic work injuries, assault cases, clients with histories of abuse) the physical and manual therapist collaborates with the client's psychologist to manage the physical and psychological recovery process. When such individuals are not receiving psychological support, and a psychiatric referral is not available nor accepted by the client, physical and manual therapists need to be cognizant of the potential difficulties that can arise with termination, the associated triggers and issues, as well as how to manage these situations. This section will briefly address some of the issues and management strategies that are particularly relevant to termination with vulnerable clients (refer to Chapter 7 for a thorough examination of recognizing psychopathology).

For the sake of efficiency, three general categories of issues are identified:

- adjustment and affective-related difficulties
- personality and behavioral vulnerabilities
- suicide.

Clients may present with adjustment or affective reactions that influence treatment, bring personality characteristics and behaviors to the therapeutic relationship that adversely influence therapy, or the threat of suicide develops or is present during the treatment. The seriousness of suicide and its unique challenge for therapists warrants a separate classification and discussion even though it could be subsumed under either of the other two categories.

Adjustment and affective-related difficulties that have an influence on treatment and its ending include anxiety, depression, inability to cope with life stress or chronic pain, and post-traumatic stress. In all these cases, the reality of termination may exacerbate symptoms, undo some of the positive changes that have occurred throughout treatment, and create new concerns for the client. As mentioned in the section on termination guidelines, for the clients who have experienced psychic trauma, the anniversary of the traumatic event (and the weeks leading up to that date) is usually significant; typically, termination dates should not coincide with that time period. Similarly, the prospect of termination for clients with post-traumatic stress symptoms may trigger a resurgence of stress symptoms such as insomnia, nightmares, cognitive dysfunction, anxiety, or depression, and this may be especially true if the client is now faced with resuming activity directly related to the traumatic event. Astute clinicians recognize the link between the affective reaction and the prospect of termination, validate clients' feelings, provide support, and may help the clients work through some of these issues. Should the clinician have concerns about the intensity of any particular reaction, a consultation with a psychologist or psychiatrist is prudent. In multidisciplinary clinic or hospital settings such consultations are readily available. For independent practitioners it is useful to establish a network of

psychologists and psychiatrists with whom these issues can be discussed. Student therapists should always bring such concerns to the attention of their supervisors.

Anxiety may also be a factor in cases other than those associated with post-traumatic stress. For example, the athlete who is physically ready to return to competition may not be psychologically ready (e.g., she may consciously or unconsciously fear re-injury). Often athletes do not work with a sport psychology consultant or a psychologist to address this issue; if the client is aware of this feeling and shares it with anyone, it will probably be the physical therapist. Again, the therapist may want to suggest that the client discuss this with someone who has expertise in sport psychology or the therapist alone may want to consult with that professional. Intense fear of re-injury may actually increase the athlete's chances of being re-injured during the course of play due to psychological conflict. Physical therapists can help athletes understand that such conflict and fear may be part of a normal reaction to injury and that assistance is available to help them address these issues. The role of the sport physiotherapist in managing stress-related issues can be important (Kolt & Kirkby 1996, Ninedek & Kolt 2000).

In certain cases, fear of re-injury may not be a factor and overzealousness to resume sports or ADLs puts the client at risk for future injury (athletes often have difficulty with the perceived slow progress of rehabilitation). The therapist will have recognized this prior to termination and probably was challenged to hold the client back from doing too much throughout treatment. This type of client behavior can be significant in repetitive strain, or cumulative trauma injuries. In such cases, therapists need to emphasize the importance of pacing throughout the termination phase and beyond. Often the client's personality and the work demands are such that these kinds of behaviors are difficult to modify. Follow-up sessions may be particularly important here, not so much for physical follow-up, but for behavioral checks on activity intensity. For example, this is especially true for clients who have lost the function of their dominant hand and have re-entered the work force in a position that demands repetitive use of their once non-preferred, and now preferred hand.

Behaviors and personality qualities are extremely difficult to change and the latter, depending on one's theory of psychology, perhaps impossible to change. Consequently, certain behaviors and personalities can be particularly challenging for therapists as termination approaches. For example, dependent clients may not feel secure or ready enough to leave the protection of therapy. In reality, they may never feel ready and behave in ways to maintain the therapeutic alliance. It is especially important for therapists to provide empathic positive regard, acknowledge the importance and meaning of the relationship, be clear and direct about an ending date, and provide sufficient time to implement very gradual step-down goals. With dependent clients, it is recommended that the therapist be contacted should they require additional assistance with specific issues. Specific guidelines may be warranted so that therapists are not contacted in regards to requests that are more appropriate for psychological services than physical or manual therapy. Some clients who seek out medical treatment may be unaware that the problem is of a psychological nature. Usually such clients can be identified by their extensive medical records and a litany of unnecessary procedures. These clients are likely to resist termination, and the most effective way to manage these clients is to be direct and clear, using clinical opinions and decisions as supportive evidence. As in all cases, sufficient time for clients to become familiar with the idea that treatment will be ending is also important at this stage.

Clients who have been exposed to early life trauma, especially physical or sexual abuse, may have developed personality and behavioral patterns that make relationship endings particularly painful. With the most sensitive and cautious therapist, the client's feelings of abandonment, rejection and worthlessness may surface as transference reactions (refer to Chapter 6). The client may become angry with the therapist or put up protective defenses and flee from therapy. Careful responses by the therapist can help the client adjust. For example, upon the termination date being set, the client voices "Well, I may as well leave now!" The therapist recognizing the transference reaction replies, "You could end treatment now if that is what you wish to do, but it would be nice to gradually wind down our sessions and get used to not seeing each other every week. So, should you change your mind, give me a call, I will be here next week". The therapist has acknowledged and respected the client's autonomy, communicated that the relationship is important to the therapist, and suggested a way to make the ending of this relationship easier to handle. Therapists need to be ever mindful of potential transference and countertransference reactions when treating clients who are known to have histories of abuse.

Cases that involve suicidal ideation or threats of suicide are always difficult. Suicide gestures may emerge during the course of termination when clients realize that their main source of social support (the therapist) will no longer be available. Such clients may have certain personality profiles, or have experienced physical or emotional abuse, or experience some level of depression. Individuals who are particularly vulnerable are those who fear abandonment and rejection, have few social supports, and who view termination as abandonment and rejection by the therapist (i.e., client's transference reaction). Regardless of the precipitating factors, *all threats and concerns of suicide need to be taken seriously*. At the very least these reactions are expressions of intense helpless feelings and at the worst, signs that a suicide attempt is imminent. It is beyond the scope of this chapter to go into detail about the management of suicidal clients; all practitioners and clients should have guidelines available to them for managing suicidal clients (see Chapter 12 of Kramer 1978). It is legally and ethically required that the therapist act in the best interest of the client and take all reasonable steps to preserve life.

SUMMARY

This chapter has described a component in the therapeutic enterprise that is often neglected, the termination phase. It is a critical part of therapy that can consolidate therapeutic achievements, or if mishandled, undo many accomplishments. A number of key issues for ending the process of termination in the most salubrious manner have been addressed. Three primary issues were covered: the importance of establishing mutually agreed upon termination goals in the beginning phase of treatment; the benefit of preparing a client-centered discharge and termination plan with step-down and termination goals; and guidelines for terminating relationships were identified in a checklist for therapists. As well, ways that a client–therapist relationship could end, and the potential for complex emotional issues to emerge for either or both the client and therapist have been discussed. Further professional responsibilities and issues related to termination (e.g., confidentiality and regulatory obligations, fiduciary, and legal obligations) have been covered. Management strategies that are particularly important when terminating vulnerable clients are also highlighted.

Terminating therapeutic relationships is a complex process, especially the longer and more psychologically involved the relationship and treatment has been. The therapist needs to guide this process with the client's best interests and vulnerabilities in mind. While acknowledging and respecting the unique responsibilities of physical and manual therapists, this chapter has offered some recommendations for terminating therapeutic relationships in the most positive way.

References

American Physical Therapy Association 1995 Criteria for standards of practice for physical therapy. American Physical Therapy Association, Alexandria, VA

Bassett S F, Petrie K J 1999 The effect of treatment goals on patient compliance with physiotherapy exercise programs. Physiotherapy 85: 130–137

Bergmann M 1988 On the fate of the intrapsychic image of the psychoanalyst after termination of the analysis. The Psychoanalytic Study of the Child 43: 137–153

British Association of Occupational Therapists 2000 College of Occupational Therapists Code of ethics and professional conduct for occupational therapists. British Association of Occupational Therapists & College of Occupational Therapies, London

Chance S 1987 Goodbye again. The Psychiatric Time/Medicine and Behavior Jan: 11, 21

Cott C, Finch E 1990 Goal setting in physical therapy practice. Physiotherapy Canada 43: 19–22

Di Fabio R P, Mackey G, Holte J B 1995 Disability and functional status in patients with low back pain receiving workers compensation: A descriptive study with implications for the efficacy of physical therapy. Physical Therapy 75(3): 180–193

Epstein L 1980 Helping people: The task-centered approach. Mosby, St. Louis, MO

Eisenberg D M, Kessler R C, Foster C et al 1993 Unconventional medicine in the United States: Prevalence, costs, and patterns of use. New England Journal of Medicine 328: 246–252

Firestein S K 2001 Termination in psychoanalysis and psychotherapy, revised edn. International Universities Press, New York

Gilbourne D, Taylor A H 1998 From theory to practice: The integration of goal perspective theory and life development approaches within an injury-specific goal setting programme. Journal of Applied Sport Psychology 10: 124–139

Kagel J D, Giebelhausen P N 1994 Dual relationships and professional boundaries. Social Work 39(2): 213–218

Kirk-Sanchez N J, Roach K E 2001 Relationship between duration of therapy services in a comprehensive rehabilitation program and mobility at discharge in patients with orthopedic problems. Physical Therapy 81(3): 888–895

Kramer S A 1990 Positive endings in psychotherapy. Jossey-Bass, Oxford, UK

Kramer E 1978 A beginning manual for psychotherapists, 2nd edn. Grune & Stratton, New York

Kolt G S, Kirkby R J 1996 Injury in female competitive gymnasts: A psychological perspective. Australian Journal of Physiotherapy 42: 121–126

Levenson E A 1976 Problems in terminating psychoanalysis: The aesthetics of termination. Contemporary Psychoanalysis 12(3): 338–342

Mainwaring L 1999 Restoration of self: A model for the psychological response of athletes to severe knee injuries. Canadian Journal of Rehabilitation 12: 145–156

Ninedek A, Kolt G S 2000 Sports physiotherapists' perceptions of psychological strategies in sport injury rehabilitation. Journal of Sport Rehabilitation 9: 191–206

Rangell L 1980 Some notes on the postanalytic phase. International Journal of Psychoanalytic Psychotherapy 8: 165–170

Ross C E, Duff R S 1982 Returning to the doctor: The effect of client characteristics, type of practice, and experiences with care. Journal of Health and Social Behavior 23: 119–131

Teyber E 2000 Interpersonal process in psychotherapy: A relational approach, 4th edn. Wadsworth, London

Siporin M 1975 Introduction to social work practice. Macmillan, New York

Weddington W W, Cavenar J O 1979 Termination initiated by the therapist: A countertransference storm. American Journal of Psychiatry 136(10): 1302–1305

Wiese D M, Weiss M R 1987 Psychological rehabilitation and physical injury: Implications for the sports medicine team. The Sport Psychologist 1: 318–330

Udry E 1996 Social support: Exploring its role in the context of athletic injuries. Journal of Sport Rehabilitation 5: 151–163

SECTION **3**

Working with specific client populations

SECTION CONTENTS

Chapter 13

Traumatic brain injury and stroke

Joseph H. Ricker

INTRODUCTION

Traumatic brain injury (TBI) and stroke are among the most frequent reasons for admission to rehabilitation facilities. Given the common primary organ system involved (i.e., the brain), the rehabilitation of these two populations certainly necessitates the input and involvement of psychology. This chapter will examine the various key aspects of relevance to physical and manual therapists treating individuals and families who are faced with these forms of neurologic compromise.

PHYSICAL AND MEDICAL CONSIDERATIONS

OVERVIEW OF BRAIN INJURY PATHOPHYSIOLOGY

Defining traumatic brain injury

For the present chapter, the definition of traumatic brain injury (TBI) to be used will be that of the Traumatic Brain Injury Model Systems National Database (Harrison-Felix et al 1996). Harrison-Felix et al (1996) defined TBI as "Damage to brain tissue caused by an external mechanical force, as evidenced by loss of consciousness due to brain trauma, post-traumatic amnesia, skull fracture, or objective neurological findings that can reasonably be attributed to TBI on physical examination or mental status examination" (p 1).

Epidemiology of traumatic brain injury

TBI has become one of the primary diagnostic entities in medical rehabilitation throughout the world. In Australia, there is a high incidence of TBI: at 322 head injuries per 100 000 of population annually, it exceeds studies (with comparable methodologies) in communities in the United States and Europe (Hillier et al 1997). In the United States, estimates of the occurrence of traumatic brain injury range from 100 to 392 per 100 000 (Centers for Disease Control 1997, Kraus & McArthur 1998), with the most typically cited statistic of 200 per 100 000 of the US population. A recent analysis of data from the United States, The Netherlands, and the United Kingdom (Murray et al 1999) demonstrated similarities in incidence of brain injury, but with some variability in admissions and treatment that might reflect differences in policy and pathways for care.

TBI is associated with a variety of demographic and etiologic variables. The peak age ranges for TBI are between 15 and 24, and then again at over 75 years (Centers for Disease Control 1997). Approximately two to three times as many men compared to women sustain traumatic brain injury. Although it has generally been accepted that there is significantly greater incidence of TBI in ethnic minority populations (Cooper et al 1983, Whitman et al 1984), concerns have been raised about the accuracy of such data due to inconsistent hospital reporting procedures (Kraus & McArthur 1998). Lower socioeconomic status has been, however, a more consistent risk factor in the incidence of TBI. The primary etiologies for traumatic brain injury include motor vehicle accidents, physical assault, other accidents (e.g., falls), and injuries related to recreation or sports.

Of increased relevance to psychologists and other rehabilitation practitioners is the consistent observation that many individuals who experience a TBI are not representative of the general population (Rosenthal & Ricker 2000). The prevalence of positive blood alcohol levels in people with TBI following motor vehicle accidents and violence is clearly a risk factor (Kraus et al 1989). In addition, a disproportionate number of individuals that have TBI also have a significant pre-injury history of criminal prosecution (e.g., 19.5% of 327 consecutive TBI admissions reported by Kreutzer et al 1996a), or other significant problems with the legal system (e.g., 50% of the sample in Thomsen 1987).

Types of brain injury

It is clearly not the role of the rehabilitation psychologist, neuropsychologist, or other rehabilitation practitioners, to determine the nature of the underlying neuropathology following known or putative brain injury. There are no neuropsychological tests or patterns that are specific to any particular neuropathology following TBI. Instead, psychologists and other rehabilitation professionals might integrate neuroanatomic concerns and hypotheses when formulating cognitive, emotional, and functional status after brain injury. Thus, it is important for psychologists that work with survivors of TBI to have a basic understanding of the potential neurobiological substrates of brain injury. The principal neuropathological sequelae of TBI can be grossly distinguished as anatomic or biochemical. Such a distinction might not be useful clinically, as anatomic and biochemical changes covary and, of course, interact.

The brain is suspended within the skull, essentially floating in cerebrospinal fluid, and is surrounded by three layers of meninges. Thus, it is generally well protected from normal mechanical forces. Mechanical trauma to the head may, however, cause the brain to become injured through penetration (e.g., gunshot wound) or through mechanical deceleration (e.g., from the head striking a resilient surface at a high speed). Penetrating injuries often result in prominent neurologic effects that are consistent with their anatomic focus, but there may also be widespread effects in other brain regions. In mechanical deceleration events (e.g., from a fall or motor vehicle accident), the physical forces to which the brain could be subjected might cause structural injury to the brain itself in the absence of significant injury to the skull or dura.

A head in motion that experiences a sudden stop may result in the brain coming into abrupt contact with one or more internal surfaces of the skull, usually in the anterior aspects of the brain (i.e., frontal lobes and poles of the temporal lobes). Primary contusion injuries in the posterior portions of the brain are unusual in deceleration events, given the relative smoothness of those interior regions of the skull case. In addition to primary contusions, the brain can move within the skull, which may result in twisting of ascending and descending axonal pathways. Commissural fibers (e.g., the corpus callosum) and other fiber tracts (e.g., the fornices) may also become stretched or torn as the result of differential deceleration of the brain within the skull case. This widespread potential disruption of axonal fibers is usually referred to as "diffuse axonal injury" (DAI), and is hypothesized to underlie many of the chronic neurocognitive and neurobehavioral consequences of brain injury. Earlier conceptualizations of DAI assumed that axonal injuries were immediate and were solely the outcome of direct mechanical tearing or shearing forces that immediately disconnected shear axons. Contemporary histopathological investigations have established, however, that the permanent neuropathology of DAI occurs many hours to days following the event as the result of progressive biochemical cascades (Novack et al 1996).

Presentation and natural history

In general, loss of consciousness is a typical finding following significant TBI. Exceptions may occur in instances of very focal injuries, and loss of consciousness does not always occur in the presence of a primarily penetrating injury. Formal "coma" (defined as absence of eye opening, no following of commands, and no understandable speech; also defined by a Glasgow Coma Scale score of 8 or less) does not need to be present for a diagnosis of TBI, but the depth and length of loss of consciousness is a generally accepted indicator of brain injury severity, particularly in cases of suspected diffuse cerebral injury (Rosenthal & Ricker 2000).

Approximately 20% of individuals who survive an initially severe TBI remain unresponsive at 30 days postinjury (Braakman et al 1988). The term "coma" is used frequently, but is often misused when unresponsiveness lasts longer than 1 month.

The correct descriptor for individuals who have spontaneous sleep–wake cycles but no apparent level of conscious awareness is "persistent vegetative state" (PVS). In PVS, individuals appear to maintain relatively normal sleep–"wake" patterns (Giacino et al 2002). This can be particularly troubling for families, who observe that the patient "appears" awake but does not interact in any meaningful manner.

Upon emergence from unconsciousness, most individuals with TBI experience some degree of post-traumatic amnesia (PTA). PTA refers to the time period after brain trauma during which a conscious individual demonstrates disorientation to time and other aspects of consciousness. It has been suggested that length of PTA is a very useful clinical indicator of outcome when used in combination with immediate injury severity variables (Levin et al 1982). Although PTA is useful when properly measured and tracked regularly during the course of recovery (e.g., using the Galveston Orientation and Amnesia Test; Levin et al 1979), retrospective estimates of PTA by patients or clinicians are unreliable in the absence of formal documentation (Gronwall & Wrightson 1981). Furthermore, many factors that are independent of the primary brain injury may either exacerbate PTA, or interfere with formal assessment of PTA. Such factors include alcohol or other substances, pain, metabolic disruption, emotional trauma or shock, or even the retelling of the event, with inaccuracies in "recollection" that accumulate over time and then become incorporated in the individual's account of the event.

Medical management and traumatic brain injury recovery

In addition to the primary brain injury itself, it is important for rehabilitation clinicians to be aware that there are many medical problems that frequently co-occur. Comorbid complications can exacerbate the primary brain injury, and may also interfere with goal attainment in the rehabilitation process. Such factors include intracranial edema, cardiac and respiratory injuries (which develop from co-occurring chest injuries or from post-traumatic hypertension), infection, metabolic disorders (particularly if the liver or pancreas is also injured), and seizure (Whyte et al 1998). For additional reviews of medical aspects of TBI, the reader is referred to Hammond & McDeavitt (1999) and Zafonte et al (1999).

Even a brain injury that is described initially as severe does not invariably result in total and permanent disability. Of note, is the degree of variability in outcome that may occur. For example, a brain injury that is classified initially as severe may result in a variety of outcomes, from death to surprisingly good recovery. Prolonged impairments in consciousness are common following severe TBI. Approximately 30–50% of individuals who sustain an initially severe TBI die within the first hours to weeks after their injury. Of those that do not expire, approximately 20% remain in an unresponsive state 30 days postinjury (Braakman et al 1988). The initial recovery process may be prolonged, and individuals might not be able to tolerate extensive psychometric assessment or higher-level rehabilitation interventions (e.g., cognitive rehabilitation) during their initial rehabilitation hospitalization.

People that are classified as having a moderate TBI often demonstrate a great deal of variability in their presentation. As an example, individuals that sustain relatively mild brain injuries (in terms of Glasgow Coma Scale score) but that also have focal lesions or discrete penetrating injuries are typically classified as having sustained moderate TBI, but such individuals typically have good recovery relative to individuals who are diagnosed with a moderate TBI resulting from diffuse injury throughout the brain (Williams et al 1990).

Mild head trauma has been of growing interest, as well as controversy. The increased attention paid to mild head trauma has been fueled, at least in part, by increased research, increased numbers of outpatient brain injury rehabilitation programs, and increased personal injury litigation in some areas. From a prospective and empirical viewpoint, the literature suggests that the usual course following mild head impact is that of complete or nearly complete recovery (Binder 1997). There is, however, a small percentage of individuals with symptoms that persist well beyond what clinical and scientific research would predict relative to initial injury status. In a meta-analytic review, Binder et al (1997) found that little of the neurobehavioral symptoms reported following mild head impact could be directly attributed to brain damage. Yet, there appears to be a minority of individuals who continue to report symptoms and disability for many months or years following mild head trauma. Cullum & Thompson (1997) provided an insightful review of the literature, and concluded that there are many factors that must be taken into consideration when interpreting persisting emotional, functional, and cognitive symptoms after mild head impact.

OVERVIEW OF STROKE PATHOPHYSIOLOGY

Defining stroke

Stroke usually refers to the sudden onset of lateralized or focal neurologic signs (Sacco 2000). It is usually applied to situations of cerebrovascular origin, although there are other less frequent etiologies for stroke-like presentations (e.g., some types of focal tumors).

Epidemiology of stroke

Stroke is typically the most frequent single cause of admissions to rehabilitation units, and is the leading cause of disability in many countries (Mayo 1993). Although acute stroke invariably results in some form of cognitive or motor impairment, at least one third of individuals that experience a stroke will sustain permanent reduction or loss of some aspect of cognition or mobility (Stineman et al 1997). These impairments are frequently associated with significant difficulty in returning to competitive employment, increased need for assistance in the home, and reduced participation in community activities (Wolf 1990). Although nearly 80% of stroke survivors recover a great deal of motor function, only half achieve sufficient recovery to reintegrate within the community without significant assistance (Friedman 1990). The inability to achieve even limited community participation has a high social and economic impact, and the importance of facilitating recovery of even simple motor functions cannot be overestimated (Duncan et al 1997).

Types of stroke

There are two distinct types of stroke: ischemic and hemorrhagic. Ischemic stroke occurs when there is a partial or full reduction of blood flow to a particular brain region. The initial effects of ischemic stroke are a function of reduced oxygen and glucose to the affected region. Such effects may be transient if blood flow is restored relatively soon. Long-term effects, however, are a function of actual tissue death, and may not be reversible. Recovery of function may occur if other brain regions take over the primary function (Pizzamiglio et al 2001). Ischemic strokes can be caused by multiple factors, but are most frequently the outcome of longstanding vascular disease (e.g., hypertension, atherosclerosis). Acute embolic events can occur, however, usually as the result of recent intracardial infection, which sometimes occurs after cardiac surgery, or following some types of invasive dental surgery.

Hemorrhagic stroke occurs when there is actual bleeding into tissue or into extracerebral intracranial space. The initial effects can be multifaceted and may result from decreased or depleted flow to proximal or distal brain regions, increased intracranial pressure, decreased cerebral perfusion pressure, or biochemical changes caused by the effects of intraparenchymal blood on glia and neural membranes. Hemorrhagic stroke is often considered a more critical acute event, as blood loss or increased intracranial pressure may result in coma or death. Hemorrhagic stroke has a variety of causes. It is most frequently the result of rupture in a preexisting aneurysm, but sudden increases in blood pressure may also herald the occurrence of hemorrhagic stroke (Mayer et al 2000).

Cerebrovascular distributions and stroke presentation

Strokes can arise from the middle, anterior, or posterior cerebral arteries.

Middle cerebral artery strokes The middle cerebral artery (MCA) is a branch of the internal carotid artery, and is responsible for the perfusion of 75% of the brain. Thus, disruption of blood flow in this artery or its branches can be functionally devastating. Specific deficits can include impairment in speech, motor function, spatial processing, and several aspects of cognition. Given the magnitude of perfusion by the MCA, there is the possibility of death if there is sufficient edema resulting in anatomical shift and compression of brain structures (Sacco 2000).

Anterior cerebral artery strokes The anterior cerebral artery (ACA) and its branches perfuse the anterior brain structures such as the prefrontal cortex and anterior cingulate cortex. The ACA system also perfuses basal forebrain structures and anterior aspects of the hippocampus. Thus, stroke that affects the ACA system is most likely to dramatically impact on primarily cognitive functions (e.g., new learning, planning, and problem-solving).

Posterior cerebral artery strokes The posterior cerebral artery (PCA) and its branches perfuse the structures that mediate many basic brain functions, including some aspects of sensorimotor functioning (e.g., some thalamic regions, and the cerebellum).

Branches of the PCA also perfuse the posterior hippocampus, thus making PCA strokes potentially devastating with reference to cognitive functions such as memory.

Medical management and stroke recovery

Acute medical management of stroke involves the identification of its nature (e.g., hemorrhagic, ischemic), stabilization of the acute medical condition, and in some cases the deployment of pharmacological or neurosurgical interventions to prevent further cerebral compromise (in the case of tissue plasminogen activator) or death (in the case of intracranial bleeds or herniation). Postacute medical procedures involve ensuring medical stabilization and determining discharge disposition. In some settings, early rehabilitation procedures are implemented before transfer to a specialized rehabilitation unit or facility. In others settings, rehabilitation services are provided within the context of a more general medical or neurological unit.

The mechanisms leading to functional improvement after stroke are not well understood. Cognitive recovery is certainly more likely if perfusion returns to brain regions that mediate activities such as learning, problem-solving, and language use. When brain regions that mediate these activities become permanently compromised (e.g., from tissue necrosis that may result from ischemia) mechanisms of brain reorganization might be suggested.

Neurofunctional recovery from stroke is complex (Ricker in press). Using speech-language recovery as an exemplar, one can state that some degree of recovery is expected following stroke, irrespective of treatment. Recovery of speech and language are mediated by either recruitment of homologous contralesional cortex, or by reorganization of non-language cortex (Cappa 1998). Recent studies of speech-language recovery have suggested that a better outcome was more likely in the presence of greater amounts of intact perilesional tissue, rather than actual recruitment of contralesional homologous resources (Warburton et al 1999). Several studies (Heiss et al 1997, 1999, Karbe et al 1998) provide strong evidence indicating that left perisylvian regions of cortex are quite necessary for adequate recovery of language, with homologous right hemisphere regions contributing to recovery only when left hemisphere regions are irrevocably compromised. If left perisylvian regions are unaffected, there is a fairly close relationship between increasing metabolic activity and functional improvement

(Ohyama et al 1996, Warburton et al 1999, Zahn et al 1999). If these same left hemisphere regions remain chronically compromised, recovery does then appear to be related to increased metabolic activity in the right hemisphere (Calvert et al 2000). Activation of homologous "language" cortex in the right hemisphere is certainly the result of the lesion that caused the stroke, but this is not necessarily evidence for "reorganization" or the emergence of novel functioning in these regions (Herholz & Heiss 2000, Pizzamiglio et al 2001). Given the fact that language recovery is virtually never complete, it has been proposed that the right hemisphere activation in language tasks may actually represent a maladaptive process that is responsible for the persistence of residual deficits rather than for the amount of recovery realized (Belin et al 1996). Similar models have been proposed for visuospatial recovery (Pantano et al 1992, Pizzamiglio et al 1998).

PSYCHOLOGICAL CONSIDERATIONS IN BRAIN INJURY AND STROKE REHABILITATION

Psychological practice in neurological rehabilitation settings involves the application of psychological principles and procedures (i.e., standardized testing, measurement, structured observation, behavioral intervention, psychotherapy) in the evaluation and treatment of people with neurological and/or orthopedic compromise. Neuropsychological services can provide both a unique and necessary component to the evaluation and rehabilitative treatment of the multitude of potential cognitive and emotional compromises following stroke, traumatic brain injury, brain tumor, and other types of central neurologic dysfunction (Ricker 2003).

Traditional medical tests and examinations provide information on gross anatomic structure and physiology. Because of its psychometric and comprehensive nature, a detailed neuropsychological evaluation can assist in identifying and quantifying the potential functional effects of central neurological dysfunction. Such deficits include impairments in attention, language, memory, spatial skills, problem-solving, psychomotor abilities, and emotional functioning (Caplan & Moelter 2000). This information is critical in the context of medical rehabilitation because, more often than not, the primary diagnosis (e.g., stroke or brain injury) is already known. The unique contribution comes with providing information that will help an individual regain as much independent functioning as possible.

TRAUMATIC BRAIN INJURY AND PSYCHOLOGICAL FUNCTIONING

Given the variety of etiologies and the often diffuse nature of brain dysfunction following a given TBI, it is difficult to predict the specific neuropsychological sequelae for a given individual. In general, the following types of cognitive impairments are often observed following TBI: deficits in arousal, attention, and capacity for new learning; problems in initiating, maintaining, organizing, or engaging in goal-directed behavior; reduced abilities in self-monitoring and awareness of deficits; impaired language and/or communication; visuoperceptual deficits; and agitation, aggression, disinhibition, and depression (Rosenthal & Ricker 2000). The nature, severity, and chronicity of these deficits are highly variable between individuals, and dependent on the interaction between a variety of factors including the nature of the brain dysfunction, time since injury, pre-injury neuropsychological and psychological status, family support, and receptivity of the physical, psychological, and social environments. A challenge for psychologists in TBI rehabilitation is to select those measures that are both sensitive and specific to the effects of TBI and show the strongest predictive relationship with acute and long-term outcome.

Neuropsychological assessment

In the context of rehabilitation, neuropsychological assessment can provide a wealth of information to the treating team, patient, and family. It is important to recognize that formal neuropsychological assessment in a rehabilitation setting is rarely purely diagnostic (i.e., TBI or non-TBI). Typically, the diagnosis is already established. Rather, neuropsychological assessment can assess the level of disability, assist in formulating realistic rehabilitation goals, assess changes in status, and assist in making realistic discharge plans (Ricker 2003). The information gained from such assessment is useful for the entire rehabilitation team.

The formal assessment may derive from a fixed battery of tests, or it may derive from tests that are selected based on the patient's working diagnosis and symptoms. The most widely used formal battery of neuropsychological tests is the Halstead-Reitan Neuropsychological Test Battery (HRNTB; Reitan & Wolfson 1993) (see Box 13.1), although the majority of psychologists by no means use this battery in its complete form. Given its length and heavy reliance on sensorimotor functioning, however, the HRNTB may not be the most appropriate battery for TBI inpatients in the rehabilitation setting.

In the US, the National Institute on Disability and Rehabilitation Research (NIDRR) Traumatic Brain Injury Model Systems of Care (Ragnarsson et al 1993) has also established a "fixed" battery of neuropsychological tests, but it has been specifically designed for use during both inpatient and outpatient TBI rehabilitation. This battery (see Box 13.2) includes: the Galveston Orientation and Amnesia Test (Levin et al 1979); Symbol Digit Modalities Test (Smith 1991); the Token Test (Benton et al 1994); Wechsler Memory Scale – Revised Logical Memory I & II (Wechsler 1987); WAIS-R Digit Span and Block Design (Wechsler 1981); Grooved Pegboard (Matthews & Klove 1964); Visual Form Discrimination Test (Benton et al 1983); Controlled Oral Word Association Test (Benton et al 1994); Rey Auditory Verbal Learning Test (Rey 1964); Trail Making Test (Army Individual Test Battery 1941); and the Wisconsin Card Sorting Test (Grant & Berg 1948). Some psychometrically based assessment tools may also have limitations with the TBI population (Martin et al 2000). Of note, however, is that in spite of clinical lore suggesting that maximal recovery and improvement is achieved within the first 1 to 2 years after injury, prospective research from the NIDRR TBI Model Systems project has demonstrated improvements in neuropsychological

---

Box 13.2 The National Institute on Disability and Rehabilitation Research (NIDRR) Traumatic Brain Injury Model Systems of Care Neuropsychological Test Battery (Ragnarsson et al 1993)

Galveston Orientation and Amnesia Test (Levin et al 1979)

Symbol Digit Modalities Test (Smith 1991)

Token Test (Benton et al 1994)

Wechsler Memory Scale – Revised Logical Memory I & II (Wechsler 1987)

WAIS-R Digit Span and Block Design (Wechsler 1981)

Grooved Pegboard (Mathews & Klove 1964)

Visual Form Discrimination Test (Benton et al 1983)

Controlled Oral Word Association Test (Benton et al 1994)

Rey Auditory Verbal Learning Test (Rey 1964)

Trail Making Test (Army Individual Test Battery 1941)

Wisconsin Card Sorting Test (Grant & Berg 1948)

---

functioning at 1-year follow-up, and over the course of up to at least 8 years, with the greatest improvement noted in the domains of attention, concentration, and verbal learning (Millis et al 2001).

Emotional and behavioral functioning

Emotional dysfunction following TBI is common, and is the result of both direct (i.e., neurophysiological) and indirect (i.e., psychosocial) causes. Emotional dysfunction is a broad construct and its manifestations may occur in many ways.

Acutely, agitation is often reported, but the term "agitation" actually has very specific meaning in the TBI literature, and the term is often incorrectly applied to several forms of undesired behavior (Bogner et al 2001). The generally accepted definition of "agitation" is a phenomenon that occurs within the context of PTA. Thus, patients who exhibit outbursts, non-compliance, or anger, but are not in PTA, cannot be truly classified as "agitated" in the formal sense.

Blunting of affect is common after TBI, and is noted particularly in the early phases of recovery. This is often accompanied by unawareness of deficit, which is commonly considered to be a hallmark feature of moderate and severe TBI. Impaired

---

Box 13.1 The Halstead–Reitan Neuropsychological Test Battery (Reitan & Wolfson 1993)

Aphasia Screening Test

Seashore Rhythm Test

Speech Sounds Perception Test

Finger Oscillation Test

Trail Making Test

Category Test

Tactual Performance Test

Reitan-Klove Sensory-Perceptual Examination

Hand Dynamometer

awareness after TBI is most likely a function of impaired cognition rather than being a specific cognitive deficit in and of itself (Trudel et al 1998). Improvement in self-awareness is critical for functional gains, but improvement in self-awareness alone is not a guarantee of recovery (Malec & Moessner 2000).

As recovery from the initial neuromedical impact of TBI progresses, emotional status may evolve into a more formal clinical depression. Such depression shares many features with major depression encountered in non-neurological populations, and may possess many similar neurophysiological substrates. Whether TBI per se (as opposed to depression that emerges from TBI) results in an increased incidence of suicidality is somewhat controversial. It is clear, however, that approximately 3–4% of individuals who survive an initial brain injury later commit suicide (Teasdale & Engberg 2001).

Sexual functioning

The combination of neurological, pharmacological, physical (e.g., fractures in TBI; hemiplegia or spasticity in stroke and TBI), cognitive, psychological, behavioral, and social sequelae following TBI result in a variety of social disabilities, including the challenges of re-establishing meaningful social relationships, particularly those involving intimacy and sexuality. It is often the case that self-image is significantly impaired following TBI, even in cases where changes in physical appearance or movement may be minor (Zasler 1995). Inaccurately perceiving and expressing emotion, as well as physical limitations, can pose obstacles for individuals attempting to engage in sexual behavior. On a more basic level, feelings of unattractiveness and awareness of one's disability may impede the capacity to establish satisfying intimate relationships. Sexual education, assertiveness training, and couples counseling are some of the techniques that are useful in assisting the person with TBI to re-establish their identity as a "sexual being" (Griffith & Lemberg 1993).

Clinicians in rehabilitation typically make the presumption that all individuals in rehabilitation programs are heterosexual, often without having directly inquired as to the individual's affectional orientation. Such presumably benign neglect of matters relevant to affectional orientation might contribute to poor progress or distrust of the rehabilitation team and may indirectly or directly contribute to depression, decreased self-esteem, and decreased self-confidence (Mapou 1990). Although rehabilitation considerations per se certainly should be informed by evidence-based assessment intervention, it remains imperative for rehabilitation clinicians to consider all forms of couples and familial relationships, and to educate themselves about – and remain open to – the diversity of affectional orientations and identifications such as lesbian, gay, bisexual, and trangendered, all of which present among individuals and families in the context of neurological rehabilitation.

STROKE AND PSYCHOLOGICAL FUNCTIONING

Neuropsychological functioning may be variably impaired following stroke. Although it is certainly the case that some individuals who experience a stroke may have minimal cognitive or communication impairment, most individuals sustain a cerebrovascular event will demonstrate at least short-term effects that are of relevance to neuropsychological functional status.

Neuropsychological assessment

A detailed review of each type of potential neuropsychological deficit is beyond the scope of this chapter. Rather, it is important for clinicians to realize that many (if not most) "classical" neurocognitive phenomena might occur in individuals that have sustained a cerebrovascular event. A comprehensive review of the neurocognitive sequelae of stroke of particular relevance to rehabilitation may be found in Caplan & Moelter (2000).

Given the typically lateralized nature of stroke, discrepancies in psychomotor functioning are frequently identified. Such impairments are most frequently manifested through aphasia, hemiplegia, and apraxia. Because the MCA provides blood flow to 75% of each cerebral hemisphere, including those territories that mediate the comprehension and production of speech and language, speech-language impairments are common. The MCA also perfuses the parietal lobes, as well as the geniculostriate projections, thus it should not be surprising that visuospatial impairments are not uncommon following stroke. Memory impairment may follow stroke because of direct involvement of medial temporal lobe structures, but is more frequently the result of compromise in brain structures that mediate the processing of information during registration and thus prior to consolidation (Ricker et al 1994). Nonetheless both focal and generalized cerebrovascular compromises may result in impairments that cause impaired retrieval in new information. Executive control deficits may also follow from stroke. These may result from direct frontal lobe compromise, or may be related to the more diffuse status of cerebral compromise (Kramer et al 2002).

Brief assessment may be quite predictive of outcome. For example, Stewart et al (2002) demonstrated that the Wechsler Abbreviated Scale of Intelligence (WASI; Psychological Corporation 1999) and the Hopkins Verbal Learning Test – Revised (HVLT-R; Brandt & Benedict 1998) were predictive of cognitive discharge scores on the Functional Independence Measure (FIM; Hamilton et al 1987) and need for supervision upon discharge. The Mini-Mental State Examination (Folstein et al 1975), although often criticized for its relative simplicity, has also been demonstrated to be predictive of functional status at discharge (Zwecker et al 2002).

Emotional and behavioral functioning

The prevalence of poststroke depression in acute and rehabilitation settings has been estimated to be 40–50% (Robinson 1998). On discharge, a third of patients present symptoms of depression, while a year after the stroke the figure rises to 67% (Carod-Artal et al 2002). The risk factors most consistently associated with poststroke depression are a previous history of depression, previous psychiatric history, language impairment, functional impairment, and returning to live at home alone (Ouimet et al 2001). Risk factors not associated with poststroke depression are dementia and cognitive impairment. Controversial risk factors are age, socio-economic status, prior social distress, dependency in regard to activities of daily living, and gender (Ouimet et al 2001). Depression may be an important mediator in treatment effectiveness. Depression following stroke can impede recovery and rehabilitation and is associated with higher mortality. Randomized trials show that antidepressants, especially selective serotonin uptake inhibitors, are effective in the treatment of this condition. Despite the evidence available, a large number of patients remain undertreated. Early identification and treatment can reduce the functional impairment and mortality related to poststroke depression (Gupta et al 2002). In cases of significant language or cognitive impairment the meaningful completion of traditional instruments such as the Beck Depression Inventory (Beck 1996) or the Center for Epidemiological Studies – Depression Scale (CES-D) (Radloff 1977) is precluded. The use of mood assessment instruments that do not require reading (e.g., the Visual Analog Mood Scales; Stern 1997) can be used in these cases.

The presence of fatigue is also a significant problem following stroke, but it is difficult to study psychometrically. A survey of 88 people with acute stroke found that 68% of the sample complained of fatigue compared to 40% of an age-matched control group (Ingles et al 1999). Many (40%) of the patients in this study also reported that fatigue was the worst symptom of their illness. In another study, van der Werf et al (2001) reported similar findings with 51% of their sample reporting fatigue compared to 16% in the control group. Interestingly, the prevalence of depression was similar in both groups (i.e., 20% and 16%, respectively). Although fatigue may be a feature of depression, depression and fatigue may represent separate constructs. Hence, it may be important to consider both conditions in the assessment of individuals with stroke.

Several functional neuroimaging studies have implicated the involvement of various limbic, prefrontal, striatal, and thalamic structures in disturbances of mood (Drevets 2000). These structures have also been implicated in neuropsychological and neuroimaging studies of mood following stroke (Ricker in press). For example, it has been demonstrated that after ischemic stroke, individuals that present with depression have decreased blood flow in the frontal lobes and striatum (Mayberg et al 1988, Starkstein et al 1996). Temporal lobe structures have also, but less commonly, been implicated in some aspects of poststroke depression (Grasso et al 1994). Disruptions of serotonin-rich regions of the brain are also implicated by positron emission tomography (PET) studies of poststroke depression (Mayberg et al 1988).

Although the existence of hemispheric theories of depression might suggest that poststroke depression differs from major depression in general, this may not be the case. Nicholl et al (2002) showed that poststroke depression does not differ qualitatively from general depression and that general theories and thus treatments for depression may be valid within the stroke population.

True agitation following stroke is an unusual phenomenon, although emergent agitated behavior over the early course of recovery may occur (Schreiner & Morimoto 2002). Behavioral decreases are more common following stroke. Motor impairment is an obvious contributor to behavioral suppression, but there are additional factors including fatigue and depression (Jongsma & Rusin 2001). Behavioral compliance with therapies and self-care are of great importance following stroke. This also becomes particularly critical after discharge, when there is likely to be an increased need to either eliminate behaviors (e.g., smoking) or increase behaviors (e.g., exercise) that will impact on the individual's risk for having another stroke.

Social functioning

Given that acute and early rehabilitation concerns in stroke focus on medical stabilization, restoration or enhancement of functional abilities, and discharge planning, there has not been much written on the topic of social functioning in the early recovery phase of stroke. Following discharge, however, resumption of prestroke social roles and interests may be compromised. For example, Mackenzie & Chang (2002) demonstrated that social support, functional ability, psychological, and physical symptoms at 2 weeks poststroke explained almost half of the variance in functional impact at 3 months after stroke. In another study (O'Connell et al 2001), the absence of organized ongoing psychosocial and rehabilitative support was found to be predictive of poorer outcome.

Sexual functioning

By its very nature, stroke may cause sexual dysfunction in women and men through alterations in sensory and/or motor abilities. Medications that are used in the prevention or treatment of stroke (e.g., antihypertensives) may also interfere with sexual functioning. In a recent survey of a cohort of stroke survivors (Cheung 2002), investigators demonstrated a poststroke decrease in libido, coital frequency, sexual arousal, orgasm, and sexual satisfaction. As was previously stated in the context of TBI, it is critical that rehabilitation clinicians consider the wide variety of potential significant relationships that can present within the stroke population.

PSYCHOLOGICAL INTERVENTIONS IN BRAIN INJURY AND STROKE

In the acute setting, the primary focus of care is medical stabilization, and often in sustaining life. Psychologists and other rehabilitation practitioners can, however, play an important role at this stage in recovery. Psychologists often employ early assessment instruments such as the Galveston Orientation and Amnesia Test (GOAT; Levin et al 1979) and the Coma-Near-Coma Scale (Rappaport et al 1992). These tools can assist other healthcare professionals (e.g., physical therapists) in making realistic early treatment plans. Psychologists also may provide support and education for families during the acute phase of brain injury and stroke recovery. Psychologists may contribute significantly to rehabilitation on inpatient rehabilitation units. For example, it has been demonstrated that the intensity of psychological services is actually the greatest predictor of successful multidisciplinary inpatient rehabilitation outcome, even after controlling for factors such as age, admission status, and length of stay (Heinemann 1995).

BEHAVIORAL APPROACHES

Patients who sustain brain injury or stroke often have behavioral disturbances. Although some aspects of their behavior may be related to "nonbehavioral" factors (e.g., biologically mediated agitation), many other issues may be at least partially addressed through the application of behavior modification approaches. It must be noted, however, that traditional approaches to behavior modification are based heavily upon learning theory, and learning is typically impaired among individuals with cerebral dysfunction. Thus, successful behavior management with many rehabilitation populations may need to focus more on stimulus control (i.e., environmental factors) than operant learning (i.e., recalling relationships between behaviors and their consequences). Environmental management and stimulus control techniques are often effective, and do not involve complicated contracting or excessive commitment of staff resources. For example, room doors designating certain types of rooms or functions can be painted in distinctive colors. Temporary signage can also be utilized for specific individuals' needs (e.g., "This is Mary's Room"). Traditional behavioral management approaches may be applied, but cognitive compromise can limit the success of outcomes (Turnbull 1988). Several useful manuals have been published which detail the application of behavior management techniques with neurological rehabilitation populations (Jacobs 1993, Matthies et al 1997). For further details on behavioral interventions refer to Chapter 8.

GROUP APPROACHES

Groups may help individuals with processing the emotional impact of their experience, and in promoting psychological and social adjustment within the context of their changed cognitive and physical circumstances (Barton et al 2002). It has also been demonstrated that group program interventions and home visits together contribute to increases in confidence in knowledge and the use of active coping strategies (van den Heuvel et al 2002). In the van den Heuvel et al (2002) study, the amount of social support remained stable in the intervention groups, whereas it decreased in the no-treatment control group.

PSYCHOTHERAPEUTIC APPROACHES

As indicated earlier in this chapter, an evaluation to assess for the cognitive and emotional impact of brain trauma is often an important early step in the rehabilitation process. When the neurocognitive sequelae result in significantly decreased self-awareness, the types of psychological supports and interventions typically offered to patients and their families may need to be modified. As described by Ricker (2003), traditional insight-oriented therapy approaches may be hampered by the presence of cognitive deficits in the patient's presentation. Such approaches generally depend upon the patient's ability to understand, at least on a basic level, their recent experience and their current situation, to use abilities such as insight and awareness to monitor their own reaction and communicate their reaction to others, and to use abstraction to think about how their current situation may affect their future. Indeed, the patient's ability to monitor and communicate about their internal states is key to many psychotherapeutic approaches to grief and adjustment counseling. As a result, intervention strategies that rely heavily on external stimulus control strategies and family participation may be most useful in many cases of significant brain injury or illness (Matthies et al 1997).

Emotional symptoms and adjustment reactions in the patient with cerebral compromise can take different courses. As indicated earlier, a patient with significant brain injury may present initially with emotional symptoms secondary to brain trauma itself, and only later, as they recover some degree of self-awareness, present with emotional symptoms secondary to a sense of loss. As a result, treatment approaches for emotional symptoms in these patients will often differ at various times in the process of their recovery. The patient who presents acutely with emotional and behavioral symptoms of brain trauma, may benefit from a quiet, structured, and consistent environment. Individuals who have recovered some level of self-awareness and begin to verbalize feelings of loss may increasingly benefit from more traditional psychotherapeutic approaches.

Another issue related to the psychological treatment of the brain-injured patient is that patients must deal with loss regarding not only cognitive functions, but also psychosocial functions. The patient's physical trauma and immediate cognitive losses are often the initial focus of grief for both the patient and family. As the patient is encouraged to become increasingly independent of the rehabilitation unit and in the community after discharge, the presence of emotional and personality changes may become increasingly apparent. Intervention aimed at assisting the patient and family to cope with loss must attend not only to the objective loss of cognitive function, but also to reports that the patient has somehow "changed" with reference to personality or role within the family.

FAMILY THERAPY

Psychologists and other rehabilitation practitioners working in neurological rehabilitation are often asked to provide education and support to TBI survivors and their families. Survivors of TBI and stroke may become more dependent upon family members, and this perceived level of burden may not decrease even as time passes (Rosenthal & Ricker 2000). Patient and family education may occur through a variety of approaches, ranging from formal interdisciplinary family conferences and educational groups, to supportive counseling and formal family therapy (Ricker 2003).

Most research on the impact of neurological compromise on the family has dealt with psychosocial effects over the long term, but early effects are also critical. While the severity of stroke is of importance, the individual's perception of the disease and its potential impact on future activities, in conjunction with the spouses' own coping capacity, is of great significance in the perception of quality of daily life (Forsberg-Warleby et al 2002).

COGNITIVE REHABILITATION

The implementation of behavioral or learning-based procedures to improve cognitive functioning has a long history (see Boake 1991), but systematic studies are of far more recent origin. It is arguably one of the more controversial areas within TBI rehabilitation (Bergquist & Malec 1997, Sohlberg & Mateer 1989), although recent reviews (e.g., Cicerone et al 2000) have presented evidence-based support for certain cognitive rehabilitation interventions in specific situations. The term "cognitive rehabilitation" is broad, and typically encompasses endeavors including cognitive retraining, cognitive remediation, and compensatory strategy training. Cognitive rehabilitation is often divided into two major approaches: restorative and compensatory. Restorative approaches focus on intervening at the level of areas of impaired cognitive functioning, while compensatory approaches are focused on functional goals and are designed to teach the individual how to reach goals using residual abilities and relative strengths.

Direct retraining techniques are based primarily on practice, with the assumption that practicing various cognitive tasks will result in general improvements in cognition. Examples include having individual's memorize lists or generate solutions to hypothetical problems. Although patients generally show improvement on tasks that they are required to practice, there is insufficient evidence to support generalization to real-world tasks or functional domains apart from the specific target areas. Potential exceptions to this are process-specific training approaches that derive from direct training, but specific skills are targeted for improvement. Some skills that have been shown to be positively impacted by intervention include visual scanning, attention and concentration, and spatial organization (Cicerone et al 2000).

The most common approaches to compensatory device training involve the use of cognitive memory "orthoses" such as planners, tape recorders, or calendars. Although their functional effectiveness is fairly well established, there is little evidence that the use of such devices results in a meaningful improvement in the underlying core cognitive abilities (Parente & Stapleton 1997). Such orthoses can prove useful during rehabilitation to assist with adherence. In addition, the efficacy and benefit of personal organization and time management products are hardly limited to individuals with acquired cerebral impairment.

Although cognitive rehabilitation is often applied as a specific intervention for impairments, some centers have taken a more programmatic approach. In such programs, cognitive rehabilitation is seen as a process that occurs within the context of a therapeutic milieu (i.e., treatment is seen as "holistic") rather than in the context of specific time-delimited sessions. The results of many programmatic approaches are generally in a positive direction, but improvement has been difficult to attribute solely to specific cognitive interventions (Rosenthal & Ricker 2000).

REMOTE SERVICE DELIVERY

In recent years, attention has been directed toward the provision of rehabilitation services remotely (i.e., "telerehabilitation"). Telerehabilitation is the application of telecommunication technology to provide distance support, assessment, and intervention to individuals with disabilities, and is a subcomponent of the broader area of telemedicine (Burns et al 1998). Although telecommunications is by no means a new industry, recent developments in telecommunication and its related technology are leading to advances in postacute and rehabilitative care. Using a telephone or cable modem hookup, along with either a personal computer or piece of dedicated-use remote hardware, physicians and other clinicians could presumably provide ongoing, real-time care to patients at either remote clinics or in their own homes (Palsbo & Bauer 2000). Telerehabilitation may hold particular promise for individuals who live in remote or underserved areas. Among consumers with brain injury or stroke, there have been several positive investigations, including providing telephone intervention with family caregivers of stroke survivors following traditional rehabilitation (Grant et al 2002), teleconferencing-based psychotherapy and behavioral training with individuals who have sustained traumatic brain injury (Schopp et al 2000), and examining computer and internet utilization among people with traumatic brain injury (Ricker et al 2002).

INTEGRATED MANAGEMENT APPROACHES

INTEGRATING THE TREATMENT TEAM

In medical rehabilitation, much of the assessment and treatment planning process is multidisciplinary. Findings from evaluations are increasingly described in terms of uniform functional status ratings (e.g., the FIM; Hamilton et al 1987), with treatment and discharge plans being formulated with a treatment team model (e.g., team rounds or chart rounds). Effective communication between the rehabilitation team, the patient, and the family facilitates optimal care and provides the stroke survivor with the opportunity to reach his or her maximal functional potential (Zorowitz et al 2002).

Within the context of a rehabilitation medicine setting, psychologists may typically be viewed as the primary "mental health" professionals. This may represent a different relationship when compared to psychiatric settings. In such settings, the psychiatrist is more likely to be seen as the senior mental health professional, and other professionals (e.g., social workers) may be seen as equivalent to psychologists.

For neuropsychologists, however, there may be a different phenomenon in the rehabilitation setting of having to work closely with individuals from other health professions (e.g., physical therapists, speech-language pathologists, and occupational therapists) that also assess domains of functioning such as memory, language, problem-solving, motor skills, etc. (Ricker 2003). Furthermore, in some settings, psychologists (along with other professionals, such as speech-language therapists and occupational therapists) provide services focused upon ameliorating acquired cognitive problems. Services may also be provided to assist patients with learning new strategies to compensate for acquired cognitive impairments. Such cognitive rehabilitation approaches, although in wide use, vary greatly from facility to facility, and have only recently been subject to more rigorous empirical research. There are certainly procedures that have demonstrated effectiveness in well-controlled, well-designed, and suitably monitored programs (e.g., Attention Process Training, Sohlberg & Mateer 1989), but it is incorrect to assume that anything that is done under the broad rubric of cognitive rehabilitation is thereby also effective (Ricker 1998). In addition, many activities and procedures that are conducted within the context of rehabilitation may not be uniquely "rehabilitative" in the most literal sense. For example, training someone to use a personal calendar or planner may certainly increase his or her time management skills and adherence to rehabilitation tasks, but this is not cognitive rehabilitation per se. When considering a referral for such services (regardless of the discipline that offers the service), it is important to consider the empirical basis for the intervention, the likely improvement in function arising from the passage of time alone (i.e., spontaneous recovery), the rationale for the intervention (e.g., retraining versus teaching compensatory strategies), the effects of practice, and the qualifications and experience of the provider.

Although all rehabilitation specialties represent different disciplines and approaches to assessment and intervention, it is critical that clinicians from all fields make every effort to approach cases from the same perspective, both conceptually and practically. That is, it may cause unwarranted confusion and conflict if one discipline views a patient from a strict test score-based or numeric "cut-off" perspective, while another discipline views the same patient in the context of the patient's education, life experience, effort, personal goals, and values. As important as it is for all disciplines to know their professional limits, it is equally important for referral source, professional colleagues, and interdisciplinary teams also to recognize these limits. For example, to a colleague or payer source not familiar with the differences, an occupational therapy or speech-language evaluation of higher cognitive functions and a neuropsychological evaluation might appear very similar. It is critical that each discipline educates consumers as to the unique contributions of their discipline's approach to assessment and intervention.

This should hold for not only cognitive therapies, but also physical therapies and non-cognitive aspects of occupational therapies. It is imperative that physical and occupational therapists make use of the psychologist in order to examine ways in which patients' compliance with treatment can be enhanced (see Chapter 4). There may be problems or situations which initially appear to be purely physical in their focus, but upon closer examination psychological issues might be responsible for mediating or maintaining aspects of non-compliance with therapies. For example, a patient might make fewer gains in physical therapy than would be predicted based on injury status, and initial examination might suggest that the individual is giving less than full physical effort during treatment sessions and attributes their own behavior to pain or fatigue. Upon closer examination and consultation between the physical therapist and the psychologist, however, it might be determined that the patient is fearful of returning home in a "changed" status, and is either intentionally or unintentionally not putting forth full effort in order to delay their return home. This is but one example of a situation in which a psychologist might assist another therapist in enhancing participation in therapy (and hopefully subsequent participation in the community after discharge).

As most rehabilitation psychologists are typically trained as clinical, health, or counseling psychologists, they are uniquely qualified to formally assess emotional states and to intervene using applied principles of psychology. This is not to say that other rehabilitation professionals have no input into such issues, as their observations may be of great utility in assisting with the formulation of a hypothesis regarding a patient's status, treatment, or outcome. It is within the scope of practice for other rehabilitation professionals to train and counsel patients, family members, educators, employers, and other rehabilitation professionals in adaptive strategies for managing cognitive-communication disorders. Other rehabilitation professionals must also integrate behavior modification treatment techniques (see Chapter 8) as appropriate for the management of associated problems, such as self-abusive and combative behaviors and agitation. Ultimately, the use of behavioral techniques and strategies should be viewed not as a psychological intervention, but rather as a way in which all team members might maximally increase each patient's participation in rehabilitation. Furthermore, therapists should not hesitate to request the assistance of a psychologist in facilitating this participation. In some settings, this might occur through direct referral from individual therapists. In other settings, such a referral might have to be requested as a formal order through the attending physician.

INPATIENT MANAGEMENT

Interdisciplinary team dynamics must be considered (Kreutzer & Sander, 1997), and psychologists can help to facilitate adaptive professional relations among team members and across disciplines. In an inpatient rehabilitation setting, the efficient provision of clinical services is critical. This is an important issue not only for patient care (patients and families, having already gone through an acute care hospitalization, do not want an unnecessarily long rehabilitation stay), but also for third party payers. For example, in the US, within inpatient rehabilitation, neuropsychologists commonly encounter the requirement of the "3-hour rule" with most third party payment providers. Essentially, this is a policy of the Health Care Finance Administration (HCFA), stating that if a patient is in an inpatient rehabilitation facility, they must receive 1 hour each of physical therapy, occupational therapy, and/or speech-language therapy each day. As no aspect of psychological or neuropsychological services is included in this 3-hour provision, psychologists find themselves competing with other disciplines (and outside consultants) for patient time and access, even though the psychologists might not be reimbursed for these services. In such an environment, it is recommended that team members adopt a patient-centered approach. In other words, the focus is on the needs of the patient, not on "which discipline does what." Thus, it should be seen as appropriate for a physical therapist to request a psychologist's assistance in increasing a patient's participation in gait training. Although the psychologists may know little or nothing about the mechanics or restoration of gait, he or she brings a wealth of information on analyzing what triggers or inhibits behavior, and can design strategies to increase desired activity while decreasing that which is not desired.

Extensive neuropsychological testing in the acute care setting immediately following the onset or exacerbation of cerebral impairment may be of minimal or no benefit given the possibility of delirium, post-traumatic amnesia, psychological shock, agitation, anxiety, transient aphasic presentations, significant motoric compromise, or other injuries (Ricker 2003). Brief focused testing (to be followed-up later with a more comprehensive neuropsychological evaluation) can, however, be of benefit in identifying and quantifying residual impairments, as well as in making appropriate recommendations. This is critical for effective rehabilitation programming given the need to determine the individual's functional capacities that are available for compensatory strategies, as well as those areas that may need to be targeted for improvement. Neuropsychological testing can help in formulating plans for community reintegration following cerebral compromise, such as return to work or school. Such testing is also useful in identifying and quantifying areas of improvement, which may be required for certain aspects of reintegration after brain impairment (e.g., re-establishing legal independence following appointment of a guardian). Documentation of improvement is likely to be of comfort to individuals (and to the families of these individuals) who have sustained central neurological dysfunction. Formal assessment is also useful when formulating individual behavioral management plans, given the fact that such plans rely heavily on an individual's ability to learn and follow directions. Neuropsychological assessment can also, in some instances, be utilized as an index of efficacy for some types of treatment, such as interventions designed to improve or compensate for cognitive impairments (sometimes referred to as cognitive rehabilitation, remediation, or retraining). Neuropsychological testing may also be used to index changes following certain medical interventions (e.g., pharmacotherapy).

Documentation within a medical rehabilitation context is likely to differ from a traditional neuropsychiatric setting. Given the treatment and ongoing assessment orientation of most accredited rehabilitation programs, reports are likely to be briefer, more frequent, and functionally based with recommendations for treatment (rather than simply listing a series of impaired test scores). In addition, greater emphasis may be placed on daily assessment reports and treatment notes. Given the interactive and multidisciplinary nature of medical rehabilitation, it is critical that the psychologist has excellent consultative and interactive skills. This is of particular importance when the psychologist is interacting with disciplines more physical in nature, as the potential contributions of a psychologist to the enhancement of factors such as balance or gait might not be directly apparent.

Even as an outside consultant to a rehabilitation team, a psychologist can provide an informative perspective. This may be especially true in the context of a rehabilitation setting that is accustomed to patients without prominent cognitive impairment (e.g., a spinal cord injury or orthopedic setting). In terms of assessment, many events that can lead to other medical rehabilitation conditions (e.g., spinal cord injury, complicated fractures) may also result in traumatic brain injury (e.g., motor vehicle accidents, assaults, and falls). Although moderate and severe TBI are not likely to be "overlooked" clinically, co-existing mild or mild-to-moderate TBI may be missed upon initial examination of the SCI patient in the acute trauma setting (Ricker & Regan 1999).

Treating the individual with cognitive compromise may pose special challenges for rehabilitation professionals accustomed to working primarily with individuals who have sustained non-brain injuries or illnesses. Although the acute rehabilitation process for any individual can be stressful to the primary consumer (i.e., the patient), family, and team members, the rehabilitation process for someone with multiple conditions (e.g., a SCI and brain injury) is multiply compounded. For example, many aspects of medical rehabilitation involve educating patients about self-care procedures (e.g., medication regimen training, bowel training, bladder management, transfers). The team's approach to education and training may have to be modified for the patient who presents with significant cognitive symptoms. Such patients may exhibit multiple difficulties in advancing through the rehabilitation program, including difficulties retaining new information over time, sequencing information during multistep tasks, making judgments about safety, problem solving in novel situations, and initiating self-care behavior. Thus, psychologists can have a favorable impact on patient care by assisting in the modification of the actual treatment program. For instance, the team may need to emphasize caregiver training more heavily than patient training, at least initially. Training may also need to be approached using simple and concrete communication. The individual with cognitive inefficiencies may become "overloaded" with new information more easily than non-brain-compromised persons.

Even in the context of an injury or illness that clearly involves the brain, rehabilitation teams may still require significant input from the neuropsychologist. Cerebral compromise is, by any definition, a potentially catastrophic and life-changing event. Immediately after the injury, medical practitioners and family are often most concerned with the patient's acute medical condition and chances of survival. Once survival appears likely, individuals and family often become more aware of and focused on issues of functional loss. A grieving process often begins during the acute medical stage and continues through the rehabilitation process and beyond (Hainsworth 1998). In brain injury and stroke, emotional adjustment may take a somewhat different course as compared to rehabilitation populations that experience non-brain-based impairments. Accurate assessment of emotional functioning requires that the patient demonstrates some degree of insight and awareness regarding their recent experiences and their emotional functioning. Unfortunately, individuals that sustain TBI and stroke often experience deficits in these areas. Thus, individuals might be truly unaware of their situation and may lack many common symptoms of grief and readjustment. Indeed, these individuals may report little or no emotional reaction or changes in functioning. This type of presentation may be misinterpreted by staff as representing a purely "psychological" process such as denial. As individuals recover from their acute event and self-awareness improves, they may develop "delayed" emotional symptoms or behavior problems that were not present or apparent more proximal to the onset of their injury or stroke. Thus, it is important for psychologists to assist team members in differentiating what problems are "really" psychological in origin, and which might be more primarily physiological.

In contrast to the individual who initially presents with a lack of emotional symptoms, some individuals will alternatively present with notable emotional symptoms and personality change. They may exhibit a variety of symptoms including increased irritability, impatience, agitation, and fatigue, as well as decreased frustration tolerance and motivation (Matthies et al 1997). These symptoms may be misinterpreted by staff as either maladaptive psychological reactions to catastrophic injury or simply as the presentation of a "noncompliant" patient. Staff who are either unaware of the presence of brain trauma in the patient, or that are not accustomed to working with individuals that have cerebral involvement, may become easily frustrated with the level of attention, encouragement, and structure required by these patients in combination with their apparent non-compliance with aspects of the rehabilitation program. Behavioral approaches with patients and staff can often help in these situations.

Thus, an accurate understanding of the patient's initial presentation in inpatient rehabilitation, including an understanding of the extent to which brain trauma has occurred, can greatly assist staff in understanding aspects of the patient's emotional presentation and in addressing issues related to the course of adjustment. This understanding will also assist team members in interpreting and monitoring their own emotional responses to the situation.

PHARMACOLOGICAL ADJUNCTS TO BEHAVIORAL MANAGEMENT

Although psychologists and most other rehabilitation practitioners do not directly prescribe medications or directly recommend specific psy-

chopharmacological regimens for patients, it is important to have familiarity with the drugs that are currently used in the treatment and management of TBI. A comprehensive review of psychopharmacological treatment following brain injury can be found in Zafonte et al (1999).

Psychostimulants such as methylphenidate (best known under the brandname of Ritalin), amantadine, and bromocriptine are used with TBI and stroke patients. This drug may be of particular use in increasing the tonic (i.e., general) arousal of individuals with neurologic compromise, and may also assist in increasing speech initiation in individuals with aphasia (Zafonte et al 1999).

Antiseizure medications are, of course, used as seizure prophylaxis or to control a known seizure disorder. They are also used in some TBI patients to manage agitation, regardless of whether the cause is seizure-related. Antiseizure medications are also gaining popular use in the non-TBI populations as well as a primary or adjunctive treatment for mood disorders (e.g., bipolar disorder, American Association of Neurological Surgeons 2000).

Antipsychotic medications are often used to decrease agitated behavior in non-TBI populations. Their use in the TBI population has been historically controversial given assumptions about the effects of antipsychotics on post-TBI neurobehavioral symptoms and negative impact on the rehabilitation process. Much of the caution derives from animal studies (and limited human data). Of note, however, are potential beneficial uses of the newer generation of atypical antipsychotics. Since these agents have different mechanisms of action as well as different neurotransmitter targets, concerns about exacerbation of agitation might be fewer (Elovic et al 2003).

OUTPATIENT MANAGEMENT

Given the nature of training and practice of clinical neuropsychology (i.e., typically lengthy batteries of psychometric tests), neuropsychologists involved in rehabilitation may find it easier to practice "traditional" battery-based neuropsychology in an outpatient setting. Of note, however, is the fact that such batteries and approaches were developed irrespectively of known or suspected diagnosis, and were not developed within the context of the needs of contemporary medical rehabilitation. In fact, batteries that are heavily dependent upon sensorimotor input and output functions may be of little incremental utility with many neurorehabilitation populations (Rosenthal & Ricker 2000). In addition, it is important to note that normative databases are rarely equivalent, and are virtually never identical. For example, one group used to norm one particular test may differ dramatically and in clinically meaningful ways from the normative group used for another test. In clinical psychology and neuropsychology, an excellent example is the Wechsler Adult Intelligence Scale – Revised (WAIS-R). The WAIS-R and the WAIS-III are well standardized in the sense of having large normative databases across age ranges (Ricker 2003). Beyond the Wechsler scales, however, there are no additional cognitive test data obtained from the original standardization sample. Otherwise stated, there are data as to how the standardization sample performs on the WAIS-R or WAIS-III, but no data widely available addressing how these individuals perform in other cognitive domains or on other neuropsychological tests. Clinically, however, psychologists routinely use the WAIS-R/III IQ scores as a "baseline" for comparison, and then proceed to compare additional tests to these scores as if all scores were comparable. Furthermore, as the population ages and the number of individuals who experience some period of disability in their lives increases, it will be critical to develop tests and normative data that take normal aging into account. Having said this, however, it should be noted that most practicing neuropsychologists do not utilize a rigid fixed-battery approach (Sweet et al 2000).

Psychologists can certainly provide useful information to patients, families, and to other professionals. First, clinical neuropsychologists can provide neuropsychometric assessment. This refers to the use of various tests and measures designed to allow for inferences about brain–behavior relationships. This type of data can provide information about a client's cognitive functioning and psychosocial issues. A formal neuropsychological evaluation can provide patients and healthcare providers with estimates of a client's abilities across many areas of neurocognitive functioning including attention, language, memory, visuospatial abilities, planning, problem-solving, and emotional status. Comprehensive neuropsychological evaluations may also allow for predictions to be made regarding a client's cognitive capacity to return to work, and about the client's motivation to do so. Clinical neuropsychologists can also assist in estimating a client's actual pre-injury or pre-illness level of functioning or adaptation. Because most clinical neuropsychologists are trained not only in brain–behavior relationships but also in clinical, health, or counseling psychology, they are also able to take into account factors other than a primary brain injury that may contribute to abnormal neuropsychological test findings. Such factors can include emotional disruption, age, premorbid psychiatric history, substance abuse, learning disability, decreased motivation, or even secondary gain.

Although many clinical neuropsychologists focus primarily or exclusively on neuropsychometric assessment, many provide direct intervention in the form of behavior management, client education, psychotherapy, or guidance in vocational pursuits. Community reintegration may be cognitively difficult and emotionally stressful for clients, and short-term psychological interventions can be quite useful in facilitating adaptive functioning.

Within the context of outpatient rehabilitation, a major focus of psychological practice for the majority of adults is vocational reintegration. Clinical neuropsychologists may provide consultation to vocational counselors, employers, and state vocational rehabilitation services (referred to as job commissions in some areas). This is particularly important in light of the Americans With Disabilities Act (1990), which, among many things, emphasizes accommodations that can assist individuals with successful return to work. Clinical neuropsychologists can be of great utility in assisting institutions and organizations in fulfilling the spirit and letter of this legislation.

OUTPATIENT PROGRAMMING

Perhaps the most pervasive forms of postacute rehabilitation are outpatient therapy and day treatment. Outpatient therapy can consist of a single or combination of therapies (e.g., physical therapy, occupational therapy, speech-language therapy, psychotherapy) that an individual may receive at a rehabilitation center or specialized neurological rehabilitation program. In all but the mildest of cases, a period of outpatient therapy is recommended after inpatient rehabilitation to assist individuals in reaching their highest level of physical and psychological functioning. This is often accompanied by periodic medical monitoring, usually by a physiatrist, and follow-up psychological or neuropsychological evaluation after 6 months or longer to assess the level of recovery and residual impairments. Day treatment is a form of outpatient treatment in which a full array of treatment services is provided to individuals who often attend 3–5 days per week for 4–6 hours per day. The duration of day treatment programs is generally 3–6 months. These programs, which in the US are often accredited by the Commission for the Accreditation of Rehabilitation Facilities (CARF) as "community-integrated programs," provide the standard array of rehabilitation services with ongoing medical supervision, cognitive rehabilitation, case management, vocational rehabilitation services, and individual, family, and group psychotherapy. Many of these programs are psychologist-led or managed and are termed "holistic" or "neuropsychological rehabilitation" programs and have produced very positive outcomes (see Malec & Basford 1996).

Transitional living programs are designed for higher functioning individuals who are ready to learn independent living skills in a community setting. Often, such individuals have completed an extensive therapy program and are medically stable. Usually, transitional living programs are located in single or multi-family dwellings in the community, staffed by counselors or therapists who may be affiliated with a brain injury rehabilitation program. Due to a variety of cognitive and/or behavioral problems, residents in a transitional living program need some training to develop or regain skills in community mobility, shopping, managing personal finance, job-seeking, use of leisure time, and developing appropriate interpersonal relationships.

For individuals with chronic, severe behavior problems, a neurobehavioral residential treatment program is often a desired placement. This type of program may be hospital-based with a focus on a high degree of structure, systematic use of behavioral management, physical management, and/or psychopharmacology. Individuals who exhibit severe disinhibition, agitation (beyond the acute phase of recovery), and antisocial behavior (including the threat of potential harm to self or others) are likely candidates to receive treatment in these settings.

PSYCHOSOCIAL MANAGEMENT

Family reintegration

Families are often characterized as the "second victim" of TBI or stroke. The typically sudden onset of the event, and its residual sequelae, creates difficulties in acceptance and coping. The family is a critical component of successful community integration (Perlesz et al 1999). Individuals often return to their family, which then assumes the role of caregiver. This can pose a considerable burden on the family, who are unaccustomed to their new roles and experience a great deal of "burden" which may even increase over the years after TBI or stroke (Brooks et al 1986). For example, a person with a TBI returns to a spouse, who may quite accurately perceive their partner as a significantly different person or even as a "child." This can create tremendous stress on the caregiving spouse, and in some cases, parent–child relationships. As Serio et al (1995) found in their study of family needs following brain injury, the need for emotional support is most frequently "unmet," in comparison to needs for medical information, professional support, and instrumental support.

Vocational reintegration

Given that the majority of stroke survivors are older individuals, including many retirees, return to work is not as pressing an issue as it is in the TBI population. For many survivors of brain injury, the process of re-entering competitive employment is one of the greatest obstacles and likely factors contributing to a sense of quality of life. Despite the catastrophic nature of TBI, many survivors have sufficiently recovered basic physical and cognitive skills within 6–12 months postinjury to begin the process of vocational rehabilitation. The first step is usually a referral from the rehabilitation facility to a vocational rehabilitation agency. In the US, many state vocational rehabilitation agency offices have counselors that specialize in TBI. After establishing eligibility for services, an individualized written rehabilitation plan may be established, consisting of a variety of elements:

- comprehensive extended evaluation, which may include up-to-date medical, neuropsychological, and vocational interest/aptitude examinations
- referral to a specialized brain injury rehabilitation program which has a vocational rehabilitation component
- contact with pre-injury employer and attempts to assist the client to return to pre-injury employment in the same or, more typically, reduced job
- referral to a supported employment program, which may be administered by the state agency or by a vocational rehabilitation company or brain injury rehabilitation program.

The supported employment model, which is known as a "place-train" model is one in which clients are placed in a competitive work setting with a job coach, who works alongside the employee until the employee no longer needs the cueing or guidance which has been provided. Initially developed with the psychiatric population, it has appeared to be an effective model for the brain injury population as well (Wehman et al 1989). For some individuals, the level of residual deficit is so severe that return to work is not feasible. In these cases, the client is referred to the Disability Determination Service in the US situation for evaluation of eligibility for long-term disability payments through the social security system. Similar systems also exist in other countries.

Academic reintegration

For children or young adults that experience brain injury, an important goal is resumption of school or academic activities. In the past decade, the US federal and state education agencies have recognized traumatic brain injury as a distinct entity. Using the US as an example, children and adolescents that experience any disabling neurological condition are eligible to receive special education services under the Individuals with Disabilities Education Act (Americans With Disabilities Act 1990), which was initially enacted in 1990 and revised in 1997. In some rehabilitation programs, educational tutoring is initiated during the inpatient hospitalization. When discharge approaches, the rehabilitation team (frequently the psychologist or social worker) often works directly with the individual's local school district to develop a transition plan to enable a person to re-establish an educational program. An individualized educational plan is developed, which may include homebound tutoring, part-time schedule, use of compensatory strategies or devices, modified curriculum, assistive technology, special transportation and similar services. This plan is subject to review on a yearly basis, or more often as needed. For young adults, many universities around the world offer services for students with disabilities.

Substance abuse

A major risk factor for successful community reintegration following TBI is the use and abuse of alcohol and/or drugs. A recent study from the TBI Model Systems examined cross-sectional data for up to 4 years postinjury (Kreutzer et al 1996b). The investigators found that those who used alcohol excessively prior to the injury remained heavy drinkers at follow-up several years postinjury. Other investigators have identified substance abuse as a major impediment to participation in supported employment programs and job retention (Sale et al 1991). A recent study demonstrated the effectiveness of a community-based model, termed the "TBI Network," in increasing the productivity and decreasing the level of substance use in individuals who sustained severe traumatic brain injury (Bogner et al 1997). Although many rehabilitation psychologists do not have advanced training in substance abuse treatment, it is important to utilize screening measures, such as the Michigan Alcoholism Screening Test (MAST, Pokorney et al 1972) or the Ewing questionnaire (usually referred to as the "CAGE," representing the "Cutting down," "Annoyance," "Guilt," and "Eye-Opener" items of the question list, Ewing 1984) to correctly identify those who used substances excessively and may be likely to abuse substances following discharge into the community. It is also important for the rehabilitation psychologist to identify, educate and/or refer to community providers who can treat substance abuse problems in persons with TBI. The technique of motivational interviewing during the inpatient stay has been shown to be of some utility in reducing later drinking behavior among individuals with TBI that have a history of alcohol abuse (Bombardier & Rimmele 1999). Rehabilitation practitioners other than psychologists can play an important role in identifying symptoms of the abuse of alcohol and other drugs.

SUMMARY

This chapter has provided a brief overview of the nature of TBI and stroke, and their cognitive, neurobehavioral, and psychosocial consequences. Descriptions have been provided to understand the multiple roles of psychologists and other rehabilitation practitioners in assessing and managing impairments and issues encountered in the rehabilitation process, both for the survivor and significant others. Brain injury and stroke have become core programs in many, if not most, rehabilitation programs. Psychologists have been instrumental in establishing innovations in clinical practice and in engaging in critical research to establish the validity of new techniques of assessment (e.g., neuropsychological assessment) and rehabilitation treatment (e.g., cognitive rehabilitation). In addition, psychologists have been actively involved in treatment efficacy research, which has become of increased relevance in the era of healthcare reform and, in the US and many other countries, managed care. It has also been the case that psychologists have been at the forefront in model systems of care, and also in the policy and legislative arena in developing standards of care.

Even with greater external constraints being placed on rehabilitation practice, there may be greater numbers of patients that are referred for services. Recent publications suggest the effectiveness of some physical (e.g., constraint induced therapy; van der Lee et al 1999) and cognitive (Cicerone et al 2000) interventions. As empirical support grows for medical rehabilitation, third party payers may be more inclined to approve longer stays or to approve referral to comprehensive rehabilitation services in the first place. A recent National Institute of Health Consensus Conference (held in 1998) also heavily emphasized the beneficial role that psychologists and neuropsychologists can play in the assessment and rehabilitation of survivors of neurologic injury. Such influential support will benefit the "front-line" clinical practitioner.

Recent research suggests that rehabilitation services can have the greatest impact on functional outcomes when they are implemented early. The effect of this is that patients are admitted to rehabilitation settings much earlier than in previous years. Thus, the nature of the neuropsychological services that can – and should – be provided is likely to become increasingly different. The provision of multi-hour standardized testing batteries is more likely to be reserved as an outpatient service, with cognitive screening and behavioral management being the focus of inpatient rehabilitation.

As with all practice environments for psychologists, the medical rehabilitation setting poses many challenges, but also offers many rewards. The capacity for neuropsychologists to interact directly and regularly with multiple healthcare professionals is, although not unique, almost a cardinal feature of rehabilitation neuropsychology. As advances have occurred in acute medical interventions (e.g., improvements in managing acute intracranial pressure in brain injury, or early pharmacological interventions following stroke), rehabilitation psychology has seen an increase in the number of patients, but has also had to look for ways to continue to make contributions in the face of a very different healthcare reimbursement market. A large percentage of one's patients will demonstrate improvement and make meaningful reintegration into their communities. The information that the neuropsychologist can communicate, and the interventions that psychologists provide, contribute positively to the process of rehabilitation, and ultimately to the functional outcome of patients and their families.

ACKNOWLEDGMENTS

Preparation of this chapter was supported, in part, by funding awarded to the author from the National Institute on Disability and Rehabilitation Research (NIDRR) and the National Institutes of Health (NIH).

References

American Association of Neurological Surgeons: The Joint Section on Neurotrauma and Critical Care 2000 Role of antiseizure prophylaxis following head injury. Journal of Neurotrauma 17(6–7): 549–553

Americans With Disabilities Act 1990 42 U.S.C.A. ss. 12101 et seq. United States Government, Washington, DC.

Army Individual Test Battery 1941 The trail making test. Department of Defence, Washington, DC

Barton J, Miller A, Chanter J 2002 Emotional adjustment to stroke: A group therapeutic approach. Nursing Times 98(23): 33–35

Beck A T 1996 The Beck Depression Inventory – II. The Psychological Corporation, San Antonio, TX

Belin P, van Eeckhout P, Zilbovicius M et al 1996 Recovery from nonfluent aphasia after melodic intonation therapy: A PET study. Neurology 47: 1504–1511

Benton A L, Hamsher K deS, Varney N R et al 1983 Contributions to neuropsychological assessment. Oxford University Press, New York

Benton A L, Hamsher K deS, Sivan A B 1994 Multilingual aphasia examination, 3rd edn. AJA Associates, Iowa City, IA

Bergquist T F, Malec J F 1997 Current practice and training issues in treatment of cognitive dysfunction. Neurorehabilitation 8: 49–56

Binder L M 1997 A review of mild head trauma. Part II: Clinical implications. Journal of Clinical and Experimental Neuropsychology 19(3): 432–457

Binder L M, Rohling M L, Larabee G J 1997 A review of mild head trauma. Part I: Meta-analytic review of neuropsychological studies. Journal of Clinical and Experimental Neuropsychology 19(3): 421–431

Boake C 1991 History of cognitive rehabilitation following head injury. In: Kreutzer J S, Wehman P H (eds) Rehabilitation for persons with traumatic brain injury. Paul H. Brookes, Baltimore, MD, p 3–12

Bogner J A, Corrigan J D, Spafford D E et al 1997 Integrating substance abuse treatment and vocational rehabilitation after traumatic brain injury. Journal of Head Trauma Rehabilitation 12(5): 57–71

Bogner J A, Corrigan, J D, Fugate L et al 2001 Role of agitation in prediction of outcomes after traumatic brain injury. American Journal of Physical Medicine and Rehabilitation 80(9): 636–644

Bombardier C H, Rimmele C T 1999 Motivational interviewing to prevent alcohol abuse after traumatic brain injury: A case series. Rehabilitation Psychology 44(1): 52–67

Braakman R, Jennett W B, Minderhoud J M 1988 Prognosis of the posttraumatic vegetative state. Acta Neurochirgica 95: 49–52

Brandt J, Benedict R H B 1998 Hopkins Verbal Learning Test – Revised. Psychological Assessment Resources, Odessa, FL

Brooks N, Campsie L, Symington C et al (1986) The five year outcome of severe blunt head injury: A relative's view. Journal of Neurology, Neurosurgery and Psychiatry 49: 764–770

Burns R B, Crislip D, Davious P et al 1998 Using telerehabilitation to support assistive technology. Assistive Technology 10: 126–133

Calvert G A, Brammer M J, Morris R G et al 2000 Using fMRI to study recovery from acquired dysphasia. Brain and Language 71: 391–399

Caplan B, Moelter S 2000 Stroke. In: Frank R, Elliott T (eds) Handbook of rehabilitation psychology. American Psychological Association Press, Washington, DC, 75–108

Cappa S F 1998 Spontaneous recovery from aphasia. In: Whitaker H, Stemmer B (eds) Handbook of neurolinguistics. Academic Press, San Diego, CA, p 534–545

Carod-Artal F J, Gonzalez-Gutierrez J L, Egido-Herrero J A et al 2002 Post stroke depression: Predictive factors at one year follow up. Revue Neurologique 35(2): 101–106

Centers for Disease Control (1997) Traumatic brain injury – Colorado, Missouri, Oklahoma, and Utah, 1990–1993. Morbidity and Mortality Weekly Report 48(1): 8–11

Cheung R T 2002 Sexual functioning in Chinese stroke patients with mild or no disability. Cerebrovascular Disorders 14(2): 122–128

Cicerone K D, Dahlberg C, Kalmar K et al 2000 Evidence-based cognitive rehabilitation: Recommendations for clinical practice. Archives of Physical Medicine and Rehabilitation 81: 1596–1615

Cooper K D, Tabbador K, Hauser W A et al 1983 The epidemiology of head injury in the Bronx. Neuroepidemiology 2: 70–88

Cullum C M, Thompson L L 1997 Neuropsychological diagnosis and outcome in mild traumatic brain injury. Applied Neuropsychology 4(1): 6–16

Drevets W C 2000 Functional anatomical abnormalities in limbic and prefrontal cortical structures in major depression. Progress in Brain Research 126: 413–431

Duncan P, Samsa G, Weinberger M 1997 Health status of individuals with mild stroke. Stroke 28: 740–745

Elovic E P, Lansang R, Li Y et al 2003 The use of atypical antipsychotics in traumatic brain injury. Journal of Head Trauma Rehabilitation 18(2): 177–195

Ewing J A 1984 Detecting alcoholism: The CAGE Questionnaire. Journal of the American Medical Association 252(14): 1905–1907

Folstein M F, Folstein S E, McHugh P R 1975 Mini-mental state: A practical method for grading the state of patients for the clinician. Journal of Psychiatric Research 12: 189–198

Forsberg-Warleby G, Moller A, Blomstrand C 2002 Spouses of first-ever stroke patients: Their view of the future during the first phase after stroke. Clinical Rehabilitation 16(5): 506–514

Friedman P 1990 Gait recovery after hemiplegic stroke. International Disability Studies 12: 119–122

Giacino J T, Ashwal S, Childs N et al 2002. The minimally conscious state: Definition and diagnostic criteria. Neurology 58(3): 349–353

Grant D A, Berg E A 1948 A behavioural analysis of the degree of reinforcement and ease of shifting to new responses in a Weigl-type card sorting problem. Journal of Experimental Psychology 38: 404–411

Grant J S, Elliott T R, Weaver M et al 2002 Telephone intervention with family caregivers of stroke survivors after rehabilitation. Stroke 33(8): 2060–2065

Grasso M G, Pantano P, Ricci M et al 1994 Mesial temporal cortex hypoperfusion is associated with depression in subcortical stroke. Stroke 25(5): 980–985

Griffith E R, Lemberg S 1993 Sexuality and the person with traumatic brain injury: A guide for families. FA Davis, Philadelphia

Gronwall D, Wrightson P 1981 Memory and information processing after closed head injury. Journal of Neurology, Neurosurgery and Psychiatry 44: 889–895

Gupta A, Pansari K, Shetty H 2002 Post-stroke depression. International Journal of Clinical Practice 56(7): 531–537

Hainsworth D S 1998 Reflections on loss without death: The lived experience of acute care nurses caring for neurologically devastated patients. Holistic Nursing Practice 13(1): 41–50

Hamilton B B, Granger C V, Sherwin F S et al 1987 A uniform national data system for medical rehabilitation. In: Fuhrer M (ed) Rehabilitation outcome analysis and measurement. Paul Brookes, Baltimore, MD, p 137–147

Hammond F M, McDeavitt J T 1999 Medical and orthopedic complications. In: Rosenthal M, Griffith J S, Kreutzer, Pentland B (eds) Rehabilitation of the adult and child with traumatic brain injury, 3rd edn. F A Davis, Philadelphia, p 53–73

Harrison-Felix C, Newton N, Hall K et al 1996 Descriptive findings from the traumatic brain injury model systems national data base. Journal of Head Trauma Rehabilitation 11(5): 1–14

Heinemann A W, Hamilton B, Linacre J M et al 1995 Functional status and therapeutic intensity during inpatient rehabilitation. American Journal of Physical Medicine and Rehabilitation 74: 315–326

Heiss W D, Karbe H, Weber-Luxenburger G et al 1997 Speech-induced cerebral metabolic activation reflects recovery from aphasia. Journal of Neurological Sciences 145: 213–217

Heiss W D, Kessler J, Thiel A et al 1999 Differential capacity of left and right hemispheric areas for compensation of poststroke aphasia. Annals of Neurology 45: 430–438

Herholz K, Heiss W D 2000 Functional imaging correlates of recovery after stroke in humans. Journal of Cerebral Blood Flow and Metabolism 20(12): 1619–1631

Hillier S L, Hiller J E, Metzer J 1997 Epidemiology of traumatic brain injury in South Australia. Brain Injury 11(9): 649–659

Ingles J, Eskes G, Phillips S 1999 Fatigue after stroke. Archives of Physical Medicine and Rehabilitation 80: 173–178

Jacobs H E 1993 Behavior analysis guidelines and brain injury rehabilitation. Aspen Publishers, Gaithersburg, MD

Jongsma A E, Rusin M J 2001 The rehabilitation psychology treatment planner. Wiley, New York

Karbe H, Thiel A, Weber-Luxeburger G et al 1998 Brain plasticity in post stroke aphasia: What is the contribution of the right hemisphere? Brain and Language 64: 215–230

Kramer J H, Reed B R, Mungas D et al 2002 Executive dysfunction in subcortical ischaemic vascular disease. Journal of Neurology, Neurosurgery and Psychiatry 72(2): 217–220

Kraus J S, McArthur D L 1998 Incidence and prevalence of, and costs associated with, traumatic brain injury. In: Rosenthal M, Griffith E, Kreutzer J, Pentland B (eds) Rehabilitation of the adult and child with traumatic brain injury, 3rd edn. F A Davis, Philadelphia, p 3–18

Kraus J, Fife D, Conroy C et al 1989 Alcohol and brain injuries: Persons blood-tested, prevalence of alcohol involvement, and early outcome following injury. American Journal of Public Health 79: 294–299

Kreutzer J S, Sander A 1997 Issues in brain injury evaluation and treatment. Rehabilitation Psychology 42(3): 231–239

Kreutzer J S, Marwitz J H, Witol A D 1996a Interrelationships between crime, substance abuse, and aggressive behaviors among persons with traumatic brain injury. Brain Injury 9(8): 757–768

Kreutzer J S, Witol A D, Sander A M et al 1996b A prospective longitudinal multicenter analysis of alcohol use patterns among persons with traumatic brain injury. Journal of Head Trauma Rehabilitation 11(5): 58–69

Levin H S, O'Donnell V M, Grossman R G 1979 The Galveston Orientation and Amnesia Test: A practical scale to assess cognition after head injury. Journal of Nervous and Mental Diseases 167(11): 675–684

Levin H S, Benton A L, Grossman R G 1982 Neurobehavioral consequences of closed head injury. Oxford University Press, New York

Mackenzie A E, Chang A M 2002 Predictors of quality of life following stroke. Disability Rehabilitation 24(5): 259–265

Malec J F, Basford J S 1996 Post-acute brain injury rehabilitation. Archives of Physical Medicine and Rehabilitation 77: 198–207

Malec J F, Moessner A M 2000 Self-awareness, distress, and postacute rehabilitation outcome. Rehabilitation Psychology 45(3): 227–259

Mapou R L 1990 Traumatic brain injury rehabilitation with gay and lesbian individuals. Journal of Head Trauma Rehabilitation 5(2): 67–72

Martin T A, Donders J, Thompson E 2000 Potential of and problems with new measures of psychometric intelligence after traumatic brain injury. Rehabilitation Psychology 45(4): 402–408

Matthews C G, Klove H 1964 Instruction manual for the Adult Neuropsychology Test Battery. University of Wisconsin Medical School, Madison, WI

Matthies B K, Kreutzer J S, West D D 1997 The behavior management handbook: A practical approach to patients with neurological disorders. Therapy Skill Builders, San Antonio, TX

Mayberg H S, Robinson R G, Wong D F et al 1988 PET imaging of cortical S–2 serotonin receptors after stroke: Lateralized changes and relationship to depression. American Journal of Psychiatry 145(8): 937–943

Mayer S A, Bernardini G L, Brust J C M et al 2000 Subarachnoid hemorrhage. In: Lewis R P (ed) Merritt's neurology, 10th edn. Lippincott Williams & Wilkins, Philadelphia, p 260–267

Mayo N 1993 Stroke epidemiology and recovery. Physical Medicine and Rehabilitation: State of the Art Reviews 7: 1–25

Millis S R, Rosenthal M, Novack T A et al 2001 Long-term neuropsychological outcome following traumatic brain injury. Journal of Head Trauma Rehabilitation 16(4): 343–355

Murray G D, Teasdale G M, Braakman R et al 1999 The European Brain Injury Consortium survey of head injuries. Acta Neurochirgica (Wien) 141(3): 223–236

Nicholl C R, Lincoln N B, Muncaster K et al 2002 Cognition and post-stroke depression. British Journal of Clinical Psychology 41(3): 221–231

Novack T A, Dillon M C, Jackson W T 1996 Neurochemical mechanisms in brain injury and treatment: A review. Journal of Clinical and Experimental Neuropsychology 18: 685–706

O'Connell B, Hanna B, Penney W et al 2001 Recovery after stroke: A qualitative perspective. Journal of Qualitative Clinical Practice 21(4): 120–125

Ohyama M, Senda M, Kitamura S et al 1996 Role of the nondominant hemisphere and undamaged area during word repetition in poststroke aphasics. Stroke 27: 897–903

Ouimet M A, Primeau F, Cole M G 2001 Psychosocial risk factors in poststroke depression: A systematic review. Canadian Journal of Psychiatry 46(9): 819–828

Palsbo S E, Bauer D 2000 Telerehabilitation: Managed care's new opportunity. Managed Care Quarterly 8(4): 56–64

Pantano P, Guariglia C, Judica A et al 1992 Pattern of cerebral blood flow in the rehabilitation of visuospatial neglect. International Journal of Neuroscience 66: 153–161

Parente R, Stapleton M 1997 History and systems of cognitive rehabilitation. Neurorehabilitation 8: 3–11

Perlesz A, Kinsella G, Crowe S 1999 Impact of traumatic brain injury on the family: A critical review. Rehabilitation Psychology 44(1): 6–35

Pizzamiglio L, Perani D, Cappa S F et al 1998 Recovery of neglect after right hemispheric damage: $H_2^{(15)}O$ positron emission tomographic activation study. Archives of Neurology 55(4): 561–568

Pizzamiglio L, Galati G, Committeri G 2001 The contribution of functional neuroimaging to recovery after brain damage: A review. Cortex 37(1): 11–31

Pokorney A D, Miller B A, Kaplan H B 1972 The Brief MAST: A shortened version of the Michigan Alcoholism Screening Test. American Journal of Psychiatry 129: 342–345

Psychological Corporation 1999 Wechsler Abbreviated Scale of Intelligence. The Psychological Corporation, San Antonio, TX

Radloff L S 1977 The CES-D scale: A self-report depression scale for research in the general population. Applied Psychological Measurement 1: 385–401

Ragnaarson K T, Thomas J P, Zasler N D 1993 Model systems of care for individuals with traumatic brain injury. Journal of Head Trauma Rehabilitation 8: 1–11

Rappaport M, Dougherty A, Kelting D 1992 Evaluation of coma and the vegetative states. Archives of Physical Medicine and Rehabilitation 73: 628–634

Reitan RM, Wolfson D 1993 Halstead-Reitan Neuropsychological Test Battery: Theory and clinical interpretation, 2nd edn. Neuropsychology Press, Tucson, AZ

Rey A 1964 L'examen clinique en psychologie. Presses Universitaires de France, Paris

Ricker J H 1998 Traumatic brain injury rehabilitation: Is it worth the cost? Applied Neuropsychology 5(4): 184–193

Ricker J H 2003 Neuropsychological practice in medical rehabilitation. In: Lamberty G J, Courtney J, Heilbronner R J (eds) The practice of neuropsychology. Swets & Zeitlinger, The Netherlands, p 305–317

Ricker J H in press Functional neuroimaging in medical rehabilitation populations. In: DeLisa J, Gans B (eds) Rehabilitation medicine, 4th edn. Lippincott, Philadelphia

Ricker J H, Regan T 1999 Neuropsychological and psychological factors in the rehabilitation of individuals with both spinal cord injury and traumatic brain injury. Topics in Spinal Cord Injury Rehabilitation 5(2): 76–82

Ricker J H, Keenan, P A, Jacobson M 1994 Visuoperceptual-spatial abilities and visual memory in vascular dementia and dementia of the Alzheimer type. Neuropsychologia 32(10): 1287–1296

Ricker J H, Rosenthal M, Garay E et al 2002 Telerehabilitation needs: A survey of persons with traumatic brain injury. Journal of Head Trauma Rehabilitation 17(3): 242–250

Robinson E 1998 The clinical neuropsychiatry of stroke: Cognitive, behavioral, and emotional disorders following vascular brain injury. Cambridge University Press, Cambridge

Rosenthal M, Ricker J H 2000 Traumatic brain injury. In: Frank R G, Elliott T R (eds) Handbook of rehabilitation psychology. American Psychological Association Press, Washington, DC, p 49–74

Sacco R L 2000 Pathogenesis, classification, and epidemiology of cerebrovascular disease. In: Lewis R P (ed) Merritt's neurology, 10th edn. Lippincott Williams & Wilkins, Philadelphia, p 217–228

Sale P, West M, Sherron P et al 1991 Exploratory analysis of job separations from supported employment for persons with traumatic brain injury. Journal of Head Trauma Rehabilitation 6(3): 1–11

Schopp L H, Johnstone B R, Merveille O C 2000 Multidimensional telecare strategies for rural residents with brain injury. Journal of Telemedicine and Telecare 6: S146–149

Schreiner A S, Morimoto T 2002 Factor structure of the Cornell Scale for Depression in Dementia among Japanese poststroke patients. International Journal of Geriatric Psychiatry 17(8): 715–722

Serio C D, Kreutzer J S, Gervasio A H 1995 Predicting family needs after brain injury: Implications for intervention. Journal of Head Trauma Rehabilitation 10(2): 32–45

Smith A 1991 Symbol Digit Modalities Test. Western Psychological Services, Los Angeles, CA

Sohlberg M M, Mateer C A 1989 Introduction to cognitive rehabilitation: Theory and practice. Guilford Press, New York

Starkstein S E, Sabe L, Vazquez S et al 1996 Neuropsychological, psychiatric, and cerebral blood flow findings in vascular dementia and Alzheimer's disease. Stroke 27(3): 408–414

Stern R 1997 Visual Analog Mood Scales manual. Psychological Assessment Resources, Odessa, FL

Stewart K J, Gale S D, Diamond P T 2002 Early assessment of post-stroke patients entering acute inpatient rehabilitation: Utility of the WASI and HVLT-R. American Journal of Physical Medicine and Rehabilitation 81(3): 223–228

Stineman M, Maislin G, Fiedler R et al 1997 A prediction model for functional recovery in stroke. Stroke 28: 550–556

Sweet J J, Moberg P J, Suchy Y 2000 Ten-year follow-up survey of clinical neuropsychologists. The Clinical Neuropsychologist 4(4): 479–495

Teasdale G, Engberg I 2001 Completed suicide after traumatic brain injury. Journal of Head Trauma Rehabilitation 12: 16–28

Thomsen I V 1987 Late psychosocial outcome in severe blunt head trauma. Brain Injury 1(2): 131–143

Trudel T M, Tryon W W, Purdum C M 1998 Awareness of disability and long-term outcome after traumatic brain injury. Rehabilitation Psychology 43(4): 267–281

Turnbull J 1988 Perils (hidden and not so hidden) for the token economy. Journal of Head Trauma Rehabilitation 3: 46–52

van den Heuvel E T, Witte L P, Stewart R E et al 2002 Long-term effects of a group support program and an individual support program for informal caregivers of stroke patients: Which caregivers benefit the most? Patient Education and Counseling 47(4): 291–299 van der Lee J H, Wagenaar R C, Lankhorst G J et al 1999 Forced use of the upper extremity in chronic stroke patients: Results from a single-blind randomized clinical trial. Stroke 30: 2369–2375

van der Werf S, van den Broek H, Bleijenberg G 2001 Experience of severe fatigue long after stroke and its relation to depressive symptoms and disease characteristics. European Neurology 45: 28–33

Warburton E, Price C J, Swinburn K et al 1999 Mechanisms of recovery from aphasia: Evidence from positron emission tomography studies. Journal of Neurology, Neurosurgery and Psychiatry 66(2): 155–161

Wechsler D 1981 Wechsler Adult Intelligence Scale – Revised. The Psychological Corporation, San Antonio, TX

Wechsler D 1987 Wechsler Memory Scale – Revised. The Psychological Corporation, San Antonio, TX

Wehman P, Kreutzer J, West M et al 1989 Employment outcomes of persons following traumatic brain injury: Preinjury, postinjury and supported employment. Brain Injury 3(4): 397–412

Whitman S, Coonley-Hoganson R, Desai B T 1984 Comparative head trauma experience in two socioeconomically different Chicago-area communities: A population study. American Journal of Epidemiology 4: 570–580

Whyte J, Hart T, Laborde A et al 1998 Rehabilitation of the patient with traumatic brain injury. In: DeLisa J, Gans B M, Bockenek W L et al (eds), Rehabilitation medicine: Principles and practice, 3rd edn. Lippincott-Raven, Philadelphia, p 1191–1239

Williams D H, Levin H S, Eisenberg H M 1990 Mild head injury classification. Neurosurgery 27(3): 422–428

Wolf P 1990 An overview of the epidemiology of stroke. Stroke 21: 14–16

Zafonte R D, Elovic E, O'Dell M et al 1999 Pharmacology in traumatic brain injury: Fundamentals and treatment strategies. In: Rosenthal M, Griffith E R, Kreutzer J S, Pentland B (eds) Rehabilitation of the adult and child with traumatic brain injury, 3rd edn. F A Davis, Philadelphia, p 536–555

Zahn R, Huber W, Eberich S, Kemeny S et al 1999 Recovery of auditory comprehension in a case of acute transcorticalsensory aphasia: An fMRI study. NeuroImage 6: S720

Zasler N D 1995 Traumatic brain injury and sexuality. Physical Medicine and Rehabilitation: State of the Art Reviews 9: 361–375

Zorowitz R D, Gross E, Polinski D M 2002 The stroke survivor. Disability and Rehabilitation 24(13): 666–679

Zwecker M, Levenkrohn S, Fleisig Y et al 2002 Mini-Mental State Examination, cognitive FIM instrument, and the Loewenstein Occupational Therapy Cognitive Assessment: Relation to functional outcome of stroke patients. Archives of Physical Medicine and Rehabilitation 83(3): 342–345

Chapter 14

Spinal cord injuries

Beth L. Dinoff, J. Scott Richards

INTRODUCTION

Spinal cord injury (SCI), fortunately, is a rare event. When it does occur, however, SCI can have a devastating impact on the individual who is paralyzed, as well as their family members and friends. We do not currently have the ability to greatly undo the damage that is done neurologically and functionally when SCI occurs, although recent research has been more encouraging in that regard (e.g., Stover 1995). Thus, for the present, SCI effectively means permanent paralysis, the extent of which varies depending on the location and the degree of neurological damage. As could be expected, the impact of such an injury to a person's emotional, behavioral, and social functioning can be substantial. Accordingly, psychologists for many years have been providers of clinical services to people who receive this kind of injury.

In this chapter we have assumed that the reader has little familiarity with SCI or the role of the psychologist in the management of such conditions. In this chapter we describe the basic medical outcomes of SCI, the secondary complications that can occur across that individual's subsequent lifetime, and the role of the psychologist in evaluating and facilitating coping and adjustment, a lifetime process.

WHAT IS SPINAL CORD INJURY?

Spinal cord injuries are the result of significant trauma to the central nervous system. Often the injuries are complex, and the functional outcomes vary considerably due to unpredictable factors such as the amount of hemorrhage or swelling within the spinal canal. Most SCIs are caused by blunt trauma to the spinal cord.

Initially a thorough neurological assessment is conducted using the International Standards for Neurological and Functional Classification of Spinal Cord Injury (Bonica 1990). The neurological level of injury is determined by examining the sensory and motor levels of impairment. People with tetraplegia experience loss of feeling and/or movement throughout the body including the hands and/or arms. In people with paraplegia, arm and hand function are preserved with motor and sensory functions diminished or absent at or below the level of injury.

EPIDEMIOLOGY

In the United States the incidence of SCI is roughly 40 cases per million population, indicating that there are approximately 10 000 new cases of SCI per year (DeVivo 2003). Incidence rates in other countries are consistently lower than in the United States. The rate outside the United States is around 20 new cases per million population annually (DeVivo 2003). Based on information derived from the SCI Model Systems national database, risk factors for SCI in the US include age, gender, and ethnicity. The highest incidence rates are in males and people in their late teens through early thirties. African Americans represent 20% of the SCI population even though they only form 12% of the general population (Go et al 1995).

Automobile accidents account for more than 30% of SCIs. In the US, falls (22%), gunshot wounds (17%), diving injuries (almost 5%), and motorcycle crashes (almost 5%) are also common causes of SCI. Causes of SCI vary considerably by race. Among whites, automobile accidents remain the major cause of SCI (DeVivo 2003). Among African Americans, the major cause of SCI is gunshot wounds. Motor vehicle accidents frequently result in tetraplegia whereas acts of violence usually result in paraplegia (DeVivo 1997). As a result, overall costs for treatment of people injured via motor vehicle accidents are much higher than for people who are injured via violent acts (DeVivo 1997).

More than half of all people who incur SCI had never been married at the time of injury. One-third of those injured were married when injured. Being unmarried at the time of injury is predictive of never marrying, as more than a third of those over the age of 15 when injured had not married two decades after SCI (DeVivo 2003). Individuals with SCI are more likely to marry if they are college educated, had been married before, had paraplegia, and are independent in activities of daily life (DeVivo 2003). Over 60% of people with SCI were employed at the time of injury. However, the figure drops substantially when examining people post-SCI as only 27% become gainfully employed (DeVivo 2003). Life expectancy after SCI depends on age at injury. For a 30-year-old individual with tetraplegia, life expectancy is approximately 60% of normal; for a 50-year-old person life expectancy is close to 48% that of normal (DeVivo 1997).

MEDICAL MANAGEMENT

In this section, medical management of conditions secondary to or concomitant with SCI will be described. In particular, those complications that may be related to psychological factors or amenable to psychological interventions will be the focus. These will include concomitant traumatic brain injury (TBI), cardiovascular and respiratory conditions, endocrine and metabolic disturbances, gastrointestinal and urinary conditions, pressure ulcers, and spasticity. Also, the impact of aging and the areas of sexual functioning, fertility, and pregnancy will be discussed.

CONCOMITANT TRAUMATIC BRAIN INJURY

As noted above, SCIs are frequently the result of blunt insults to the body caused by rapid deceleration (e.g., motor vehicle accidents and falls). An injury of sufficient severity to cause damage to the spinal cord itself is likely to produce concomitant or co-occurring injuries, such as TBI (Trieschmann 1992). Recently, it has been noted that people who sustain an SCI may also sustain mild head injuries; a fact not detected in the past (Trieschmann 1992). Studies indicate that between 40% and 60% of people with traumatic SCIs experience mild to moderate cognitive dysfunction when assessed soon after their injuries (Roth et al 1989). It is often difficult, if not impossible, to be certain that deficits typically measured by neuropsychological tests are in fact the result of a TBI. Pre-existing learning disability, prior TBI, depression and anxiety, and cognition-impairing medications can all influence test performance early on (Roth et al 1989). The presence of a substantial period of retrograde and anterograde amnesia raises the suspicion of a TBI, particularly if loss of consciousness and/or impaired cognition is well documented by emergency technicians (Roth et al 1989).

People with SCI may experience poor attention and concentration, memory disturbances, persistent headaches, and decreased problem-solving ability (Richards et al 1988). Cognitive problems may impose on the person's recovery because SCI rehabilitation requires intensive learning of new medical and self-care regimens (Richards et al 1991). However, in a longitudinal study of SCI and concomitant TBI, Richards et al (1988) found that many cognitive deficits observed at 7 weeks after SCI were resolved within 1 year. When deficits are noted, neuropsychological assessments provide an ideal opportunity to individualize treatment protocols that utilize cognitive strengths rather than weaknesses. In addition, careful education of family members and frequent follow-up of persons with a high suspicion of concomitant SCI and TBI are in order.

CARDIOVASCULAR CONSIDERATIONS

Cardiovascular functions are disturbed after SCI primarily due to autonomic nervous system complications (Campagnolo & Merli 2002, Sabharwal 2003). Immediately postinjury, cardiovascular sequelae are related directly to the neurological insult; however, indirect cardiovascular complications may occur later as a result of a sedentary lifestyle and loss of mobility (Campagnolo & Merli 2002).

Autonomic dysreflexia, hypotension, bradycardia, cardiac arrest, impaired thermoregulation, and orthostatic hypotension are among the prominent cardiovascular concerns that are monitored early in the rehabilitation course (Campagnolo & Merli 2002). Severe complications, however, can happen with people experiencing autonomic dysreflexia. Autonomic dysreflexia is a reflex response that is characterized by rapid and potentially life-threatening increases in blood pressure. Between 48% and 85% of people with SCI at the thoracic level of T6 or above experience complications from autonomic dysreflexia (Campagnolo & Merli 2002). Symptoms of autonomic dysreflexia can include anxiety, papillary dilation, flushing, and bladder sphincter contraction, all of which need to be closely observed (Campagnolo & Merli 2002). Guidelines for the clinical management of autonomic dysreflexia have been published by the Consortium for Spinal Cord Medicine (1997).

Indirect or secondary cardiovascular complications are linked to lifestyle changes that coincide with SCI. Deconditioning syndromes result from reduced exercise capacity. As a result, individuals with SCI are at risk for developing cardiovascular diseases earlier than their able-bodied counterparts (Campagnolo & Merli 2002). Thromboembolic disorders related to stasis and increased platelet aggregation have been reported to occur in 47% to 100% of people with acute SCI (Campagnolo & Merli 2002). Cigarette smoking, lipid abnormalities, obesity, and diabetes contribute independently to the risk of developing cardiovascular disease. Psychological factors such as chronic life stress, social isolation, and depression are significant cardiovascular disease risk factors (Sabharwal 2003). Psychological interventions such as relaxation training (see Chapter 9) or smoking cessation interventions may be warranted in a subset of people with SCI to help prevent cardiovascular complications. However, there are no published intervention/outcome studies to aid the rehabilitation psychologist in this area.

RESPIRATORY CONSIDERATIONS

Respiratory complications are the leading cause of mortality in people with paraplegia and tetraplegia (Peterson & Kirshblum 2002). Approximately 67% of people with acute SCI develop respiratory conditions during the initial hospitalization (Jackson & Groomes 1994). Because complications from respiratory disorders have been found to increase the length of initial hospitalization by as long as 27 days (Tator et al 1993), such complications need to be monitored carefully. Respiratory complications post-SCI include atelectasis, pneumonia, pleural effusion, and aspiration (Peterson & Kirshblum 2002). People with SCI should also be assessed for sleep apnea, which can lead to respiratory and cognitive compromise (DeVivo et al 1993). Although older individuals are at significantly greater risk for respiratory problems than their younger counterparts (Ragnarsson et al 1995), young people with SCI should still be monitored carefully. Due to loss of muscle control, increases in respiratory congestion, and decreased lung capacity, people with SCI need to develop compensatory skills while in the acute rehabilitation environment. Education should focus on promoting and protecting respiratory health. During initial inpatient rehabilitation, emphasis should be on weight control, smoking cessation, and correct wheelchair posture. Many of these risk factors are preventable through lifestyle changes and may be addressed by the psychologist using behavioral or cognitive behavioral interventions both individually or in groups. Again, however, there are no published studies to guide the rehabilitation psychologist in this area.

ENDOCRINE AND METABOLIC CONSIDERATIONS

SCI impacts on the endocrine system resulting in a wide range of metabolic disorders. Disorders of the thyroid, pituitary, calcium metabolism, and lipid absorption can have a profound effect on the quality of life of people with SCI. Initially, weight loss occurs as a result of muscle atrophy (Ragnarsson et al 1995), insulin production (Bauman & Spungen 2000), and water diuresis that can persist for weeks to months (Staas et al 1998). Due to permanent alterations in the basic metabolic rate and energy output, obesity usually develops at a later point in time. Obesity is a threat to the longevity of people with SCI (Ragnarsson et al 1995) and increases the risk of developing diabetes, pressure ulcers, problems in self-care, and restrictions in mobility.

Chen et al (2002) conducted a pilot weight management study on four white males with SCI. The SCI EatRight program consists of 12 weekly classes covering exercise, nutrition, stress reduction, and behavior modification with documented success in the general population. In the initial pilot study, SCI participants lost on average 3 kg while in the program. In a follow-up study on 11 people with SCI, similar findings were found. On average, participants lost 10 pounds and reduced their blood cholesterol levels by 13.7 mg/dl. Clearly, goals of rehabilitation should address the implementation of active exercise programs whenever appropriate. Such programs can involve a variety of rehabilitation practitioners.

A further complication of SCI is altered bone and calcium metabolism. Calcium, which is generally reduced in the bone structures in the paralyzed areas of the body, can result in hypercalciuria or high levels of calcium in the urine. In general, however, reduction of calcium intake does not appear to reduce the amount of calcium in the urine (Bauman & Spungen 2000). Loss of bone mass requires increased effort by the kidney (Bauman & Spungen 2000), which can result in hypercalcemia. In addition, osteoporosis is frequently observed in this population due to the lack of weight bearing. Bone mineral depletion occurs over time, with bone mineral loss of 20% to 50% found in women (Garland et al 2001).

GASTROINTESTINAL AND URINARY CONSIDERATIONS

Voluntary bowel and bladder control are disrupted or lost with SCI depending on the level and extent of injury. Research by Glickman & Kamm (1996) indicated that 95% of people with SCI in their sample required at least one therapeutic method in order to defecate. Half of their participants were dependent on others for toileting, and 49% took more than 30 minutes to complete their bowel program. Of note, was that depression was correlated positively with time taken for bowel management. As people with SCI may not experience the need to defecate, they risk becoming constipated or incontinent. Krogh et al (1997) reported that 75% of people with SCI experience fecal incontinence and 80% experience constipation.

Urinary tract infections are the most commonly reported secondary condition in SCI (Cardenas et al 1995). Data collected by the US Model Systems program revealed that urinary tract infections were found in just over 80% of their sample (Cardenas et al 1995). People with SCI may not perceive the typical signs and symptoms of urinary tract infections such as pain or urgency, however, they may experience new-onset urinary incontinence, fever, flushing, lower-extremity spasms, and autonomic dysreflexia (Cardenas et al 1995). Untreated urinary tract infections may lead to chronic renal dysfunction and ultimately kidney failure or death (Cardenas et al 1995).

Management should focus on prevention of gastrointestinal and genitourinary complications. Therapeutic goals include the implementation of bowel and bladder programs. The bowel program usually consists of routinizing evacuation of the bowel at a time that is appropriate for each individual. Intermittent catheterization is usually recommended for urinary control and has been found to be superior to chronic indwelling Foley catheterization

(Weld et al 2000). Dietary changes often consist of increasing the consumption of fiber, grains, fruit, and vegetables. Caffeine and spicy or fatty foods may cause diarrhea in some individuals and, if so, should be avoided. Fluid intake, particularly water, is important to both proper bowel and bladder function. With the dramatic lifestyle changes that the individual with SCI has to incorporate, compliance with medical regimens may become problematic. The psychologist or the physical therapist may address compliance within group sessions as well as in individual behavior therapy (Trieschmann 1988).

PRESSURE ULCERS

Pressure ulcers are localized areas of cellular necrosis usually located between a prominent bone and the bed or wheelchair (Donovan et al 1993). Pressure ulcers are thought to be preventable, but continue to affect up to 66% of people hospitalized for SCI (Priebe et al 2003). Behavioral risk factors for pressure ulcers include smoking, alcohol use, and low average cognitive functioning (Priebe et al 2003). Pressure sore prevention education is needed throughout rehabilitation. Management consists of turning regimens, skin assessment and care, and pressure relief at appropriate intervals. The success of such programs, however, is based on adherence to the new regimen.

SPASTICITY

Increased muscle tone or spasticity often accompanies SCI. Spasticity is associated with uncontrolled limb movements that may result in chronic pain, fractures, and joint dislocations (Nance 2003). On the positive side, spasticity can be beneficial in retaining muscle tone and assisting with transfers. Maynard et al (1990) found that up to 78% of people with SCI required treatment for spasticity within the first year postinjury. In another study, 41% of individuals with SCI reported that spasticity resulted in restricted daily activities or pain (Levi et al 1995). Spasticity may be treated with an array of oral and intrathecal medications (e.g., valium, baclofen). Compliance with range-of-motion exercises to reduce the incidence of spasticity may be addressed with behavior modification. There have been some clinical reports of improvements in spasticity from relaxation training and hypnosis (Baer 1960) although there is very limited research in this area.

AGING

With advances in medical science and rehabilitation, the life expectancy of people with SCI is increasing. Cross-sectional studies have indicated that, with aging, people with SCI experience increased pain, bowel and urinary complications, pressure ulcers, nursing care admissions, and medical costs (see Weitzenkamp et al 2001 for review). Studies also demonstrate decreased independence in self-care, decreased mobility, and decreased participation in social roles. In contrast with these findings, aging has been positively associated with improved life satisfaction in some people with SCI (see Weitzenkamp et al 2001 for review).

People with SCI face multiple injury-related challenges (e.g., wear and tear from transfers and wheelchair use) in addition to the normal effects of aging that everyone experiences. Thus, normal aging and duration of disability offer unique contributions to our understanding of long-term health outcomes following SCI (Pentland et al 1995). Pentland et al (1995) found that, in men, aging was significantly related to increased fatigue, decreased physical activity due to pain, and greater satisfaction with life. Duration of disability measures indicated that the longer people lived with SCI, the more physical symptoms and illnesses they experienced, and they perceived themselves to be less secure financially. In this study of males only, aging and duration of disability interacted to compound the negative effects of financial security.

A study of females with SCI found that aging women often feel isolated and believe that their key concerns are not addressed effectively by healthcare providers (Pentland et al 2002). Studies such as these reiterate the need for people with SCI to be followed longitudinally by multidisciplinary teams in order to prevent psychosocial and medical complications that may occur with aging. Early identification, education, and intervention may minimize or eliminate age-related difficulties (Charlifue & Lammertse 2003).

SEXUAL FUNCTIONING, PREGNANCY, AND FERTILITY

SCI may affect sexual functioning both physiologically and psychologically. The physical aspects of sexual functioning are directly related to the injury. Individuals with incomplete injuries and upper motor neuron injuries have a better prognosis than do people with lower motor neuron injuries (Elliott 2003). Having a concomitant TBI may further increase sexual dysfunction or produce inappropriate sexual responses (Elliott 2003). Nevertheless, all people retain the ability to function sexually in some way. Returning to an active sex life can be related to perceptions of self-esteem and body image, all of which can be addressed within the multidisciplinary team.

Women with SCI may return to enjoying an active sex life in time. Menses may cease temporarily, only returning to normal after several months, but the need for birth control does not decrease (Ducharme et al 1993). The choice of birth control needs to be considered carefully as each method may present complications. Condoms and spermicide have been found to be consistently effective with the fewest complications. Of course, this method requires partner cooperation. Regarding sexual responsiveness, vaginal lubrication and vasocongestion occur both psychogenically and via reflex so that many women are not impaired sexually even when they lose sensation (Harrison et al 1995). Jackson (2003) reported that 54% of SCI women experienced orgasm and an additional 30% were able to have extragenital pleasure similar to orgasms. Women with SCI are able to become pregnant and carry a healthy baby to full term. Some difficulties in pregnancy, however, are noted (e.g., autonomic dysreflexia and spasticity). Frequently a cesarean section will be recommended even though uterine contractions are not typically impaired.

As stated earlier, males represent 80% of the SCI population and hence more is known about their sexual functioning (Elliott 2003). Men can be assured that sexual function and pleasure may be enjoyed again with some variations. Research suggests that between 54% and 87% of men are able to experience erections (Crooks & Baur 2002). Men may experience psychogenic erections, which are stimulated through afferent stimuli in the brain. Reflex erections are mediated by an arc in the sacral spinal column (S2–S4). Men with SCI above T6 should be able to experience reflex erections. Men with SCI in the sacral region may experience psychogenic erections. However, in both cases men may have difficulty maintaining erections and often fail to ejaculate. Further, semen quality is diminished as concentration of sperm and sperm motility decline (Elliott 2003). These problems may be addressed with any number of new technologies and drug treatments, such as Viagra.

Psychologically, sexual dysfunction may have a profound impact on the individual in the wake of an acute SCI. Rehabilitation programs should address sexual functioning early in rehabilitation so that the individual may feel comfortable enough to raise questions. Body image changes need to be addressed openly. People with SCI should be encouraged to expand their sexual repertoire and focus on non-coital expression of sexuality. Inclusion of the sexual partner in the education process is important as perceived partner satisfaction and relationship quality are significantly related to sexual satisfaction in men with SCI (Phelps et al 2001). Clinicians can play a significant part in facilitating resumption of sexual roles (Burns & Jackson 2001).

PSYCHOLOGICAL CONSIDERATIONS

SCI is most often the result of trauma leaving the individual with no opportunity to "prepare" for such an event, as might be the case with some progressive neurological or other chronic diseases. Therefore, onset of SCI may be accompanied by substantial emotional and behavioral responses, some of which require clinical intervention. We have reviewed how SCI affects physical mobility and, therefore, independence and access to employment, recreation, and work activities. People who receive an SCI, in addition, face both physical and social barriers when trying to reintegrate into society. People with SCI might also have some of their own internal attitudinal barriers to overcome. The early adjustment and coping literature for SCI emphasizes a "stage of adjustment model" (Buckelew et al 1991). Such stage theories may provide a convenient framework for understanding what can happen in the adjustment process, but recent research fails to support their validity (Buckelew et al 1991). That is, there is no evidence for a necessary or invariable sequence of adjustment steps that one "should" go through, and that individual differences in coping with SCI are at least as evident as commonalities. In this section, we will focus on the common emotional and behavioral responses to SCI that occur or may occur in the coping and adjustment process and describe interventions that have been used by psychologists in that process. Such responses include depression and suicide, anxiety and post-traumatic stress disorders, substance abuse, stress appraisal and coping, and pain. Cognitive behavioral interventions are described when they are relevant to each section with a more complete explanation of cognitive and behavioral interventions afterward.

DEPRESSION AND SUICIDE

Assessment of depression is challenging in people with SCI as a number of the symptoms of a major depression overlap with physical consequences of SCI. According to the Diagnostic and Statistical Manual – IV (American Psychiatric Association 1994), major depression is characterized by the experience of five or more of the following symptoms for a period of at least two weeks:

- depressed mood most of the day
- markedly diminished interest in pleasurable activities
- significant weight loss or decrease in appetite
- insomnia or hypersomnia
- psychomotor agitation or retardation
- fatigue or loss of energy
- feelings of worthlessness or excessive guilt
- diminished ability to think or concentrate.

Therefore, unless an individual was experiencing depression prior to the SCI, it is problematic to be diagnosed with clinical depression early in the acute phase of treatment. Adjustment reactions with depressed mood are more likely to be observed during this period than a clinical depression. The diagnosis of "adjustment disorder with depressed mood" is assigned when the development of emotional or behavioral symptoms are a response to an identifiable stressor and occur within 3 months of the onset of the stressor (American Psychiatric Association 1994).

Over time, the vast majority of people with SCI will experience some symptoms of distress, such as tearfulness, irritability, and grief that may last for years. However, diagnosable major depression is found in only 20–45% of people with SCI. Depression scores are highest when people with SCI enter the initial phases of rehabilitation (Kennedy & Rogers 2000). For example, as people move from the bed to the wheelchair, they may become aware of the challenges that they are facing in rehabilitation. Typically depressive symptoms resolve within 3 months postdischarge (Richards 1986), but this is not always the case. In some people

with SCI (up to 30%), depression remains constant as much as 2 years later (Hancock et al 1993).

Depression has been linked to several poor outcomes, including long-term health consequences. Depressed people with SCI need more medical assistance, spend more hours in bed, and enjoy fewer hours out of the house than do non-depressed people with SCI (Tate et al 1994). Suicide rates are two to six times higher in people with SCI than in the able-bodied community (Charlifue & Gerhart 1991).

Individual differences are found among people with SCI with regard to the development of depression. People with SCI and low educational levels (i.e., high school or less) tend to experience depression more frequently than do people with higher education levels (Scivoletto et al 1997). Females with SCI are more likely to become depressed than are males with SCI (Tate et al 1994). Older individuals experience depression more frequently than do younger individuals (Krause et al 2000). Persons of minority status are at higher risk for depression than are other people with SCI (Krause et al 2000). Of note, however, is that people with tetraplegia are no more likely to be depressed than those with paraplegia (Hancock et al 1993).

Scivoletto et al (1997) suggested that depression may be related to obstacles in social role fulfillment and reduction of autonomy. Indeed, rates of divorce for both pre-existing and post-SCI marriages are higher in people with SCI than in the general population (DeVivo et al 1995). Vocational and other social roles are affected too (Buckelew et al 1991). For example, alterations in financial security, material assets, and meaningful social roles decrease perceptions of quality of life (Duggan & Dijkers 2001). Participation in sporting activities has improved life quality and maintained role function while reducing medical complications (Stiens et al 2002). Hanson et al (2001) found that SCI athletes scored significantly higher on physical independence, mobility, occupational status, and social integration as compared to non-athletes with SCI.

As stated earlier, rates of suicide in the SCI population are two to six times higher than in the general population (DeVivo et al 1995). Approximately half of people with SCI express suicidal thoughts. A recent Danish study (Hartkopp et al 1998) using data from 888 individuals revealed that the suicide rate among individuals with SCI was five times higher than expected in the general population, with suicide rates being higher for women than for men. Hartkopp et al (1998) also found that the suicide rate doubled from the 1970s to the 1990s. Additionally, people who were marginally disabled were twice as likely to commit suicide as the people with functionally complete tetraplegia. It is important to recognize that suicide rates may be underestimated as some accidental deaths or drug-related deaths may be socially acceptable forms of suicide. Rehabilitation providers are in a prime position to assess suicidality. Fichtenbaum & Kirshblum (2002) provide a good review of assessing suicidality. They suggest that suicidality assessments should include questions about suicidal ideation, plan, intent, current access to lethal means, any possible prior attempt(s), and comorbid alcohol or drug use. Questions that are useful in assessing suicidal ideation include: "Is life still worth living?," "Do you feel like going to sleep forever?," and "Are you having thoughts of hurting yourself?" If the patient answers in the affirmative to any questions about suicidal ideation, the suicidal plan should be discussed. A question such as "How would you commit suicide?" would be appropriate as a follow-up to assess the suicidal plan. Intent to commit suicide may be assessed with a question like "Do you think that you would really harm yourself?," or "What is there in your life preventing you from harming yourself?" Follow-up questions should address the availability of the means to commit suicide, such as does the person have access to a gun or lethal doses of medications. Thus, in this way, suicidality may be assessed in a stepwise fashion. When suicidal ideation is noted, a more thorough suicide assessment and appropriate referral and/or treatment by a psychologist are warranted (see suicide assessment above).

ANXIETY AND POST-TRAUMATIC STRESS DISORDERS

Additional psychological consequences of SCI may include the anxiety disorders such as generalized anxiety disorder, adjustment disorder with anxiety, acute stress disorder, and post-traumatic stress disorder (PTSD). Anxiety disorders have not been as thoroughly investigated as depression, and as such, their prevalence and incidence are not well delineated (Richards et al 2000). Anxiety disorders are often comorbid with depressive disorders, making the diagnosis difficult at best.

Hancock et al (1993) found that anxiety levels were higher in people with SCI as compared to their control group. Approximately 25% of the SCI group experienced anxiety whereas only 5% of the control group was anxious. Furthermore, anxiety levels remained elevated in the same group as long as 2 years later (Craig et al 1994).

The Diagnostic and Statistical Manual – IV (American Psychiatric Association 1994) characterizes PTSD as resulting when a person has been exposed to a traumatic event and responded with intense fear, helplessness, or horror. Also characteristic of PTSD is that the traumatic event may be re-experienced through dreams or flashbacks, persistent avoidance of associated stimuli or generalized feelings of numbness, and symptoms of increased arousal (e.g., hypervigilance, exaggerated startle response, and sleep difficulties) (American Psychiatric Association 1994). Traumatic SCIs are typically the result of automobile accidents, violence, sports, and falls. Suddenly the injured individual must immediately address extreme physical and psychological consequences. PTSD symptoms are more likely to occur when there is a sudden event that is dangerous, uncontrollable, and unpredictable (Yule et al 1999). Thus, the very nature of traumatic SCIs places people at risk for developing PTSD.

PTSD occurs at a higher rate in people with SCI than it does in the general population. Approximately 14% of people with SCI experience trauma-related distress 6 months post-SCI (Kennedy & Evans 2001). Prior experience with trauma also increases the risk of having PTSD post-SCI (Radnitz et al 2000). Radnitz et al (2000) found that veterans with experience in direct combat were more likely to experience PTSD and had more severe symptoms following SCI than did non-combat veterans. Furthermore, all of the non-combat veterans recovered from their PTSD whereas only 26% of those people with war combat experience recovered.

SUBSTANCE ABUSE

It has been estimated that between 17% and 62% of people sustaining SCIs were intoxicated and more than 30% of individuals with traumatic SCIs were using illegal drugs at the time of injury (Kolakowsky-Hayner et al 1999). In a study of pre-injury substance abuse among people with SCI and TBI, 96% of the SCI participants reported pre-injury alcohol use, with 57% of them being heavy drinkers (Kolakowsky-Hayner et al 2002). Within the traumatic brain injury group, 81% of the participants reported pre-injury alcohol use and 42% were heavy drinkers. Given that 8–10% of the general population is estimated to abuse alcohol (Tate 1993), the percentages for the people with traumatic SCI and TBI are significant and clinically relevant.

After SCI, 73% of people return to drinking alcohol within 18 months of initial hospitalization (Heinemann et al 1990). Negative outcomes have been associated with substance use post-SCI. In the extreme, alcohol use after SCI has been found to be a leading cause of death (Smith 1990). Less severe, negative outcomes include poor rehabilitation outcomes (Tate 1993), depression, lower life satisfaction, spending less time in productive activities (Smith 1990), and development of preventable complications such as pressure ulcers (Yarkony & Heineman 1995).

STRESS APPRAISAL AND COPING

Stress refers to any event where the internal or external demands tax or exceed the adaptive resources of an individual and jeopardize well-being (Lazarus 1966). This definition accounts for the uniqueness with which we all interpret events as well as the individual differences that exist in our adaptive resources. As such, no two people will experience an event in the same way – every event is filtered through this cognitive appraisal process. Nevertheless, most people who acquire SCIs may be classified as experiencing significant events for which they were psychologically unprepared (i.e., stress). Indeed, following SCI many events may be stressful. Significant adjustment is likely to be required from the injured individual and the environment.

Coping entails efforts to master the condition that is stressful, often requiring a novel response from the individual. Coping responses can be divided into two main categories: problem-focused coping and emotion-focused coping (Lazarus 1966). Problem-focused coping includes efforts to improve the situation by taking action to change things (Lazarus 1966). For example, in the rehabilitation setting, when a person with SCI complies with treatment regimens and engages in discourse with the treatment team they are actively involved with the problem and, therefore, using problem-focused

coping. Problem-focused coping is particularly useful in situations when the person's efforts can actually modify the stressor. On the other hand, emotion-focused coping involves strategies that are utilized to relieve the emotional impact of stress (Lazarus 1966). These actions are designed, not to change the situation, but to make the person feel better about the event. Examples include prayer, talking about fears, joking, distancing, relaxation, and distraction. Thus, when a person with a complete SCI states that they will walk out of the hospital, they are using emotion-focused coping strategies to distance themselves from their fears about being paralyzed for life. Emotion-focused coping strategies are very useful in addressing aspects of stressors that are fixed or unchangeable. In people with SCI, problem-focused strategies can be most effective with situations that can change (e.g., learning bladder and bowel programs), whereas, emotion-focused approaches can be most effective in dealing with the feelings that arise from suddenly needing to learn bladder and bowel programs or situations that are more out of that individual's control (e.g., responses of other people).

Gerhart et al (1999) conducted a longitudinal study on 187 people with SCI who acquired injuries prior to 1971. Perceived stress was assessed at three points in time along with psychological measures of severity of disability, depression, life satisfaction, and well-being to assess coping and adjustment. Medical variables such as injury severity, pressure ulcers, urinary tract infections, pain, and fatigue were also measured. No relationship with stress was found for medical variables including injury severity, pain, and fatigue. Strong relationships were found between stress and ratings on psychological variables. High stress was directly related to poor psychological outcomes and depressive symptoms, and poor perceptions of well-being and low levels of life satisfaction were predictive of future stress experiences.

Hope and denial are also coping strategies that have been examined in people with SCI. Hope has been defined as a cognitive process in which people are focused on goals and the necessary planning to meet those goals (Snyder et al 1999). Pursuing goals should produce positive emotions, and experiencing barriers to goals may produce negative feelings. Initially after injury, people with SCI are likely to experience many barriers to goals and associated negative feelings. However, over time, new goals accompanied by positive feelings can develop.

Hope has been associated with positive psychological adjustment. For example, people who are high in hope feel invigorated and think positively about achieving goals (Snyder et al 1999), and they also feel good about themselves. Indeed, Elliott et al (1991) found that in people recovering from SCI, higher hope was related to less depression and better coping skills.

Denial is a normal coping mechanism that people use when facing an overwhelming situation (Fichtenbaum & Kirshblum 2002). In the short term, such as the weeks and months following SCI, denial offers people emotional detachment from the effects of trauma. This detachment allows for people to adjust in a slower, more gradual pace so as to decrease levels of arousal and anxiety that could significantly impair rehabilitation progress. Over time, as arousal in response to the trauma decreases, people will gradually confront the trauma and its consequences. Elliott & Richards (1999) found that denial was consistently associated with less distress, hostility, and perceived handicap during the first year after injury in 40 people with SCI. However, when denial becomes a long-term strategy of avoidance, negative outcomes including loneliness and increased medical complications may ensue (Elliott & Richards 1999).

Use of social support, a form of coping, has been associated with adjustment in people with SCI. Social support or lack thereof can influence both the physical and psychological outcomes of SCI (Trieschmann 1988). Social support affects individuals in two ways. First, social support can have a direct, beneficial impact on health. For example, a person with SCI may be more disposed to attend therapy sessions if a family member attends as well. Second, social support can buffer or protect us from the negative effect of serious health problems. For example, post-SCI visits from family and friends may help prevent serious depressive symptoms. Chan et al (2000) conducted a cross-sectional study on 66 people with SCI and found that the group at risk for developing psychological problems had low perceived social support.

PAIN

Pain has been defined as an unpleasant sensory and emotional experience associated with actual or potential tissue damage, or described in terms of such damage (Bonica 1990). This definition is particularly useful because it acknowledges that both physical and psychological factors play a role in the experience of pain. As such, pain is a subjective experience that is difficult to measure because we must rely exclusively on self-report. For people with SCI, pain assessment is complicated by the fact that pain may be experienced in areas of the body that are not sensitive to normal stimuli such as pin pricks.

Estimates of the prevalence of pain after SCI are reported to be between 18% and 96% (Putzke et al 2002) with up to 30% of people experiencing severe pain (Bryce & Ragnarsson 2003). The largest proportion of these patients (96%) experience acute pain while in rehabilitation (New et al 1997), but many go on to experience chronic pain. In one study, 58% of people experienced the onset of SCI-related pain within the first year after the injury (Stormer et al 1997). Post-SCI pain is difficult to classify because some of the origins of pain remain unexplained. As there have been approximately 30 classification schemes for SCI pain it can be challenging to draw conclusions across studies. Recently, Bryce & Ragnarsson (2003) proposed a systematic taxonomy for post-SCI pain that organizes pain into three levels (see Figure 14.1). The first level divides pain into two broad types: nociceptive and neuropathic. The second level is a division of pain into broad systems: under nociceptive is musculoskeletal and visceral, and under neuropathic is pain at level, below

Level	Classification	Etiologic subtype
Above level	Nociceptive	Musculoskeletal
	Neuropathic	Neuropathy
At level	Nociceptive	Musculoskeletal
		Visceral
	Neuropathic	Neuropathy
Below level	Nociceptive	Musculoskeletal
		Visceral
	Neuropathic	Central

Figure 14.1 Bryce/Ragnarsson Classification of Pain after SCI. The figure summarizes the basic elements of the Bryce/Ragnarsson Classification of Pain after SCI (Bryce & Ragnarsson 2003). The first column classifies pain (i.e., above level, at level, or below level) according to neurological level of SCI. The second column classifies pain as nociceptive or neuropathic. The third column further classifies pain into subtypes of either nociceptive or neuropathic pain types

level, and above level. The third level classifies pain into specific structures or pathology.

Nociceptive pain occurs in the muscles, bones, or abdomen. Often this pain is described as aching, cramping, dull, and constant. This type of pain may be caused by long-term overuse in a part of the body, such as may be observed in the shoulder when people use manual wheelchairs. Muscle spasm pain also would fall under the category of nociceptive pain. Nociceptive pain is usually located above the level of injury, but can be present below the level of injury in those with sensory sparing.

In contrast, neuropathic pain is caused by disruption of the central nervous system or damage to peripheral nerves. Abnormal sensations such as hyperalgesia and allodynia may be experienced. People generally describe neuropathic pain as burning, sharp, tingling, and/or electric. This pain is usually experienced at or below the level of injury. Neuropathic pain is the most common type of chronic pain reported by persons with SCI and it can be refractory to standard treatment. Accurate management of pain for people with SCI depends on recognizing that pain is not a singular construct and more than one type of pain may be experienced simultaneously. Treatment requires an understanding of the range of therapeutic options as well as factors that influence pain perception (Ragnarsson 1997). A multidisciplinary approach to pain management is the best option for long-term improvement for the person with SCI.

Pain assessment is crucial to understanding the pain experience as well as treating painful conditions. Behavioral assessments of pain used in other chronic pain populations, such as observing pain behaviors (e.g., grimacing, limping, reduced activity) may not be effective with this population due to physical function limitations. One of the simplest ways to obtain information about pain is to ask the individual to rate pain intensity on a numerical rating scale (see Chapter 11). The individual is asked to rate their pain on a scale of 0 being no pain to 10 being the worst pain imaginable (Figure 14.2). This measure of pain has been found to be sensitive to

day-to-day fluctuations in pain as well as changes related to treatment. When using this rating scale, people should be asked to rate each of their pain sites separately if they have multiple painful areas in order to obtain a full picture of the pain. It is also useful to obtain ratings of the worst and least pain experienced over the course of the past week.

Another instrument, the McGill Pain Questionnaire (Melzack & Katz 1992) is a well-established measure for evaluating pain. It consists of a checklist of 102 pain adjectives (e.g., burning, searing, dull, aching) ranked in terms of severity that are then organized into 20 categories (Figure 14.3). People select at most one from each category allowing for classification of the pain experience into three primary dimensions: evaluative/cognitive, affective, and sensory. The McGill Pain Questionnaire also contains an outline of the body to indicate pain locations. This measure has been used effectively in SCI populations revealing that people with SCI less frequently select affective components of pain and more frequently endorse sensory components when compared with people having other painful conditions (Turner et al 2001). Based on this finding, researchers suggest that people with SCI perceive their pain as less bothersome than other medical problems they are facing.

Pain perception may be altered by cognitive factors and coping strategies as described by cognitive behavioral theories. Cognitive behavioral theories as described by Turner et al (2002) and Radnitz (2002) hold that thoughts or interpretations about pain are directly related to personal adjustment. Cognitive behavioral theories regarding pain are based on Beck's (1967) cognitive behavioral theories as well as the rational emotive therapy of Ellis (1970). Turner et al (2002) define catastrophizing as the phenomenon of expecting or worrying about severe negative consequences from an event, even when it is of minor importance. Catastrophizing about the painful condition is one way for a person to think about his or her pain (e.g., I feel that I can't stand this pain anymore), such that they demonstrate an exaggerated negative view of the pain or painful stimulus. In a study of 174 community residents with SCI, Turner et al (2002) found that catastrophizing was significantly and positively related to pain ratings, psychological distress, and pain-related disability. Cognitive behavioral theories also hold that thought processes such as catastrophizing can be restructured in such a way as to bring about improved well-being (Turner et al 2002). That is,

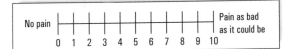

Figure 14.2 A numerical rating scale. The patient is instructed to mark the numbered vertical line as appropriate

McGill Pain Questionnaire

Patient's name _____ Date _____ Time _____ am/pm

PRI: S _____ A _____ E _____ M _____ PRI(T) _____ PPI _____
　　　(1–10)　　　(11–15)　　　(16)　　　(17–20)　　　(1–20)

1 FLICKERING	11 TIRING
QUIVERING	EXHAUSTING
PULSING	12 SICKENING
THROBBING	SUFFOCATING
BEATING	13 FEARFUL
POUNDING	FRIGHTFUL
2 JUMPING	TERRIFYING
FLASHING	14 PUNISHING
SHOOTING	GRUELLING
3 PRICKING	CRUEL
BORING	VICIOUS
DRILLING	KILLING
STABBING	15 WRETCHED
LANCINATING	BLINDING
4 SHARP	16 ANNOYING
CUTTING	TROUBLESOME
LACERATING	MISERABLE
5 PINCHING	INTENSE
PRESSING	UNBEARABLE
GNAWING	17 SPREADING
CRAMPING	RADIATING
CRUSHING	PENETRATING
6 TUGGING	PIERCING
PULLING	18 TIGHT
WRENCHING	NUMB
7 HOT	DRAWING
BURNING	SQUEEZING
SCALDING	TEARING
SEARING	19 COOL
8 TINGLING	COLD
ITCHY	FREEZING
SMARTING	20 NAGGING
STINGING	NAUSEATING
9 DULL	AGONIZING
SORE	DREADFUL
HURTING	TORTURING
ACHING	**PPI**
HEAVY	0 NO PAIN
10 TENDER	1 MILD
TAUT	2 DISCOMFORTING
RASPING	3 DISTRESSING
SPLITTING	4 HORRIBLE
	5 EXCRUCIATING

BRIEF	RHYTHMIC	CONTINUOUS
MOMENTARY	PERIODIC	STEADY
TRANSIENT	INTERMITTENT	CONSTANT

E = EXTERNAL

I = INTERNAL

COMMENTS:

Figure 14.3　McGill Pain Questionnaire. The descriptors fall into four major groups: sensory, 1–10; affective, 11–15; evaluative, 16; and miscellaneous, 17–20. The rank value for each descriptor is based on its position in the word set. The sum of the rank values is the pain rating index (PRI). The present pain intensity (PPI) is based on a scale of 0–5 (reproduced from Pain, 1, Melzack R, The McGill Pain Questionnaire: Major properties and scoring methods, pp 227–299, Copyright (1975), with permission of International Society for the Study of Pain) people can be taught strategies for reinterpreting the painful stimulus, which may enhance psychological functioning. Cognitive behavioral therapy (CBT) is based on the theory that positive thoughts, feelings, and attitudes can be acquired through skills training and practice. CBT skills may be taught to individuals or in groups and may include diverting attention or distraction, relaxation (see Chapter 9), reframing the painful experience (see Chapter 3), positive affirmation, increasing activity, humor, and prayer. Outcome studies using CBT for treating chronic pain in the SCI population are lacking. For a further discussion of pain and pain management see Chapter 11.

PSYCHOLOGICAL INTERVENTIONS

The effectiveness of CBT for people with disabilities has been well described in the literature (Radnitz 2002). CBT is based on the assumption that thoughts or cognitions are directly related to behaviors and emotions. These cognitions may be identified and altered particularly when they are no longer adaptive (cognitive distortions), and changes in thinking can then produce changes in feelings and behaviors. Central to CBT is identifying the particular cognitive distortions each individual uses. Six categories of cognitive distortions (Box 14.1) are prominent in people with SCI (Radnitz 2002). The first is an overly negative view of the world and other people in their environment, which people may describe as thinking that others are being insensitive to their needs. Second, cognitive distortions evolve around the person's sense of self-worth. For example, people with SCI may come to believe mistakenly that they are less capable of

being workers, spouses, or parents. Third, people with SCI may have distorted perceptions that lead them to anticipate poor social interactions or feel rejected. This feeling is often confirmed by reduced social contact resulting from role changes. Fourth, beliefs about hopelessness may develop as people begin to feel barriers to personal goals. As a result of despair, depression and anxiety may surface. Fifth, cognitive distortions about having a sense of entitlement emerge. People experiencing these distortions may begin to expect that other people should always extend themselves on their behalf rather than maintaining independence. Sixth, people with SCI may begin to feel overly vulnerable to life events, leading to impairments in functioning and counterproductive behaviors. CBT is used to challenge cognitive distortions through skill building, hypothesis testing, reframing, exposure, and thought stopping among others. These interventions are effective in people with chronic pain, disabling diseases, and mood disorders.

Problem-solving therapy is one type of cognitive behavioral therapy used to improve coping skills in family caregivers. One model of problem solving has been described by Elliott and colleagues (Elliott & Shewchuk 2000, Kurylo et al 2001). The components of this approach include five elements of a continuous process:

- general orientation to problem solving (i.e., admitting that a problem exists)
- problem definition including articulating the characteristics of the problem,
- generating alternatives such as brain-storming about the situation
- decision-making and implementation or selecting a solution and trying it out
- verification (i.e., reviewing the outcome).

This approach can be taught individually, in groups, or via the telephone. For a further discussion of CBT refer to Chapter 8.

QUALITY OF LIFE AND LIFE SATISFACTION

To date, no "gold standard" exists for quality of life measurement (Freeman et al 1995). For some people a good quality of life means enjoying close relationships with family and friends (requires subjective assessment). For others, a good quality of life encompasses having fast cars and beachfront homes (requires objective assessment). No matter how

---

Box 14.1 Categories of cognitive distortions in people with SCI (adapted from Radnitz 2002)

An overly negative view of the world
A distorted sense of self-worth
Anticipation of poor social interactions and feelings of rejection
Belief of hopelessness
An increased sense of entitlement
Feelings of vulnerability to life events

quality of life is defined, most people would agree that a traumatic SCI can represent a dramatic challenge to quality of life (Dijkers 1997).

In general, quality of life can be broken into four or five major domains: psychological, physical, environmental/economic, social, and, for some, spirituality. After SCI, all of these domains are likely to be vulnerable to alteration. We do not fully understand how SCI impacts life quality domains. Nor do we fully understand how subjective perceptions of these domains vary over time for people with SCI (Dijkers 1997). One thing that has been known, however, is that the average person with SCI experiences a lower quality of life than people without SCI or other disabling condition (Dijkers 1997). Life satisfaction has also been found to be somewhat lower in the SCI population when compared to the general population (Fuhrer et al 1992). In a study of 100 men and 40 women with SCI, Fuhrer et al (1992) found lowest life satisfaction scores in the financial, employment, and sex life domains and highest satisfaction ratings in family relationships, spiritual life, and activities of daily living. SCI participants reporting greater levels of social support as compared to participants with less social support also rated higher levels of life satisfaction.

INTEGRATED MANAGEMENT APPROACHES IN SPINAL CORD INJURY

A half century ago the medical system was the predominant mechanism for rehabilitation. Today, however, the prevailing model is an integrated system of multidisciplinary healthcare professionals (Stover 1995). Comprehensive rehabilitation requires a collaborative team approach capitalizing on the various skills of physicians, physical and occupational therapists, nurses, psychologists, social workers, and many other healthcare disciplines. Clinical psychologists bring additional skills to the team including assessment, behavioral interventions, and psychological counseling thereby extending the treatment options available for people with SCI (Judd & Brown 1988). Recently, the American Psychological Association Practice Directorate (1998) published guidelines for practicing psychology in hospital settings and other types of facilities that provide healthcare with the expressed goal of promoting more effective integration of psychologists within the medical

environment. This book is an excellent resource for psychologists and medical teams wishing to utilize the services of psychologists.

Gans (1987) indicated that facilitating staff–patient interactions is one of the important roles of the psychologist in rehabilitation. Non-mental health professionals such as physical and occupational therapists are the likely initial contacts for providing emotional support for the individual and their family members. However, as a general rule, these professionals have received little formal training in addressing psychological issues. The Team Attended Psychological Interview (TAPI; Gans 1987) is one type of psychiatric consultation–liaison process used to help staff members deal with psychological/behavioral issues as well as providing support for the staff members. In other words, education about psychological factors is provided to the staff members and the person with SCI simultaneously. The team is responsible for identifying patients who will benefit from such consultation. TAPIs may be requested to assist with behaviors such as manipulation, anger, and sexual provocation, to assess psychological strengths, management of unreasonable demands regarding medications, and to address "splitting" in which people unconsciously attempt to divide the treatment team. This approach has been successful in enhancing the awareness of the treatment team to psychological issues as well as providing a much-needed psychological service to the individual.

SUMMARY

Spinal cord injury can be a devastating event. Severely curtailed physical independence, lack of access to the environment, and psychological reactions to these changes are among the consequences of SCI. The ability to move around freely, take care of one's bodily physical needs, and the capacity to gain free and ready access to the social, work, and recreational environment can be severely limited. Accompanying emotional and behavioral responses in the acute rehabilitation setting and across the lifespan of these individuals represent important areas for clinical evaluation and intervention by psychologists working in rehabilitation settings. All of a psychologist's skills can be incorporated into rehabilitation. Assessment skills are needed across the diversity of issues encountered from affective disturbance to personality issues, behavioral adjustment, coping effectiveness, and pre-employment evaluation to name a few. Treatment skills can be utilized, including individual, group, family, marital, and sexuality interventions. Certainly, the consultation role is critical as well, both for helping other team members understand how the individual's psychological status can affect their response to rehabilitation interventions, and how staff can best work with such individuals. Psychologists also have a rich opportunity to engage with their medical and physical therapy colleagues in evaluating and intervening with behavioral analysis and interventions aimed at eliminating and ameliorating secondary conditions, which can have a devastatingly negative impact on quality of life.

We remain hopeful about recent advances in spinal cord injury "cure" research. Hope is important for patients and families as well as staff working with these individuals. However, until functionally significant improvements in nerve regeneration can be achieved, there is much that psychology can do to contribute to the well-being of people who receive SCIs. Further, there is abundant evidence that most of these individuals can overcome the obstacles that they face to achieve a satisfying and meaningful quality of life.

ACKNOWLEDGMENTS

Resources for production of this chapter were provided by the NIH Rehabilitation Research Training Grant: CNS Outcomes NICHD (#5T32 HDO7420–11). The authors wish to acknowledge the contributions of S Maria Meade-Pruitt and Traci Session in the preparation of the chapter.

References

American Psychiatric Association 1994 Diagnostic and statistical manual of mental disorders, 4th edn. American Psychiatric Association, Washington, DC

American Psychological Association Practice Directorate 1998 Practicing psychology in hospitals and other health care facilities. American Psychological Association, Washington, DC

Baer R F 1960 Hypnosis, an adjunct in the treatment of neuromuscular disease. Archives of Physical Medicine and Rehabilitation 41: 514–515

Bauman W A, Spungen A M 2000 Metabolic changes in persons after spinal cord injury. Physical Medicine Rehabilitation Clinics of North America 11: 109–140

Beck A T 1967 Depression: Causes and treatment. University of Pennsylvania Press, Philadelphia

Bonica J J 1990 Anatomic and physiologic basis of nociception and pain. In: Bonica J J (ed) The management of pain, 2nd edn. Lea & Febiger, Philadelphia, p 28–94

Bryce T N, Ragnarsson K T 2003 Pain management in persons with spinal cord disorders. In: Lin V W, Cardenas D D, Cutter N C et al (eds) Spinal cord medicine: Principles and practice. Demos Medical, New York, p 441–460

Buckelew S P, Frank R G, Elliott T R et al 1991 Adjustment to spinal cord injury: Stage theory revisited. Paraplegia 29: 125–130

Burns A S, Jackson A B 2001 Gynecologic and reproductive issues in women with spinal cord injury. Physical Medicine Rehabilitation Clinics of North America 12: 183–199

Campagnolo D I, Merli G J 2002 Autonomic and cardiovascular complications of spinal cord injury. In: Kirshblum S, Campagnolo D, DeLisa J A (eds) Spinal cord medicine. Lippincott Williams & Wilkins, Philadelphia, p 123–134

Cardenas D D, Farrell-Roberts L, Sipski M L et al 1995 Management of gastrointestinal, genitourinary, and sexual function. In: Stover S L, DeLisa J A, Whiteneck G G (eds) Spinal cord injury: Clinical outcomes from the Model systems. Aspen, Maryland, p 120–144

Chan R C K, Lee P W H, Lieh-Mak F 2000 The pattern of coping in persons with spinal cord injuries. Disability and Rehabilitation 22: 501–507

Charlifue S W, Gerhart K A 1991 Behavioral and demographic predictors of suicide after traumatic spinal cord injury. Archives of Physical Medicine and Rehabilitation 72: 482–487

Charlifue S, Lammertse D 2003 Spinal cord injury and aging. In: Lin V W, Cardenas D D, Cutter N C et al (eds) Spinal cord medicine: Principles and practices. Demos Medical, New York, p 829–838

Chen Y, Jackson A B, Bussey B et al 2002 SCI EatRight weight management: A pilot study. Journal of Spinal Cord Medicine 25: S33

Consortium for Spinal Cord Medicine 1997 Clinical practice guidelines: Acute management of autonomic dysreflexia. Paralyzed Veterans of America, Washington, DC

Craig A R, Hancock K M, Dickson H G 1994 A longitudinal investigation into anxiety and depression in the first 2 years following a spinal cord injury. Paraplegia 32: 675–679.

Crooks R, Baur K 2002 Our sexuality, 8th edn. Wadsworth, Pacific Grove, CA, p 431

DeVivo M J 1997 Causes and costs of spinal cord injury in the United States. Spinal Cord 35: 809–813

DeVivo M J 2003 Epidemiology of spinal cord injury. In: Lin V W, Cardenas D D, Cutter N C et al (eds) Spinal cord medicine: Principles and practice. Demos Medical, New York, p 79–85

DeVivo M J, Black K J, Stover S L 1993 Causes of death during the first 12 years after SCI. Archives of Physical Medicine and Rehabilitation 74: 248–254

DeVivo M J, Hawkins L N, Richards J S et al 1995 Outcomes of post spinal cord injury marriages. Archives of Physical Medicine and Rehabilitation 76: 130–138

Dijkers M 1997 Quality of life after spinal cord injury: A meta analysis of the effects of disablement components. Spinal Cord 35: 829–840

Donovan W H, Dinh T A, Garber S L et al 1993 Pressure ulcers. In: DeLisa J A, Gans B M (eds) Rehabilitation medicine: Principles and practice, 2nd edn. Lippincott, Philadelphia, p 716–732

Ducharme S, Gill K M, Biener-Bergman S et al 1993 Sexual functioning: Medical and psychological aspects. In: DeLisa J A, Gans B M (eds) Rehabilitation medicine: Principles and practice, 2nd edn. Lippincott, Philadelphia, p 763–782

Duggan C E, Dijkers M 2001 Quality of life after spinal cord injury: A qualitative study. Rehabilitation Psychology 46: 3–27

Elliott S 2003 Sexual dysfunction and infertility in men with spinal cord disorders. In: Lin V W, Cardenas D D, Cutter N C et al (eds) Spinal cord medicine: Principles and practices. Demos Medical, New York, p 349–365

Elliott T R, Richards J S 1999 Living with the facts, negotiating the terms: Unrealistic beliefs, denial and adjustment in the first year of acquired disability. Journal of Personality and Interpersonal Loss 4: 361–381

Elliott T, Shewchuk R 2000 Problem solving therapy for family caregivers of persons with severe physical disabilities. In: Radnitz C (ed) Cognitive-behavioral therapy for persons with disabilities. Jason Aronson, Northvale, NJ, p 309–317

Elliott T R, Witty T E, Herrick S et al 1991 Negotiating reality after physical loss: Hope, depression, and disability. Journal of Personality and Social Psychology 61: 608–613

Ellis A 1970 The essence of rational psychotherapy: A comprehensive approach to treatment. Institute of Rational Living, New York.

Fichtenbaum J, Kirshblum S 2002 Psychological adaptation to spinal cord injury. In: Kirshblum S, Campagnolo D, DeLisa J A (eds) Spinal cord medicine. Lippincott Williams & Wilkins, Philadelphia, p 300–311

Freeman A M, Westphal J R, Davis LL et al 1995 The future of organ transplant psychiatry. Psychosomatics 36: 429–437

Fuhrer M J, Rintala D H, Hart K A et al 1992 Relationship of life satisfaction to impairment disability, and handicap among persons with spinal cord injury living in the community. Archives of Physical Medicine and Rehabilitation 73: 552–557

Gans J S 1987 Facilitating staff/patient interaction in rehabilitation. In: Caplin B (ed) Rehabilitation psychology desk reference. Aspen, Rockville, MD, p 185–217

Garland D E, Adkins R H, Ashford R et al 2001 Regional osteoporosis in females with complete spinal cord injury. Journal of Bone and Joint Surgery (Am) 83A: 1195–2000

Gerhart K A, Weitzenkamp D A, Kennedy C A et al 1999 Correlates of stress in long term spinal cord injury. Spinal Cord 37: 183–190

Glickman S, Kamm M A 1996 Bowel dysfunction in spinal-cord injury patients. Lancet 347: 1651–1653

Go B K, DeVivo M J, Richards J S 1995 The epidemiology of spinal cord injury. In: Stover S L, DeLisa J A, Whiteneck G G (eds) Spinal cord injury: Clinical outcomes from the Model Systems. Aspen, Gaithersburg, MD, p 21–55

Hancock K M, Craig A R, Dickson H G et al 1993 Anxiety and depression over the first year of spinal cord injury: A longitudinal study. Paraplegia 3: 349–357

Hanson C S, Nabavi D, Yuen H K 2001 The effect of sports on level of community integration as reported by persons with spinal cord injury. American Journal of Occupational Therapy 55: 332–338

Harrison J, Glass C A, Owens R G et al 1995 Factors associated with sexual functioning in women following spinal cord injury. Paraplegia 33: 687–692

Hartkopp A, Bronnum-Hansen H, Seidenschnur A M et al 1998 Suicide in a spinal cord injured population: Its relation to functional status. Archives of Physical Medicine and Rehabilitation 79: 1356–1361

Heinemann A W, Mamott B D, Schnoll S 1990 Substance use by persons with recent spinal cord injuries. Rehabilitation Psychology 35: 217–228

Jackson A 2003 Women's health challenges after spinal cord injury. In: Lin V W, Cardenas D D, Cutter N C et al (eds) Spinal cord medicine: Principles and practices. Demos Medical, New York, p 839–849

Jackson A B, Groomes T E 1994 Incidence of respiratory complications following spinal cord injury. Archives of Physical Medicine and Rehabilitation 75: 270–275

Judd F K, Brown D J 1988 The psychosocial approach to rehabilitation of the spinal cord injured patient. Paraplegia 26: 419–424

Kennedy P, Evans M J 2001 Evaluation of post traumatic distress in the first 6 months following SCI. Spinal Cord 39: 381–386

Kennedy P, Rogers B A 2000 Anxiety and depression after spinal cord injury: A longitudinal analysis. Archives of Physical Medicine and Rehabilitation 81: 932–937

Kolakowsky-Hayner S, Gourley E V, Kteutzer J S et al 1999 Pre-injury substance abuse among persons with brain injury and persons with spinal cord injury. Brain Injury 13(8): 571–581

Kolakowsky-Hayner S A, Gourley E V, Kreutzer J S et al 2002 Post-injury substance abuse among persons with brain injury and persons with spinal cord injury. Brain Injury 16: 583–592

Krause J S, Kemp B, Coker J 2000 Depression after spinal cord injury: Relation to gender, ethnicity, aging, and socioeconomic indicators. Archives of Physical Medicine and Rehabilitation 81: 1099–1109

Krogh K, Nielson J, Djurhuus J C et al 1997 Colorectal function in patients with spinal cord lesions. Diseases of the Colon and Rectum 40: 1233–1239

Kurylo M, Elliott T, Shewchuk R 2001 FOCUS on the family caregiver: A problem-solving training intervention. Journal of Counseling and Development 79: 275–281

Lazarus R S 1966 Psychological stress and the coping process. McGraw-Hill, New York

Levi R, Hultling C, Seiger A 1995 The Stockholm Spinal Cord Injury Study 2: Associations between clinical patient characteristics and post-acute medical problems. Paraplegia 33: 585–594

Maynard F M, Karunas R, Waring W W 1990 Epidemiology of spasticity following traumatic spinal cord injury. Archives of Physical Medicine and Rehabilitation 71: 566–569

Melzack R 1975 The McGill Pain Questionnaire: Major properties and scoring methods. Pain 1: 227–299

Melzack R, Katz J 1992 The McGill Pain Questionnaire: Appraisal and current status. In: Turk D C, Melzack R (eds) Handbook of pain assessment. Guilford, New York, p 152–168

Nance P W 2003 Management of spasticity. In: Lin V W, Cardenas D D, Cutter N C et al (eds) Spinal cord medicine: Principles and practices. Demos Medical, New York, p 461–476

New P W, Lim T C, Hill S T et al 1997 A survey of pain during rehabilitation after acute spinal cord injury. Spinal Cord 35: 658–663

Pentland W, McColl M A, Rosenthal L 1995 The effect of aging and duration of disability on long term health outcomes following spinal cord injury. Paraplegia 33: 367–373

Pentland W, Walker J, Minnes P et al 2002 Women with spinal cord injury and the impact of aging. Spinal Cord 40: 374–387

Peterson W P, Kirshblum S 2002 Pulmonary management of spinal cord injury. In: Kirshblum S, Campagnolo D, DeLisa J A (eds) Spinal cord medicine. Lippincott Williams & Wilkins, Philadelphia, p 135–154

Phelps J, Albo M, Dunn K et al 2001 Spinal cord injury and sexuality in married or partnered men: Activities, function, needs, and predictors of sexual adjustment. Archives of Sexual Behavior 30: 591–602

Priebe M M, Martin M, Wuermser L A et al 2003 The medical management of pressure ulcers. In: Lin VW, Cardenas D D, Cutter N C et al (eds) Spinal cord medicine: Principles and practices. Demos Medical, New York, p 567–589

Putzke J D, Richards J S, Hicken B L et al 2002 Pain classification following spinal cord injury: The utility of verbal descriptors. Spinal Cord 40: 118–127

Radnitz C L (ed) 2002 Cognitive-behavioral therapy for persons with disabilities. Jason Aronson, Northvale, NJ

Radnitz C L, Schlein I S, Hsu L 2000 The effect of prior trauma exposure on the development of PTSD following spinal cord injury. Journal of Anxiety Disorders 14: 313–324

Ragnarsson K T 1997 Management of pain in persons with spinal cord injury. Journal of Spinal Cord Medicine 20: 186–199

Ragnarsson K T, Hall K M, Wilmot C B et al 1995 Management of pulmonary, cardiovascular, and metabolic conditions after spinal cord injury. In: Stover S L, DeLisa J A, Whiteneck G G (eds) Spinal cord injury: Clinical outcomes from the Model Systems. Aspen, Gaithersburg, MD, p 79–99

Richards J S 1986 Psychologic adjustment to spinal cord injury during first year post discharge. American Journal of Physical Medicine and Rehabilitation 67: 362–365

Richards J S, Brown L, Hagglund K et al 1988 Spinal cord injury and concomitant traumatic brain injury: Results of a longitudinal investigation. American Journal of Physical Medicine and Rehabilitation 67: 211–216

Richards J S, Osuana F J, Jaworski T M et al 1991 The effectiveness of different methods of defining traumatic brain injury in predicting post discharge adjustment in a spinal cord injury population. Archives of Physical Medicine and Rehabilitation 72: 275–279

Richards J S, Kewman D G, Pierce C A 2000 Spinal cord injury. In: Frank E G, Elliott T R (eds) Handbook of rehabilitation psychology. American Psychological Association, Washington, DC, p 11–27

Roth E, Davidoff G, Thomas P et al 1989 A controlled study of neuropsychological deficits in acute spinal cord injury patients. Paraplegia 27: 480–489

Sabharwal S 2003 Cardiovascular dysfunction in spinal cord disorders In: Lin V W, Cardenas D D, Cutter N C et al (eds) Spinal cord medicine: Principles and practices. Demos Medical, New York, p 179–192

Scivoletto G, Petrelli A, Di Lucente L et al 1997 Psychological investigation of spinal cord injury patients. Spinal Cord 35: 516–520

Smith J 1990 Substance abuse: The spiral of denial: In: Maddox S N (ed) Spinal network. Library of Congress, Washington, DC, p 238–240

Snyder C R, Cheavens J, Michael S T 1999 Hoping. In: Snyder CR (ed) Coping: The psychology of what works. Oxford University Press, New York, p 205–227

Staas W E, Formal C S, Gershkoff A M et al 1998 Rehabilitation of the spinal cord-injured patient. In: DeLisa J (ed) Rehabilitation medicine: Principles and practice. Lippincott, Philadelphia, p 635–659

Stiens SA, Kirshblum S C, Groah S L et al 2002 Spinal cord injury medicine 4. Optimal participation in life after spinal cord injury: Physical, psychosocial, and economic reintegration in the environment. Archives of Physical Medicine and Rehabilitation 83: S72–81

Stormer S, Gerner H J, Gruninger W et al 1997 Chronic pain/dysaesthesia in spinal cord injury patients: Results of a multicentre study. Spinal Cord 35: 446–455

Stover S L 1995 Review of forty years of rehabilitation issues in spinal cord injury. Journal of Spinal Cord Medicine 18: 175–182

Tate D G 1993 Alcohol use among spinal cord-injured patients. American Journal of Physical Medicine and Rehabilitation 72: 192–195

Tate D, Forcheimer M, Maynard F et al 1994 Predicting depression and psychological distress in persons with spinal cord injury based on indicator of handicap. American Journal of Physical Medicine and Rehabilitation 73: 175–183

Tator C H, Duncan E G, Edmonds V E et al 1993 Complications and costs of management of acute spinal cord injury. Paraplegia 31: 700–714

Trieschmann R B 1988 Spinal cord injuries: Psychological, social, and vocational rehabilitation. Demos Publications, New York

Trieschmann R B 1992 Psychosocial research in spinal cord injury: The state of the art. Paraplegia 30: 58–60

Turner J A, Cardenas D D, Warms C A et al 2001 Chronic pain associated with spinal cord injuries: A community survey. Archives of Physical Medicine and Rehabilitation 82: 501–508

Turner J A, Jensen M P, Warms C A et al 2002 Catastrophizing is associated with pain intensity, psychological distress, and pain-related disability among individuals with chronic pain after spinal cord injury. Pain 98: 127–134

Weitzenkamp D A, Jones R H, Whiteneck G G et al 2001 Ageing with spinal cord injury: Cross-sectional and longitudinal effects. Spinal Cord 39: 301–309

Weld K J, Graney M J, Dmochowski R R 2000 Differences in bladder compliance with time and associations of bladder management with compliance in spinal cord injured patients. Journal of Urology 163: 1228–1233

Yarkony G M, Heinemann A W 1995 Pressure ulcers. In: Stover S L, DeLisa J A, Whiteneck G G (eds) Spinal cord injury: Clinical outcomes from the Model Systems. Aspen, Gaithersburg, MD, p 100–115

Yule W, Williams R, Joseph S 1999 Post-traumatic stress disorder in adults. In: Yule W (ed) Post-traumatic stress disorders: Concepts and therapy. Wiley, Chichester, UK, p 1–24

Chapter 15

Cardiovascular and respiratory conditions

Pia B. Santiago, Robert M. Kaplan

INTRODUCTION

Cardiorespiratory conditions are the primary leading causes of mortality and morbidity among adults (Murray & Lopez 1996, National Heart Lung and Blood Institute 2002). Individuals with cardiovascular and pulmonary diseases experience significant functional impairments that consequently compromise their health-related quality of life and psychosocial functioning. Multifactorial rehabilitative care of cardiac and pulmonary patients is designed to optimize patient independent functioning through reduction and control of symptoms arising from underlying disease. Behavioral management of nutrition and exercise, smoking cessation, patient education, and psychosocial support are central components of cardiorespiratory rehabilitation. This chapter will provide an overview of the pathophysiology underlying cardiac and pulmonary conditions. We will also present a discussion of the integrative behavioral applications in multifactorial rehabilitation and relevant psychosocial outcome variables. We will conclude with a discussion of patient non-adherence, a common problem in the management of chronic illness, and the strategies providers can employ to facilitate lifestyle behavior change.

PHYSICAL AND MEDICAL CONSIDERATIONS

CARDIOVASCULAR DISEASES

Definition and pathophysiology

Cardiovascular disease (CVD), which includes coronary heart disease (CHD), hypertension, and stroke, is the leading cause of death in industrialized nations (Murray & Lopez 1996). In 1999, almost 900 000 deaths in the United States of America (US) were attributable to cerebrovascular (stroke) or heart diseases (National Heart Lung and Blood Institute 2002). Coronary heart disease is the most common form of CVD and accounts for over 520 000 deaths each year in the US (National Heart Lung and Blood Institute 2002). Clinical manifestations of CHD include stable angina pectoris, unstable angina (chest pain), acute myocardial infarction or MI (heart attack), and sudden cardiac death. Atherosclerosis, the primary disease process underlying cardiovascular disease (National Heart Lung and Blood Institute 1998, Porth 1998), is characterized by the formation of plaque lesions within blood vessels such as those supplying oxygen and nutrients to the cardiac muscle. Ischemia, or decreased blood supply to an organ, can occur when a vessel supporting an organ is significantly occluded such that the oxygen supply available is insufficient to meet the demands of the tissues. Irreversible tissue damage (necrosis) and death can occur depending on the severity and location of the ischemic event.

The exact cause(s) underlying the initiation of atherosclerosis remains a topic of active investigation. It is thought that injury to the endothelial layer lining the vessel is the initiating event that leads to atherosclerosis (Massberg et al 2003, Porth 1998, Samra et al 2002). This area of injury attracts monocytes (immune cells), platelets (clotting factors), cholesterol, and other blood components to come into contact with and stimulate the proliferation of smooth muscle cells and connective and scar tissue within the vessel wall. The physical injuries that initiate the formation of atherosclerotic plaques are hypothesized to result from contact with oxidative or injurious agents (i.e., immune factors or toxic particles from smoking), or mechanical stress such as those associated with hypertension (Dhalla et al 2000, Luscher 1994, Porth 1998). When modifiable risk factors persist (e.g., smoking, untreated hypertension), there is less time for the lesion to heal and the atherosclerotic process will progress.

Scope of impact on public health

Cardiovascular diseases are common and are associated with significant mortality. According to the National Health Interview Survey, diseases of the heart accounted for 709 894 deaths in the year 2000 among US adults (Minino & Smith 2001). In 1999, heart disease ranked as the number one cause of death for Caucasians, African Americans,

Hispanic, Asian Americans/Pacific Islanders, and Native Americans, respectively (National Heart Lung and Blood Institute 2002). However, data from the National Center of Health Statistics show that since 1970 there has been a 51% decrease in mortality attributable to CVD, suggesting improvement in the modes of care, surveillance, and prevention to address this public health problem.

Despite declines in CHD, various forms of CVD are still common. National estimates in the US suggest that 61.8 million adults have at least one condition classified under CVD (e.g., hypertension, angina pectoris, coronary heart disease, stroke, heart failure) (National Heart Lung and Blood Institute 2002). In addition to being the primary cause of death, CVD is associated with significant morbidity. Accounting for US$199.5 billion spent in healthcare expenditure in 2002, these conditions together outranked all other major chronic diseases in total direct costs for hospital care, physician visits, prescription drugs, home healthcare, and nursing home care (National Heart Lung and Blood Institute 2002).

CHRONIC OBSTRUCTIVE PULMONARY DISEASE

Definition and pathophysiology

Chronic obstructive pulmonary disease (COPD) is a set of chronic, irreversible, and progressive respiratory disorders accompanied by substantial mortality, healthcare costs, disability, and loss of quality of life (Mannino et al 2002). COPD is characterized by persistent obstructive airflow. The three main types of COPD are emphysema, chronic bronchitis, and asthma, and these result in significant shortness of breath or dyspnea and have varying etiologies.

Until recently, the diagnosis of emphysema was anatomical and typically made only at the time of autopsy. However, newer techniques in radiology, such as high resolution computed tomography (HRCT) scanning, have made it possible to separate emphysema from chronic bronchitis in living people. Emphysema is caused by the loss of elastic recoil of the lung parenchyma, resulting in over-inflation of the lung. These changes are typically associated with destruction of the alveolar walls. Emphysema is a chronic condition that develops over many years and is characterized by symptoms of progressive shortness of breath upon exertion. The disease process is largely irreversible, and results in considerable disability for affected individuals, with high morbidity and mortality.

The consequences of chronic bronchitis are similar to those of emphysema. However, chronic bronchitis is defined as the presence of a chronic cough and sputum production that lasts at least 3 months in two consecutive years (American Thoracic Society 1987), resulting in chronic inflammation of the bronchi. In some patients, the airways become obstructed, making breathing difficult.

Asthma is a condition associated with a reversible airway narrowing that may occur in response to stimuli such as infection, allergy, cold air, or cigarette smoke. The narrowing of airways may be caused by a spasm of smooth muscles, inflammation, or the oversecretion of mucus. Chronic asthma occurs when the narrowing persists over the course of time. Often, chronic asthma and bronchitis co-exist, resulting in a diagnosis of "asthmatic bronchitis".

Scope of impact on public health

Chronic obstructive lung diseases collectively have become important causes for public health concern for at least four reasons:

1. they are a major cause of death
2. they affect a large number of persons
3. incidence is increasing
4. they have a major impact upon activities of daily living (Crystal 1987).

Because COPD is insidious with a long latency period before clinical recognition, official statistics underestimate morbidity and mortality. Data from the third National Health and Nutrition Examination Survey suggested that many cases of obstructive lung disease (i.e., low lung function) remain undiagnosed (Mannino et al 2000, Petty 2000).

COPD-related mortality and morbidity are substantial and alarming. Accounting for 124 181 deaths in 1999, COPD is the fourth leading cause of death in the US in individuals over the age of 55, and has an age-adjusted death rate of 45.8 deaths per 100 000 persons (National Center for Health Statistics 1999). In addition, during the 1996 National Health Interview Survey, it was estimated that chronic bronchitis and emphysema affect 14.2 million and 1.8 million Americans, respectively (National Center for Health Statistics 1999). The 2002 surveillance report from the Centers of Disease Control documented an increasing trend in morbidity and mortality of COPD from 1971 to 2000 (Mannino et al 2002). In 2000, there were 10.5 million adults over the age of 24 with self-reported emphysema or chronic bronchitis, affecting 60 per 1000 US adults. While COPD prevalence and death rates are consistently higher among men than women, for the first time in 2000, there were more women dying of COPD than men (59 936 vs. 59 118). These changes likely reflect a shift in tobacco use patterns by men and women beginning in the 1960s and 1970s.

MULTIFACTORIAL REHABILITATION OF CARDIORESPIRATORY CONDITIONS

Comprehensive cardiac or pulmonary rehabilitation programs have been developed to provide a multidisciplinary therapeutic program tailored to the needs of the individual patient (American Association of Cardiovascular and Pulmonary Rehabilitation 1998, American College of Chest Physicians/American Association of Cardiovascular and Pulmonary Rehabilitation 1997, Cardiac Rehabilitation Guideline Panel 1995, Hodgkin et al 1993). The primary goal of rehabilitation programs for cardiorespiratory conditions is to limit the physiological and psychological effects of illness, and to optimize patient independent functioning. This goal is achieved by helping patients and significant others learn more about the disease, treatment options, and coping strategies. Patients are encouraged to become actively involved in self-care, more independent in daily activities, and less dependent on health professionals and expensive medical resources. In the case of cardiac disease, treatment goals also include modification of cardiac risk factors through secondary preventive measures involving lifestyle behavior change and medication management. These measures have been shown to reduce the likelihood of sudden death or re-infarction, and reversal of the atherosclerotic process. Successful programs can help patients to become better educated and more involved in their own care. In addition, such programs can result in reduced symptoms, improved exercise tolerance, fewer hospitalizations and physician visits, and more gainful employment.

SCIENTIFIC EVIDENCE ON CARDIORESPIRATORY REHABILITATION

Empirical evidence supports the value of multifactorial rehabilitative care in the treatment of cardiorespiratory conditions. Evidence-based clinical guidelines for cardiac rehabilitation were derived based on a critical review of 334 studies (Cardiac Rehabilitation Guideline Panel 1995). The scientific panel found that cardiac rehabilitation results in substantial functional and psychological benefits and decreased mortality. Improvements in exercise tolerance and reductions in symptoms of angina as a result of exercise training were found for both men and women with CHD and heart failure. In two meta-analyses of 21 randomized controlled trials comparing cardiac rehabilitation patients with control patients, a 25% relative reduction in mortality at 3-year follow-up was observed for patients participating in cardiac rehabilitation (O'Connor et al 1989, Oldridge et al 1988). Favorable mortality outcomes were greater in those studies implementing a comprehensive cardiac rehabilitation program (26% reduction in mortality) in contrast to those using exercise as a sole intervention (15% reduction in mortality). Several randomized controlled trials using exercise only and multifactorial programs support that participation in cardiac rehabilitation is associated with improvements in social adjustment and functioning, health-related quality of life, and psychological functioning (depression, anxiety) (Bar et al 1992, Gulanick 1991, Newton et al 1991, Oldridge et al 1991, Ott et al 1983, Stern et al 1983, Taylor et al 1986).

A growing literature also testifies to the benefits and importance of pulmonary rehabilitation programs (Bach 1996, Fishman 1996, Hodgkin et al 1993). A recent evidence-based document supports the scientific foundation of these programs (American College of Chest Physicians/American Association of Cardiovascular and Pulmonary Rehabilitation 1997). The American College of Chest Physicians/American Association of Cardiovascular and Pulmonary Rehabilitation joint panel concluded that pulmonary rehabilitation is associated with improvements in several important physical and psychological domains of health and functioning. In particular, pulmonary rehabilitation, including supervised exercise training, was shown in randomized controlled trials to result in significant improvements in patient-reported overall functional capabilities, performance of a submaximal task involving muscles of ambulation, and health-related quality of life, as well as reductions in dyspnea and healthcare utilization (Berry et al 1996, Goldstein et al 1994, Lake et al 1990, Reardon et al 1994, Ries et al 1995, Simpson et al 1992, Strijbos et al 1996, Weiner et al 1992, Wijkstra et al 1994).

Present empirical evidence regarding the psychosocial benefits of pulmonary rehabilitation are limited and not as consistent. While observational studies show that participation in pulmonary rehabilitation is associated with reductions in anxiety and depression (Emery et al 1991, Ojanen et al 1993), only one of three randomized controlled trials reported this effect (Dekhuijzen et al 1990). Randomized controlled trials of specific behavioral and psychosocial interventions (e.g., progressive muscle relaxation, stress management, dyspnea management) do not appear to be sufficient as single therapeutic modalities (Blake et al 1990, Renfroe 1988, Sassi-Dambron et al 1995). However, there is a need for further well-controlled studies utilizing validated measures of psychological and behavioral functioning to either support or refute the role of such interventions in enhancing psychosocial and behavioral outcomes.

Cardiorespiratory rehabilitation programs typically consist of several component areas requiring involvement of multiple health and psychosocial disciplines. The following section will describe each of the components of a typical multifactorial rehabilitation program.

Components of cardiorespiratory rehabilitation

Cardiorespiratory rehabilitation integrates expertise from various healthcare disciplines into a comprehensive, cohesive program tailored to the needs of each patient. Box 15.1 outlines content areas for both cardiac and pulmonary rehabilitation programs.

Exercise   Exercise training is an integral component of both cardiac and pulmonary rehabilitation programs. Evidence-based guidelines for both cardiac and pulmonary rehabilitation indicate that exercise training consistently improves measures of exercise tolerance and functional capacity (American College of Chest Physicians/American Association of Cardiovascular and Pulmonary Rehabilitation 1997, Cardiac Rehabilitation Guideline Panel 1995).

Exercise endurance training in patients with and without previous MI is associated with improvements in exercise capacity and several physiological factors related to favorable prognosis. Regular physical activity is particularly important in modification or cardiac risk profiles for patients with heart disease (e.g., higher caloric expenditure, weight loss, lipid management). Studies also document antidepressive and anxiolytic effects of exercise (Camacho et al 1991, Coats et al 1992, Curfman 1993, Siscovick et al 1984, Taylor et al 1986).

> **Box 15.1 Program content areas of cardiac and pulmonary rehabilitation programs**
>
> **Common to cardiac and pulmonary rehabilitation**
> Structured exercise training
> Psychosocial support
> Stress management and relaxation training
> Smoking cessation
> Use of medications
> Activities of daily living
>
> **Specific to cardiac rehabilitation**
> Nutrition
> Weight and blood pressure control
>
> **Specific to pulmonary rehabilitation**
> Oxygen use
> Breathing retraining
> Bronchial hygiene

Exercise intolerance due to significant breathlessness upon exertion is the primary functional limitation among patients with COPD. Physical reconditioning through exercise training during rehabilitation reduces exercise intolerance through a number of mechanisms. Progressive, successful experiences in managing symptoms of breathlessness during exercise decrease feelings of anxiety and panic as patients gain a sense of mastery over their symptoms (Toshima et al 1992b). Ries et al (1995) observed a significant increase in self-efficacy for walking among pulmonary patients as a result of participation in supervised exercise training. Other mechanisms by which physical reconditioning improves exercise tolerance can include:

1. increase in the strength and endurance of inspiratory muscles
2. improved mechanical skill (decrease in oxygen cost and ventilatory requirements for a given workload)
3. improved ventilatory pattern (larger tidal volume, lower respiratory rate) during exercise (O'Donnell 2001).

In the context of cardiorespiratory rehabilitation, exercise training is accompanied by psychosocial support and a variety of psychoeducational topics relevant to medical patients and their caregivers. The following section presents a discussion of these issues.

Education Patient education is integral to engagement of the patient in his/her own medical care. In addition to normal and disease physiology, didactic sessions typically consist of topics such as symptom management and hygiene, proper use of medications and equipment, lifestyle modification of diet and smoking, and activities of daily living. These areas will be discussed below.

Management of dyspnea An important component of education in rehabilitation is instructing patients how to manage their symptoms. Dyspnea, or shortness of breath, is the primary source of functional limitation among patients with COPD, and is also experienced by patients with cardiac disease. Dyspnea management techniques, as applied in pulmonary rehabilitation, typically consist of training in breathing techniques, self-awareness of symptoms, chest physical therapy, and proper bronchial hygiene and use of respiratory modalities.

In breathing retraining, patients with COPD are instructed on how to control and relieve breathlessness and panic through diaphragmatic and pursed-lip breathing. Diaphragmatic breathing is a maneuver in which the patient coordinates abdominal wall expansion with inspiration while purse-lip breathing is applied during the exhalation phase. Together, these techniques improve the ventilatory pattern (slowing the rate of respiration and increasing tidal volume), prevent dynamic airway compression, improve synchrony of abdominal and thoracic respiratory muscles, and improve gas exchange (Faling 1993, Rochester & Goldberg 1980).

Training in chest physical therapy and bronchial hygiene techniques ensures that patients know how to control secretions and optimize air flow. Clearance of excess secretions is important in COPD as retained mucus can potentiate the onset of a respiratory infection. Chest physical therapy techniques can alleviate symptoms during an exacerbation or aid as routine preventive measures for patients with excess mucus production (Ries 1996).

Teaching patients how to monitor changes in their symptoms is helpful for both patients and caregivers. Healthcare providers can devise a plan with patients which will help them know how to recognize the early signs of a respiratory infection, what self-care actions need to be taken, and when to consult with a nurse or doctor. The goals of symptom awareness training are to facilitate problem-solving by the patient, enhance patient self-efficacy in management of their symptoms, and increase patient familiarity with their own symptomatology.

Medication and equipment use   When initiating treatment, patients must often follow a complex regimen of self-care involving use of medications and equipment. Patients with cardiorespiratory disease must often set up dosing schedules for various medications to control or prevent symptoms. In managing this pharmacological regimen, it is helpful for health practitioners to work with the patient in drafting a written set of instructions listing the medication name, dosage, and time of dosage. Patients can keep this list on-hand which can easily be shown to other healthcare providers the patient may interact with during a routine medical or urgent care visit.

In addition to medication regimens, patients with pulmonary disease often use a variety of respiratory modalities and equipment to facilitate breathing. These can include oxygen delivery systems and aerosol therapy devices. Patients should be sufficiently educated on the proper use and maintenance of any equipment. Healthcare practitioners can also work with patients in selecting the best equipment to fit their lifestyle.

Given the complexity of treatment, open communication between providers and patients can greatly enhance the outcomes of treatment. Ongoing feedback from patients can assist the providers in troubleshooting difficulties patients may be experiencing, which in turn, can allow the providers to problem-solve, provide information to clarify, and to modify treatment regimen as necessary.

Smoking   Smoking is the most important modifiable risk factor in the development and progression of CVD and COPD. Specifically, smoking can further hasten the atherosclerotic process (Os et al 2003, Tracy et al 1997) and lung function decline (Buist 1997).

Cessation of smoking interrupts the progression of lung decline in pulmonary patients and atherosclerosis in cardiac patients, and thereby improves survival. In COPD, while cessation of smoking does not reverse lung damage, it does alter the rate of decline in lung function such that ex-smokers decline at rates comparable to non-smokers once they stop smoking (Anthonisen et al 1994, Buist 1997). Cessation of smoking can also remove further exposure to allergens and pollutants that can trigger bronchial reactivity and inflammation. However, data suggest that the benefits of smoking cessation occur early in the course of COPD (Kanner 1996) and most patients have quit smoking by the time they develop more advanced disease and participate in pulmonary rehabilitation programs (American College of Chest Physicians/American Association of Cardiovascular and Pulmonary Rehabilitation 1997). Most programs do not provide smoking cessation as a component of pulmonary rehabilitation such that patients who continue to smoke should be referred to additional behavior-based resources to aid in smoking cessation.

Among cardiac patients, smoking cessation greatly reduces risk for morbidity and mortality. After a MI, smoking cessation can reduce the expected risk of death by as much as 40–60% (Wilhelmsen 1988), and reduce symptoms of angina (Deanfield et al 1984). Education, behavioral interventions incorporating relapse prevention and stress management, nicotine replacement therapies, and individual as well as group-based counseling can augment success of smoking cessation.

Nutrition   Dietary modification and counseling are particularly important in rehabilitation and secondary prevention of cardiac disease. Lipid management can be achieved through dietary interventions in addition to medical therapies. A dietician as part of the rehabilitation program can facilitate dietary modification and resulting weight loss and lipid management by instructing patients how to monitor daily food intake, plan and prepare meals, and read food labels. Food monitoring can assist patients in increasing awareness of and targeting problematic dietary patterns (e.g., large portions of snack foods and red meats, fast food dining, food preparations that add excess saturated fats and calories). Information derived from food monitoring sheets can then be used to formulate specific dietary goals (e.g., consume at least three servings of fish per week, replace at least three snacks or dessert foods with fruit). Meal planning in conjunction with reading food labels during grocery shopping allows patients to make healthier decisions about meals ahead of time and increase availability of healthier foods in the home. Furthermore, patients can learn alternative ways of food preparation to limit addition of excess calories and fats (e.g., baking or grilling vs. frying). These dietary practices can subsequently reduce hypertension as well as risk for certain types of cancers, diabetes, and osteoporosis (Hu et al 1997, Kohlmeier et al 1997, Kushi et al 1995).

Activities of daily living   In the context of a rehabilitation program, patients typically receive instruction on how to minimize the impact of disease and symptoms on daily activities and one's lifestyle. As symptoms become more frequent and intense, patients often abandon activities of leisure, work, and daily living due to increasing discomfort or concern regarding their symptoms. However, rehabilitation instructors can teach patients specific skills that allow them to resume these activities in ways that minimize or circumvent physical discomfort, thereby limiting their disability from their symptoms and enhancing independent functioning. Techniques such as pacing of activities and energy conservation, and use of adaptive equipment, can greatly facilitate independent functioning and performance of daily activities. Cognitive strategies targeting unrealistic expectations (e.g., need to perform activity at premorbid levels of functioning) can also be identified and addressed during group sessions. Time management can prevent rushing and accompanying breathlessness by helping the patient prioritize and schedule tasks in such a way as to allow for more time for completion or travel between places. Instruction in panic control and relaxation techniques enables the patient to manage and curb the progression of acute, distressing symptoms such as breathlessness. Patient training should also include discussion focusing on specific activities that are abandoned due to presence or concern regarding symptoms (e.g., travel, work, sexual activities). Problem-solving strategies can be employed to identify ways in which the patient can still engage in these activities while avoiding overexertion. Overall, patients can exercise these skills to live more independently despite their physical limitations.

PSYCHOLOGICAL CONSIDERATIONS

Psychological and psychosocial support focuses on facilitating patient and family adjustment to the physical and psychological implications of the disease process. Patients may have difficulty coping with a growing sense of vulnerability to the impending changes in health and the resulting impact on one's social roles. Furthermore, patients may experience helplessness, frustration, hostility, and anxiety in response to feeling incapable of performing usual activities or asserting control over their health status. The following section provides a detailed discussion of common psychological and behavioral considerations in cardiorespiratory disorders.

COMMON PSYCHOLOGICAL AND BEHAVIORAL ISSUES IN CARDIORESPIRATORY DISEASES

The psychological impact of the chronic and debilitating nature of cardiorespiratory diseases on the patient and surrounding social systems are substantial. Patients with chronic illness often experience loss of independence and control over health and resulting life changes. It is common for patients with cardiac and chronic lung diseases to worry about worsening of symptoms and recurrence of pulmonary exacerbation or MI. The chronicity of symptoms inevitably compromises the patient's ability to perform occupational and social roles, leading to marked emotional distress for both the patient and family members. Patients and family members also must often face the burden of making major, difficult lifestyle changes as healthcare professionals issue complex recommendations for increased regimentation of lifestyle (i.e., compliance with medications, diet, and exercise). It becomes readily apparent that the physical consequences of chronic diseases have extensive psychological and social implications for the patient and family members. Physical and manual therapists not only have the responsibility of providing effective treatment to manage the underlying disease process, but must also deliver care in such a manner that demonstrates understanding of the physical and emotional facets of the disease and the nature of patient disability.

The following sections will discuss important psychosocial aspects of cardiorespiratory diseases and their relationship to treatment outcomes.

Health-related quality of life

Health-related quality of life (HRQOL) is now recognized as an important outcome in studies of medical care. HRQOL is conceptualized as a multidimensional construct encompassing physical, mental, social, and role functioning as well as symptoms and health perceptions (Bergner et al 1981, Ware 1995). While health status can be measured objectively using physiological measures (e.g., exercise performance, pulmonary function tests), subjective measures of HRQOL take into account an individual's expectations and beliefs about health, optimum functioning, and ability to cope (Testa & Simonson 1996). The degree to which one perceives important domains of functioning are impacted by physical status will determine one's HRQOL such that two individuals with similar physiological measures can have two different ratings of HRQOL.

HRQOL is an important outcome among chronic illness, such as cardiac and respiratory disorders, as the clinical manifestations of disease (e.g., breathlessness, chest pain) inevitably impact on one's social, occupational, and emotional roles, and capacity to live independently over extended periods of time. As discussed earlier in this chapter, cardiorespiratory rehabilitation and secondary prevention measures can improve objective measures of functioning such as exercise performance. However, in the case of COPD, while physiological assessments of lung function do not improve with rehabilitation, measures of HRQOL do (Ries et al 1995), indicating that interventions such as rehabilitation can limit the effects of disability and symptoms from illness on important domains of functioning.

HRQOL can be either disease-specific, focusing on the particular symptoms experienced during illness or general, representing overall functioning. In research of COPD and other respiratory diseases, disease-specific HRQOL measures emphasize dyspnea as this is the primary clinical manifestation and functional limitation in lung disease (Eakin et al 1993). A dyspnea measure developed by our research group at the University of California, San Diego pulmonary rehabilitation program is the UCSD Shortness of Breath Questionnaire (SOBQ). The SOBQ is a 24-item measure listing 21 activities of daily living and requires the participant to rate his/her level of dyspnea while doing each of the activities. As well, three items require the participant to rate how shortness of breath, fear of "hurting myself" or overexertion, and fear of shortness of breath limit him/her in daily life. Scores on the SOBQ have been shown to correlate with exercise tolerance, disease severity, depression, and Borg scale ratings of dyspnea following a 6-minute walk (Eakin et al 1998). The Chronic Respiratory Questionnaire (CRQ) developed by Guyatt et al (1987) is another instrument used to measure HRQOL in respiratory diseases and measures four domains of functioning: dyspnea, fatigue, emotional function, and perception of mastery over illness.

Global or generic measures of HRQOL are assessments that can be used for both medical and non-medical populations, and measure dimensions of health that have been determined to be important to people in general. The Sickness Impact Profile (SIP)

(Bergner et al 1981), RAND Health Status Measure (Stewart et al 1978), and Quality of Well-Being Scale (QWB) (Kaplan et al 1993) have been used to assess HRQOL within cardiac (Goss et al 2002, Ott et al 1983) and respiratory populations (Johnson et al 2000, Kaplan et al 1984b, Low & Gutman 2003, Moorer et al 2001, Orenstein et al 1989).

The QWB is a general health status index and a utility-weighted measure that classifies patients according to observed levels of functioning of mobility, physical activity, and social activity. In addition to classification according to observable function, individuals are also classified by their chief symptom or problem. Symptoms or problems may be severe (e.g., serious chest pain) or minor (e.g., taking medications or a prescribed diet for health reasons). Preferences or values are used to map function states and symptoms onto a "quality continuum ranging between 0.0 (for death) and 1.0 (for optimum function)" yielding an overall score. The quality-adjusted life year (QALY) is defined as the equivalent of a completely well year of life or a year of life free of any symptoms, problems, or health-related disabilities. The QWB is particularly useful in quantifying cost utility as it accounts for both HRQOL and mortality outcomes over time, making it an ideal tool for comparing treatment interventions and health policies (Kaplan & Anderson 1996).

Given the importance of HRQOL to patients as well as developers of interventions, measurement of HRQOL (disease-specific and general) should be integrated into program evaluation and pre- to post-rehabilitation measurements to ensure that the treatment (i.e., rehabilitation) is efficacious in improving overall functioning.

Depression

Depression is a common problem among patients with chronic medical conditions. It has been estimated that 20–30% of cardiac patients (Carney et al 1987, Forrester et al 1992) and about 40% of COPD patients (Isoaho et al 1995, Light et al 1985, McSweeny et al 1982, Yohannes et al 2000) experience symptoms of depression. There is also evidence suggesting that depressed COPD patients who present for emergency treatment of a respiratory exacerbation are more likely to be admitted for hospitalization or relapse within a month as compared to non-depressed patients (Dahlen & Janson 2002). It is often difficult to determine the presence of an independent psychiatric problem such as depression in the context of a debilitating chronic disease when considering the multitude of negative physical, social, and emotional consequences of such diseases and treatment on various domains of functioning. Patients may feel overwhelmed by the implications of their diagnosis and treatment. Patients who have poor coping strategies, have minimal social support, or lack the resources to obtain treatment may frequently experience feelings of hopelessness regarding the prognosis of their condition or their ability to change the course of their illness.

A possible explanation for the prevalence of depression among patients with cardiorespiratory disease is that depression is a psychological response to the limitation of activities that is common in these conditions. In COPD, the gradually deteriorating course of disease often results in numerous lifestyle changes, including the loss of many activities. In CVD, as in COPD, many patients find that they have to change or give up their jobs. As a result of disability, patients are no longer able to obtain the reinforcers that make daily life enjoyable. Ries et al (1995), however, found that although patients who participate in rehabilitation improve on functional outcomes, these benefits were not accompanied by improvements in depression. Further analyses specific to the rehabilitation condition showed that significant improvements in $VO_{2\,max}$ were made by rehabilitation patients who were initially depressed compared to those with minimal or no depression (Toshima et al 1992a). That is, the rehabilitation program was particularly useful for patients who were initially depressed. Similar findings exist supporting improvements in measures of depression as a result of exercise participation among cardiac patients (Newton et al 1991, Taylor et al 1986).

The measurement of depression for patients with COPD is difficult because most assessments are based on the general population. For example, items on the Center for Epidemiological Studies for Depression (CES-D) scale and other depression measures assess decreased sleep, poor appetite, decreased energy, and so on. These are often symptomatic experiences of lung disease. It is not uncommon for patients with COPD to have trouble sleeping or decreased energy because of dyspnea. Further, many patients with COPD report decreased appetite because of the discomfort associated with a full stomach pressing on the diaphragm. Therefore, scores on depression measures may not accurately reflect the level of clinical depression in patients experiencing chronic diseases such as COPD. Currently, there are no data available concerning disease-appropriate depression-associated variables, so it is impossible to determine how many patients who report depression-like symptoms actually have a major affective disorder.

Given the high prevalence of depression in cardiorespiratory patients, assessment of depression should be a standard procedure in the assessment protocol. There is growing evidence from prospective studies documenting that depression can affect post-MI prognosis. Post-MI depression is associated with higher rates of infarction and rehospitalization (Frasure-Smith et al 1993, 1995). Furthermore, depressed patients, as clinically diagnosed using validated measures, had at least a 4-fold increase in mortality following an acute MI even after controlling for left ventricular dysfunction, tobacco use, or history of MI. While underlying biochemical mechanisms for this are not clear, severe levels of depression may interfere with the patient's ability to adhere to complex medical regimens. Difficulty in concentrating, fatigue, and lack of motivation may also make it difficult for patients to benefit from cardiorespiratory rehabilitation programs. In a meta-analysis of 12 studies of various medical populations, DiMatteo et al (2002) found that, compared to non-depressed patients, depressed patients were three times more likely to be non-compliant with medical treatment recommendations (DiMatteo et al 2000). In the case of severe depression, it may be necessary to refer the patient to a mental health professional prior to initiating rehabilitation.

Anxiety and negative physiological states

Anxiety is a common symptom among patients with cardiac (Moser & Dracup 1996) and pulmonary conditions (Karajgi et al 1990, Yellowlees et al 1987), and is often associated with concerns about underlying disease states (e.g., heart attack, inability to breathe). Physiological states of increased heart rate and breathlessness can trigger feelings of anxiety, which, in turn, can exacerbate the physiological symptoms.

Patients with COPD experience severe dyspnea or shortness of breath. Dyspnea, the primary clinical manifestation in COPD, is the subjective sensation of labored or difficulty in breathing, and represents a complex interplay of physiological and psychological mechanisms. This sensation is often accompanied by fear and anxiety, and usually perceived as life-threatening. Dyspnea or breath-lessness is usually experienced during exertion. The subjective distress caused by dyspnea can lead to a fear of future attacks of breathlessness and subsequent avoidance of activities and situations that trigger breathlessness. Consequently, individuals with COPD, in efforts to minimize dyspnea, begin to limit or avoid activities that involve exertion. Losses in musculoskeletal and cardiorespiratory functioning that accompany physical decondition-ing from an increasingly sedentary lifestyle further compound the consequences of COPD (impaired maximum ventilation and gas exchange capabilities). This cycle eventually leads to further breath-lessness, leaving the patient even more debilitated and furthering the course of deterioration and loss of independent functioning. This series of events characterizes the anxiety–dyspnea cycle (see Figure 15.1) that leads to progressive debilitation among patients with COPD.

Given the associations between anxiety, dyspnea, and functional capacity among patients with COPD as posited by this model, we evaluated the efficacy of a dypsnea management program consisting of training in progressive muscle relaxation, breathing exercises, pacing, self-talk, and panic control in reducing anxiety and improving other psychological and functional outcomes (Sassi-Dambron et al 1995). Eighty-nine patients with COPD were randomly assigned to either 6 weeks of treatment or to a general health education program. Following the 6-week intervention, although there was a significant group difference at 6-month follow-up on a dyspnea index (Mahler & Wells 1988), there were no other differences observed on measures of anxiety, depression, or health-related quality of life. The results of this study suggest that management of dyspnea alone is not enough to produce significant changes in anxiety or other psychological and func-tional outcomes for patients with COPD. As a result of this experience, we believe that behavioral com-ponents such as exercise are integral to the design of any program (Sassi-Dambron et al 1995).

In a randomized controlled trial, Emery et al (1998) compared a combined program of exer-cise, stress management, and education (EXESM) to stress management and education only (ESM) and also to wait list control condition (WL). Their find-ings showed that only participants in the EXESM sustained improvements in anxiety and exercise performance. These results are consistent with the belief that while psychosocial interventions can be designed to target anxiety and dyspnea, exercise training plays an important role in reducing anxiety and enhancing exercise capacity.

Among cardiac patients, anxiety is especially salient as the warning signs of a heart attack closely resemble those symptoms which also occur in the context of severe anxiety (e.g., chest discomfort or pain, discomfort in areas of the upper body, short-ness of breath, cold sweat, and lightheadedness or feeling faint). Cardiac patients with a history of MI are conditioned to watch for any of these warning signs that may precede a heart attack in order that they may get timely help.

While hypervigilance to signs of a heart attack can be life-saving for cardiac patients when there is an underlying disease-related process responsible for the symptoms, this chronic state of hyperarousal may also be detrimental for the patient's emotional and physical health. The primary clinical implication for healthcare providers is that comprehensive diag-nostic tests using electrocardiography (ECG) should be performed to determine the presence of cardiac abnormalities. This information should then be clearly discussed with the patient in addition to guidelines describing the steps the patient should take to respond to these warning signs and differenti-ate between anxiety symptoms and a life-threatening emergency.

Another second implication is that both cardiac and pulmonary patients will benefit greatly from techniques that allow them to reduce and alleviate symptoms of anxiety. Behavioral interventions are important in decreasing symptoms of anxiety and dyspnea. Strategies that include diaphragmatic breathing, imagery (see Chapter 10), and muscle

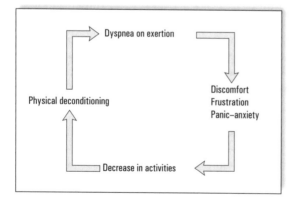

Figure 15.1 The anxiety–dyspnea cycle that leads to progressive debilitation among people with COPD

relaxation techniques (see Chapter 9) can displace the physical and psychological manifestations of anxiety (muscle tension, excessive worry or fear, shallow breathing) and can restore normal heart rate and respiratory patterns. Furthermore, instructing patients on how to distinguish symptoms of dyspnea, angina, and accompanying anxiety from clinically significant warning signs warranting immediate medical treatment is crucial in helping patients cope with fluctuations in their physical symptoms. Healthcare practitioners can work with patients in formulating a plan to respond to these symptoms (e.g., initiate relaxation and breathing techniques and if pain or discomfort persists, contact a medical professional).

Self-efficacy

One model that has been widely used and investigated in the study of exercise participation is Bandura's (1986) social cognitive theory which posits that individuals regulate their own behavior by setting goals, monitoring their own progress toward these goals, and actively intervening to make their social and physical environments supportive of these goals. Self-efficacy is hypothesized to be an important determinant of behavior, including actual attempts and persistence of behavior before giving up. The four influences on self-efficacy are personal experience of mastery or failure, vicarious experience, verbal persuasion, and physiological state. Among these four influences, personal experience of mastery is considered the most important. Interventions based on social cognitive theory have emphasized the use of feedback, goal-setting, and monitoring techniques that allow the individual to define the target behavior(s) and quantify his/her performance and mastery of specific tasks, which in turn increases his/her sense of self-efficacy. It is widely recognized that behavior and self-efficacy reciprocally influence one another such that increases in self-efficacy also lead to increased likelihood of performance of the target behavior.

In the context of pulmonary rehabilitation of COPD, self-efficacy for exercise performance has been traditionally operationalized as one's perceived ability to perform walking given increasing levels of duration (e.g., walk one block in approximately 5 minutes, walk two blocks in approximately 10 minutes . . . walk 3 miles in 90 minutes) and/or intensity (e.g., maximum treadmill speed and grade for which patient had confidence he/she

can walk for 5 minutes). Increases in self-efficacy have been observed with exercise training (Celli 1995, Gormley et al 1993, Kaplan et al 1984a, Scherer & Schmieder 1997, Scherer et al 1998, Toshima et al 1990). As well, self-efficacy expectation for exercise performance was found to be an important predictor of 5-year survival (Kaplan et al 1994) and was related to increases in maximum exercise performance (Gormley et al 1993) and exercise endurance (Toshima et al 1992b).

Many authors have cited the relationship between dyspnea and behavioral avoidance of exertion in patients with COPD. Toshima et al (1992b) suggested that individuals with COPD, as a result of years of debilitation and increased breathlessness upon exertion, learn to focus on negative physiological reactions to exertion, and rely on these signals to terminate, continue, or avoid participation in a given activity. However, with successful mastery of breathlessness during activities involving exertion (e.g., supervised exercise sessions during rehabilitation), patients receive feedback about their performance and learn to shift their focus onto the positive aspects of their physical capabilities (e.g., increased endurance and stamina) and away from distressing physiological states (e.g., dyspnea or muscle fatigue). These experiences consequently increase one's expectations of self-efficacy for performing physical activity despite sensations of dyspnea.

There is also evidence that self-efficacy plays a role in cardiac risk profile modification and functional outcomes among cardiac patients. In a population-based study of individuals diagnosed with newly documented heart disease (the Groningen Longitudinal Aging Study), higher premorbid levels of self-efficacy were associated with less functional decline 8 weeks after diagnosis of congestive heart failure after controlling for age, gender, and disease severity (Kempen et al 2000).

Carlson et al (2000, 2001) compared a modified cardiac rehabilitation protocol (MP) to a traditional clinic-based cardiac rehabilitation protocol in enhancing self-efficacy, actual performance of independent exercise, and physiological outcomes at 6-month follow-up. Based on principles from Bandura's self-efficacy theory the modified protocol was designed to promote independent exercise behavior through ongoing weekly education/support groups focusing on overcoming barriers to behavioral change with accompanying reductions in facility-based exercise sessions. Their findings indicated that while physiological outcomes were not different between conditions, patients in the MP condition had significantly higher levels of self-efficacy for independent exercise over 3 months and higher rates of independent exercise over 6 months (Carlson et al 2000). Furthermore, self-efficacy was the only significant predictor of independent exercise at 3 and 6 months (Carlson et al 2001). These findings provide additional support for the relationship between performance of health behaviors and self-efficacy. It is apparent that future behavioral interventions that promote improvements in self-efficacy can facilitate long-term maintenance of behavior change.

Patient non-adherence

Most medical encounters result in a physician or other healthcare professional advising a patient to follow a specific regimen. For example, patients are instructed to take medication on a specific schedule, to exercise, or to engage in a type of self-care routine. Non-adherence occurs when this advice is not followed by the patient. It is widely believed that many patients fail to attain the optimal benefits from therapy as a result of non-adherence. Most authors agree that patient non-adherence is a common problem with non-adherence rates ranging between 15% and 93% depending on patient population and definition of non-adherence (Becker 1985, Becker & Maiman 1980). Studies that have examined non-adherence by disease state have consistently shown that chronically ill individuals comply less than those with acute illnesses (Sackett 1979, Sackett & Snow 1979). A recent meta-analysis of 63 studies examining the relationship between adherence and medical outcomes found that 26% more patients experience a favorable treatment outcome if they adhere versus do not adhere (DiMatteo et al 2002). DiMatteo et al (2002) also found that the association between adherence and outcome is higher in studies of chronic conditions than acute, and those involving behavioral rather than medication-based regimens. As cardiorespiratory disorders are both chronic and employ several behavioral practices as part of the treatment regimen, adherence to treatment is particularly salient to outcomes of treatment.

Non-adherence is a common problem in behaviorally based treatment programs for chronic disease. A recent meta-analysis by Cooper et al (2002) found that cardiac patients who failed to attend cardiac rehabilitation were more likely to be older, to have lower income/greater financial hardship, to deny the severity of their illness, are less likely to believe they can influence its outcome, or to perceive that their physician recommends cardiac rehabilitation. In a study of 91 patients with obstructive lung disease, Young et al (1999b) reported that patients who refused or failed to complete a pulmonary rehabilitation program were more likely to be widowed/divorced/unmarried, to live alone, to reside in rented accommodations, to be currently smokers, to be dissatisfied with disease-specific social support, and to be less compliant with inhaled corticosteroid therapy. It is clear that non-adherence is related to a host of physical, psychological, and socio-economic factors.

In considering the problem of non-adherence, it is important to recognize that many factors influence adherence behavior. Some regimens are easy to follow, such as taking only one pill per day. Other treatments may be more complex if, for instance, they involve side effects or frequent dosing schedules (for medications) or lifestyle changes that can be time-consuming (e.g., exercise) or painful (e.g., regular monitoring blood glucose levels). Although most physicians believe that their patients satisfactorily comply with prescribed treatments, the evidence does not support these beliefs. Physicians typically overestimate the extent to which their patients comply and overstate the extent to which the patient behaviors correspond with their orders (Norell 1981).

Lifestyle behavioral changes underlie the treatment of chronic conditions such as cardiac and pulmonary diseases. As previously described, rehabilitative care involves patient education geared towards making key lifestyle changes including cessation of smoking, modification of dietary intake, adoption of regular exercise, proper use of medications and/or oxygen, and use of techniques to manage dyspnea and/or stress. Adoption and maintenance of these behaviors within and beyond rehabilitation are expected to limit patient disability from underlying disease processes and attenuate declines in functioning.

With respect to cardiovascular diseases, patient adherence to these behavioral measures has even been shown to reverse disease as indicated by important biomarkers of coronary artery disease (CAD) as well as improve measures of self-reported physical and psychological symptoms. In the Lifestyle Heart Trial (Ornish et al 1990), 48 patients with CAD were randomized to either a 1-year lifestyle change program (targeting areas of diet, inactivity, smoking, and stress) or routine medical care. The lifestyle change program resulted in substantial increases in exercise participation and use of stress management techniques, a significant reduction in angina and coronary stenoses, decreases in anger and hostility, and increases in feelings of well-being. Meanwhile, patients in the control condition experienced almost a two-fold increase in frequency of angina and almost a 50% increase in level of coronary stenoses. Findings from this trial are particularly important in that it demonstrated that for some patients with CAD, regression of coronary atherosclerosis can be achieved by a comprehensive lifestyle management program without the use of lipid-lowering medications.

Despite well-established support for lifestyle modification in improving health and psychological outcomes, lifelong behavioral patterns are difficult to change. Education is not sufficient in initiating and maintaining lifestyle behavior changes. The presence of salient negative health consequences may initially motivate changes in behavior, but maintenance is not guaranteed. Individuals must continue and maintain participation in the behavior to obtain the concurrent benefits in physical and psychological health. Healthcare practitioners can apply the following behavioral strategies to enable patients to modify their risk factors through adoption and maintenance of changes in lifestyle health habits.

Facilitating behavior change   Patients with cardiorespiratory disorders develop their symptoms as a result of lifelong patterns of poor health practices. Smoking, poor nutrition, and physical inactivity have been shown to hasten the development of heart disease. It is also well-recognized that individuals who smoke greatly increase their risk for developing and dying from COPD (Doll 1999, Doll et al 1994, Lam et al 1997). Given the importance of behavioral patterns in the development of cardiorespiratory disorders, measures to curb or reverse disease progression must involve modifications of these unhealthy lifestyle habits.

Rehabilitation succeeds in improving patient well-being and physical functioning through behavioral change. For an older adult with cardiac or pulmonary disease, adopting and maintaining changes in numerous domains of health behavior such as nutrition, tobacco use, and exercise, in addition to taking medications, can be difficult if not overwhelming. Some patients may succeed in

adopting one or more behavioral changes during rehabilitative care, but may find it difficult to sustain these changes without the structured environment of a clinic and ongoing support from peers and staff. Patients with cardiorespiratory disease may also face a host of physical, psychosocial, and practical obstacles that interfere with efforts to change health behaviors. These obstacles may include perceived lack of social support, lack of adequate information to perform behavior change, poor self-efficacy for performing target behaviors, low valuation of benefits of making changes, limited financial resources, and perceived lack of fitness or poor health status (Woodard & Berry 2001).

There is evidence suggesting that the patient–provider relationship can impact on patient compliance and outcomes of treatment (Hall et al 1988, Sherbourne et al 1992, Stewart 1995). Fostering a professional relationship that invites open communication from patients and their families can allow providers to identify obstacles to treatment and problem-solve with patients and family members when encountering barriers to adherence. Patients and family members should also be encouraged to ask questions regarding concerns about treatment and possible side effects as these can potentially impact on adherence. In developing an individualized program of self-care, healthcare professionals must perform comprehensive testing measures to quantify the patient's physical strengths and limitations. Similarly, providers must also assess patients' notions and expectations about the benefits of complying with recommendations and ensure that these expectations about the treatment are reasonable. With the goal of collaboration with patients and their family members, healthcare professionals can enlist several behavioral strategies to improve patient adherence to a lifestyle behavioral management program.

Providing rationale for behavior change   Healthcare providers must assist the patient to understand why he/she is being instructed to engage in new behaviors. The health belief model (Rosenstock 1974) postulates that an individual's health behavior is primarily influenced by two cognitive factors:

1. the degree to which the individual perceives a personal health threat
2. the perception that a particular health practice will be effective in reducing that health threat.

A patient will be less likely to follow through with the recommended measures if he/she does not perceive a threat and/or does not believe that engaging in the health behavior(s) will be beneficial.

Using information and terminology understandable to the patient, a rationale for a new behavior can be presented by:

- defining a direct association between the patient's current health practices and health risk
- identifying expected benefits for the patient as a result of participating in new health practices.

For example, a patient who is a current smoker receives laboratory findings regarding elevated blood lipids, hypertension, and moderate obstruction in expiratory airflow. In communicating laboratory results to the patient, providers can relate the presence of a health threat by discussing patient results in comparison to healthy/normal values expected for the patient's age and gender. Providers can address specific poor health practices (e.g., smoking) in this context by highlighting the role of the unwanted health behavior (i.e., smoking) in increasing the risk for development and progression of his/her cardiorespiratory disease (i.e., smoking induces the heart to work harder, hastens the decline of lung function, promotes constriction of blood vessels that leads to hypertension, increases rate of blockage of arteries, and negatively impacts blood cholesterol levels). In addition, providers can emphasize how adoption of the new health practice (i.e., cessation of smoking) can lower the risk for or reverse disease progression as monitored by physiological measures) and lead to less breathlessness and angina.

Enhancing personal motivation for behavior change

The transtheoretical model (TTM) postulated by Prochaska & DiClemente (1983) provides a conceptual framework with which to understand how individuals change behavior. This model describes the process of behavior change as a series of steps, moving through precontemplation (no intention to change), contemplation (seriously thinking about change), preparation (intention to change in the near future), action (modifying behavior) and maintenance (continuing a healthy lifestyle practice). Incorporating a theory based on decision-making (Janis & Mann 1977), TTM predicts that individuals who perceive more positive aspects of change as compared to negative aspects of change will be more likely to transition through stages of change, moving closer to action and maintenance. Similarly, the TTM posits that individuals who are at the precontemplation and contemplation stages have more

negatives than positives while those at later stages have more positives than negatives. The goal is then to facilitate identification of valuable benefit by the patient while also acknowledging the presence of negative aspects of change.

Patients with COPD frequently limit or abandon activities they value as a result of shortness of breath and accompanying decreased tolerance for physical exertion. These activities can include work, household chores, sexual activities, interacting with others, participating in sports, and performing errands. Exercise has been identified in a large number of scientific investigations (Benzo et al 2000, Emery et al 1991, Ries et al 1995, Young et al 1999a) as important in improving health-related quality of life, exercise tolerance, and breathlessness, which can consequently help patients resume valuable and pleasurable activities. While exercise can bring about acute shortness of breath, a primary obstacle in performing regular exercise, practitioners can work with patients to meet goals focused on previously abandoned activities. Patients who recognize personally significant reasons for exercising despite initial discomfort (e.g., being able to play with grandchildren, travel, return to golf) will be more likely to change their behaviors and maintain these changes.

Ambivalence is a feeling frequently encountered by individuals in the precontemplation and contemplation stages of change. While the positive aspects of change can be easily identifiable (e.g., reduced likelihood of an invasive, high-risk surgical procedure in the immediate future), the individual may feel reluctant about changing due to the amount of effort such change will require of them (e.g., exercising five times a week, eating more fresh fruits and vegetables, giving up sweets and high-fat foods).

Motivational interviewing as developed by Miller & Rollnick (1991) is a directive, client centered counseling approach to assist the client in exploring and resolving ambivalence about behavior change. The primary assumption of this approach is that the patient is inherently responsible for changing his/her behavior. Using techniques of reflection of patient's statements and feedback, the goal is to create a dissonance between the patient's current behavior and important personal goals. Enabling the patient to state personal concerns about his/her behavior and how it impacts on his/her health status is crucial in getting the patient to assume responsibility for the presence of a problem and their ability to resolve it. In addition to expressing empathy and highlighting the dissonance between the patient's goals and current behaviors, the provider should guard against argumentation. When met with resistance, the provider can help the patient discuss his/her concerns underlying the resistance and simply acknowledge the patient's personal responsibility and freedom of choice (Miller 1995). Providing the patient with a menu of options also supports the patient's sense of personal freedom of choice in that he/she has made the decision about the course of action to take.

Defining the target behavior   Before patients can perform a new health behavior, they must clearly understand what is expected of them. Communicating the treatment recommendations in as clear and simple a manner as possible can assist patients' understanding of what they need to do. After receiving recommendations verbally from the clinician, patients should be asked to repeat back the specific steps they should be doing to comply with treatment to confirm their understanding of the recommendations. Additionally, verbal instructions should be supplemented with written information detailing a plan of action, with specific instructions on what the patient should do. This prevents patients forgetting instructions and also avoids the miscommunication that can occur when patients are given general instructions they do not know how to follow. Like a prescription, the target behavior or plan of action should be written out clearly for the patient to take home so that he/she can use it as a prompt to engage in the necessary behaviors and refer to it when he/she needs clarification. A written plan is also useful for family members as well as other providers involved in patient care in facilitating collaboration towards common goals and minimizing confusion about what is being recommended as part of the patient's treatment.

Setting concrete and attainable goals   Goal setting can greatly facilitate lifestyle behavior change. In defining the targeted behavior, it is helpful to employ concrete terms in describing patient goals for performing the behavior. For instance, stating a general goal of "exercising more" is often not sufficient. Patients may not know what to do and how much they should be doing. A more specific manner of restating this goal would be to "walk for 15 minutes twice a day for at least 5 days of the week." Framing the goal in specific, concrete terms will easily inform the patient and the provider that the goal was attained.

In addition to being specific, goals should also be tailored to the patient as much as possible. Typically, when cardiorespiratory patients begin rehabilitation, they may often feel overwhelmed with new information or feel initially compelled or enthusiastic to make drastic lifestyle changes immediately. Providers may also have high expectations for their patients in instituting these lifestyle changes simultaneously within a short period of time. However, if expectations are initially set too high, patients may be unable to begin or sustain new behaviors. Being overwhelmed by a goal that seems impossible may make it difficult for some people to take any steps toward that goal. Patients can also easily become discouraged and frustrated about their abilities to make changes. In looking at failed attempts at making behavioral changes, patient self-efficacy becomes compromised. With poor sense of self-efficacy, patients will be less likely to undertake future efforts at changing their lifestyles (Bandura 1986). Providers may also become frustrated with the patient, attributing the patient's non-adherence to patient resistance or lack of motivation or will power.

Healthcare practitioners should interview patients and determine a realistic place to start given various factors that might affect performance of new behavior. When initiating a new and complex behavior (e.g., an exercise program) it can be helpful to break the behavior into small, realistic, and attainable goals. If a patient cannot sustain prolonged activity beyond 30 minutes, the provider can recommend that the patient starts with doing two bouts of continued activity such as walking for at least 5 minutes each time. Patients can then be encouraged to increase duration as they become more comfortable. Others may find it difficult to perform an activity on a daily basis. Setting small, attainable goals allows the person to gain confidence (increase self-efficacy) and have a number of experiences with success, thus making it more likely that he/she will continue to work toward the larger goal.

Promoting self-monitoring behaviors   Patients in rehabilitative care find it easier to practice new behaviors under the close supervision of clinical staff and with support from peers. However, many find it difficult to maintain behavioral changes after completion of rehabilitation when they must assume greater responsibility for performing these new behaviors. Self-regulation becomes a key issue and can determine whether the patient will be able to integrate these new behaviors into their daily lifestyle. Self-monitoring of new behaviors promotes self-regulation and can enhance long-term maintenance of behavioral changes.

Self-monitoring serves two regulatory functions:

1. confirms attainment of specific goals and
2. instills accountability for performing behaviors.

In conjunction with goal setting, patients can monitor their specific habits and compare their actual behaviors to the targeted behavior. They can then determine if they have consistently succeeded in meeting their goals, thereby enhancing self-efficacy, or whether they need to modify their goals to become more attainable (e.g., break up long bouts of exercise into shorter bouts). Self-monitoring of behavior also promotes feelings of accountability to oneself, thereby increasing the likelihood of performing the desired behavior and discouraging relapse into old behavioral patterns. There is evidence supporting that when used on an ongoing basis self-monitoring can enhance compliance and facilitate weight-loss outcomes (O'Neil 2001).

Evaluating obstacles   Non-adherence to treatment recommendations is often easily linked to obstacles in performing the targeted behaviors. In formulating an action plan for behavioral change, providers should inquire if patients can foresee obstacles that will interfere with adherence. Patients may not be able to maintain a dosing schedule for a medication if one dose must be taken in the middle of the night when they are asleep. A patient with limited financial resources may not be able to join a gym. Another patient with arthritis of the knee may not be able to walk for long periods of time. Some patients referred to rehabilitation may be just transitioning from acute care units. Others may feel apprehensive as they have never had any premorbid experience with the new targeted behavior. Non-adherence under these conditions provides the provider with an opportunity to problem solve with patients and circumvent these obstacles.

Plans for behavior change should take into account current personal, physical, and environmental promoters and limitations specific to each patient to ensure attainment of goals. Types of recommended activities should be ones that the patient can enjoy or has had previous experience with. However, patients should be cautioned to not overdo it nor expect that they can perform the same activity with similar vigor, ease, or endurance relative to premorbid functioning. Pragmatic factors can also pose challenges in making lifestyle changes. Does the patient have the financial (e.g., join a gym, own a treadmill) or proximal resources (e.g., nearby park) to perform the behavior? Providing patients with several options to meet goals can ensure success such that if one activity is not possible (e.g., cannot walk in inclement weather), there is an alternative behavior that can be performed to meet the targeted goal for exercise (e.g., walk around an indoor mall). Designing an individually tailored program by selecting activities and options that are realistic given the patient's circumstances and abilities can greatly optimize patient adoption of and long-term adherence to new behavioral patterns.

Formulating a plan to handle lapses to old behaviors
Occasional lapses are normal and expected when changing one's lifestyle. Patients may forego doing any physical activity on some days for reasons such as fatigue, more significant shortness of breath, or travel. Other patients may deviate from daily dietary plans during the holidays or when entertaining guests. Relapse is defined as "a breakdown or failure in a person's attempt to change a particular habit pattern" (Marlatt & George 1998). Frequent lapses may signal a relapse when the patient has returned to old behaviors and has ceased to take any steps in adhering to behavioral recommendations for treatment.

Relapse prevention is based on Bandura's (1986) social learning theory and combines behavioral and cognitive techniques to help prevent or intervene in the relapse process after one has begun implementing the new behavior(s) (Marlatt & George 1998). Lapse and relapse are anticipated in the process of change. These instances are frequently followed by reductions in perception of self-efficacy and feelings of self-blame and guilt for transgressing an absolute rule (e.g., exercising everyday). The patient's reaction to this transgression is called an "abstinence violation effect." The individual consequently feels helpless and often passively succumbs to the violation which is perceived as irreparable (Marlatt & George 1998). The goal of relapse prevention is to increase one's awareness of environmental, cognitive, and affective antecedents that comprise a high-risk situation (conducive to lapse) in order to learn and practice coping skills necessary to prevent or limit the duration of future relapses.

It is important to discuss these lapses or relapses with patients to:

1. determine the event or obstacle that initiated the lapse(s)

2. assist the person in coming up with solutions to address the obstacle if it is a recurring one (e.g., modify time of walking if it often conflicts with work schedule)
3. help the person deal with the negative emotions and thoughts that arise with slips (e.g., disappointment, uncertainty about one's abilities).

Lapses can undermine future efforts at making behavioral changes when the patients begin to question their abilities to ultimately succeed. Others may give up efforts completely. It is helpful for providers to remind the patient that lapses can and do occur and that the most important behavior they can do is simply to resume their plan of action following the lapse. Providers and patients can work together to address frequent lapses or prevent full relapse by revisiting the action plan and specific goals. Together they can determine if breaking down goals further into smaller steps will assist patients in gaining mastery over their behaviors and work towards the overall goal of changing health habits.

Patients can easily slip back into formerly sedentary behaviors following hospitalization or treatment for a reinfarction or pulmonary exacerbation. Rehabilitative care following recovery may be necessary to help transition patients back into independent functioning. Providers can work with patients in coming up with a safe plan to resume physical activity and help increase their sense of self-efficacy for performing physical tasks. These efforts can prove to be valuable in preventing future deconditioning for patients.

Engaging social support systems   Social support has positive and functional purposes when it reinforces behaviors that are compatible with optimal health outcomes. Significant others in the support environment can encourage adherence to the medical regimen and the adoption of appropriate health behaviors. For example, family members can model health behaviors for the patient. If at least one person in the patient's immediate support system is making the same lifestyle changes concurrently, outcomes may be enhanced through mutual encouragement, mutual modeling, and a reduction in the perceived difficulty of making lifestyle changes (Burke et al 2002).

Social support can also have negative functional effects on health outcomes when members of the support system reinforce behaviors that are incompatible with desired health outcomes. Family members who do not understand the rationale or know the specific details of behavioral recommendations may inadvertently interfere with the patient's ability to carry out these recommendations. For example, patients with COPD need to comply with regimens that are often difficult, painful, or burdensome. A caring and empathetic support-giver may reinforce comfortable but nonadherent behaviors. A spouse may feel that exercise is "harmful" to the patient, thereby discouraging the activity. This is most likely to occur when the support-giver believes that any suffering should be avoided. For these reasons, it is important that providers communicate well with family members who participate in the patient's care.

For patients with poorer health, caregivers can be particularly instrumental in facilitating behavior change as they are usually charged with preparing meals, scheduling and coordinating medical appointments, and overseeing the patient's daily schedule and activities. Ensuring that caregivers are fully aware of appropriate prescriptions for exercise will ease their concerns that physical activity might "harm" the patient. In addition, providers can also educate caregivers on healthier food selection and preparation that will allow the patient to meet the dietary requirements of their treatment. In these situations, caregivers play a pivotal role in modifying the patient's environment to promote lifestyle changes.

INTEGRATED MANAGEMENT APPROACHES

Integrated management approaches to chronic disease are characterized by practices designed to address the patient's presenting physical condition while recognizing the importance of psychological sequelae of disease and treatment. Given the impact of diagnosis and treatment of cardiorespiratory disease on social, emotional, and occupational functioning, emotional reactions that include anger, sadness, helplessness, guilt, and anxiety are common. However, despite the presence of these reactions, both patients and providers may not readily perceive the patient–provider relationship as a forum for discussion of concerns about loss of health and independence. Patients may see the provider in an authoritative role who merely provides information and whose recommendations they must follow. Likewise, providers' perceptions of patients may be limited to the physical and clinical manifestations of disease.

Providers can be more integrative in their approach to patient care by asking questions, eliciting patient feedback and concerns about their condition and treatment, and validating emotional reactions experienced by the patient. Questions about how symptoms and treatment are impacting on the patient's ability to work, maintain social roles, and perform activities of daily living can help the provider obtain a sense of the patient's HRQOL and overall functioning. Open-ended and follow-up questions are particularly helpful in getting the patient to elaborate on concerns and difficulties in adjustment. Reflective statements commenting on, or questions regarding how the patient might be feeling (e.g., during review of laboratory results or discussion of treatment procedures), can help the provider explore how well the patient is adjusting emotionally to his/her condition and engage the patient in discussing his/her difficulties. Based on the information gathered, providers can determine if the patient might benefit from psychoeducational or support groups where they can further interact with others with the same physical condition.

SUMMARY

Cardiorespiratory disorders are prevalent, chronic, and often debilitating conditions that impact on physical, social, emotional, and occupational domains of patient functioning. Declines in physical health lead to inevitable changes in lifestyle and decreased levels of independence, with subsequent negative emotional responses that limit one's ability to effectively cope with the symptoms of disease and comply with treatment recommendations.

Multifactorial rehabilitation programs comprised of various disciplines and targeting various areas of physical, behavioral, and psychosocial functioning can greatly enhance patient adjustment to cardiorespiratory disorders. These programs typically include individual assessment, supervised exercise training, psychosocial support, and patient education focusing on lifestyle modification, proper use of medication and equipment related to treatment, stress management and relaxation, and adjustments to activities of daily living. With the ultimate goal of restoring the patient's optimum level of independent functioning despite limitations placed by symptoms and disease, multifactorial rehabilitation has been empirically validated as a standard therapeutic modality for both cardiac and respiratory patients.

Behavioral change is central to the secondary prevention of cardiorespiratory disorders. Lifestyle behavioral modification in areas of nutrition, tobacco use, and physical activity is well recognized in modifying risk factors for disease progression and maintaining optimal health. However, non-adherence is a widespread obstacle in the effective treatment of cardiac and pulmonary disease. Long-term maintenance of behavior change is either poor or not adequately quantified in the context of chronic diseases such as diabetes, heart disease, or COPD. Behavioral strategies incorporating goal-setting, relapse prevention, self-efficacy theory, self-monitoring, and open communication between patient and provider can enhance adoption and long-term maintenance of lifestyle modification.

References

American Association of Cardiovascular and Pulmonary Rehabilitation 1998a Guidelines for pulmonary rehabilitation programs, 2nd edn. Human Kinetics Champaign, IL

American College of Chest Physicians/American Association of Cardiovascular and Pulmonary Rehabilitation 1997 Pulmonary rehabilitation: Joint ACCP/AACVPR evidence-based guidelines. ACCP/AACVPR Pulmonary Rehabilitation Guidelines Panel. Chest 112(5): 1363–1396

American Thoracic Society 1987 Standards for the diagnosis and care of patients with chronic obstructive pulmonary disease (COPD) and asthma. American Review of Respiratory Diseases 136(1): 225–244

Anthonisen N R, Connett J E, Kiley J P et al 1994 Effects of smoking intervention and the use of an inhaled anticholinergic bronchodilator on the rate of decline of FEV1. The Lung Health Study. Journal of the American Medical Association 272(19): 1497–1505

Bach J R 1996 Pulmonary rehabilitation: The obstructive and paralytic condition. Hanley & Delfus, Philadelphia

Bandura A 1986 Social foundations of thought and action. A social cognitive theory. Prentice-Hall, NJ

Bar F, Hoppener P, Diederiks J et al 1992 Cardiac rehabilitation contributes to the restoration of leisure activities and social activities after myocardial infarction. Journal of Cardiopulmonary Rehabilitation 12(2): 117–125

Becker M H 1985 Patient adherence to prescribed therapies. Medical Care 23(5): 539–555

Becker M H, Maiman L A 1980 Strategies for enhancing patient compliance. Journal of Community Health 6(2): 113–135

Benzo R, Flume P A, Turner D et al 2000 Effect of pulmonary rehabilitation on quality of life in patients with COPD: The use of SF–36 summary scores as outcomes measures. Journal of Cardiopulmonary Rehabilitation 20(4): 231–234

Bergner M, Bobbitt R A, Carter W B et al 1981 The Sickness Impact Profile: Development and final revision of a health status measure. Medical Care 19(8): 787–805

Berry M J, Adair N E, Sevensky K S et al 1996 Inspiratory muscle training and whole-body reconditioning in chronic obstructive pulmonary disease. American Journal of Respiratory and Critical Care Medicine 153(6 Pt 1): 1812–1816

Blake R L Jr, Vandiver T A, Braun S et al 1990 A randomized controlled evaluation of a psychosocial intervention in adults with chronic lung disease. Family Medicine 22(5): 365–370

Buist A S 1997 The US Lung Health Study. Respirology 2(4): 303–307

Burke V, Mori T A, Giangiulio N et al 2002 An innovative program for changing health behaviours. Asia Pacific Journal of Clinical Nutrition 11 (Suppl 3): S586–S597

Camacho T C, Roberts R E, Lazarus N B et al 1991 Physical activity and depression: Evidence from the Alameda County Study. American Journal of Epidemiology 134(2): 220–231

Cardiac Rehabilitation Guideline Panel 1995 Cardiac rehabilitation. Washington, Agency for Health Care Policy Research and the National Heart, Lung, and Blood Institute, Public Health Service, USDHHS. Clinical practice guideline no 17

Carlson J J, Johnson J A, Franklin B A et al 2000 Program participation, exercise adherence, cardiovascular outcomes, and program cost of traditional versus modified cardiac rehabilitation. American Journal of Cardiology 86(1): 17–23

Carlson J J, Norman G J, Feltz D L et al 2001 Self-efficacy, psychosocial factors, and exercise behavior in traditional versus modified cardiac rehabilitation. Journal of Cardiopulmonary Rehabilitation 21(6): 363–373

Carney R M, Rich M W, Tevelde A et al 1987 Major depressive disorder in coronary artery disease. American Journal of Cardiology 60(16): 1273–1275

Celli B R 1995 Pulmonary rehabilitation in patients with COPD. American Journal of Respiratory and Critical Care Medicine 152(3): 861–864

Coats A J, Adamopoulos S, Radaelli A et al 1992 Controlled trial of physical training in chronic heart failure. Exercise performance, hemodynamics, ventilation, and autonomic function. Circulation 85(6): 2119–2131

Cooper A F, Jackson G, Weinman J et al 2002 Factors associated with cardiac rehabilitation attendance: A systematic review of the literature. Clinical Rehabilitation 16(5): 541–552

Crystal R G 1987 Chronic obstructive pulmonary disease. Forty years of achievement in heart, lung, and blood research: A collection of essays in selected paper of biomedical research accomplishment. National Institutes of Health, National Heart Lung, Blood Institute, Bethesda, MD

Curfman G D 1993 The health benefits of exercise. A critical reappraisal. New England Journal of Medicine 328(8): 574–576

Dahlen I, Janson C 2002 Anxiety and depression are related to the outcome of emergency treatment in patients with obstructive pulmonary disease. Chest 122(5): 1633–1637

Deanfield J, Wright C, Krikler S et al 1984 Cigarette smoking and the treatment of angina with propranolol, atenolol, and nifedipine. New England Journal of Medicine 310(15): 951–954

Dekhuijzen P N, Beek M M, Folgering H T et al 1990 Psychological changes during pulmonary rehabilitation and target-flow inspiratory muscle training in COPD patients with a ventilatory limitation during exercise. International Journal of Rehabilitation Research 13(2): 109–117

Dhalla N S, Temsah R M, Netticadan T 2000 Role of oxidative stress in cardiovascular diseases. Journal of Hypertension 18(6): 655–673

DiMatteo M R, Lepper H S, Croghan T W 2000 Depression is a risk factor for noncompliance with medical treatment: Meta-analysis of the effects of anxiety and depression on patient adherence. Archives of Internal Medicine 160(14): 2101–2107

DiMatteo M R, Giordani P J, Lepper H S et al 2002 Patient adherence and medical treatment outcomes: A meta-analysis. Medical Care 40(9): 794–811

Doll R 1999 Risk from tobacco and potentials for health gain. International Journal of Tuberculosis and Lung Disease 3(2): 90–99

Doll R, Peto R, Wheatley K et al 1994 Mortality in relation to smoking: 40 years' observations on male British doctors. British Medical Journal 309(6959): 901–911

Eakin E G, Kaplan R M, Ries A L 1993 Measurement of dyspnoea in chronic obstructive pulmonary disease. Quality of Life Research 2(3): 181–191

Eakin E G, Resnikoff P M, Prewitt L M et al 1998 Validation of a new dyspnea measure: The UCSD Shortness of Breath Questionnaire. University of California, San Diego. Chest 113(3): 619–624

Emery C F, Leatherman N E, Burker E J et al 1991 Psychological outcomes of a pulmonary rehabilitation program. Chest 100(3): 613–617

Emery C F, Schein R L, Hauck E R et al 1998 Psychological and cognitive outcomes of a randomized trial of exercise among patients with chronic obstructive pulmonary disease. Health Psychology 17(3): 232–240

Faling L J 1993 Controlled breathing techniques and chest physical therapy in chronic obstructive pulmonary disease and allied conditions. In: Casaburi R, Petty T L (eds) Principles and practice of pulmonary rehabilitation. W B Saunders, Philadelphia, p 167–174

Fishman A P 1996 Pulmonary rehabilitation. Marcel Dekker, New York

Forrester A W, Lipsey J R, Teitelbaum M L et al 1992 Depression following myocardial infarction. International Journal of Psychiatry in Medicine 22(1): 33–46

Frasure-Smith N, Lesperance F, Talajic M 1993 Depression following myocardial infarction. Impact on 6-month survival. Journal of the American Medical Association 270(15): 1819–1825

Frasure-Smith N, Lesperance F, Talajic M 1995 Depression and 18-month prognosis after myocardial infarction. Circulation 91(4): 999–1005

Goldstein R S, Gort E H, Stubbing D et al 1994 Randomised controlled trial of respiratory rehabilitation. Lancet 344(8934): 1394–1397

Gormley J M, Carrieri-Kohlman V, Douglas M K et al 1993 Treadmill self-efficacy and walking performance in patients with COPD. Journal of Cardiopulmonary Rehabilitation 13: 424–431

Goss J R, Epstein A, Maynard C 2002 Effects of cardiac rehabilitation on self-reported health status after coronary artery bypass surgery. Journal of Cardiopulmonary Rehabilitation 22(6): 410–417

Gulanick M 1991 Is phase 2 cardiac rehabilitation necessary for early recovery of patients with cardiac disease? A randomized, controlled study. Heart and Lung 20(1): 9–15

Guyatt G H, Berman L B, Townsend M et al 1987 A measure of quality of life for clinical trials in chronic lung disease. Thorax 42(10): 773–778

Hall J A, Roter D L, Katz N R 1988 Meta-analysis of correlates of provider behavior in medical encounters. Medical Care 26(7): 657–675

Hodgkin J, Connors G L, Bell C W 1993 Pulmonary rehabilitation: Guidelines to success, 2nd edn. Lippincott, Philadelphia

Hu F B, Stampfer M J, Manson J E et al 1997 Dietary fat intake and the risk of coronary heart disease in women. New England Journal of Medicine 337(21): 1491–1499

Isoaho R, Keistinen T, Laippala P et al 1995 Chronic obstructive pulmonary disease and symptoms related to depression in elderly persons. Psychological Reports 76(1): 287–297

Janis I, Mann L 1977 Decision making: A psychological analysis of conflict, choice and commitment. Collier & Cassell Macmillan, London

Johnson F R, Banzhaf M R, Desvousges W H 2000 Willingness to pay for improved respiratory and cardiovascular health: A multiple-format, stated-preference approach. Health Economics 9(4): 295–317

Kanner R E 1996 Early intervention in chronic obstructive pulmonary disease. A review of the Lung Health Study results. Medical Clinics of North America 80(3): 523–547

Kaplan R M, Anderson J P 1996 The general health policy model: An integrated approach. In: Spilker B (ed) Quality of life and pharmacoeconomics in clinical trials, 2nd ed. Lippincott-Raven Publishers, Philadelphia, p 309–322

Kaplan R M, Atkins C J, Reinsch S 1984a Specific efficacy expectations mediate exercise compliance in patients with COPD. Health Psychology 3(3): 223–242

Kaplan R M, Atkins C J, Timms R 1984b Validity of a quality of well-being scale as an outcome measure in chronic obstructive pulmonary disease. Journal of Chronic Diseases 37(2): 85–95

Kaplan R M, Feeny D, Revicki D A 1993 Methods for assessing relative importance in preference based outcome measures. Quality of Life Research 2(6): 467–475

Kaplan R M, Ries A L, Prewitt L M et al 1994 Self-efficacy expectations predict survival for patients with chronic obstructive pulmonary disease. Health Psychology 13(4): 366–368

Karajgi B, Rifkin A, Doddi S et al 1990 The prevalence of anxiety disorders in patients with chronic obstructive pulmonary disease. American Journal of Psychiatry 147(2): 200–201

Kempen G I, Sanderman R, Miedema I et al 2000 Functional decline after congestive heart failure and acute myocardial infarction and the impact of psychological attributes. A prospective study. Quality of Life Research 9(4): 439–450

Kohlmeier L, Simonsen N, van 't Veer P et al 1997 Adipose tissue trans fatty acids and breast cancer in the European Community Multicenter Study on Antioxidants, Myocardial Infarction, and Breast Cancer. Cancer Epidemiology Biomarkers and Prevention 6(9): 705–710

Kushi L H, Lenart E B, Willett W C 1995 Health implications of Mediterranean diets in light of contemporary knowledge. 1. Plant foods and dairy products. American Journal of Clinical Nutrition 61(6 Suppl): 1407S–1415S

Lake F R, Henderson K, Briffa T et al 1990 Upper-limb and lower-limb exercise training in patients with chronic airflow obstruction. Chest 97(5): 1077–1082

Lam T H, He Y, Li L S et al 1997 Mortality attributable to cigarette smoking in China. Journal of the American Medical Association 278(18): 1505–1508

Light R W, Merrill E J, Despars J A et al 1985 Prevalence of depression and anxiety in patients with COPD. Relationship to functional capacity. Chest 87(1): 35–38

Low G, Gutman G 2003 Couples' ratings of chronic obstructive pulmonary disease patients' quality of life. Clinical Nursing and Research 12(1): 28–48

Luscher T F 1994 The endothelium and cardiovascular disease – a complex relation. New England Journal of Medicine 330(15): 1081–1083

Mahler D A, Wells C K 1988 Evaluation of clinical methods for rating dyspnea. Chest 93(3): 580–586

Mannino D M, Gagnon R C, Petty T L et al 2000 Obstructive lung disease and low lung function in adults in the United States: Data from the National Health and Nutrition Examination Survey, 1988–1994. Archives of Internal Medicine 160(11): 1683–1689

Mannino D M, Homa D M, Akinbami L J et al 2002 Chronic obstructive pulmonary disease surveillance – United States, 1971–2000. MMWR CDC Surveillance Summaries 51(6): 1–16

Marlatt G A, George W H 1998 Relapse prevention and the maintenance of optimal health. In: Shumaker S A, Schron E B (eds) The handbook of health behavior change, 2nd edn. Springer, New York, p 33–58

Massberg S, Gawaz M, Gruner S et al 2003 A crucial role of glycoprotein VI for platelet recruitment to the injured arterial wall in vivo. Journal of Experimental Medicine 197(1): 41–49

McSweeny A J, Grant I, Heaton R K et al 1982 Life quality of patients with chronic obstructive pulmonary disease. Archives of Internal Medicine 142(3): 473–478

Miller W R 1995 Increasing motivation for change. In: Hester R K, Miller W R (eds) Handbook of alcoholism treatment approaches, 2nd edn. Allyn & Bacon, Needham Heights, MA, p 89–104

Miller W R, Rollnick S 1991 Motivational interviewing: Preparing people to change addictive behavior. Guilford Press, New York

Minino A, Smith B 2001 Preliminary data for 2000. National Center for Health Statistics. National Vital Statistics Reports, Vol 49, no 12. NCHS, Hyattsville, MD

Moorer P, Suurmeije T, Foets M et al 2001 Psychometric properties of the RAND-36 among three chronic diseases (multiple sclerosis, rheumatic diseases and COPD) in The Netherlands. Quality of Life Research 10(7): 637–645

Moser D K, Dracup K 1996 Is anxiety early after myocardial infarction associated with subsequent ischemic and arrhythmic events? Psychosomatic Medicine 58(5): 395–401

Murray C, Lopez A 1996 The global burden of disease. World Health Organization, Geneva

National Center for Health Statistics 1999 National Vital Statistics Report 49(8)

National Heart Lung and Blood Institute 1998 Behavioral research: Report on the task force on behavioral research in cardiovascular, lung, and blood health and disease. US Department of Health and Human Services, National Institutes of Health, Rockville, MD

National Heart Lung and Blood Institute 2002 Morbidity & mortality: 2002 chartbook on cardiovascular, lung, and blood diseases. US Department of Health and Human Services, National Institutes of Health, Rockville, MD

Newton M, Mutrie N, McArthur J D 1991 The effects of exercise in a coronary rehabilitation programme. Scottish Medical Journal 36(2): 38–41

Norell S E 1981 Accuracy of patient interviews and estimates by clinical staff in determining medication compliance. Social Science and Medicine 15(1): 57–61

O'Connor G T, Buring J E, Yusuf S et al 1989 An overview of randomized trials of rehabilitation with exercise after myocardial infarction. Circulation 80(2): 234–244

O'Donnell D E 2001 Ventilatory limitations in chronic obstructive pulmonary disease. Medicine and Science in Sports and Exercise 33(7 Suppl): S647–S655

Ojanen M, Lahdensuo A, Laitinen J et al 1993 Psychosocial changes in patients participating in a chronic obstructive pulmonary disease rehabilitation program. Respiration 60(2): 96–102

Oldridge N B, Guyatt G H, Fischer M E et al 1988 Cardiac rehabilitation after myocardial infarction. Combined experience of randomized clinical trials. Journal of the American Medical Association 260(7): 945–950

Oldridge N, Guyatt G, Jones N et al 1991 Effects on quality of life with comprehensive rehabilitation after acute myocardial infarction. American Journal of Cardiology 67(13): 1084–1089

O'Neil P M 2001 Assessing dietary intake in the management of obesity. Obesity Research 9(Suppl 5): 361S–366S

Orenstein D M, Nixon P A, Ross E A et al 1989 The quality of well-being in cystic fibrosis. Chest 95(2): 344–347

Ornish D, Brown S E, Scherwitz L W et al 1990 Can lifestyle changes reverse coronary heart disease? The Lifestyle Heart Trial. Lancet 336(8708): 129–133

Os I, Hoieggen A, Larsen A et al 2003 Smoking and relation to other risk factors in postmenopausal women with coronary artery disease, with particular reference to whole blood viscosity and beta-cell function. Journal of Internal Medicine 253(2): 232–239

Ott C R, Sivarajan E S, Newton K M et al 1983 A controlled randomized study of early cardiac rehabilitation: The Sickness Impact Profile as an assessment tool. Heart and Lung 12(2): 162–170

Petty T L 2000 Scope of the COPD problem in North America: Early studies of prevalence and NHANES III data: Basis for early identification and intervention. Chest 117(5 Suppl 2): 326S–331S

Porth C 1998 Alterations in blood flow in the systemic circulation. In: Porth C M (ed) Pathophysiology: Concepts of altered health states, Lippincott, Philadelphia, p 335–362

Prochaska J O, Diclemente C C 1983 Stages and processes of self-change of smoking – toward an integrative model of change. Journal of Consulting and Clinical Psychology 51(3): 390–395

Reardon J, Awad E, Normandin E et al 1994 The effect of comprehensive outpatient pulmonary rehabilitation on dyspnea. Chest 105(4): 1046–1052

Renfroe K L 1988 Effect of progressive relaxation on dyspnea and state anxiety in patients with chronic obstructive pulmonary disease. Heart and Lung 17(4): 408–413

Ries A L 1996 Rehabilitation for the patient with advanced lung disease: Designing an appropriate program, establishing realistic goals, meeting the goals. Seminars in Respiratory and Critical Care Medicine 17(6): 451–463

Ries A L, Kaplan R M, Limberg T M et al 1995 Effects of pulmonary rehabilitation on physiologic and psychosocial outcomes in patients with chronic obstructive pulmonary disease. Annals of Internal Medicine 122(11): 823–832

Rochester D F, Goldberg S K 1980 Techniques of respiratory physical therapy. American Review of Respiratory Diseases 122(5 Pt 2): 133–146

Rosenstock I M 1974 The health belief model and preventive health behavior. Health Education Monographs 2: 354–386

Sackett D L 1979 A compliance practicum for the busy practitioner. In: Haynes R B, Taylor D W, Sakett D L (eds) Compliance in health care. Johns Hopkins Press, Baltimore, MD, p 286–294

Sackett D L, Snow J C 1979 The magnitude and measurement of compliance. In: Haynes R B, Taylor D W, Sackett D L (eds) Compliance in health care. Johns Hopkins Press, Baltimore, MD, p 11–22

Samra S S, Walwaikar P P, Morye V K et al 2002 Accelerated atherosclerosis. Journal of the Indian Medical Association 100(8): 516, 518–521

Sassi-Dambron D E, Eakin E G, Ries A L et al 1995 Treatment of dyspnea in COPD. A controlled clinical trial of dyspnea management strategies. Chest 107(3): 724–729

Scherer Y K, Schmieder L E 1997 The effect of a pulmonary rehabilitation program on self-efficacy, perception of dyspnea, and physical endurance. Heart and Lung 26(1): 15–22

Scherer Y K, Schmieder L E, Shimmel S 1998 The effects of education alone and in combination with pulmonary rehabilitation on self-efficacy in patients with COPD. Rehabilitation Nursing 23(2): 71–77

Sherbourne C D, Hays R D, Ordway L et al 1992 Antecedents of adherence to medical recommendations: Results from the Medical Outcomes Study. Journal of Behavioral Medicine 15(5): 447–468

Simpson K, Killian K, McCartney N et al 1992 Randomised controlled trial of weightlifting exercise in patients with chronic airflow limitation. Thorax 47(2): 70–75

Siscovick D S, Weiss N S, Fletcher R H et al 1984 The incidence of primary cardiac arrest during vigorous exercise. New England Journal of Medicine 311(14): 874–877

Stern M J, Gorman P A, Kaslow L 1983 The group counseling v exercise therapy study. A controlled intervention with subjects following myocardial infarction. Archives of Internal Medicine 143(9): 1719–1725

Stewart M A 1995 Effective physician–patient communication and health outcomes: A review. Canadian Medical Association Journal 152(9): 1423–1433

Stewart A L, Ware J E, Brook R H et al 1978 Conceptualization and measurement of health for adults: Vol II. Physical health in terms of functioning. Rand, Santa Monica, CA

Strijbos J H, Postma D S, van Altena R et al 1996 A comparison between an outpatient hospital-based pulmonary rehabilitation program and a home-care pulmonary rehabilitation program in patients with COPD. A follow-up of 18 months. Chest 109(2): 366–372

Taylor C B, Houston-Miller N, Ahn D K et al 1986 The effects of exercise training programs on psychosocial improvement in uncomplicated postmyocardial infarction patients. Journal of Psychosomatic Research 30(5): 581–587

Testa M A, Simonson D C 1996 Assesment of quality-of-life outcomes. New England Journal of Medicine 334(13): 835–840

Toshima M T, Kaplan R M, Ries A L 1990 Experimental evaluation of rehabilitation in chronic obstructive pulmonary disease: Short-term effects on exercise endurance and health status. Health Psychology 9(3): 237–252

Toshima M T, Blumberg E, Ries A L et al 1992a Does rehabilitation reduce depression in patients with chronic obstructive pulmonary disease? Journal of Cardiopulmonary Rehabilitation 12: 261–269

Toshima M T, Kaplan R M, Ries A L 1992b Self-efficacy expectations in chronic obstructive pulmonary disease rehabilitation. In: Schwarzer R (ed) Self-efficacy: Thought control of action. Hemisphere, New York, p 325–354

Tracy R P, Psaty B M, Macy E et al 1997 Lifetime smoking exposure affects the association of C-reactive protein with cardiovascular disease risk factors and subclinical disease in healthy elderly subjects. Arteriosclerosis, Thrombosis, and Vascular Biology 17(10): 2167–2176

Ware J E Jr 1995 The status of health assessment 1994. Annual Review of Public Health 16: 327–354

Weiner P, Azgad Y, Ganam R 1992 Inspiratory muscle training combined with general exercise reconditioning in patients with COPD. Chest 102(5): 1351–1356

Wijkstra P J, Van Altena R, Kraan J et al 1994 Quality of life in patients with chronic obstructive pulmonary disease improves after rehabilitation at home. European Respiratory Journal 7(2): 269–273

Wilhelmsen L 1988 Coronary heart disease: Epidemiology of smoking and intervention studies of smoking. American Heart Journal 115(1 Pt 2): 242–249

Woodard C M, Berry M J 2001 Enhancing adherence to prescribed exercise: Structured behavioral interventions in clinical exercise programs. Journal of Cardiopulmonary Rehabilitation 21(4): 201–209

Yellowlees P M, Alpers J H, Bowden J J et al 1987 Psychiatric morbidity in patients with chronic airflow obstruction. Medical Journal of Australia 146(6): 305–307

Yohannes A M, Baldwin R C, Connolly M J 2000 Depression and anxiety in elderly outpatients with chronic obstructive pulmonary disease: Prevalence, and validation of the BASDEC screening questionnaire. International Journal of Geriatric Psychiatry 15(12): 1090–1096

Young P, Dewse M, Fergusson W et al 1999a Improvements in outcomes for chronic obstructive pulmonary disease (COPD) attributable to a hospital-based respiratory rehabilitation programme. Australian and New Zealand Journal of Medicine 29(1): 59–65

Young P, Dewse M, Fergusson W et al 1999b Respiratory rehabilitation in chronic obstructive pulmonary disease: Predictors of nonadherence. European Respiratory Journal 13(4): 855–859

Chapter 16

Injury from sport, exercise, and physical activity

Gregory S. Kolt

INTRODUCTION

People of all ages are now being encouraged to participate in greater amounts of sport, exercise, and physical activity. Despite the many health benefits of this increased participation, exposure to these activities has potential for physical injury. Rehabilitation of people injured through sport, exercise, and physical activity is costly in terms of the loss of activity and work participation time, interventions to reduce injury vulnerability, the risk of significant long-term injury, and the associated reduced quality of life.

A growing literature has addressed sport-specific injury epidemiology across several countries (e.g., Finch et al 1998, Uitenbroek 1996, Weaver et al 1999). The varying methodologies used in such epidemiological research, however, make it difficult to compare injury incidence, prevalence, and costs across studies, let alone countries. An area of injury that those in the physical and manual therapies are only beginning to see is that associated with people participating in health-enhancing physical activity. Although encouraging people to walk 30 minutes per day on most, if not all, days of the week to satisfy the physical activity and health criteria of the US Surgeon General (United States Department of Health and Human Services 1996) appears quite simple, it often exposes people to levels of physical activity that they are unaccustomed to, and can result in musculoskeletal injury.

Injury associated with sport, exercise, and physical activity can have a psychological impact in addition to the obvious physical and performance effects. The predominant focus on musculoskeletal injury rehabilitation in the past has been on returning individuals to their pre-injury level of functioning by focusing on the physical problems. Several authors have more recently highlighted the need to manage athletes and physical activity participants more holistically, with a greater emphasis on the psychological consequences of injury and rehabilitation (Brewer 2001, Francis et al 2000, Kolt 2000, Ninedek & Kolt 2000).

This chapter will address the psychological antecedents to injury, the psychological responses to injury, and the psychological factors that can influence rehabilitation from sport, exercise, and physical activity injury. Also, several psychological approaches that can be incorporated into rehabilitation programs by physical and manual therapists will be outlined.

PSYCHOSOCIAL VARIABLES AND THE ONSET OF INJURY

The influence of psychosocial variables on injury vulnerability and resiliency has been the focus of a growing body of literature over the past 30 years. The variables that have been examined include anxiety, stress, locus of control, self-confidence, mood states, motivation, attention, coping mechanisms, and personality (Kirkby 1995, Williams & Andersen 1998).

The variables investigated early in this area included components of personality (e.g., Brown

1971, Govern & Koppenhaver 1965), and the stress resulting from major or significant life events (e.g., Bramwell et al 1975). Although this early work suggested that athletes' injuries were linked to factors such as life stress and fear of competition, the literature offered no explanations for such relationships.

STRESS–INJURY MODEL

Andersen & Williams (1988) developed a model of stress and injury that brought together many of the theoretical components suggested in the literature. Andersen & Williams (1988) posited that several psychological variables may influence the occurrence of injury through a link with stress and a resulting "stress response." Drawing on information from the large number of studies over the late 1980s and 1990s, the stress–injury model was revised (Williams & Andersen 1998). This model is shown in Figure 16.1.

The stress–injury model is based around the stress response and the three broad categories of variables hypothesized to influence this response: personality, history of stressors, and coping resources. The stress response (as seen in the central portion of the model) involves the interaction of the cognitive and physiological elements of stressful events. The impact of a stressful event or situation will be shaped by the individual's appraisal of the magnitude of the stressor, the coping processes used by the individual, and the perceptions of the resources that individuals have to manage the stressful event. That is, if an individual appraises the demands of a particular situation as outweighing the resources (e.g., the *required* coping resources

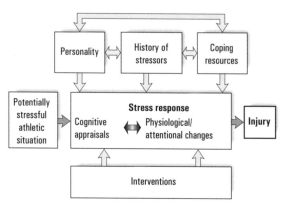

Figure 16.1   The stress and injury model (reproduced by permission from Williams & Andersen 1998, http://www.tandf.co.uk)

exceed the *available* coping resources of an individual), the stress response will increase.

In the stress–injury model, the cognitive appraisal of demands and resources is bidirectionally related to both physiological and attentional responses (Williams & Andersen 1998). An example of a physiological response to stress is generalized muscle tension. The effects of this muscle tension can include reduced flexibility and altered motor coordination, thereby increasing the risk of musculoskeletal injury. Stress can also result in attentional changes (Thompson & Morris 1994) including peripheral vision narrowing (Williams & Andersen 1997). Such changes to one's visual field can result in a failure to extract important cues from the periphery and, thereby, increase the risk of injury in some activities (Andersen & Williams 1988). Distraction is also viewed as a response to stress that can increase the likelihood of injury (Andersen & Williams 1988).

The three categories of variables (personality factors, history of stressors, coping resources) that can influence the stress response (Williams & Andersen 1998) can act either on their own or, more typically, in some complex combination. That is, the variables can have a moderating influence on each other and the resulting stress response. Substantial evidence exists to support Andersen & Williams' (1988) suggestion that an individual's history of stressors (e.g., major life events, daily hassles, previous injury) can have a significant influence on the stress response and on injury risk. A large majority of empirical studies investigating the association between life stress and injury in sport has found a positive relationship (e.g., Andersen & Williams 1999, Kolt & Kirkby 1996, Petrie 1993a, 1993b, Thompson & Morris 1994).

Daily hassles are another form of stressors suggested in the stress–injury model to influence the stress response (Williams & Andersen 1998). Despite the early failure of studies to show a link between daily hassles and injury (e.g., Blackwell & McCullagh 1990), Fawkner et al's (1999) prospective study showed that athletes were more likely to incur an injury if they had experienced significant increases in daily hassles during the week of, and week prior to, their injury.

Previous injury is a further category of stressor thought by Andersen & Williams (1988) to affect future injury. For example, if an athlete returns to sport when physically, but not psychologically, prepared, they could be worried about their ability to perform, still have concerns about their level of recovery, and be worried about their lack of sport-specific training over the rehabilitation period. Such negative self-evaluations could distract the athlete from important aspects of safe participation in their sport. Further, as Williams & Andersen (1998) suggested, fear of re-injury can be a substantial stressor, and thus, can increase injury risk. There is, however, mixed support for this component of the model (Hanson et al 1992, Lysens et al 1984).

Personality (e.g., competitive trait anxiety, locus of control) is the second category of variables suggested to influence the stress response. Positive associations have been found between injury and variables such as locus of control (Kerr & Minden 1988, Kolt & Kirkby 1996), and trait anxiety (Kerr & Minden 1988, Petrie 1993b). Other personality factors linked to injury in sport include negative states of mind, tough mindedness, defensive pessimism, and state anxiety (see Williams & Andersen 1998).

In the stress–injury model, an individual's coping resources are also thought to influence the stress response. Such resources include social support, stress management skills, general coping behaviors (e.g. sleep habits, nutrition), and other psychological coping skills. Williams & Andersen (1998) presented a great deal of evidence indicating that coping resources are related to injury outcome, or at least moderate the effects of life stress on vulnerability to injury. For example, low levels of social support have been shown to influence stress responsivity and injury vulnerability (Andersen & Williams 1999).

INTERVENTIONS TO REDUCE INJURY VULNERABILITY

Given the extensive literature suggesting that variables such as stress can increase the risk of injury, it is logical to believe that interventions aimed at reducing stress levels, or teaching people to cope better with stress, might decrease the risk of injury. Research in this area, however, is limited: only six published empirical studies have taken this approach (Davis 1991, Kerr & Goss 1996, Kolt & Hume 2003, May & Brown 1989, Perna et al 2003, Schomer 1990). May & Brown (1989) reported that a program of imagery, attention control, and other mental practice skills resulted in a reduced rate of injury, increased confidence, and enhanced self-control in US Olympic alpine skiers at the Calgary

Olympic Games. Schomer (1990) taught marathon runners how to use attentional strategies (i.e., associative thought processes) over a 5-week period and found that heavy training could be facilitated without injury. The findings of both of these studies, however, should be viewed with caution as neither incorporated a control group or used statistical comparisons to examine changes.

Four more recent studies examined the effects of stress management programs on injury prevention in athletes (Davis 1991, Kerr & Goss 1996, Kolt & Hume 2003, Perna et al 2003). Davis (1991) used a program of sport skill imagery and progressive muscular relaxation with college-level swimmers and football players and reported a 52% and 33% reduction in injuries, respectively. In a later study, Kerr & Goss (1996) investigated the effects of a 16-session stress management program on national- and international-level Canadian gymnasts over an 8-month period. The intervention program included a range of stress management skills such as relaxation exercises, imagery, thought stopping, and evaluating and changing thought processes. Compared to a matched control group, gymnasts in the stress management group reported significantly lower levels of negative athletic stress from the mid-part of the season to the peak of the season. In relation to injury, no statistically significant difference between the two groups was found. Andersen & Stoové (1998), in critiquing the Kerr & Goss paper, suggested that Kerr & Goss probably showed a clinically significant effect in injury reduction from their stress management intervention despite statistical significance not being met.

Two more recent studies have looked at stress management and injury in athletes (Kolt & Hume 2003, Perna et al 2003). Kolt & Hume (2003) investigated the effects of a 12-session stress management program on injury in competitive gymnasts. They found that gymnasts in the stress management group and control group did not differ significantly in stress scores after the intervention. Those in the stress management group, however, missed or modified 43% fewer hours of training due to injury compared to those in the control group. It could be that the intervention, although not reducing stress, taught the gymnasts how to cope better with stress and injury, and hence resulted in less time missed from training. The best evidence to date for using stress management techniques to reduce risk of injury comes from Perna et al (2003). Perna et al (2003) found, through a randomized controlled trial, that a cognitive behavioral stress management program contributed to reductions in the number of injury and illness days for competitive collegiate rowers when compared to a control group.

Despite the mixed support for the role of psychological interventions to reduce the risk of injury in sport, physical and manual therapists are in an ideal environment to discuss such issues with sport, exercise, and physical activity participants. Physical and manual therapists often identify issues related to stress and coping abilities brought up by their clients. Identifying such matters during rehabilitation may provide an opportunity to teach people ways of coping with stressful events, reaching goals, and identifying and overcoming barriers. The techniques commonly recommended for such purposes include relaxation techniques (see Chapter 9), imagery (see Chapter 10), the teaching of coping mechanisms, social support, and the use of more positive self-talk. Some of these techniques will be described later in this chapter.

PSYCHOLOGICAL RESPONSES TO INJURY

When injured or ill, people display a range of psychological responses. In the context of sport, exercise, and physical activity, the meaning of such activities to individuals can influence the quality and extent of such psychological responses. These responses range from those that can improve the chance for more effective and speedy rehabilitation (productive responses) to those that hinder effective rehabilitation and return to pre-injury activity (unproductive responses). It is necessary for those involved in the physical and manual therapies to have an understanding of both the productive and unproductive responses that people can display, and to consider these carefully in planning and implementing rehabilitation programs. Psychological responses that people display in relation to injury can be categorized as cognitive, emotional, or behavioral.

COGNITIVE RESPONSES TO ACTIVITY-RELATED INJURY

Many of the responses athletes experience when injured are cognitively based. For example, when a professional basketball player sustains a significant knee injury, some common thoughts could be "Will I ever make it back onto the court?," "Are my playing days over?," and "How will I ever continue without my basketball income?" At the other end of the physical activity participation spectrum, when a 70-year-old person who has only recently increased their physical activity levels with a 20-minute walk each day sustains an ankle sprain, they may ask themselves "Will I ever be able to get back to this walking routine again?" or comment to themselves, "I will never be able to maintain my new fitness levels so important for my heart condition now that my ankle is sprained." More specifically, the many cognitive responses and factors that have been linked with injury include increases in negative thoughts and self-talk, and changes in self-esteem and self-confidence. Self-esteem is the cognitive factor that has been most extensively researched in relation to injury in sport. Although some studies have shown that global self-esteem is not influenced by injury (Brewer & Petrie 1995, Smith et al 1993), others have reported decreases in global self-esteem after injury (Leddy et al 1994) or differences according to injury status (i.e., injured or non-injured) (Leddy et al 1994, McGowan et al 1994). When considering self-esteem that is domain-specific (i.e., self-esteem for particular sports activities), Leddy et al (1994) found evidence that injured athletes report lower levels than their non-injured counterparts.

Several other cognitive responses have also been demonstrated to be linked to injury. For example, Quinn & Fallon (1999) reported that, for athletes with significant injuries, sport self-confidence was high at the commencement of rehabilitation, decreased throughout rehabilitation, and then increased again in the latter phase of rehabilitation. The same group of athletes reported constant high levels of self-confidence in adhering to their rehabilitation programs.

Cognitive responses to injury often present as irrational and unrealistic beliefs, negative thought processes, and unwarranted worry about problems beyond the control of the individual. For example, a tennis player might present to a physical therapist with a relatively minor sprain on the medial collateral ligament of the knee. Within the examination, they may indicate that this injury is "the worst thing that has happened to them" (irrational belief) and that they feel they will "never be able to play tennis again" (negative thought process). In this case, the meaning of the injury to that person has been exaggerated and catastrophized. Another response to this injury could be worrying about how a competitor will see this injury as an opportunity to gain better rankings than the injured individual (unwarranted worry about problems beyond the control of the individual). These thoughts and beliefs can influence emotions and, subsequently, self-esteem and confidence. The tendency of injured athletes to worry about things outside of their control can have the effect of taking their focus away from rehabilitation activities that they can control.

EMOTIONAL RESPONSES TO ACTIVITY-RELATED INJURY

Depression, anger, fear, frustration, and confusion are common emotional responses to injury, particularly in the early phases of rehabilitation (Bianco et al 1999, Chan & Crossman 1988, Shelley & Sherman 1996, Smith et al 1990a, Udry et al 1997, Weiss & Troxel 1986). Although many of these emotional responses to injury are considered normal, and do not reach clinical levels, Brewer et al (2002a) summarized the literature and indicated that up to 24% of injured athletes do experience clinically meaningful levels of psychological distress. At the extreme of the continuum, some injured athletes with severe depression consider attempting suicide (Smith & Milliner 1994).

Most research indicates that negative emotions decrease and positive emotions increase as rehabilitation and recovery progress (Dawes & Roach 1997, Macchi & Crossman 1996, Miller 1998, Quinn & Fallon 1999). Some studies have shown, however, that as rehabilitation is ending and return to sport or activity is approaching, emotions related to fear of re-injury increase (Bianco et al 1999, Johnston & Carroll 1998). Such increases in fear have been found particularly with long-term rehabilitation from reconstructive knee surgery (Morrey et al 1999). In the Morrey et al (1999) study, athletes showed high negative and low positive mood states around the time of the surgery, more positive and less negative mood during the first few weeks post-surgery, and then more negative and less positive mood as they were about to return to sporting activity.

BEHAVIORAL RESPONSES TO ACTIVITY-RELATED INJURY

Behavioral responses to injury in sport and exercise often stem from the cognitive and emotional responses that people experience. The main behavioral responses to injury of importance and relevance to physical and manual therapists relate to rehabilitation adherence (see later in this chapter) and the use of coping mechanisms throughout rehabilitation. People who participate in sport, exercise, and physical activity use a range of coping behaviors including social support, avoidance, distraction, and isolation. For example, Gould et al (1997) reported that skiers with major injuries that precluded further participation for that competitive season used social support, distraction, avoiding others and isolating oneself, and "driving through" (e.g., working hard towards rehabilitation goals) to cope with their injuries. In another study (Udry 1997), athletes recovering from knee surgery most commonly used instrumental coping behaviors (i.e., those aimed at dealing directly with a stressor). It has been suggested (Gould et al 1997, Smith et al 1990b) that athletes tend to prefer active coping strategies (i.e., coping behaviors that are dependent on their own input) rather than passive strategies (i.e., behaviors that are reliant on others).

Most physical and manual therapists would have experienced cases of malingering. Malingering, as a behavioral response to injury, can be displayed in a variety of ways including exaggerating injury symptoms and prolonging return to sport through various methods. Rotella et al (1999) described malingering as an adjustment to negative circumstances that requires an external incentive for being injured. Athletes who repeatedly display malingering behavior may do so for fear of re-injury on return to sport or for the attention that they may otherwise not receive (Rotella et al 1999). Other common reasons for malingering include poor performance, personal realizations of limited ability, an escape from the pressure of sport, and a way of rationalizing a change of status in their sport.

POSITIVE RESPONSES TO INJURY

Although a common practice of physical and manual therapists is to focus on the negative responses to injury and plan rehabilitation programs around such responses, on many occasions positive emotional benefits emerge from sport and exercise injuries. For example, Udry (1997) found that 95% of injured athletes they interviewed reported positive consequences of their injuries: these included personal growth consequences, psychologically

based performance enhancements, and physical–technical development opportunities. More specifically, some athletes indicated that they became "mentally tougher" and learned more about their own psychological limitations; some indicated that they learned to be more empathetic toward other injured athletes, and some took the opportunity to develop skills and interests outside of their sports. Another positive response reported was that injury provided athletes with time to spend time on other physical and technical aspects of their sports that were not contraindicated during the rehabilitation program.

To gain maximum benefit from rehabilitation, physical and manual therapists should attempt to highlight the positive consequences of injury as a way of minimizing the impact of the negative consequences. Udry (1999) suggested five recommendations for facilitating positive consequences from athletic injuries:

1. Recognize that deriving positive consequences takes effort – injured athletes need to work on deriving positive consequences rather than simply assuming a passive role.
2. Recognize the different problem-solving strategies that can be used – these include converting negative situations into positive situations (or at least less negative) and encouraging athletes to voluntarily relinquish problematic roles.
3. Recognize that reframing may not occur immediately – athletes may require considerable time to counterbalance the negative aspects of their injuries.
4. Avoid secondary victimization – ensure that those who come into contact with injured athletes (e.g., families, coaches, team members) do not trivialize or minimize the experiences of the injured athlete.
5. Acknowledge that positive consequences may extend beyond the individual athlete – individuals whose lives are related to the injured athlete must often also work to counterbalance the negative impact of injury.

PSYCHOLOGICAL ASPECTS OF INJURY REHABILITATION

Recent research has focused on the impact of psychological variables on the way people respond to injury and the rehabilitation process that follows.

THEORETICAL EXPLANATIONS OF PSYCHOLOGICAL FACTORS IN INJURY REHABILITATION

Theoretical models can be used to explain and summarize the psychological reactions athletes and exercise participants experience when injured, and their impact on rehabilitation. It is useful for physical and manual therapists to consider the range of responses shown by a client and to be able to place those responses in a coherent model. This process allows the therapist to interpret why many reactions are occurring and how these reactions may influence the rehabilitation process. The two types of models commonly used to explain injury as a result of sport, exercise, and physical activity, are psychological models and the biopsychosocial model.

Psychological models

A range of psychological models has been suggested in the literature as an explanation of injury and rehabilitation in sport, exercise, and physical activity. In particular, the grief response model and cognitive appraisal models have been widely adopted.

Grief response model Kubler-Ross' (1969) grief response model has been used to explain responses to injury in sport. Although this model was initially developed to explain significant loss (e.g., death of a family member), it has been applied to sport injury rehabilitation based on suggestions that such injuries involve a loss of an aspect of the self (Gordon et al 1991, Macchi & Crossman 1996). The original model is based on the premise that individuals typically progress through five stages of grieving: denial, anger, bargaining, depression, and acceptance. Each "stage" of the grief response model is characterized by particular moods and behaviors that athletes may move through during the recovery and rehabilitation period. For example, an injured exercise participant may initially show *denial* of the injury, possibly rejecting the diagnosis and refusing to abide by the activity restrictions placed on them by the physical or manual therapist. After this stage, the exercise participant may experience *anger*, possibly towards someone considered responsible for the injury. On some occasions, the physical or manual therapists can be the focus of anger, as may be perceived as being responsible for the diagnosis. The next stage in the grief response model involves the exercise participant entering a

bargaining stage. This stage could involve bargaining with the physical or manual therapist over when they can return to their usual exercise regime. The fourth stage of the grief response model is symptoms of *depression*, often occurring when people comprehend the extent of their injuries and the actual limitations it may put on them. The final stage involves *acceptance* of the extent and implications of the injury. Table 16.1 shows examples of some typical thought processes and their corresponding behaviors at each stage of the grief response model in the case of an exercise-related injury.

Stage models such as the grief response model have received some level of criticism, in that athletes do not usually progress through the injury and rehabilitation period in a structured and staged manner (Brewer 1994). In reality, progression through rehabilitation varies considerably and can be influenced by both personal and situational factors (Brewer 1994, Wiese-Bjornstal et al 1998). Theoretical explanations that consider individual differences, whilst also recognizing some staged responses to grief, have been developed.

Cognitive appraisal models Cognitive appraisal models are based around stress, coping, and emotional responsivity theories. In sport, exercise, and physical activity, several theories have been developed (e.g., Gordon 1986, Weiss & Troxel 1986). In one example, Weiss & Troxel (1986) suggested that an individual's experience of stress emanating from an injury is a function of more general thoughts they may have about stressful situations. That is, a stressful situation such as an injury is cognitively appraised in relation to the situational and personal resources that the person developed to deal with the situation, as well as the possible outcomes of the injury. Then, an emotional response (consisting of both psychological and attentional components) follows the appraisal. Stemming from the emotional responses are the behavioral consequences.

A more comprehensive cognitive appraisal model is that proposed by Wiese-Bjornstal et al (1998), the Integrated Model of Psychological Response to the Sport Injury and Rehabilitation Process (Figure 16.2). This model suggests that an athlete's response to a sport-related injury is influenced by pre-injury variables such as history of stressors, coping resources, personality, and preventative interventions, as well as postinjury variables. During the postinjury phase, it is proposed that an individual's cognitive appraisal of the injury influences the behavioral responses they have (e.g., use

Table 16.1 Examples of typical thoughts and corresponding behaviors during each stage of the grief response model as it relates to exercise-based injury

Stage	Thoughts	Corresponding behaviors
1. Denial	"I can continue on my walking program despite my knee injury. It's not going to stop me"	Continues on walking program of 30 minutes per day despite the knee injury
2. Anger	"Why did my trainer make me increase from 3 to 5 days per week of walking" "Just my luck to get injured when I was finally seeing some fitness and weight loss results from it"	Leaves physical therapy rehabilitation session before the end in an angry state
3. Bargaining	"If I do more knee exercise than I've been asked to do at home, maybe I can begin back on my power walking a week earlier than the physical therapist said I could. He really doesn't know what I am going through"	Failure to follow the advice of the physical therapist regarding rehabilitation exercise and return to walking activity
4. Depression	"This exercise program is no good. I'm not getting anywhere with it. Why should I even bother going to rehabilitation any more"	Lack of motivation Lethargy Withdrawal from rehabilitation involvement
5. Acceptance	"I can now see why the physical therapist was giving me those rehabilitation exercises. I really should continue to follow the instructions"	Positive self-talk Showing commitment to the rehabilitation program Adhering to rehabilitation advice

of social support, use of psychological skills, rehabilitation adherence), their emotional responses (e.g., depressed mood, frustration, fear of the unknown), and the physical and psychosocial recovery outcomes. In this model, both personal (e.g., injury history, pain tolerance, coping skills) and situational factors (e.g., type of sport, coach influences, rehabilitation environment) can affect the cognitive interpretation and appraisal of the injury.

To date, not much research has addressed the interactional aspects of cognitive appraisal models, although some aspects of such models have gained strong support (see review by Brewer 2001). Nevertheless, models such as Wiese-Bjornstal et al's (1998) provide a strong framework from which to explain the psychological responses to injury in sport, exercise, and physical activity.

Biopsychosocial model

A recent model of sport injury rehabilitation and its outcomes was developed by Brewer et al (2002a). The Biopsychosocial Model of Sport Injury Rehabilitation combines elements of medical and psychological approaches to sport injury rehabilitation (Figure 16.3). The components of the model are injury, sociodemographic factors, biological factors,

psychological factors, social/contextual factors, intermediate biopsychological outcomes, and sport injury rehabilitation outcomes. In this model, both the characteristics of injury (e.g., type, course, severity, location, history) and sociodemographic factors (e.g., age, gender, race/ethnicity, socio-economic status) are suggested to influence the biological, psychological, and social/contextual factors. In turn, biological, psychological, and social/contextual factors affect the intermediate biopsychological outcomes (e.g., range of motion, strength, joint laxity, pain, endurance, recovery rate), and hence, rehabilitation outcomes (e.g., quality of life, readiness to return to activity, functional performance).

The strength of the biopsychosocial model (Brewer et al 2002a) is its relevance and applicability to the physical and manual therapies; it proposes links between medically focused models and psychological models.

ADHERENCE TO INJURY REHABILITATION

Adherence has been defined in many ways, but most comprehensively as "active, voluntary collaborative involvement of the client in a mutually acceptable course of behavior to produce a desired

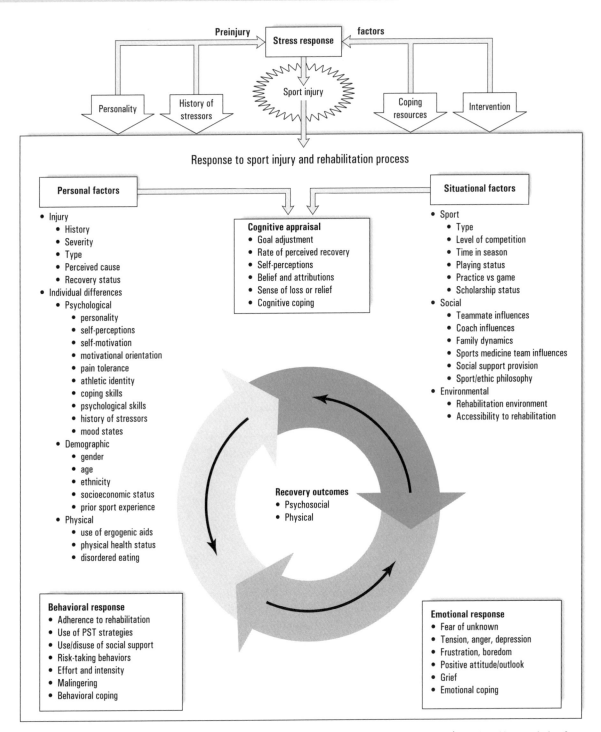

Figure 16.2   Integrated model of psychological response to the sport injury and rehabilitation process (reproduced by permission from Wiese-Bjornstal et al 1998, http://www.tandf.co.uk)

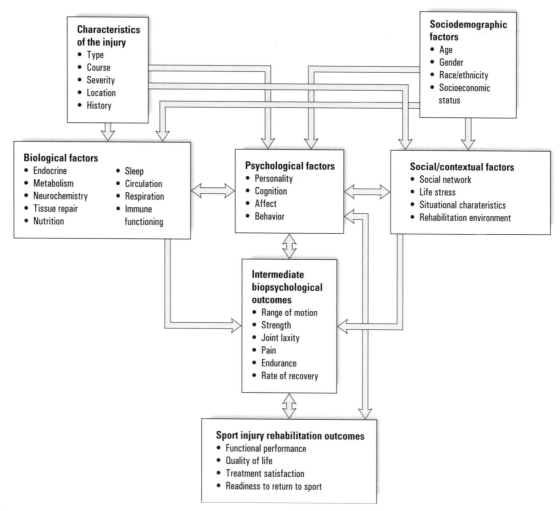

Figure 16.3 The biopsychosocial model of sport injury rehabilitation (reproduced from Brewer et al 2001b by permission of Fitness Information Technology)

preventative or therapeutic result" (Meichenbaum & Turk 1987, p 20). Due to the breadth of the physical and manual therapies, many components of rehabilitation programs require adherence by clients. These include attendance at rehabilitation appointments, completion of home-based and clinic-based rehabilitation exercises, adherence to advice given by physical and manual therapists (e.g., activity restriction), cryotherapy usage, and adherence to advice given and changes made to rehabilitation programs during clinic appointments. Studies of rehabilitation adherence in sport injury settings show a range of adherence from 40–91% (Almekinders & Almekinders 1994, Daly et al 1995, Laubach et al 1996, Taylor & May 1996).

Chapter 4 includes a detailed discussion of rehabilitation adherence including measurement issues and theoretical explanations. Although focused on adherence to rehabilitation for a variety of conditions seen by physical and manual therapists, the information in Chapter 4 can readily be applied to rehabilitation adherence for injuries from sport, exercise, and physical activity. Much of the literature on rehabilitation adherence stemmed from research on sport injury. The current chapter will, therefore, focus more on the psychological factors that can influence rehabilitation adherence and methods that can be used to enhance adherence.

The underlying assumption in most sport injury and musculoskeletal injury research is that adherence to rehabilitation activities is in some way related to rehabilitation outcome. Empirical support for this relationship is, in most cases, limited. Only a few studies have concluded that higher levels of adherence were related to a better sport injury rehabilitation outcome (e.g., Brewer et al 2000a, Derscheid & Feiring 1987, Kolt & McEvoy 2003, O'Reilly et al 1999, Schoo 2002, Treacy et al 1997). See Chapter 4 for more detail on the adherence–outcome relationship.

MEASUREMENT OF REHABILITATION ADHERENCE

A range of adherence measures have been developed for, and used in, sport injury rehabilitation. These measures address attendance at clinic-based rehabilitation sessions, client behavior during clinic sessions, and adherence to home-based components of rehabilitation.

Attendance at rehabilitation

Attendance at rehabilitation sessions is the most commonly used measure of adherence in most musculoskeletal rehabilitation programs (e.g., Brewer et al 2000a, Daly et al 1995, Fields et al 1995, Kolt & McEvoy 2003). Attendance is most commonly calculated as a ratio of rehabilitation sessions attended to sessions scheduled. This measure has been criticized on the basis that it only captures one aspect of rehabilitation (i.e., attendance) and does not tap what people do during their clinic-based rehabilitation sessions (Brewer 1998, Spetch & Kolt 2001). It is suggested that attendance measures be used in combination with other adherence measures that capture further aspects of rehabilitation behaviors.

Adherence to clinic–based rehabilitation

Measuring the behaviors of clients during clinic-based rehabilitation sessions is important to physical and manual therapists, and assists them in implementing aspects of the program. The Sport Injury Rehabilitation Adherence Scale (SIRAS, Brewer et al 2000b) can be used to rate the intensity with which participants complete rehabilitation exercises, the frequency of following practitioner instructions and advice, and the receptivity to changes in the rehabilitation program during that day's appointment (see Chapter 4, and specifically Figure 4.1 for a further description). The SIRAS has been used extensively in sport and exercise injury

rehabilitation, and has sound psychometric properties (Brewer et al 2000b, 2002b, Kolt et al 2001).

Another instrument that can be used to measure clinic-based rehabilitation behavior is the Sports Medicine Observation Code (SMOC, Crossman & Roch 1991). The SMOC involves systematic coding of behaviors displayed in rehabilitation into 13 categories (e.g., active rehabilitation, waiting, nonactivity). These categories are grouped into productive behaviors (i.e., those behaviors that have a high probability of facilitating rehabilitation from injury), unproductive behaviors (i.e., those behaviors that have little or no potential of facilitating rehabilitation from injury), and concurrent behaviors (i.e., those behaviors that have a moderate potential of facilitating the rehabilitation process). The SMOC may be useful in measuring adherence, and its productive behaviors score has been shown to correlate significantly with SIRAS scores (Kolt et al 2001). In terms of utility, the SMOC is quite labor intensive and, therefore, is not often used in clinical settings.

Adherence to home–based rehabilitation

Equally important to behaviors carried out by clients in the clinic, are the rehabilitation behaviors they carry out at home. Measurement of non-clinic-based adherence usually involves self-reporting and has been criticized for that reason (Dunbar-Jacob et al 1993, Meichenbaum & Turk 1987). Self-reports, often carried out retrospectively, can be distorted, biased, and inaccurate. Typical methods used include single retrospective reports of adherence over the course of home-based rehabilitation or the completion of daily logs or diaries. As discussed by Brewer in Chapter 4, a number of objective methods of assessing home exercise completion include the use of accelerometers to detect movement (Schlenk et al 2000), a motion sensor embedded in an ankle exerciser (Belanger & Noel 1991), and an electronic counting device attached to a splint for individuals after tendon surgery (Dobbe et al 1999).

PSYCHOLOGICAL FACTORS RELATED TO REHABILITATION ADHERENCE

A variety of personal, situational, and cognitive and emotional factors can influence rehabilitation adherence (Brewer 2001). Personal factors that have been shown to have positive associations with sport injury rehabilitation adherence include health locus of control (Murphy et al 1999), pain tolerance (Byerly et al 1994, Fields et al 1995, Fisher et al 1988), self-motivation (Brewer et al 2000a, Duda et al 1989, Fields et al 1995, Fisher et al 1988), tough-mindedness (Wittig & Schurr 1994), and task involvement (Duda et al 1989).

Evidence exists for a number of situational variables being positively related to sport injury rehabilitation adherence. For example, a higher belief in the efficacy of the treatment has been linked to higher levels of adherence (Duda et al 1989, Taylor & May 1996). The importance or value of the rehabilitation to the athlete (Taylor & May 1996), the convenience of the rehabilitation appointment scheduling (Fields et al 1995, Fisher et al 1988), the social support for rehabilitation (Byerly et al 1994, Duda et al 1989, Finnie 1999), the perceived injury severity (Taylor & May 1996), the comfort of the clinical environment (Fields et al 1995, Fisher et al 1988), and perceived exertion during rehabilitation (Fisher et al 1988) all have demonstrated positive associations with rehabilitation adherence.

Adherence levels can also be influenced by the variety of cognitive and emotional responses people have to injury in sport, exercise, and physical activity. For example, Daly et al (1995) reported that those athletes with a higher coping ability for their injuries tended to adhere better to post-surgical knee rehabilitation programs. Further, Taylor & May (1996) found that athletes with high rehabilitation self-efficacy were more likely to adhere to rehabilitation programs than their counterparts with lower self-efficacy in relation to rehabilitation. Lampton et al (1993) reported that, compared to athletes who attributed their recovery to factors that were outside of their control, those who attributed their recovery to stable and personally controllable factors adhered to higher levels.

METHODS TO ENHANCE REHABILITATION ADHERENCE IN ATHLETES, EXERCISERS, AND PHYSICAL ACTIVITY PARTICIPANTS

Several strategies have been outlined in Chapter 4 to enhance rehabilitation adherence in a range of musculoskeletal and other medical conditions. This section will discuss the methods that are directly related to rehabilitation of injuries associated with sport, exercise, and physical activity. The main methods used to enhance rehabilitation adherence include education, communication and rapport building, social support, goal setting, treatment efficacy and tailoring, threats and scare tactics, and athlete responsibility.

Education

Physical and manual therapists, compared to other healthcare practitioners, tend to spend longer periods of time with their clients. Given these longer periods, physical and manual therapists often dedicate time to educating their clients about their injuries, the rationale behind treatment approaches and injury management, and in establishing realistic expectations. Despite these efforts, however, one study showed that 77% of injured athletes interviewed misunderstood some aspect of their rehabilitation, and only 14% were given any written instructions (Webborn et al 1997). In another study, Schneiders et al (1998) found that clients who were given written exercise instructions adhered to 77% of their home exercise program compared to 38% for those who received exercises via verbal instructions alone. The Schneiders et al (1998) study demonstrates the importance of supplementing education regarding exercises with written material.

Communication and rapport building

A standard in probably all physical and manual therapy training programs is the message that practitioners should try to establish rapport with their clients, and communicate in ways suited to the individual. This ideal, however, cannot solely be taught from textbooks, but must be developed through experience. A number of investigators have indicated that athletes who perceive that medical professionals are genuinely interested in their health and well-being, and are aware of the psychological manifestations relating to their injuries, may be more highly motivated to adhere to rehabilitation programs (Byerly et al 1994, Duda et al 1989, Ford & Gordon 1993). Little research, however, has specifically examined the relationship between adherence and practitioner–client communication and rapport.

Social support

Providing social support through injury support groups and peer modeling has been recommended for sport injury rehabilitation (Wiese et al 1991). Peer modeling involves linking a currently injured individual with an athlete who has undergone successful rehabilitation and returned to pre-injury functioning (preferably from a similar injury). Given the difficulty of setting up such links in some clinical settings (particularly after discharge of clients), it is often possible to use a person who is still in rehabilitation but at a more advanced stage. Setting up appointment times that coincide is one method of introducing peer modeling. Modeling has been shown to improve adherence to postsurgical knee rehabilitation (Flint 1991).

Injury support groups are sometimes used for people undergoing long periods of rehabilitation, where a possibility exists for the development of negative and malproductive psychological manifestations. These groups are useful in providing a forum for clients to discuss their injuries and rehabilitation. Injury support groups can also assist in motivating injured athletes (Weiss & Troxel 1986).

Goal setting and attainment

Goal setting in rehabilitation is commonplace (see Chapter 8). Research has focused on goal setting as a strategy to enhance adherence (Penpraze & Mutrie 1999, Scherzer et al 2001). Setting specific rehabilitation goals has been shown to result in greater time spent doing rehabilitation exercises and a greater knowledge of the rehabilitation program in injured people at a sports injury clinic (Penpraze & Mutrie 1999). In a more recent study, Scherzer et al (2001) found that goal setting was positively associated with home exercise completion in people undergoing rehabilitation following anterior cruciate ligament surgical reconstruction.

Three important elements should be considered when using goal setting. First, the practitioner and client should establish challenging (yet realistic and positive) goals in a collaborative manner. These goals should be recorded and measurable (Wiese & Weiss 1987). Second, to encourage a sense of control by the client, strategies for achieving goals should be negotiated between the practitioner and client. Finally, the agreed goals should be closely monitored and evaluated throughout rehabilitation, and modified if and when necessary.

Treatment efficacy and tailoring of rehabilitation programs

Perception of the efficacy of the rehabilitation program is important to a client's belief that they will be able to achieve the rehabilitation goals. This often involves tailoring of rehabilitation programs to the needs of individual clients. Duda et al (1989) suggested that perceived treatment efficacy has an important impact on rehabilitation adherence behaviors. Therefore, in building a sense of treatment efficacy in clients, physical and manual therapists should ensure that athletes are capable of performing the assigned rehabilitation tasks and identifying the context of their rehabilitation as meaningful and worthwhile to the individual. Of note, is that Sluijs et al (1993) found that complex rehabilitation programs (i.e., those that contain skills beyond the abilities of the client) resulted in lower levels of adherence.

Athlete responsibility

Fisher et al (1993) reported that athletes like to feel responsible for their own rehabilitation, and this sense of control over rehabilitation can increase commitment and adherence to the behaviors required for a successful outcome. This concept has been supported by Laubach et al (1996) who reported a positive relationship between personal control and rehabilitation adherence in athletes following knee surgery. Physical and manual therapists could, therefore, use approaches to rehabilitation that encourage some level of independence for clients, and provide them with a better sense of control over rehabilitation activities.

Threats and scare tactics

A further method that can be used to improve rehabilitation adherence (albeit only with suitable clients) is to increase an athlete's perception of injury severity and susceptibility to poor rehabilitation, re-injury, or more serious debilitation (Taylor & May 1996). Clearly, care must be taken when using methods such as these, as threats or ultimatums can harm rapport with clients (Fisher et al 1993).

PSYCHOLOGICAL INTERVENTIONS

COGNITIVE BEHAVIORAL INTERVENTIONS FOR INJURED ATHLETES

Chapter 8 is dedicated to cognitive and behavioral interventions that have utility in rehabilitation. Many of the techniques outlined in that chapter have obvious application to injuries associated with sport, exercise, and physical activity. The current chapter will not, therefore, provide a detailed account of the large number of cognitive behavioral techniques that can be used with injured athletes during rehabilitation, but rather, focus on a smaller number of techniques that can be of direct use to physical and manual therapists during rehabilitation. These techniques include relaxation, cognitive rehearsal, goal setting, social support, and cognitive restructuring. For further information on cognitive behavioral interventions refer to Chapter 8 and other specific references (e.g., Heil 1993, Kolt 2000, Pargman 1999, Ray & Wiese-Bjornstal 1999, Taylor & Taylor 1997).

Relaxation techniques

A large number of relaxation techniques are used in healthcare. Depending on their focus, relaxation techniques achieve their goals by different means. For example, injury can lead to pain and a sense of stress, which in turn, can elicit muscle tension. Such muscle tension can restrict blood flow and hence, increase pain (Cousins & Phillips 1985). In this case, it would be logical to implement a relaxation technique that directly targets muscle and aims to reduce muscle tension. Alternately, if it was established that muscle tension in an individual was being caused by cognitive stress, techniques that target the cognitive aspects of relaxation could be used.

An important model in explaining relaxation is the multiprocess theory (Davidson & Schwartz 1976). Davidson & Schwartz (1976) suggested three effects of relaxation: somatic, cognitive, and attentional. The somatic response to relaxation refers to effects on physiological parameters (e.g., heart rate, muscle tension). The cognitive effects apply to mental activity. The attentional component relates to a continuum from active, self-regulating behavior (e.g., breathing control) to passive awareness of a pre-existing behavior without any overt attempt to modify it (e.g., observing your breathing). The multiprocess theory includes a "specific-effects" hypothesis. That is, relaxation techniques have different effects depending on the relative cognitive and somatic components involved in each. For example, a technique that predominantly focuses on somatic functioning (e.g., progressive relaxation, Jacobson 1938) is likely to influence somatic outcomes, whereas a technique that focuses predominantly on cognitive functions (e.g., Benson's relaxation response, Benson 1975) is more likely to affect cognitive aspects of stress.

A common form of muscular (somatic) relaxation is progressive relaxation (Jacobson 1938). Progressive relaxation (see Chapter 9 for further detail and scripts) involves a systematic relaxation of major skeletal muscle groups by firstly recognizing the muscle tension present (often achieved by contracting the muscles), and then by relaxing those muscle groups. It has been suggested that the role of muscle contraction before relaxation allows clients to recognize the feeling of muscle tension, so that they can then learn the sensations of a relaxed muscle. With technique familiarity, the individual can simply relax muscle groups from whatever condition they are at rest, without having to contract the muscle group first. Divided opinion exists regarding the usefulness of muscle contraction before relaxation (Lucic et al 1991, O'Bannon et al 1987, Payne 2000). Physical and manual therapists must be careful when using progressive relaxation on clients with pain, and monitor carefully the level of muscle contraction used in the exercise, so that pain symptoms are not aggravated. Progressive relaxation has been shown to have a variety of benefits including reducing somatic anxiety (e.g., Kolt et al 2002, Maynard et al 1995, Weinstein & Smith 1992), rheumatic pain (Stenstrom et al 1996), and muscle tension (e.g., Jacobson 1938, Lehrer 1982)

Benson's relaxation response (Benson 1975) is another common form of relaxation used in rehabilitation. The relaxation response is based on four principles:

1. a quiet environment, which allows for the reduction of external distractions
2. adopting a comfortable position to reduce undue muscular tension
3. an object to dwell on, such as the repetition of a word (e.g., "relax")
4. a passive attitude that allows emptying all other thoughts from one's mind, and letting distracting thoughts that do return pass on while returning to a focused state.

In summary, the relaxation response evolved from transcendental meditation, and involves a focus on breathing and repetition of a word in time with the individual's breathing. In more recent adaptations, there has been the use of imagery on an object that moves in time with the client's breathing (Kolt & McConville 2000).

The relaxation response works mainly on the premise that distracting or drawing focus away from stressors associated with injury, allows the person to focus on more relevant activities for the rehabilitation process. Taylor & Taylor (1998) suggested that the relaxation response provides a greater sense of control over pain, and a reduction in the negative emotions associated with pain and injury.

What is obvious from the literature is the lack of an evidence base for the wide variety of relaxation techniques used in health care. Clearly this is an area for future research. For a more detailed account of relaxation techniques refer to Chapter 8 and Payne (2000).

Cognitive rehearsal

Cognitive rehearsal refers to the broad range of skills such as imagery, mental rehearsal, visualization, and mental practice. Chapter 10 describes a range of imagery-based skills used across healthcare. Cognitive rehearsal techniques relate to practicing a skill in one's mind that mimics real experience. Cognitive rehearsal relies on the ability to feel a movement, see a movement, and bring in other senses in rehearsing an activity without actually carrying out the physical skill (i.e., re-creation of an activity in one's mind).

Athletes most commonly use cognitive rehearsal to practice skills and techniques, focus on relevant cues for performance, and enhance learning and performance (Vealey & Greenleaf 2001), as well as a method to enhance self-confidence (McKenzie & Howe 1997) and decrease anxiety (Savoy 1997). Only recently, however, has cognitive rehearsal been used in rehabilitation (see Chapter 10 and Graham 1995). Some possible practical applications of cognitive rehearsal as part of physical and manual therapy regimes include techniques to help maintain a positive outlook, to control stress, to encourage positive self-talk, and to encourage self-efficacy regarding the rehabilitation process (Shaffer & Wiese-Bjornstal 1999). Cognitive rehearsal may also be used during rehabilitation to cope with pain and maintain physical skill levels in the absence of physical practice (Hall 2001, Richardson & Latuda 1995).

Physical and manual therapists, as well as other healthcare professionals, have begun to use forms of imagery (or cognitive rehearsal) to assist their clients in managing pain (Whitmarsh & Alderman 1993). General forms of imagery involve imagining oneself in a relaxing environment (i.e., an environment that has a relaxing meaning for the individual), and focusing on the feeling of being in that environment. The aim of this type of imagery is to distract the individual from the sensation of pain or from other stressors associated with the injury. From clinical experience, the more complex the scene to be imaged or rehearsed, and the more detail the client is asked to attend to (e.g., using tactile and auditory senses, as well as visual), the more likely they are to be distracted from their pain or other stressors.

Some investigators have developed specific types of imagery for different aspects of rehabilitation. For example, Ievleva & Orlick (1999) described pain management imagery, where clients imagine the pain being washed away or see cool blue colors running through the painful area to reduce the pain and inflammation. Despite the many suggestions for practical use of imagery in rehabilitation, and the increasing practice in this field, specific research is needed to establish the effectiveness of such interventions.

Goal setting

Goal setting has been described in general in Chapter 8 and some principles have been covered earlier in this chapter in relation to enhancing rehabilitation adherence. The use of goal setting in rehabilitation is not dissimilar from goal setting for other activities. That is, it is important when setting goals to identify the attributes the client has to contribute to the goals, identify any possible obstacles to achieving the goals, secure a commitment from the client to work towards the goals, develop an action plan, provide feedback on goal attainment, evaluate goal attainment, and reinforce achievement of goals. Rehabilitation providers are fortunate in that many people involved in sport, exercise, or physical activity are accustomed to setting goals and working towards them as part of their physical activity regime. This experience can assist the goal-setting process in rehabilitation. Danish et al (1993) suggested that teaching goal setting is a means of encouraging athletes to take greater responsibility for their return to activity following injury. As discussed earlier in this chapter, goal setting has been shown to be an effective strategy to enhance adherence to rehabilitation activities (Penpraze & Mutrie 1999, Scherzer et al 2001).

Social support

Social support in injury rehabilitation has been widely investigated (Brewer 2001). Udry (1996) referred to social support in the rehabilitation context as the quantity, quality, and type of interactions that athletes have with other people. A variety of forms of social support exist, including listening support, emotional support, emotional challenge, task appreciation, task challenge, reality confirmation, material assistance, and personal assistance

(Richman et al 1993). Physical and manual thera-pists, because of their work, spend long periods of time with clients during rehabilitation. Some clients see this relationship as providing an important form of social support during their recovery and return to physical activity. In a review of the literature, how-ever, Brewer (2001) reported that injured athletes perceive family members and team-mates as better social support providers than medical professionals and coaches. In one study, Johnston & Carroll (1998) found that the need for different levels of social sup-port changes throughout rehabilitation; the need for emotional support decreases as rehabilitation pro-gresses and then increases as the athlete returns to sport participation.

Cognitive restructuring

During rehabilitation it is not unusual for people to experience negative or irrational thoughts regard-ing their injuries, subsequent rehabilitation, and return to sporting or physical activity. The process of cognitive restructuring involves reframing or changing negative and irrational thoughts into more positive, rational thoughts. Physical and man-ual therapists often play a role in identifying nega-tive attitudes that people are experiencing towards their injuries and rehabilitation. Often, through informal discussions during treatment, they have the ability to encourage clients to reframe their thoughts in a more positive way that may be bene-ficial to rehabilitation and return to full function. Ievleva & Orlick (1991) reported that injured ath-letes who healed at a slow rate compared to those who healed faster were more likely to use self-talk that was positive and encouraging.

INTEGRATED MANAGEMENT APPROACHES TO REHABILITATION OF INJURIES FROM SPORT, EXERCISE, AND PHYSICAL ACTIVITY

Approaches to healthcare have begun to focus more on interdisciplinary practice in recent times, rather than discrete field of care delivered by separate disciplines. In encouraging physical and manual therapists to be more aware of the psychological aspects of injury and rehabilitation, I am suggesting that they integrate basic cognitive behavioral approaches into their existing management strate-gies. Of course, physical and manual therapists are not expected to act as qualified psychologists, but having an understanding of how psychological

issues can inflence injury and the rehabilitation process is valuable in being able to design and implement the most effective rehabilitation pro-grams. For several reasons, physical and manual therapists are in ideal positions to provide some form of psychological assistance to people injured through sport, exercise, or physical activity (Francis et al 2000, Gordon et al 1998, Kolt 2000, Ninedek & Kolt 2000, Pearson & Jones 1992). First, physical and manual therapists are closely involved with injured athletes during rehabilitation and tend to spend longer periods of time with them than many other health professionals. Given this relationship, clients may be more likely to raise psychological issues with them. The second reason is that with the use of touch as part of many physical and manual therapy techniques, people are more likely to disclose psy-chosocial matters (Nathan 1999). Dealing with such matters at the time may be beneficial, especially if these issues are affecting the recovery and rehabili-tation progress. Third, due to the many possible psychological reactions to injury, it appears logical that such issues are discussed concurrently with the physical aspects of rehabilitation. The final reason relates to perceptions held by athletes. Pearson & Jones (1992) found that the injured athletes they studied reported that physical therapists are ideally positioned to provide them with basic psychologi-cal and counseling support.

Despite the strong arguments for physical and manual therapists to integrate basic psychological approaches into their work, their ability and will-ingness to do so needs to be established. In two recent surveys (Francis et al 2000, Ninedek & Kolt 2000), physical therapists reported that using posi-tive and sincere communication, having knowledge about setting realistic goals, understanding stress, anxiety, and motivation, being able to encourage positive self-thoughts and self-confidence, and being able to reduce symptoms of depression were important skills for them to have when working with people injured through sport and exercise. Similar findings have been reported for other physi-cal and manual therapy disciplines (e.g., athletic trainers, Wiese et al 1991).

Only a limited amount of literature has assessed the ability of physical and manual therapists to deal with basic psychological issues as they relate to rehabilitation. In an early study (Gordon et al 1991), physical therapists suggested that they were limited in their ability to deal with psychosocial aspects of the recovery process and suggested further practical training in appropriate skills. In a more recent study, Potter et al (2003) reported that physical therapists found it difficult to manage both behavioral problems in their clients and client expectations during rehabilitation. Interestingly, the Potter et al (2003) study also identified differences between more experienced and less experienced physical therapists. For example, the more experienced physical therapists specifically distinguished between clients with diagnosed psychological problems and clients with psychosocial concerns, whereas their less experienced counterparts did not.

There appears to be adequate justification for physical and manual therapists to play a greater role in managing some of the basic psychological consequences of sport, exercise, and physical activity injuries. A clear need exists, however, for more standardized and advanced psychological training for physical therapists. Where more severe psychological difficulties are encountered, clients should be referred to other relevant professionals (e.g., sport and exercise psychologists, clinical psychologists, health psychologists, psychiatrists) for specialized intervention.

SUMMARY

Research on psychological aspects of injury and rehabilitation is growing, especially in the area of sport, exercise, and physical activity. By using the models and theoretical explanations developed for the psychology of injury and rehabilitation, physical and manual therapists now have a framework in which to integrate psychological and physical care. More recently, clinical and theoretical research has focused on adherence to rehabilitation, with many suggestions on methods that may be appropriate to enhance adherence. One area that requires further research is the effectiveness of cognitive behavioral techniques as part of rehabilitation. To date, much of the evidence for this practice has been based on anecdotal evidence.

For physical and manual therapists to include basic psychological and behavioral techniques into their rehabilitation practices, they must ensure that they are appropriately trained in the use of such skills, and are able to recognize when more serious pathology presents that requires referral to specialized professionals.

References

Almekinders L C, Almekinders S V 1994 Outcome in the treatment of chronic overuse sports injuries: A retrospective study. Journal of Orthopaedic & Sports Physical Therapy 19: 157–161

Andersen M B, Williams J M 1988 A model of stress and athletic injury: Prediction and prevention. Journal of Sport & Exercise Psychology 10: 294–306

Andersen M B, Williams J M 1999 Athletic injury, psychosocial factors, and perceptual changes during stress. Journal of Sports Science 17: 735–751

Andersen M B, Stoové M A 1998 The sanctity of $p < .05$ obfuscates good stuff: A comment on Kerr and Goss. Journal of Applied Sport Psychology 10: 168–173

Belanger A Y, Noel G 1991 Compliance to and effects of a home strengthening exercise program for adult dystrophic patients: A pilot study. Physiotherapy Canada 43(1): 24–30

Benson H 1975 The relaxation response. William Morrow, New York

Bianco T, Malo S, Orlick T 1999 Sport injury and illness: Elite skiers describe their experiences. Research Quarterly for Exercise and Sport 70: 157–169

Blackwell B, McCullagh P 1990 The relationship of athletic injury to life stress, competitive anxiety and coping resources. Athletic Training 25: 23–27

Bramwell S T, Masuda M, Wagner N N et al 1975 Psychosocial factors in athletic injuries: Development and application of the Social and Athletic Readjustment Rating Scale (SARRS). Journal of Human Stress 1: 6–20

Brewer B W 1994 Review and critique of models of psychological adjustment to athletic injury. Journal of Applied Sport Psychology 6: 87–100

Brewer B W 1998 Adherence to sport injury rehabilitation programs. Journal of Applied Sport Psychology 10: 70–82

Brewer B W 2001 Psychology of sport injury rehabilitation. In: Singer R N, Hausenblas H A, Janelle C M (eds) Handbook of sport psychology, 2nd edn. John Wiley, New York, p 787–809

Brewer B W, Petrie T A 1995 A comparison between injured and uninjured football players on selected psychosocial variables. Academic Athletic Journal 10: 11–18

Brewer B W, Van Raalte J L, Cornelius A E et al 2000a Psychological factors, rehabilitation adherence, and rehabilitation outcome following anterior cruciate ligament reconstruction. Rehabilitation Psychology 45: 20–37

Brewer B W, Van Raalte J L, Petitpas, A J et al 2000b Preliminary psychometric evaluation of a measure of adherence to clinic-based sport injury rehabilitation. Physical Therapy in Sport 1: 68–74

Brewer B W, Andersen M B, Van Raalte J L 2002a Psychological aspects of sport injury rehabilitation: Toward a biopsychosocial approach. In: Mostofsky D I, Zaichkowsky L D (eds) Medical and psychological aspects of sport and exercise. Fitness Information Technology, Morgantown, WV, p 41–54

Brewer B W, Avondoglio J B, Cornelius A E et al 2002b Construct validity and interrater agreement of the Sport Injury Rehabilitation Adherence Scale. Journal of Sport Rehabilitation 11: 170–178

Brown R B 1971 Personality characteristics related to injury in football. Research Quarterly 42: 133–138

Byerly P N, Worrell T, Gahimer J et al 1994 Rehabilitation compliance in an athletic training environment. Journal of Athletic Training 29: 352–355

Chan C S, Crossman H Y 1988 Psychological effects of running loss on consistent runners. Perceptual and Motor Skills 66: 875–883

Cousins M J, Phillips G D 1985 Acute pain management. Clinics in Critical Care Medicine 8: 82–117

Crossman J, Roch J 1991 An observation instrument for use in sports medicine clinics. The Journal of the Canadian Athletic Therapists Association April: 10–13

Daly J M, Brewer B W, Van Raalte J L et al 1995 Cognitive appraisal, emotional adjustment, and adherence to rehabilitation following knee surgery. Journal of Sport Rehabilitation 4: 23–30

Danish S J, Petitpas A J, Hale B D 1993 Life development interventions for athletes: Life skills through sports. Counseling Psychologist 21: 352–385

Davidson R J, Schwartz G E 1976 The psychobiology of relaxation and related states: A multi-process theory. In: Mostofsky D E (ed) Behavioural control and modification of physiological activity. Prentice-Hall, Englewood Cliffs, NJ, p 399–442

Davis J 1991 Sports injuries and stress management: An opportunity for research. The Sport Psychologist 5: 175–182

Dawes H, Roach N K 1997 Emotional responses of athletes to injury and treatment. Physiotherapy 83: 243–247

Derscheid G L, Feiring D C 1987 A statistical analysis to characterize treatment adherence of the 18 most common diagnoses seen at a sports medicine clinic. Journal of Orthopaedic & Sports Physical Therapy 9: 40–46

Dobbe J G, van Trommel N E, de Freitas Baptista J E et al 1999 A portable device for finger tendon rehabilitation that provides an isotonic force and records exercise behaviour after finger tendon surgery. Medical and Biological Engineering and Computing 37: 396–399

Duda J L, Smart A E, Tappe M L 1989 Predictors of adherence in the rehabilitation of athletic injuries: An application of personal investment theory. Journal of Sport & Exercise Psychology 11: 367–381

Dunbar-Jacob J, Dunning E J, Dwyer K 1993 Compliance research in pediatric and adolescent populations: Two decades of research. In Krasnegor N A, Epstein L, Johnson S B, Yaffe S J (eds) Developmental aspects of health compliance behavior. Erlbaum, Hillsdale, NJ, p 29–51

Fawkner H J, McMurray N E, Summers J J 1999 Athletic injury and minor life events: A prospective study. Journal of Science and Medicine in Sport 2: 117–124

Fields J, Murphey M, Horodyski M et al 1995 Factors associated with adherence to sport injury rehabilitation in college-age recreational athletes. Journal of Sport Rehabilitation 4: 172–180

Finch C, Valuri G, Ozanne-Smith J 1998 Sport and active recreation injuries in Australia: Evidence from emergency department presentations. British Journal of Sports Medicine 32: 220–225

Finnie S B 1999 The rehabilitation support team: Using social support to aid compliance to sports injury rehabilitation programs. Paper presented at the annual meeting of the Association for the Advancement of Applied Sport Psychology, Banff, Canada

Fisher A C, Domm M A, Wuest D A 1988 Adherence to sports injury rehabilitation programs. Physician and Sportsmedicine 16(7): 47–51

Fisher A C, Mullins S A, Frye P A 1993 Athletic trainers' attitudes and judgments of injured athletes' rehabilitation adherence. Journal of Athletic Training 28: 43–47

Flint F A 1991 The psychological effects of modeling in athletic injury rehabilitation. Unpublished doctoral dissertation, University of Oregon, Eugene

Ford I W, Gordon S 1993 Social support and athletic injury: The perspective of sport physiotherapists. Australian Journal of Science and Medicine in Sport 25: 17–25

Francis S R, Andersen M B, Maley P 2000 Physiotherapists' and male professional athletes' views on psychological skills for rehabilitation. Journal of Science and Medicine in Sport 3: 17–29

Gordon S 1986 Sport psychology and the injured athlete: A cognitive-behavioral approach to injury response and injury rehabilitation. Science Periodical on Research and Technology in Sport March: 1–10

Gordon S, Milios S, Grove J R 1991 Psychological aspects of the recovery process from sport injury: The perspective of sports physiotherapists. Australian Journal of Science and Medicine in Sport 23: 53–60

Gordon S, Potter M, Ford I W 1998 Towards a psychoeducational curriculum for training sport-injury rehabilitation personnel. Journal of Applied Sport Psychology 10: 140–156

Gould D, Udry E, Bridges D et al 1997 Stress sources encountered when rehabilitating from season-ending ski injuries. The Sport Psychologist 11: 361–378

Govern J W, Koppenhaver R 1965 Attempt to predict athletic injuries. Medical Times 93: 421–422

Graham H 1995 Mental imagery in health care: An introduction to therapeutic practice. Chapman & Hall, London

Hall C R 2001 Imagery in sport and exercise. In: Singer R N, Hausenblas H A, Janelle C M (eds) Handbook of sport psychology, 2nd edn. John Wiley, New York, p 529–549

Hanson S J, McCullagh P, Tonymon P 1992 The relationship of personality characteristics, life stress, and coping resources to athletic injury. Journal of Sport & Exercise Psychology 14: 262–272

Heil J 1993 Psychology of sport injury. Human Kinetics, Champaign, IL

Ievleva L, Orlick T 1991 Mental links to enhanced healing: An exploratory study. The Sport Psychologist 5: 25–40

Ievleva L, Orlick T 1999 Mental paths to enhanced recovery from a sports injury. In: Pargman D (ed) Psychological bases of sport injuries, 2nd edn. Fitness Information Technology, Morgantown, WV, p 199–220

Jacobson E 1938 Progressive relaxation. University of Chicago Press, Chicago

Johnston L H, Carroll D 1998 The provision of social support to injured athletes: A qualitative analysis. Journal of Sport Rehabilitation 7: 267–284

Kerr G, Goss J 1996 The effects of a stress management program on injuries and stress levels. Journal of Applied Sport Psychology 8: 109–117

Kerr G, Minden H 1988 Psychological factors related to the occurrence of athletic injuries. Journal of Sport & Exercise Psychology 10: 167–173

Kirkby R J 1995 Psychological factors in sport injuries. In: Morris T, Summers J (eds) Sport psychology: Theories, applications and issues. John Wiley, Milton, Australia, p 456–473

Kolt G S 2000 Doing sport psychology with injured athletes. In: Andersen M B (ed) Doing sport psychology. Human Kinetics, Champaign IL, p 223–236

Kolt G S, Hume P 2003 Injury and stress levels in gymnastics: The effects of a stress management program. Medicine & Science in Sports & Exercise 35(5 Suppl): S51

Kolt G S, Kirkby R J 1996 Injury in Australian female competitive gymnasts: A psychological perspective. Australian Journal of Physiotherapy 42: 121–126

Kolt G S, McConville L C 2000 The effects of a Feldenkrais Awareness Through Movement program on state anxiety. Journal of Bodywork and Movement Therapies 4: 216–220

Kolt G S, McEvoy J F 2003 Adherence to rehabilitation in patients with low back pain. Manual Therapy 8: 110–116

Kolt G S, Pizzari T, Schoo A M M et al 2001 The Sport Injury Rehabilitation Adherence Scale: A reliable and valid measure of clinic-based injury rehabilitation. In: Papaioannou A, Goudas M, Theodorakis Y (eds) Proceedings of the 10th World Congress of Sport Psychology (Vol 4, p 144–146). Christodoulidi, Thessaloniki, Greece

Kolt G S, Gill S, Keating J 2002 An examination of the multi-process theory: The effects of two relaxation techniques on state anxiety [Abstract]. Australian Journal of Psychology 54(Suppl): 39

Kubler-Ross E 1969 On death and dying. Macmillan, New York

Lampton C C, Lambert M E, Yost R 1993 The effects of psychological factors in sports medicine rehabilitation adherence. Journal of Sports Medicine and Physical Fitness 33: 292–299

Laubach W J, Brewer B W, Van Raalte J L et al 1996 Attributions for recovery and adherence to sport injury rehabilitation. Australian Journal of Science and Medicine in Sport 28: 30–34

Leddy M H, Lambert M J, Ogles B M 1994 Psychological consequences of athletic injury among high-level competitors. Research Quarterly for Exercise and Sport 65: 347–354

Lehrer P M 1982 How to relax and how not to relax: A re-evaluation of the work of Edmund Jacobson. Behavior Research and Therapy 20: 417–428

Lucic K S, Steffen J J, Harrigan J A et al 1991 Progressive relaxation training: Muscle contraction before relaxation? Behavior Therapy 22: 249–256

Lysens R, Steverlynk A, Vanden Auweele Y et al 1984 The predictability of sports injuries. Sports Medicine 1: 6–10

Macchi R, Crossman J 1996 After the fall: Reflections of injured classical ballet dancers. Journal of Sport Behavior 19: 221–234

McGowan R W, Pierce E F, Williams N et al 1994 Athletic injury and self-diminution. Journal of Sports Medicine and Physical Fitness 34: 299–304

McKenzie A, Howe B L 1997 The effect of imagery on self-efficacy for a motor skill. International Journal of Sport Psychology 28: 196–210

May J R, Brown L 1989 Delivery of psychological services to the U.S. alpine ski team prior to and during the Olympics in Calgary. The Sport Psychologist 3: 320–329

Maynard I W, Hemmings B, Warwick-Evans L 1995 The effects of a somatic intervention strategy on competitive state anxiety and performance in semiprofessional soccer players. The Sport Psychologist 9: 51–64

Meichenbaum D, Turk D C 1987 Facilitating treatment adherence: A practitioner's guidebook. Plenum, New York

Miller W N 1998 Athletic injury: Mood disturbances and hardiness of intercollegiate athletes [Abstract]. Journal of Applied Sport Psychology 10 (Suppl): S127–S128

Morrey M A, Stuart M J, Smith A M et al 1999 A longitudinal examination of athletes' emotional and cognitive responses to anterior cruciate ligament injury. Clinical Journal of Sport Medicine 9: 63–69

Murphy G C, Foreman P E, Simpson C A et al 1999 The development of a locus of control measure predictive of injured athletes' adherence to treatment. Journal of Science and Medicine in Sport 2: 145–152

Nathan B 1999 Touch and emotion in manual therapy. Churchill Livingstone, London

Ninedek A, Kolt G S 2000 Sports physiotherapists' perceptions of psychological strategies in sport injury rehabilitation. Journal of Sport Rehabilitation 9: 191–206

O'Bannon R M, Rickard H C, Runcie D 1987 Progressive relaxation as a function of procedural variations and anxiety level. International Journal of Psychophysiology 5: 207–214

O'Reilly S C, Muir K R, Doherty M 1999 Effectiveness of home exercise on pain and disability from osteoarthritis of the knee: A randomized controlled trial. Annals of the Rheumatic Diseases 58: 15–19

Pargman D (ed) 1999 Psychological bases of sport injury, 2nd edn. Fitness Information Technology, Morgantown, WV

Payne R A 2000 Relaxation techniques. A practical handbook for the health care professional, 2nd edn. Churchill Livingstone, Edinburgh

Pearson L, Jones G 1992 Emotional effects of sports injuries: Implications for physiotherapists. Physiotherapy 78: 762–770

Penpraze P, Mutrie N 1999 Effectiveness of goal setting in an injury rehabilitation programme for increasing patient understanding and compliance [Abstract]. British Journal of Sports Medicine 33: 60

Perna F M, Antoni M H, Baum A et al 2003 Cognitive behavioral stress management effects on injury and illness among competitive athletes: A randomized clinical trial. Annals of Behavioral Medicine 25: 66–73

Petrie T A 1993a The moderating effects of social support and playing status on the life stress–injury relationship. Journal of Applied Sport Psychology 5: 1–16

Petrie T A 1993b Coping skills, competitive trait anxiety, and playing status: Moderating effects of the life stress–injury relationship. Journal of Sport & Exercise Psychology, 15: 261–274

Potter M, Gordon S, Hamer P 2003 The difficult patient in private practice physiotherapy: A qualitative study. Australian Journal of Physiotherapy 49: 53–61

Quinn A M, Fallon B J 1999 The changes in psychological characteristics and reactions of elite athletes from injury onset until full recovery. Journal of Applied Sport Psychology 11: 210–229

Ray R, Wiese-Bjornstal D M (eds) 1999 Counseling in sports medicine. Human Kinetics, Champaign, IL

Richardson P A, Latuda L M 1995 Therapeutic imagery and athletic injuries. Journal of Athletic Training 30: 10–12

Richman J M, Rosenfeld L B, Hardy C J 1993 The Social Support Survey: A validation study of a clinical measure of the social support process. Research on Social Work Practice 3: 288–311

Rotella R J, Ogilvie B C, Perrin D H 1999 The malingering athlete: Psychological considerations. In: Pargman D (ed) Psychological bases of sport injuries, 2nd edn. Fitness Information Technology, Morgantown, WV, p 111–122

Savoy C 1997 Two individual mental training programs for a team sport. International Journal of Sport Psychology 28: 259–270

Scherzer C B, Brewer B W, Cornelius A E et al 2001 Psychological skills and adherence to rehabilitation after reconstruction of the anterior cruciate ligament. Journal of Sport Rehabilitation 10: 165–172

Schlenk E A, Dunbar-Jacob J, Sereika S et al 2000 Comparability of daily diaries and accelerometers in exercise adherence in fibromyalgia syndrome [Abstract]. Measurement and Evaluation in Physical Education and Exercise Science 4: 133–134

Schneiders A G, Zusman G, Singer K P 1998 Exercise therapy compliance in acute low back pain patients. Manual Therapy 3: 147–152

Schomer H H 1990 A cognitive strategy training programme for marathon runners: Ten case studies. South African Journal of Research in Sport, Physical Education and Recreation 13: 47–78

Schoo A M M 2002 Exercise performance in older people with osteoarthritis: Relationships between exercise adherence, correctness of exercise performance and associated pain. Unpublished doctoral dissertation, La Trobe University, Bundoora, Australia

Shaffer S M, Wiese-Bjornstal D M 1999 Psychological intervention strategies in sports medicine. In: Ray R, Wiese-Bjornstal D M (eds) Counseling in sports medicine. Human Kinetics, Champaign, IL, p 41–54

Shelley G A, Sherman C P 1996 The sport injury experience: A qualitative case study [Abstract]. Journal of Applied Sport Psychology 8(Suppl): S164

Sluijs E M, Kok G J, van der Zee J 1993 Correlates of exercise compliance in physical therapy. Physical Therapy 73: 771–786

Smith A M, Milliner E K 1994 Injured athletes and the risk of suicide. Journal of Athletic Training 29: 337–341

Smith A M, Scott S G, O'Fallon W M et al 1990a Emotional responses of athletes to injury. Mayo Clinic Proceedings 65: 38–50

Smith A M, Stuart M J, Wiese-Bjornstal D M et al 1993 Competitive athletes: Preinjury and postinjury mood state and self-esteem. Mayo Clinic Proceedings 68: 939–947

Smith R E, Smoll F L, Ptacek J T 1990b Conjunctive moderator variables in vulnerability and resiliency research: Life stress, social support and coping skills, and adolescent sport injuries. Journal of Personality and Social Psychology 58: 360–369

Spetch L A, Kolt G S 2001 Adherence to sport injury rehabilitation: Implications for sports medicine providers and researchers. Physical Therapy in Sport 2: 80–90

Stenstrom C H, Arge B, Sundbom A 1996 Dynamic training versus relaxation training as home exercise for patients with inflammatory rheumatic diseases: A randomized controlled study. Scandinavian Journal of Rheumatology 25: 28–33

Taylor A H, May S 1996 Threat and coping appraisal as determinants of compliance with sports injury rehabilitation: An application of protection motivation theory. Journal of Sports Sciences 14: 471–482

Taylor J, Taylor S 1997 Psychological approaches to sports injury rehabilitation. Aspen, Gaithersburg, MD

Taylor J, Taylor S 1998 Pain education and management in the rehabilitation from sports injury. The Sport Psychologist 12: 68–88

Thompson N J, Morris R D 1994 Predicting injury risk in adolescent football players: The importance of psychological variables. Journal of Pediatric Psychology 19: 415–429

Treacy S H, Barron O A, Brunet M E et al 1997 Assessing the need for extensive supervised rehabilitation following arthroscopic ACL reconstruction. American Journal of Orthopedics 26: 25–29

Udry E 1996 Social support: Exploring its role in the context of athletic injuries. Journal of Sport Rehabilitation 5: 151–163

Udry E 1997 Coping and social support among injured athletes following surgery. Journal of Sport & Exercise Psychology 19: 71–90

Udry E 1999 The paradox of injuries: Unexpected positive consequences. In: Pargman D (ed) Psychological bases of sport injuries, 2nd edn. Fitness Information Technology, Morgantown, WV, p 79–88

Udry E, Gould D, Bridges D et al 1997 Down but not out: Athlete responses to season-ending injuries. Journal of Sport & Exercise Psychology 19: 229–248

Uitenbroek D G 1996 Sports, exercise, and other causes of injuries: Results of a population survey. Research Quarterly for Exercise and Sport 67: 380–385

United States Department of Health and Human Services 1996 Physical activity and health. A report of the Surgeon General. National Center for Chronic Disease Prevention and Health Promotion, Atlanta, GA

Vealey R A, Greenleaf C A 2001 Seeing is believing: Understanding and using imagery in sport. In: Williams J M (ed) Applied sport psychology: Personal growth to peak performance, 4th edn. Mayfield Publishing, Moutainview, CA, p 247–272

Weaver N L, Marshall S W, Spicer R et al 1999 Cost of athletic injuries in 12 North Carolina high school sports [Abstract]. Medicine and Science in Sports and Exercise 31(Suppl): S93

Webborn A D, Carbon R J, Miller B P 1997 Injury rehabilitation programs: What are we talking about? Journal of Sport Rehabilitation 6: 54–61

Weinstein M, Smith J C 1992 Isometric squeeze relaxation (progressive relaxation) US meditation: Absorption and focusing as predictors of state effects. Perceptual and Motor Skills 75: 1263–1271

Weiss M R, Troxel R K 1986 Psychology of the injured athlete. Athletic Training 21: 104–109, 154

Whitmarsh B G, Alderman R B 1993 Role of psychological skills training in increasing athletic pain tolerance. The Sport Psychologist 7: 388–399

Wiese D M, Weiss M R 1987 Psychological rehabilitation and physical injury: Implication for the sports medicine team. The Sport Psychologist 1: 318–330

Wiese D M, Weiss M R, Yukelson D P 1991 Sport psychology in the training room: A survey of athletic trainers. The Sport Psychologist 5: 15–24

Wiese-Bjornstal D M, Smith A M, Shaffer S M et al 1998 An integrated model of response to sport injury: Psychological and sociological dimensions. Journal of Applied Sport Psychology 10: 46–69

Williams J M, Andersen M B 1997 Psychosocial influences on central and peripheral vision and reaction time during demanding tasks. Behavioural Medicine 26: 160–167

Williams J M, Andersen M B 1998 Psychosocial antecedents of sport injury: review and critique of the stress and injury model. Journal of Applied Sport Psychology 10: 5–25

Wittig A F, Schurr K T 1994 Psychological characteristics of women volleyball players: Relationships with injuries, rehabilitation, and team success. Personality and Social Psychology Bulletin 20: 322–330

Chapter 17

Arthritides

Melainie Cameron

INTRODUCTION

The arthritides are chronic, progressive diseases, for which the causes are mostly unknown, and cures remain elusive. All forms of arthritis and connective tissue diseases (over 100 diseases) are grouped together as the arthritides. Arthritis is generally characterized by pain and joint damage, and may be accompanied by organ and system degradation. Connective tissue diseases are similarly painful and destructive, but damage soft tissue (e.g., skin, ligament, muscle) rather than joint structures. Consistent features of arthritides include pain and stiffness (impairment) and reduced function (disability). People with arthritis may experience both the general psychological consequences of chronic illness, pain, and disability, and psychological issues specific to the condition.

The Arthritis Foundation of the USA reported that osteoarthritis (OA), the most common form of arthritis, is a universal problem directly affecting approximately 1% of adults (Klippel 1997). This broad-based statistic (incidence in adults) is somewhat misleading because the incidence of OA increases with age, and varies according to body site. Incidence is an estimate of the number of new cases of a disease at a point in time (i.e., the percentage of the population that are developing OA at a particular point in time). In a large-scale population study in the USA, Oliveria et al (1995) reported the incidence of OA in the hand, when standardized for age and sex, as 100 per 100 000 person years. Put simply 0.1% of the population developed new cases of OA in the hand every year. From the same study, incidence estimates for OA varied from 0.08% for the hip to 0.24% for the knee. Incidence increased with age, and at ages over 50 years this increase was more pronounced in women than men, such that at 70 years or older, new cases of knee OA among women peaked at 1% per year.

Because OA is a chronic and progressive condition, measures of lifetime prevalence (i.e, the percentage of the population that have ever had OA in their lifetime) provide a picture of the burden of OA in the community. The nature of this disease, and indeed the majority of arthritides, is such that if a person has developed OA at some time in the past, that person will have OA now. In the Framingham Study, a population-based study in Britain, the prevalence of symptomatic OA of the knee was estimated at 9.5% of elderly adults (Felson et al 1987). Peyron & Altman (1992) demonstrated that the prevalence of OA varies between racial groups. Their epidemiological investigation identified that in British Caucasians aged over 35 years, 70% of women and 69% of men displayed diagnostic features of OA, while in Alaskan Eskimos aged over 40 years, the same features were identified in only 24% of women and 22% of men.

Rheumatoid arthritis (RA) has a worldwide distribution and involves people of all ethnic groups. Depending upon the stringency of the diagnostic criteria used in population-based studies, lifetime prevalence estimates vary between 0.3% and 1.5% of the North American adult population (Klippel 1997). Regardless of the precise epidemiology, there is consensus that arthritides are a significant international health problem with considerable impact on the quality of human life (Lorig & Fries 2000).

PHYSICAL AND MEDICAL CONSIDERATIONS

CLASSIFICATION OF THE ARTHRITIDES

The diversity of the arthritides necessitates some classification of diseases to simplify this area of medical practice. Arthritides may be primary (idiopathic, of unknown cause), or secondary to another disease process. For example, primary OA is eventual, age-related "wearing out" of the weightbearing synovial joints of almost everyone who lives long enough. An example of secondary OA is that which occurs in the synovial joints of people with hemophilia following hemarthroses (Flores & Hochberg 1998). Arthritides may be classified as monoarthritic or localized (one or very few types of joints), polyarthritic or generalized (three or more types of joints), or systemic (multiple organs or systems). Classification of arthritides based on the radiographic appearance of joints has limitations, and is not always clinically useful. Arthritides may be further classified according to the pathophysiological mechanisms active in each disease. These mechanisms, however, are not always well understood, and a single disease may fit more than one classification. An overview and comparison of several of the arthritides is shown in Table 17.1.

In pathophysiological classifications, RA is identified as an inflammatory arthritide because it involves a prostaglandin-mediated inflammatory process, and thereby produces joints that are red, hot, swollen, painful, and dysfunctional (Ferrari et al 1996). Some inflammatory arthritides, including RA, are concomitantly classed as autoimmune diseases, in which the immune system fails to differentiate self from non-self tissue and mounts an inflammatory response to its own articular tissues (Shephard & Shek 1997). In other arthritides (e.g., Lyme disease, reactive enteropathic arthritis, Reiter's arthritis) the inflammatory process is triggered by an infection or infestation (Yu & Kuipers 2003).

OA is usually categorized as a degenerative arthritide, which occurs when abnormal physical forces (e.g., macrotrauma or repeated microtrauma) damage articular cartilage. Although the precise mechanism of inflammation is unclear, a moderate inflammatory process follows cartilage damage in OA. It is likely that the by-products of cartilage breakdown stimulate synovitis (Ferrari et al 1996). Radiographically, osteoarthritis is demonstrated by loss of functional joint space, sclerosis and osteophytic outgrowths at joint margins, roughened articular cartilage, and subchondral cyst formation (Yochum & Rowe 1996). OA in the hands produces characteristic nodal formation; Heberden's nodes at the distal interphalangeal joints and Bouchard's nodes at the proximal interphalangeal joints.

Table 17.1   Comparison of types of arthritides

Arthritide	Gender ratio	Age[1]	Location	Distribution	Current understanding of pathophysiology
Ankylosing spondylitis	1F:10M	15–30	Sacroiliac joint, thoracic and lumbar spine, ascending with progression	Polyarticular	Inflammatory, autoimmune
Diffuse idiopathic skeletal hyperotosis (DISH)	Men > women	50+	Spine, enthuses	Polyarticular	Degenerative
Enteropathic	Women > men	15–30	Lumbar spine, hips, sacroiliac joints	Polyarticular	Inflammatory, secondary to gastroenteritis
Erosive osteoarthritis	Women > men	40–50	Distal end proximal interphalangeal joint, small joints of hands and feet	Polyarticular	Inflammatory, inflammatory mediators unknown
Gout	1F:20M	40–50	Metacarpophalangeal joints, metatarsophalangeal joints, great toe, thumb	Monoarticular	Metabolic, crystal deposition disease
Jaccoud's	1F:1M	Variable	Small joints of hands and feet	Polyarticular	Inflammatory, secondary to Streptococcal infection
Lupus (discoid form)	Women > men	15–35		Localized connective tissue disease	Inflammatory, inflammatory mediators unknown
Systemic lupus erythematosis	Women > men	15–35	Hands, face, lungs, soft tissues	Systemic connective tissue disease	Inflammatory, autoimmune
Lyme disease				Polyarticular	Inflammatory, secondary to infection with *Borrelia burgdorferi* (bacterium)
Neuropathic	Varies as per disease	Varies as per disease	Asymmetrical distribution in joints of affected limb/s	Polyarticular	Degenerative, secondary to loss of afferent neurology
Osteoarthritis	Women > men	40+	Asymmetrical distribution in weightbearing joints	Monoarticular	Degenerative, secondary to joint trauma
Osteoarthritis	Women > men	40+	Weightbearing joints, hips, knees	Polyarticular	Degenerative, age related joint function loss
Pseudogout	1F:1M	30–60	Knees, toes	Monoarticular	Metabolic, crystal deposition disease
Reiter's	1F:50M	15–30	Spine, lower limbs	Polyarticular	Inflammatory, secondary to urinary tract infection
Rheumatoid	3F:1M	20–30	Metacarpophalangeal, proximal interphalangeal joints, bilateral, symmetrical distribution in small joints of hands	Polyarticular	Inflammatory, autoimmune

Continued

Table 17.1 Comparison of types of arthritides — cont'd

Arthritide	Gender ratio	Age[1]	Location	Distribution	Current understanding of pathophysiology
Rheumatoid	3F:1M	20–30	Bilateral, symmetrical distribution in small joints of hands	Systemic connective tissue disease	Inflammatory, autoimmune
Scleroderma	Women > men	20–50	Small joints of hands and feet, lungs, gut, soft tissues	Systemic connective tissue disease	Inflammatory, autoimmune

[1]Age is typical age in years at onset of symptoms.

A less common form of osteoarthritis demonstrates erosions of the articulating surfaces in the small joints of the hands, and thus is classed as distinctly inflammatory. This type, known as erosive OA, is typified by the absence of Heberden's and Bouchard's nodes, and may render the interphalangeal joints unstable (Flores & Hochberg 1998).

Table 17.1 highlights that arthritides are not, as frequently assumed, exclusively diseases of the elderly. The symptoms of many arthritides (e.g., joint pain, muscle pain, weight loss) commence in adolescence or early adulthood, and continue through life. Some arthritides are progressively destructive, worsening with increasing age (e.g., OA, RA). In other types, symptoms are somewhat static but persistent (e.g., postinfectious arthropathies such as Lyme disease, Ross River fever, or Reiter's syndrome). Regardless of the type, extent, or location of arthritis, the resultant pain, tissue atrophy, and tissue damage may reduce health-related quality of life (HRQOL) and contribute to the development of disability (Centers for Disease Control and Prevention 2000). Social and psychological sequelae may include social withdrawal, loss and grief, anxiety, depression, and reduced well-being.

DIAGNOSES AND DIAGNOSTIC CRITERIA

Rheumatology is a complex and specialist area of medical practice. Most people with arthritis experience a gradual onset of symptoms, although acute onset of symptoms can occur. Typically, at early stages of arthritis symptoms may be vague, radiographs and serology negative, and the diagnosis unclear. The diagnostic dilemma of early arthritic disease may give way to two equally unfortunate scenarios: people with early arthritic symptoms may be told that they have a range of innocuous musculoskeletal conditions (e.g., bursitis, tendonitis, metatarsalgia), or they may be subject to extensive, but often pointless, tests to investigate for arthritis. As arthritides progress, the clinical markers listed above (symptom picture, radiography, serology) become clearer and the diagnosis apparent.

The American College of Rheumatology (ACR) and American Rheumatism Association, in conjunction with other experts in the field, developed explicit diagnostic criteria for most arthritides (Ferrari et al 1996). ACR criteria for the diagnosis of RA are presented in Table 17.2.

ACR criteria for the diagnosis and classification of OA differ between body regions. The criteria for

Table 17.2 ACR criteria for rheumatoid arthritis (Arnett et al 1988)

1. Morning stiffness lasting longer than 1 hour
2. Arthritis in at least three types of joints
3. Arthritis of the hand joints
4. Symmetrical distribution of arthritis
5. Rheumatoid nodules
6. Rheumatoid factor
7. Joint erosions on radiographs of wrist and hand

Must have at least four items for diagnosis of RA.
Items 1–4 must be present for at least 6 weeks, because polyarthritis of shorter duration may not be due to rheumatoid arthritis, and may resolve spontaneously without a diagnosis.

Table 17.3 ACR criteria for osteoarthritis of the knee (Flores & Hochberg 1998)

Clinical[1]
1. Knee pain for most days of prior month
2. Crepitus on active joint motion
3. Morning stiffness < 30 minutes duration
4. Age > 38 years
5. Bony enlargement of the knee on examination

Clinical, laboratory, and radiographic[2]
1. Knee pain for most days of prior month
2. Osteophytes at joint margins (X-ray spurs)
3. Synovial fluid typical of OA (laboratory)
4. Age > 40 years
5. Morning stiffness < 30 minutes
6. Crepitus on active joint motion

[1]OA present if items 1–4, or 1, 2, 5, or items 1, 5, are present. Sensitivity is 89% and specificity is 88%.
[2]OA present if items 1, 2, or items 1, 3, 5, 6, or items 1, 4, 5, 6, are present. Sensitivity is 94%, and specificity is 88%.

the diagnosis of OA of the knee are presented in Table 17.3.

To assist non-rheumatologists in the diagnosis of arthritis, Ferrari et al (1996) developed a diagnostic algorithm for use in conjunction with ACR criteria (see Figure 17.1). This stringent approach to diagnosis gives the primary contact practitioner confidence in diagnosis and prevents established arthritic disease from being overlooked. ACR criteria provide consistency in diagnosis adequate for participant selection into clinical trials.

MEDICAL MANAGEMENT OF ARTHRITIDES

The pathogeneses of arthritic diseases are not well understood (Ferrari et al 1996, Simon 2000), and although some disease-modifying drug therapies might slow disease progression, no cures have been discovered or developed to date. Typically, outpatient (non-hospitalized) medical care for people with arthritides comprises an array of medications, usually provided under the care of a rheumatologist (Kavanaugh 1999, Klippel 1997, Simon 2000). Commonly used pharmaceutical agents can be grouped into four classes, each with a different therapeutic purpose:

- analgesics, to reduce or limit pain (Simon 1999)

- non-steroidal anti-inflammatory drugs (NSAIDs) to reduce inflammation in joints and surrounding soft tissue
- corticosteroids, used to reduce severe inflammation (Simon 1999)
- disease-modifying antirheumatic drugs (DMARDs), to slow the course of the disease by preventing joint and tissue damage (Kavanaugh 1999). The aims of drug therapy in arthritis are to reduce symptoms and simultaneously prevent, limit, or control, joint damage. Combinations of drugs may be required to achieve these dual aims. Several generations of each drug type are now available. Individuals with arthritis may trial different drug regimes before settling upon the combination that is most effective for them.

If drug therapy is inadequate to control joint destruction then surgical procedures may be used to repair, reconstruct, or replace a damaged joint. Joint debridement, resurfacing, and cartilage grafts are used to repair articulating joint surfaces. Osteotomies, stabilization procedures, and resection arthroplasties (partial joint replacements) are used to realign joints, to improve stability, or maximize congruency between joint surfaces. Joint replacement arthroplasty is used in people with arthritis when a particular joint has become so extensively damaged as to prevent normal function. Total joint replacement is an established surgical procedure for the hip, knee, elbow, shoulder, and interphalangeal joints of the hands, and experimental procedures for other joints are under development (Knutson 1998).

Decisions about surgery are of considerable importance for people with arthritis. In a recent survey of 1024 Norwegian adults with RA, Heiberg & Kvien (2002) asked participants to identify the areas of their own health in which they would most like to see improvement. Hand and finger function (44.6%), walking and bending (33.3%), and mobility (23.9%) were rated as the three priorities immediately behind pain (68.6%). Joint surgeries are undertaken for the express purpose of improving health in these priority areas, but typically require general anesthesia for the surgery, and weeks to months of rehabilitation to gain anticipated function. Both the extent of most arthritides, and the risk of complications from major surgery increase with age (Knutson 1998). People with arthritis will often seek the advice of physical or manual therapists about when to proceed with joint surgery.

THE ALGORITHM

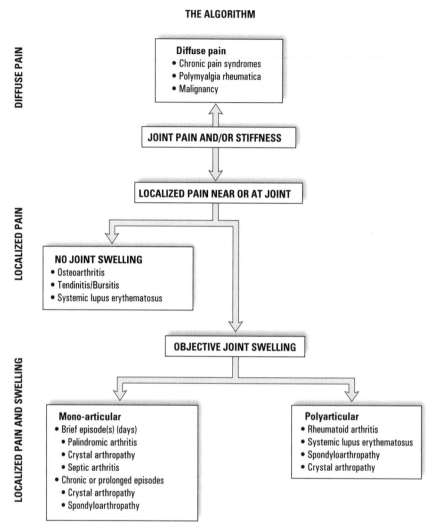

Figure 17.1   Diagnostic algorithm to use in conjunction with American College of Rheumatology criteria for the diagnosis of RA (reproduced from Ferrari et al 1996 with permission of BIOS Scientific Publishers Ltd)

ALLIED MEDICAL, COMPLEMENTARY, AND ALTERNATIVE THERAPIES

Allied medical, complementary, and alternative therapies are often used by people with arthritis (Ramsey et al 2001, Rao et al 1999), and may sometimes be recommended by rheumatologists and other medical personnel (Klippel 1997). Not all complementary and alternative therapies used by people with arthritis are physical or manual therapies (e.g., herbal supplements). Neither will all physical and manual therapists see themselves as alternative or complementary, but for the purposes of organization in this chapter, physical and manual

therapies of all disciplines will be grouped under this heading.

Physical and manual therapies may be divided into two types: active therapies, in which the client takes a driving role, and passive therapies, in which the therapy cannot proceed unless driven by a therapist. This division requires an understanding of how therapy is delivered, and is important from a psychological perspective (Mitchell & Cormack 1998). Some physical therapies used by people with arthritis do not fit neatly into the active/passive subdivisions (e.g., wax therapy, exercise in a group, portable transcutaneous electrical nerve stimulation). These therapies may be active if investigated, sought out, and administered by the client, or somewhat passive if adopted exclusively on the recommendation of a therapist. A broad distinction between physical and manual therapies is that most physical therapies, other than the use of electrophysical agents, are active, and most manual therapies are passive.

Active therapies include exercise and movement programs. Arthritis associations the world over recommend exercise and movement as a self-management strategy for arthritis. Lorig & Fries (2000) have recommended many exercise programs for arthritis management, including aerobic exercise (land-based, water-based, and chair-based), bicycling, flexibility and strengthening exercises for use in the home, and weight training. Movement-based programs recommended for use by people with arthritides include various forms of Tai chi and Qigong (Lam & Horstman 2002).

The evidence for exercise programs as specific therapy for arthritis is somewhat lacking, but the positive effects of exercise on general health and physical function are well documented. Clearly, people who do resistance training become stronger (Maurer et al 1999), people who do aerobic exercise on a regular basis improve their cardiorespiratory capacity. People with arthritis are not exempt from these training-related gains of exercise. Philbin et al (1995) demonstrated that even in elderly people with very advanced and severe OA, regular tailored training programs led to improvements in cardiovascular fitness and muscle strength without exacerbation of arthritic symptoms.

Van den Ende et al (1998, 2002) completed a systematic review of the evidence for dynamic exercise in treating rheumatoid arthritis and concluded that dynamic exercise at 60% of maximal heart rate for 20 minutes, twice per week, for at least 6 weeks, was effective in increasing aerobic capacity and muscle strength in people with RA. Furthermore, this level of training produced no detrimental effects on RA progression. The evidence was inadequate for Van den Ende et al (1998, 2002) to comment on whether such exercise programs had any detrimental effects on joint stability or radiological markers of RA progression, or produced any improvements in functional ability. The paradoxical outcome possible from this review is that people with RA who undertake regular, dynamic exercise may become physically fitter, but not necessarily more able.

Further evidence of the efficacy of exercise came from Thomas et al (2002) who demonstrated, in a clinical trial of 786 people aged over 45 years with self-reported knee pain, that home-based exercise was consistently better than no exercise in controlling pain over 6-, 12-, and 18-month follow-up.

Passive manual therapies used in arthritis management include manipulative physical therapy (physiotherapy), osteopathy, chiropractic, massage, and craniosacral therapy. There is a dearth of evidence as to whether these manual therapies influence arthritis progression or symptoms, but they are widely used by people with arthritis (Lorig & Fries 2000). In Ramsey et al's (2001) analysis of the use of alternative therapies by 124 older adults (aged 55–75 years) with OA, the most commonly used therapies were massage therapy (57%) and chiropractic manipulation (20.7%).

Very few studies provide evidence of efficacy of manual therapies in the treatment of arthritides. Hallas et al (1997) investigated rats with artificially induced OA in the hind limb and found that rats treated with a combination of manual therapy and exercise improved in a range of physical markers, including joint swelling and stride length. Although these findings are not automatically applicable to the human situation, they suggest that manual therapy and exercise may be useful to redress some of the pathophysiological changes induced by articular cartilage destruction.

Many manual therapists consult with people who have arthritic diseases, receive referrals from rheumatologists, and consider the arthritic diseases to be within their field of practice. Professional associations representing manual therapists promote manual therapies to people with arthritic pain, sometimes making claims of efficacy in the absence of evidence of the same from clinical trials. Because "the absence of evidence does not equal evidence of absence," professional associations argue that when clinical trials are conducted it is likely they will demonstrate the efficacy of manual therapy in arthritis management. Clients rarely use published clinical trails as a yardstick by which to evaluate therapy. Anecdotal evidence from years of continued client use suggests that some improvements in HRQOL may be derived from alternative and complementary therapies.

Astin (1998) compared three explanations of why Americans use complementary and alternative medicines:

- dissatisfaction with conventional treatment
- a need to control their own health care

- agreement with the philosophy and ideas of alternative therapies.

He found that the most common reason people sought alternative healthcare was philosophical congruence. These therapies appeal ideologically to clients. Astin's results, interpreted alongside Rao et al's (1999) and Ramsey et al's (2001) reports that manual therapies (chiropractic, osteopathy, massage) are among the alternative therapies most commonly sought by people with arthritis, indicate that it is likely that clients will continue to seek manual therapies for arthritis care regardless of the paucity of research demonstrating efficacy or effectiveness.

PSYCHOLOGICAL CONSIDERATIONS

Arthritic disease correlates to a variable extent with several psychological constructs and markers of psychological dysfunction. Well-documented associations have been found between physical function and depression (Katz & Yelin 1995), and depression and bodily pain (Dexter & Hayes 1998) in people with arthritis. Furthermore, satisfaction with self and abilities (Katz & Neugebauer 2001), self-efficacy (Brekke et al 2001a), internal health locus of control (Norman et al 1998), and positive social support (Riemsma et al 2000) go some way to buffering the negative psychological correlates of arthritic disease.

In most studies of the association between psychological and physical variables in arthritic disease, a temporal relationship has not been established, and so causality cannot be demonstrated. Put simply, we know that depression and pain are linked in rheumatoid arthritis. What we don't know is which causes the other, or even if the relationship is strictly causal. Clinically, sorting out these "chicken and egg" quandaries matters very little (Dexter & Hayes 1998). It is important, however, that physical and manual therapists do not overlook the psychological aspects of arthritic disease. A person with arthritis, who concomitantly is depressed, will be inadequately served by a physical or manual therapist who skirts around (or fails to recognize) depressive symptoms.

PSYCHOLOGICAL CONSTRUCTS IMPORTANT IN ARTHRITIS CARE

Several psychological constructs are of relevance to the management of people with arthritides. Among these are locus of control, self-efficacy, dependence, depression, and anxiety.

Locus of control

Health locus of control (HLC) is one of the most widely researched constructs in health psychology (Norman et al 1998). Studies of HLC are driven by, and investigate the assumption that, people who believe they have control over their own health are more likely to engage in health-promoting behaviors and consciously avoid health-damaging behaviors. The Multidimensional Health Locus of Control Scale (Wallston et al 1978) can be used to measure beliefs about health control along three dimensions, that is, the extent to which individuals believe that their health:

- results from their own actions (internal locus of control)
- is under the control of other powerful people such as doctors and other clinicians (powerful others locus of control)
- is due to fate (chance locus of control).

Norman et al (1998) applied this measure to a stratified sample of 11 632 people representative of the general population of Wales (UK). Their results indicated that each of the HLC dimensions correlated with health behavior. A strong belief that health was under one's own control was significantly correlated with engagement in a greater number of positive health behaviors. As well, a negative correlation was found between chance HLC and health-promoting behaviors. Applying this finding to the arthritides, clients who demonstrate chance locus of control over illness would not be expected to regularly engage in positive health behavior such as an arthritis self-management program. They may commence such a program, but discontinue it within a few weeks, explaining this behavior with a statement such as "The program wasn't helping me."

Self-efficacy

Self-efficacy refers to an individual's perceived ability to do things for him- or herself. People with high self-efficacy feel able to effect their own recovery through action, deliberate rest, and engagement in positive health behaviors. Self-efficacy has been shown to be negatively correlated with the severity of pain (Brekke et al 2001b, Lefebvre et al 1999), and clients with high self-efficacy display fewer pain behaviors than those with low self-efficacy (Lorig

1998). Because of the close relationship between self-efficacy and physical symptoms (e.g., pain) improvement in self-efficacy should be an explicit goal of physical therapy programs for people with arthritis (Rejeski et al 1998).

Dependence

Manual therapies are considered passive because they are practitioner-driven. Clients attend, and often pay for treatment, but are not responsible for developing, planning, or conducting the therapy. Manual therapies draw criticism that they may reinforce behavior patterns of dependency and learned helplessness in clients (Mitchell & Cormack 1998). This criticism is particularly valid when working with clients who, because they experience chronic illness, seek therapy over many years.

Not all people who seek manual therapy display dependent behaviors. Ideally, the client reports consistent improvement over the course of therapy, and ceases to receive manual therapy when they and the therapist agree that satisfactory gains have been made. Mitchell & Cormack (1998) argued that the client who becomes dependent on a manual therapist may either:

- not acknowledge gains in functional ability to avoid discharge from care, or
- resist discharge from care claiming inability to cope with symptoms without the therapist.

Furthermore, dependent clients may experience exacerbation of symptoms or declining functional ability if the therapy is curtailed (i.e., therapist or client moves, relationship ceases). Manual therapists need to be aware of the hallmarks of dependency and conduct therapy in a manner that does not cultivate dependency.

Stages of change

Prochaska and DiClemente (1983) developed a Transtheoretical Model of Change to explain the stages a person moves through to change health behaviors. The stages of change, in chronological order, are:

- precontemplation
- contemplation
- preparation
- action
- maintenance.

This model has been used as the basis for developing interventions to effect health behavior change, both ceasing health-damaging behaviors (e.g., smoking, heroin addiction) and commencing health-promoting behaviors (e.g., regular exercise). Prochaska & DiClemente (1998) have since developed a series of Stage of Change questionnaires to identify the stage of change a client is in at a point in time with regard to a given health behavior.

Kerns & Rosenberg (2000) identified that client-driven (active) therapies may fail to engage a portion of the targeted population, and are associated with high drop-out and relapse rates. They found that in a group of people with chronic pain, the Pain Stages of Change questionnaire could be used to discriminate between those who would complete a course of client-driven treatment, and those who would not. Further, Kerns & Rosenberg (2000) suggested that increased commitment to self-management for chronic pain might improve the probability of therapeutic success.

In another study, Keefe et al (2000) specifically applied the Transtheoretical Model of Change to people with RA and OA, and reported that 55% of respondents identified themselves in the precontemplation and contemplation stages of change. People in these early stages of change are unlikely to participate in client-driven therapies for arthritis. For example, these clients are likely to respond to an invitation to join an arthritis exercise class with comments such as "That's not something I have thought about before" or "I'll consider it and let you know." Information gathering and deliberation need to occur before these clients will be prepared to undertake the life change of commencing a client-driven therapy.

An example of applying the Transtheoretical Model of Change to the promotion of positive health behaviors for arthritic care is shown in Figure 17.2.

LIFE EVENTS, DISEASE ONSET, DIAGNOSIS, AND PSYCHOLOGICAL HEALTH

Allowing for differences in personality type and coping strategies, arthritides are stressful for people because of the life changes associated with all stages of an arthritic disease (Dekkers et al 2001). The course of an arthritic disease may extend 30 years or more, dominating long periods of peoples' lives. Over that time, clients experience symptoms, seek a diagnosis, receive a diagnosis, accept and disclose that diagnosis to others, seek assistance for pain and

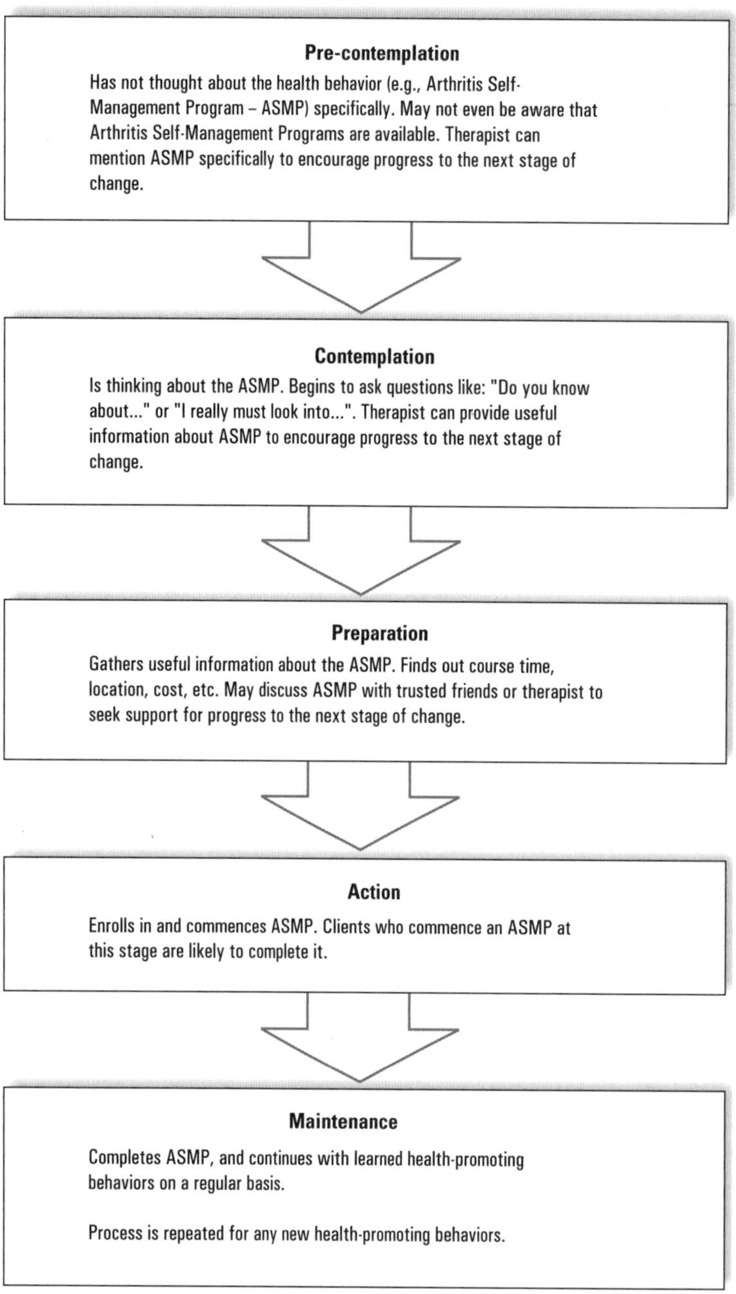

Figure 17.2 Application of the transtheoretical model of change to positive health behaviors for arthritic care (modified from Prochaska & DiClemente 1983)

Pre-contemplation

Has not thought about the health behavior (e.g., Arthritis Self-Management Program – ASMP) specifically. May not even be aware that Arthritis Self-Management Programs are available. Therapist can mention ASMP specifically to encourage progress to the next stage of change.

Contemplation

Is thinking about the ASMP. Begins to ask questions like: "Do you know about..." or "I really must look into...". Therapist can provide useful information about ASMP to encourage progress to the next stage of change.

Preparation

Gathers useful information about the ASMP. Finds out course time, location, cost, etc. May discuss ASMP with trusted friends or therapist to seek support for progress to the next stage of change.

Action

Enrolls in and commences ASMP. Clients who commence an ASMP at this stage are likely to complete it.

Maintenance

Completes ASMP, and continues with learned health-promoting behaviors on a regular basis.

Process is repeated for any new health-promoting behaviors.

declining function, and progressively adapt activities to accommodate these changes.

Life events, both major events (e.g., death of a loved one, marriage, divorce) and daily hassles (e.g., arguments, losing things), affect psychological and physical health, but interrelationships between these variables are far from clear cut (Dohrenwend et al 1984). Diagnosis with a serious or chronic illness is usually considered a major life event. The process of managing a chronic illness (e.g., appointments with health practitioners, medication regimes) may contribute to daily hassles. In one study, Dekkers et al (2001) investigated the relationships between major life events, daily hassles, psychological well-being, and biological markers of disease activity in 54 people with a recent diagnosis of RA. They found that major life events and daily hassles were significantly correlated and that major life events and daily hassles were correlated with psychological distress but not with disease activity.

Arthritides may be acute, subacute, or chronic in onset. Acute arthritides are easily identified and diagnosed according to ACR criteria, but often carry a poor prognosis. Acute-onset rheumatic disease can have a major impact on an individual as they may be required to cease working, be confined to bed, and commence major drug therapy in the period of a few days. People with acute-onset arthritis can experience considerable distress associated with these rapidly ensuing major life changes.

Alternatively, the onset of arthritis may be slow, commencing with arthralgia (joint pain) or stiffness. Chronic-onset arthritis is a diagnostic dilemma, because the symptoms and signs may be non-specific, and serology and radiographic imaging are often negative (Ferrari et al 1996). Stringent adherence to the ACR criteria is not without problems. Harrison et al (1998) studied a cohort of people in rural England with inflammatory polyarticular arthritis and concluded that the ACR criteria do not well identify those people with early arthritis who will go on to develop RA. There is consensus among rheumatologists that the ACR criteria allow diagnostic certainty, but adherence to these criteria forces clients to wait until their clinical signs are obvious before diagnoses are confirmed.

Prognostically, chronic-onset arthritis is better than any other presentation because joint damage occurs later in the disease, and sometimes may be prevented. Clients with chronic-onset arthritides have time to adapt to this major life event, however, they may complain that it took a long time for a diagnosis to be found. The uncertainty of the "waiting game" can have negative psychological consequences, including self-doubt (e.g., "maybe it's all in my head") and fear of the unknown (e.g., "what if it's. . ."), which may lead to catastrophizing, blaming of health practitioners, or avoidance of health practitioners (a form of denial). The process of continuing to seek a diagnosis may exacerbate daily hassles.

Given the conclusions of Dekkers et al (2001) that major life events and daily hassles were linked to psychological stress, it is in the interest of clients'

psychological well-being that arthritic diagnoses should be made accurately, and as early in the disease course as possible, regardless of the nature of symptom onset. The ACR criteria for the diagnosis of RA were last reviewed in 1987 (Arnett et al 1988), and Visser et al (2002) recently suggested that a review of these criteria be undertaken in light of new investigative techniques for arthritis.

DMARDs are expensive drugs, with considerable side effects. In the late 1980s people with arthritides were no better served by early diagnosis than by waiting until their symptoms fulfilled the ACR criteria because DMARDs were prescribed only for those clients with advanced joint destruction. DMARDs were reserved as "second-line" therapy because of the expense and side effects (e.g., liver toxicity) of their use, and because the understanding at that time was that erosion and joint damage were long term consequences of synovitis, inflammation, and swelling. Current understanding is that joint damage occurs far earlier than previously believed. Joint erosions in RA may occur within the first year (Van der Heijde 1995), and early instigation of drug therapy considerably improves long-term outcomes (Symmons et al 1998). Three recent independent clinical trials have demonstrated that treatment with DMARDs early in the course of RA is superior to delaying DMARDs for as little as 8–12 months (Egmose et al 1995, Tsakonas et al 2000, Van der Heide et al 1996). In the current climate, clients with RA are likely to be prescribed powerful pharmacological agents with many side effects soon after diagnosis, and consequently are likely to experience rapid life changes, and psychoemotional distress associated with these changes.

PAIN

Pain is a highly subjective phenomenon, and may produce emotional as well as physical responses (Kugelmann 2000). There is no single type of arthritic pain. Pain is a feature of all types of arthritic disease, but is not a consistent marker of any one physiological or pathological process (Klippel 1997). Kugelmann (2000) conducted a qualitative investigation of pain, and demonstrated that the experience of pain differed little according to cause, making it pointless to differentiate between biological and psychological pain.

Heiberg & Kvien (2002) surveyed 1024 Norwegians with RA. These participants reported that pain was their highest priority for health improvement. The preference for pain as the most desired area of health improvement was consistent across all subgroups. It follows that pain is probably the central feature of reduced quality of life for people with arthritis. Ironically, one-third of those participants with a preference for improvement in pain were not using analgesic medication. Reasons for this finding were not explored within the study, but many medications used in arthritis management have substantial side effects. For example, NSAIDs are prescribed to reduce inflammation and reduce pain within joints, but are associated with the development of upper gastrointestinal tract toxicity (e.g., nausea, ulcer formation, and upper gut hemorrhage) (Hogan et al 1994, Smalley et al 1996). Furthermore, dyspepsia is a symptom that decreases quality of life for people with arthritis (Parr et al 1989). In using NSAIDs to control pain, it is possible that people with arthritis might improve one aspect of HRQOL and sacrifice another.

Pain is related to several areas of psychological health. For example, pain is consistently positively correlated with depression in people with arthritis (Salaffi et al 1991, Wolfe & Hawley 1993), and in some studies the strength of this correlation is such that depression may more accurately predict pain variability than objective disease measures (e.g., radiographic signs, painful joint count, erythrocyte sedimentation rate) (Dexter & Hayes 1998).

Although the type and stage of arthritis may influence the nature of pain (e.g., people with RA experience episodic "flares" of symptoms, in which painful joints become tender, hot, and red), the vast majority of people with arthritic diseases experience chronic pain as well as episodes of acute pain, and in due course, may adopt pain behaviors associated with chronic pain states.

Pain behavior

Avoidance of pain is a primitive human response. Retraction from a painful stimulus is a reflex that is preserved even partly into unconsciousness. In arthritic disease, pain can be chronic but variable, and may be aggravated by a range of activities. A particularly common pain behavior of people with arthritic disease is to avoid those activities that aggravate pain. Initially, this pain behavior seems logical and reasonable, but avoidance of an activity may worsen arthritis over the long term despite the short-term benefit of reduced pain.

Despite evidence that regular, low-impact exercise (e.g., walking, water aerobics, tai chi) is of long-term benefit for pain (Maurer et al 1999, Thomas et al 2002), many people with arthritis experience increased joint pain when attempting activities that mechanically stress joints (Lorig & Fries 2000). When daily activities aggravate pain, negative self-talk and reluctance to exercise may follow. For example, people with arthritis may comment that "It hurts just putting on my sports shoes, how will I ever manage to go for a walk?", or "I can't turn door handles or taps without pain. I couldn't possibly use a hand-held weight for exercises." The paradox in this pain behavior is that lack of physical activity leads to further physical deterioration such as reduced muscle strength and cardiovascular fitness. Furthermore, avoidance of an activity may not resolve pain entirely.

In one approach to modifying pain behavior Multon et al (2001) tested the effect of stress management training on pain behaviors in 131 people with RA. Although participants in the intervention group reported reduced pain and reduced stress, their pain behaviors (e.g., grimacing, active rubbing of muscles, sighing) did not alter significantly from the non-intervention or attention control groups. Multon et al (2001) suggested that these pain behaviors are not necessarily a direct response to pain, but a more complex pattern of behaviors, a product of disease activity, age, and disease duration.

Refer to Chapter 11 for a more detailed description of pain and pain behavior.

THE SICK ROLE: JOINT PROTECTION AS A CASE STUDY

Adoption of the sick role is a psychobehavioral part of the illness process. At its simplest level, adoption of the sick role occurs when a person with an acute viral infection takes to bed for a couple of days. The behavior (bedrest) is an illness behavior. It marks the person as "sick," but it also affords recovery. The sick role is not so simple in chronic illness.

Adoption of the sick role in arthritic disease is much more complicated because illness behavior does not necessarily promote recovery. Regardless of illness behavior, people with arthritic diseases are likely to remain sick. Strategic use of illness behavior may prevent deterioration, but it will not reverse the disease process. Poorly used illness behavior may exacerbate arthritic disease. It is important that people with arthritides understand the sick role and adopt it wisely.

Consider joint protection as an illness behavior widely promoted for people with arthritis. In a joint protection program the sick role is used for the purpose of preventing joint damage. Joint protection comprises avoiding joint movements that are particularly painful, mechanically stressful on joints, and render joints vulnerable to injury (Klippel 1997). Gait aids (e.g., walking sticks) and orthotic devices such as splints may be used to prevent loading of joints. These highly visible items label the client as "sick."

Joint protection is an intuitively logical therapy. If a joint can be protected from mechanical stress, and thereby from inflammation, that joint is unlikely to deteriorate. Hammond et al (1999) conducted a cross-over trial comparing two programs of joint protection education in 35 people with RA. Results indicated that adherence to joint protection strategies was greater following one educational strategy rather than the other, but no significant physical or psychological improvements were identified at any point post-intervention. Measures of pain, functional disability, grip strength, self-efficacy, and helplessness did not change significantly from the pre-intervention state. If joint protection does not improve physical or psychological well-being, why is it taught?

When the sick role is publicly visible, as is often the case in joint protection, a variety of reactions may follow. Some clients abhor the idea of being seen as sick, reject the sick role outright, deny any benefits the sick role may offer, and continue to engage in activities that may worsen their health. For example, people may turn down the opportunity to use a disabled parking permit and aggravate their condition by having to walk greater distances than necessary for activities of daily living (e.g., shopping for food). Persistence with health-damaging behaviors is not a likely explanation of Hammond et al's (1999) findings, because they measured adherence to joint protection and found it to be increased when strong educational strategies were employed.

As part of a joint protection program, a person who enjoyed running, but had osteoarthritis in the knees, would be discouraged from jogging on land, and encouraged to participate in activities that load less mechanical force on the joints (e.g., jogging in water, swimming, cycling). If acceptable alternative exercise could not be found, the client might refrain from exercise altogether, and detraining effects (i.e., reduced aerobic capacity, reduced endurance, decreased muscle strength, muscle atrophy) could follow. Although the client could be said to have "protected" his or her joints, the net value of this type of joint protection is highly questionable.

Some people enjoy the "benefits" of a visible sick role (e.g., use of a walking stick may result in preferential treatment in shopping queues). Adoption of the sick role is not usually a deliberate manipulation to seek benefit. Rather, when secondary gain arises from the sick role the client's motivation to adopt the sick role becomes blurred. A client with pain and swelling in her small finger joints, who happens not to enjoy her job as a word processor due to interpersonal conflict in her workplace, experiences considerable secondary gain (e.g., avoiding the interpersonal conflict) when she takes time off work for her pain. Similarly, family, friends, and concerned loved ones, may leap to the assistance of a person with arthritic disease, taking on unpleasant duties usually done by that person. This behavior affords secondary gain to the sick role and decreases the likelihood of relinquishing that role (Gatchel & Turk 1999).

It is beholden upon therapists who prescribe joint protection strategies to do so in a way that minimizes the deleterious effects of the sick role. Try to use joint protection as a way of continuing with activities of daily living. For example, say: "Use this brace/stick/orthosis when you walk/run/play sport" rather than "Don't run, it's bad for your knees."

DEPRESSION

Depression is common among people with arthritides. Depression rates in people with OA and RA do not differ substantially from those in other chronic disease populations, but more people with arthritis are depressed than in the general population (Hawley & Wolfe 1993).

Pain and depression are positively correlated in arthritic disease (Salaffi et al 1991, Wolfe & Hawley 1993). It is unclear whether arthritis contributes to depression, or depression to arthritis, or both. There is overlap between the symptoms associated with arthritides and symptoms of depression (e.g., fatigue, insomnia, weight loss) (American Psychiatric Association 1994). Bodily pain is an inherent feature of arthritis, but is also a symptom of psychological pain in people without arthritis (Kugelmann 2000). Regardless of whether the client is a depressed person who has arthritis, or a person with arthritis who becomes depressed, the symptom pictures interplay (Wolfe & Hawley 1993).

Depression following a diagnosis of arthritis often appears exogenous, that is external to the physiology of the individual, arising as a psychological consequence of physical and social loss. However, the pathophysiology of the arthritides is poorly understood, and there is room to question whether associated depression may be endogenous (Scammell & Brown 1998), possibly a response to some unidentified chemical mediator. This endogenous theory of depression in people with arthritis may help explain why depression is so common in this client group, and why depression does not always resolve in those people who regain physical function (Dexter & Hayes 1998). If depression is an inherent feature of arthritis, as Scammell & Brown (1998) suggested, then appropriate treatment of arthritis necessitates management of depression. It would be grossly inadequate, and possibly unethical, to offer therapy only to ameliorate joint pain.

If depression in arthritis is endogenous, then depression should be a clinical feature, to a greater or lesser extent, in all clients with arthritis. The counter to this argument is evidence that not everyone with arthritides appears depressed (Dexter & Hayes 1998). Advice to therapists at this time is to be aware of the signs and symptoms of depression and to establish appropriate referral networks to facilitate screening and diagnosis where necessary.

Antidepressant medications are sometimes used in the management of depression with arthritides, particularly when depressive symptoms include disturbed sleep patterns. Adequate sleep is vital for pain control in arthritis (Lorig & Fries 2000). Conversely, poor sleep patterns can fuel a downward spiral of pain, causing fatigue and reduced function, which leads to altered levels of daily activity, and thus to further disturbance of sleep patterns. Antidepressant drugs may help break into this cycle, and even clients who do not recognize their own depression may be willing to use low-dose antidepressants to rectify sleep patterns (Ferrari et al 1996).

It is important to identify and manage depression in people with arthritis, because depression may aggravate pain, compromise activities of daily living, and promote social withdrawal (Dexter & Hayes 1998). Put simply, depression can exacerbate many of the negative consequences of arthritis. Clients have a far greater chance of success in managing their arthritis if they are not concomitantly depressed (Dexter & Hayes 1998).

ANXIETY

Conceptually, anxiety and depression differ, but clinically, there is much symptom overlap between these conditions (American Psychiatric Association 1994). Much of the time anxiety and depression occur together (Dexter & Hayes 1998). Anxiety is to be expected in people with arthritis as they worry about their future health, well-being, and function (Lorig & Fries 2000). One example of an anxiolytic event for people with RA has been reported to be worries over intra-articular corticosteroid injections and first hospital admissions (Edwards et al 2001).

There is little evidence that mild anxiety exacerbates arthritis, except if concurrent depression aggravates pain. In fact the astute clinician may use mild anxiety associated with the contemplation stage of change to motivate the client to manage their disease responsibly in order to shore up some certainty for the future (Prochaska & DiClemente 1998). For example, a client who is worried (mildly anxious) about future lung function in systemic sclerosis (scleroderma) may be encouraged to stop cigarette smoking. That said, tapping into health-related anxiety to motivate clients to change should be used with some caution, because of recent evidence that the process of thinking about personal health risks may increase anxiety and the need for reassurance (Lister et al 2002).

Moderate to severe anxiety may compromise the care of a person with arthritic disease by limiting appropriate engagement with the processes of management. The person who is worried about side effects of medication may either not take medication as prescribed, or identify side effects in themselves, whether or not such side effects are actually present (hypochondriasis). Because of the potentially stifling nature of moderate to severe anxiety, it needs to be identified and treated, possibly via anxiolytic medication, as part of the overall management of arthritis.

LOSS AND GRIEF

General losses associated with arthritides include loss of bodily function and body image, loss of social role, and loss of social support. These losses are experienced psychologically as any significant loss, and produce grief responses. Grief may comprise shock, displays of emotion, depression, physical symptoms of distress, guilt, hostility, resentment, and an inability to continue usual activities. Because these losses may be protracted, grief may be experienced over a prolonged period.

Individuals also experience specific and unique losses. For example, in a case I have managed, Jean, a retired music teacher and accomplished musician, struggled to come to terms with the loss of the dexterous hand function required to play piano. When Jean moved from her own home into a serviced room in an aged care center, she sold or gave away most of her furniture. Because she was not ready to admit the loss of her ability to play music, Jean did not dispose of her piano, but negotiated with the aged care center to house her piano in the dining and function room of the center. Jean cannot play the piano anymore, but the piano stands in the function room as a reminder of her previous abilities.

LOSS OF BODILY FUNCTION

Over the long term, all arthritides reduce body function, and produce impairment (Lorig & Fries 2000). Physical impairments consistent in arthritis are loss of joint range of motion and loss of muscle strength. Persistence of these impairments leads to reduced capacity for activity and exercise, which produces further impairments such as loss of cardiovascular endurance and loss of bone density. Loss of bodily function in arthritis can be delayed by early and judicious drug therapy (Symmons et al 1998), but it cannot be prevented altogether. Even people with mild or static forms of arthritis will eventually face issues associated with loss of bodily function, even if it occurs as a result of the interaction of mild arthritis with the frailty of old age (Philbin 1995).

As an example of the impact of arthritis on bodily function, and hence other capacities, Turner et al (2002) interviewed 12 ex-professional football (soccer) players about their experiences of developing OA. Of the 12 participants, five had retired early, from all paid employment, not just football, due to OA. Recurrent themes emerging from these interviews were of physical impairment producing loss of bodily function and negative social consequences including reduced work capacity, lowered income, and loss of both self-image and self-worth.

LOSS OF SOCIAL ROLE

Social role is partly determined by physical function and work capacity (Turner et al 2002) and allows people to identify their place in society, and to contribute to the structure and life of the community. Because social roles attract status, people may draw self-esteem from them.

People with arthritis often experience a decline in social roles because the damage to their joints, weakness and atrophy of their muscles, and fatigue and lack of endurance that characterize arthritis prevents them from participating in the physical tasks required in such roles. Social rules which may diminish in this way range from manual-based employment to caring for family members. Loss of social roles may occur slowly, with a gradual realization that the person with arthritis is simply "not keeping up" with everyone else. One of Turner et al's (2002, p 293) ex-footballers described his gradual loss of work-related social role thus: "I have got an FA coaching badge, which has got me work over in Norway, Iceland and South Africa, and I coached a few clubs here [UK]. But nobody wants you with a bad limp. You know it is embarrassing. Like if you are a coach you've got to demonstrate. You don't want to be stood there with a walking stick. So in 1992, I had to really call it a day."

People with arthritis, like almost everyone else, are reluctant to reduce involvement in social roles they enjoy, and so they may try to prevent these losses by modifying the way they perform physical tasks. This strategy is successful in many situations, and clinicians are well placed to assist clients in adapting activities (Lorig & Fries 2000).

Barlow et al (2001) assessed the effectiveness of the Into Work Personal Development (IWPD) program with people with arthritis (all types). The IWPD program is aimed at preventing work disability by reducing the internal and external barriers to employment presented by disease. In this study, 79 people with arthritis were divided (not randomized) into intervention and control groups, and assessed pre- and post-delivery of the program via self-report questionnaires and in-depth interviews. Participants in the IWPD program demonstrated significant decreases in measures of anxiety, depression, negative mood, and improvements in positive mood, satisfaction with life, and self-esteem. A glaring omission in Barlow et al's study, however, is that they failed to measure how many participants actually entered work of any kind. Furthermore, not all of the post-intervention gains were maintained at 6-month follow-up. Removing perceived barriers to employment for people with arthritis is only part of the issue. Physical capacity to do work must also be addressed if people with arthritis are to be in gainful employment.

ECONOMIC LOSS

Due to the diversity and far-reaching effects of arthritides, broad-based estimates of the public health impact of arthritic diseases are difficult to ascertain. Economic costs of arthritis are both direct (i.e., money spent on medical care) and indirect (e.g., wages lost through reduced capacity for paid work). Yelin & Callahan (1995) reported that the economic impact of all forms of arthritis on the economy in the United States of America during 1992 was $US15.2 billion in direct medical costs and $US49.6 billion in indirect costs.

Arthritis seriously impairs work ability and leads to reduced individual and household incomes. Meenan et al (1981) found that people with RA had a 50% decline in earnings over a 9-year period, accounting for an average 37% reduction in family income.

Lapsley et al (2001) conducted an investigation to determine the "out of pocket" expenses associated with living with OA. Because the study was conducted in Sydney, Australia, all costs were reported in Australian dollars. Women spent significantly more than men on arthritis care, a mean of $537.15 per annum compared with $258.31, and higher expenditure was also related to more advanced disease. Most of the additional expenditure by women was on prescription and non-prescription medications and "private services." It is reasonable, in the Australian healthcare context, to assume that "private services" were allied health services such as physiotherapy or osteopathy, that are not covered under the Australian government universal free access medical scheme (i.e., Medicare). Lapsley et al's (2001) data are consistent with general data on the use of health services in Australia; that women use both public and private health services to a greater extent than men. Against the backdrop of the Australian healthcare system that provides heavily subsidized health services and a pharmaceutical benefits scheme, Lapsley et al's findings emphasize the personal cost of OA.

LOSS OF SOCIAL SUPPORT

Social roles offer social support. Employed people have the social role of employees, and by meeting other people in the workplace are afforded the social support of colleagues. People who are unable to maintain a social role may experience reduced social support. Rarely are communities so generous as to support those who do not contribute to the life of the community, so a corollary of social withdrawal is loss of social support. Drawing again on the Lapsley et al (2001) study, 33% of women identified reduced opportunities for sporting and outdoor activities as a mode by which OA affected family and other close relationships.

Social support may be positive if it provides affirmation or timely assistance, or problematic if it is neither desired nor needed, or if the support offered does not match the client's needs. Riemsma et al (2000) demonstrated, in a study of 229 people with RA, that positive social support counters feelings of depression, but problematic social support correlates positively with depression. Problematic and positive social support also interact with each other, such that "the negative aspects of problematic support may be partly diminished by positive support" (p 221).

When people with arthritis become socially disabled, they may seek social support from a small circle of family members and intimate friends. Sometimes professional carers and clinicians are recruited into this social network, but the burden of social support is primarily borne by those who live with the individual. Burnout and illness are common amongst those who care for chronically ill people with arthritis (Pollard 2000).

It is unreasonable to expect all an individual's social and emotional needs to be satisfied by a single relationship. Unfortunately, many people with arthritis behave in precisely this fashion when they become housebound. To protect the health of carers, and to provide adequate positive social support for themselves, people with arthritis are encouraged to keep up whatever social roles they can, for as long as they can, and if socially disabled, to seek social support from more than one person (Lorig & Fries 2000).

LOSS OF BODY IMAGE

It is intuitively logical that potentially disfiguring arthritides might influence clients' body image, but this topic has received little coverage in published literature. Since 1987, six English language studies on the effects of arthritides on body image have been published in peer-reviewed medical literature, and four of these studies focused only on female participants. It appears that researchers and practitioners alike tend to overlook the negative effects of arthritides on body image, especially for male clients. For example, Lorig & Fries (2000) discussed many of the feelings that clients with arthritis report, but did not mention distress specifically over body image. In Turner et al's (2002) study, one participant reported feelings of embarrassment, but none spoke specifically of body image.

Body image is linked to arthritic disease profile, and also to age and self-esteem, but the relationships between these variables are unclear. People with RA very rarely describe themselves as "attractive" (Skevington et al 1987). Attractiveness tends to be included in the self-concept of people with high self-esteem, and is therefore unlikely in people who are in pain or chronically ill.

The studies that have looked at body image in the arthritides report interesting and relevant findings. For example, Cornwell & Schmitt (1990) compared the perceived health status, self-esteem, and body image of women with RA or systemic lupus erythematosis (SLE) with healthy controls. They found that perceived health status was significantly related to self-esteem, but not to body image. Further, women with SLE had lower mean body image scores than women in the other two groups. A client with SLE typically develops a red, butterfly-shaped facial rash (across cheeks and nose), and may develop photosensitive rashes on the face and arms. These highly visible signs of arthritic disease present a considerable affront to even the most robust body image. According to Cornwell & Schmitt (1990), a woman with SLE may see herself as quite healthy yet have poor body image, while conversely, a woman with RA may see herself as sick but have positive body image.

In another study, Hider et al (2002) investigated men and women with ankylosing spondylitis (AS). They found that, unlike healthy adults, those with AS did not report a positive effect on body image from engagement in regular exercise. Packham & Hall (2002) conducted a long-term follow-up of 246 adults with juvenile idiopathic arthritis (JIA) of 28.3 years average duration. JIA had a detrimental effect on body image in 50.7% of participants, and negatively affected intimate relationships in 28.2%.

It could be that JIA has a greater influence on body image than other arthritides because it develops in childhood and persists through adolescence. In a further study, Vamos et al (1990) surveyed 80 women with RA and found that body image (particularly negative feelings about the hands) was a significant predictor of these women seeking RA-related surgery. It can be seen, therefore, that practitioners should carefully consider the range of effects on body image that the arthritides can have during treatment and rehabilitation.

PSYCHOLOGICAL INTERVENTIONS

Physical and manual therapists are ideally placed to encourage clients to see things in a different light. Discussion with clients often occurs during treatment sessions. The physical or manual therapy provides both the setting for the discussion, and adequate distraction if the discussion becomes too confronting at any stage (Kolt 2000). Therapists' language, and behavior towards clients can be used to reinforce the consideration of psychological issues.

Take for example, a client who has experienced some loss (e.g., inability to continue with a favorite activity) due to arthritic disease. Progress can be made through the loss associated with arthritis if the client is able to consciously distinguish the loss from self-image and self-worth. The therapist can engage the client in discussion about the sources from which the client draws self-image and self-worth, and encourage the client to shape self-esteem in new and appropriate ways. As the therapist treats the client with respect, this behavior reinforces the message that clients are valuable in and of themselves.

Physical and manual therapists are in a powerful position to influence uptake or rejection of the sick role. As discussed earlier, the sick role is to be encouraged in so far as it prevents progression of disease and protects against further joint damage, however, the sick role should be discouraged when its adoption would allow disease progression or the development of comorbidities. A delicate balance between simultaneously adopting and rejecting the sick role is required, so that the sick role might be used to promote health rather than undermine it.

Relationship and discussion are not always adequate to bring about psychological change in clients. Explicit psychological interventions demonstrated to be effective in arthritis care include relaxation, electromyographic (EMG) biofeedback, counseling, and cognitive behavioral therapy (Astin et al 2002). Specifically, these interventions impacted positively on pain, functional disability, psychological status, coping, and self-efficacy (Astin et al 2002). An important trend emerging from Astin et al's work was that psychological interventions appeared to be more effective in clients who had shorter illness duration. If needed, physical or manual therapists may recommend direct psychological interventions for clients by referral to an appropriately qualified practitioner (e.g., psychologist).

A more specific account of psychological interventions can be found in Chapter 8 (Cognitive and behavioral interventions), Chapter 9 (Relaxation techniques), Chapter 10 (Imagery), and Chapter 11 (Pain and its management).

INTEGRATED MANAGEMENT STRATEGIES

No therapies clearly and consistently arrest the natural course of arthritic diseases (Ferrari et al 1996). Usually, people with the arthritides experience chronic, incurable, progressive illnesses, and must adapt their lives and daily activities accordingly (Lorig & Fries 2000). Improvements in quality of life and functional ability are usually the main goals of treatment. Kavanaugh (1999) suggested that improvement in quality of life is a key goal of therapy for people with RA. Simon (1999, p 26) argued the same case for people with OA, and summarized the ethos of current care approaches: "Given that most patients must learn to live with a disease that may significantly alter their earning potential, basic function, and lifestyle, it is important to develop a treatment system that views the patient as a whole, using methods enlisting the patient's enthusiasm for therapy and allowing them to participate in their own care."

PSYCHOLOGICAL INTERVENTION IN MANUAL THERAPIES

Many physical and manual therapies have been inadequately researched, and because of the physical contact component of these therapies, they do not fit well into the double-blind clinical trial model of efficacy research (Chambless & Hollon 1998). This issue makes it difficult to determine the "effective ingredients" in the therapeutic encounter.

The therapist–client relationship may be one of the prime therapeutic aspects of treatment (Mitchell & Cormack 1998, Petitpas et al 1999) and for clients with arthritic disease, who experience loss of social support, this aspect of therapy is likely to be particularly important. For people not ready (i.e., not in the appropriate stage of change) to adopt self-management approaches, practitioner-driven manual therapies may offer rational, but largely untested, approaches to pain management. Physical and manual therapists are well advised to employ passive therapies judiciously. The purpose of physical and manual therapy in arthritis care is at least partly as a vehicle of communication with the client, to encourage the client to move towards self-management of chronic illness.

CARE CONTRACT

A care contract is a simple agreement between the client and the therapist that covers the goals of therapy, an estimate of when those goals will be achieved, and a process for measuring whether the goals are achieved. It is possible to maintain a verbal care contract, but written contracts are less likely to be neglected. Because a care contract is a mutual agreement, the goals of therapy are at least partly set by the client.

A mutually agreed care contract can be used in passive therapies to enlist the client's enthusiasm, allow client participation in care, and encourage progress towards self-management. The care contract is not a new idea, but it is a particularly useful one for clients with chronic illnesses who are at risk of becoming dependent upon their therapists. It is also a useful disciplinary strategy for therapists, who have vested financial interest in not discharging clients from care (Mitchell & Cormack 1998). Various forms of care contract are regularly used in institutional settings (e.g., hospitals) and are required by third parties (e.g., workers' compensation bodies) to determine how many treatment sessions will be paid for. The use of care contracts in private physical and manual therapy practice is somewhat lax.

Hammond et al's (1999) study of joint protection programs demonstrated that an educational program comprised of goal-setting, contracts, and other educational reinforcements resulted in considerably greater use of joint protection than an "ordinary" program. This increase in use occurred in people who gleaned no physical or psychological benefits from joint protection (e.g., reduced pain). Clearly, care contracts are powerful tools for motivating client behavior, and therapists are well advised to use contracts to encourage behaviors that are demonstrated to be beneficial (e.g., a graduated strength training program).

PHYSICAL ACTIVITY AS PSYCHOLOGICAL THERAPY

The relationship between exercise (physical activity) and health, in both clinical and non-clinical populations, has been widely researched and well documented (Paluska & Schwenk 2000). Physical activity is associated with improvement in key markers of psychological well-being and HRQOL, including mood, self-perception, health perception, and self-efficacy (Rejeski et al 1998), as well as anxiety, depression, and subjective well-being (Morgan 1997). The exact processes by which exercise promotes changes in psychological well-being and HRQOL are uncertain, but the value of exercise for enhancing both mental and physical health is well supported by research.

Physical inactivity leads to substantial negative effects on health, including muscle weakness, atrophy, and fatigue. Leading a sedentary life may compound the loss of quality of life associated with chronic illness. Inactivity is well correlated with depressed mood, reduced sociability, and a decline in well-being (Morgan 1997).

In summary, exercise is of benefit for people with arthritis. Exercise improves muscle strength, lessens pain, and reduces joint stiffness (Maurer et al 1999). Further, exercise in a group or with an individual therapist may also offer important social support.

ARTHRITIS SELF-MANAGEMENT PROGRAM

One approach to self-management in arthritis is the Arthritis Self-Management Program (ASMP) developed in 1979 by Kate Lorig at Stanford University in the US which has been widely adopted internationally (Australia, New Zealand, Denmark, Canada, South Africa, Iceland, Finland, Norway, Hong Kong, UK, Lithuania, Czech Republic, and The Netherlands) (Lorig & Fries 2000). The ASMP is typically conducted for small groups (tutorial classes of between ten and 20 participants) in 2-hour weekly sessions for 6 weeks. Participation in regular gentle exercise (e.g., hydrotherapy/warm-water exercise, tai chi, low-impact land-based aerobics, seated aerobics/exercise in a chair), without altering typical drug therapy, education about arthritis, and cognitive behavioral therapy, are the mainstays of this program. The ASMP includes direct psychological intervention. Participants are instructed in the nature and transmission of pain, and made aware of pain behaviors, illness behaviors, and the sick role. Participants are encouraged to take responsibility for their own illness behaviors (i.e., move to a more internal HLC) and to make deliberate and considered choices about when and how they will adopt the sick role (i.e., self-efficacy).

Clinical trials investigating the medium- (4 months) and long-term (12 months) outcomes of the ASMP in the UK (Barlow et al 1998) and US (Lorig & Holman 1989, Lorig et al 1981, 1989, 1993) have consistently shown that people with arthritis derive substantial and prolonged benefits in their perceived ability to manage arthritis, reduction in pain, and improved psychological well-being (Barlow et al 1998). Preliminary data from a similar study currently underway in Australia (G McColl, unpublished work, 2001) add weight to the suggestion that the ASMP is useful across cultural boundaries. Local Arthritis Foundations will usually hold details of ASMPs available for your clients.

A caution is necessary at this juncture. The ASMP is an active, client-driven, therapy. Only people near the end of preparation, or in the action or maintenance stages of change with regard to this health-promoting behavior, are likely to complete the program or derive benefits from it (Keefe et al 2000, Kerns & Rosenberg 2000). Furthermore, not completing the ASMP may contribute to clients' feelings of incompetence or failure. Therapists should listen carefully to clients for indications of their stage of change (see Figure 17.2), and reserve deliberate promotion of the ASMP for those clients ready to proceed.

MULTIDISCIPLINARY CARE

Given the diversity within the arthritides and the absence of any certain cure, solo manual and physical therapists are likely to find the management of people with arthritis beyond their scope. Physical and manual therapists are well advised to develop a network of colleagues with diverse skills to contribute to the management of people with arthritis.

Multidisciplinary health care teams usually have one leader – the primary care practitioner – and other practitioners who contribute to specific areas of healthcare as required. Physical or manual therapists might lead healthcare teams, but more likely team leaders are family physicians (general practitioners) and rheumatologists. Bidaut-Russell et al (2002) investigated the relationship between patient satisfaction with healthcare and the type of practitioner (general practitioner versus specialist rheumatologist) delivering that care in 86 adults with RA. They found that patients' overall satisfaction with healthcare delivery was unaffected by practitioner type.

In a study of clinical outcomes in people with RA, Yelin et al (1998) found that patients of rheumatologists were less likely to progress in disability compared with patients of general practitioners.

Given the potential effects of anxiety and depression on people with arthritis, links with psychologists and mental health practitioners may be particularly useful. People with arthritis may require either specific psychological counseling or medication for anxiety or depression. If depressive symptoms are severe (e.g., delusions, suicidal tendencies, etc.) in people with arthritis, referral to an appropriately qualified practitioner is necessary (Dexter & Hayes 1998).

Given the considerable evidence in favor of exercise as a psychological as well as physical therapy, a multidisciplinary care team might include someone to prescribe appropriate exercises. In addition to the skills of professionals such as physical therapists in this area, other practitioners that go by a variety of names (e.g., exercise leader, athletic trainer, coach, personal trainer, rehabilitation officer), can be of use in this area of healthcare.

Weighing the evidence together, satisfactory healthcare teams may be led by either specialist or generalist practitioners. Involvement of a rheumatologist at some level in any healthcare team may be necessary to provide the best-quality physical care over the long term. Healthcare teams comprised of practitioners from many disciplines may be better able to cover all the aspects of healthcare delivery that are important to patients.

SUMMARY

The effects of arthritis are complex and largely interdependent. Pain may produce physical disability, which in turn can produce social disability and changes in HRQOL. Joint and muscle disuse resulting from physical disability produces muscle atrophy, bone density loss, and may lead to further pain.

People with arthritis should be encouraged to manage their own illness and take responsibility for their own care in the long term. Both physical and manual therapies may be appropriate for people with arthritis, depending upon their readiness to adopt self-management strategies.

ASMPs, based on Lorig's work, are offered through arthritis foundations in many countries around the world. These programs have been well evaluated, and shown to improve both physical and psychological well-being in people with arthritis. Furthermore, these programs appear to reduce the direct healthcare costs associated with arthritis care (Lorig et al 1993). ASMPs are of greatest use to people in the action and maintenance stages of change (Kerns & Rosenberg 2000).

Therapists can use consultations as a vehicle for communication with clients, and to assist them in the transition from practitioner-driven to client-driven care, from the early to later stages of change. Practitioners of the passive (usually manual) therapies are advised to use deliberate tactics such as mutually agreed care contracts to prevent client dependence.

ACKNOWLEDGMENTS

Through her life, my mother, Carrolle Cowdery, taught me a great deal about the psychological effects of arthritic disease. With gratitude and love, I dedicate this work to her memory.

References

American Psychiatric Association 1994 Diagnostic and statistical manual of mental disorders, 4th edn. American Psychiatric Association, Washington, DC

Arnett F C, Edworthy S M, Bloch D A et al 1988 The American Rheumatism Association 1987 revised criteria for the classification of rheumatoid arthritis. Arthritis and Rheumatism 31: 315–324

Astin J A 1998 Why patients use alternative medicine: Results of a national study. Journal of the American Medical Association 279: 1548–1553

Astin J A, Beckner W, Soeken K et al 2002 Psychological interventions for rheumatoid arthritis: A meta-analysis of randomized controlled trials. Arthritis and Rheumatism 47(3): 291–302

Barlow J H, Turner A P, Wright C C 1998 Long-term outcomes of an arthritis self-management programme. British Journal of Rheumatology 37(12): 1315–1319

Barlow J, Wright C, Kroll T 2001 Overcoming perceived barriers to employment among people with arthritis. Journal of Health Psychology 6(2): 205–216

Bidaut-Russell M, Gabriel S E, Scott C G et al 2002 Determinants of patient satisfaction in chronic illness. Arthritis and Rheumatism 47(5): 494–500

Brekke M, Hjortdahl P, Kvien T K 2001a Involvement and satisfaction: A Norwegian study of health care among 1024 patients with rheumatoid arthritis and 1509 patients with chronic noninflammatory musculoskeletal pain. Arthritis Care and Research 45: 8–15

Brekke M, Hjortdahl P, Kvien T K 2001b Self efficacy and health status in rheumatoid arthritis: A two-year longitudinal observational study. Rheumatology 40: 387–392

Centers for Disease Control and Prevention 2000 Health-related quality of life among adults with arthritis: Behavioral risk factor surveillance system, 11 states, 1996–1998. Morbidity and Mortality Weekly Report 49: 366–369

Chambless D L, Hollon S D 1998 Defining empirically supported therapy. Journal of Consulting and Clinical Psychology 66: 7–18

Cornwell C J, Schmitt M H 1990 Perceived health status, self-esteem and body image in women with rheumatoid arthritis or systemic lupus erythematosis. Research in Nursing & Health 13(2): 99–107

Dekkers J C, Geenan R, Evers A W M et al 2001 Biopsychosocial mediators and moderators of stress–health relationships in patients with recently diagnosed rheumatoid arthritis. Arthritis Care and Research 45: 307–316

Dexter P A, Hayes J R 1998 Depression in osteoarthritis. In: Brandt K D, Doherty M, Lohmander L S (eds) Osteoarthritis. Oxford University Press, Oxford, UK, p 338–349

Dohrenwend B S, Dohrenwend B P, Dodson M 1984 Symptoms, hassles, social support, and life events: Problem of confounded measures. Journal of Abnormal Psychology 93: 222–230

Edwards J, Mulherin D, Ryan S et al 2001 The experience of patients with rheumatoid arthritis admitted to hospital. Arthritis Care and Research 45: 1–7

Egmose C, Lund B, Borg G et al 1995 Patients with rheumatoid arthritis benefit from early 2nd line therapy: 5-year followup of a prospective double blind placebo controlled study. Journal of Rheumatology 22: 2208–2213

Felson D T, Naimark A, Anderson J et al 1987 The prevalence of knee osteoarthritis in the elderly. Arthritis and Rheumatism 30(8): 914–918

Ferrari R, Cash J, Maddison P 1996 Rheumatology guidebook: A step-by-step guide to diagnosis and treatment. BIOS Scientific, Oxford, UK

Flores R H, Hochberg M C 1998 Definition and classification of osteoarthritis. In: Brandt K D, Doherty M, Lohmander L S (eds) Osteoarthritis. Oxford University Press, Oxford, p 1–12

Gatchel R J, Turk D C (eds) 1999 Psychosocial factors in pain: Critical perspectives. Guilford Press, New York

Hallas B, Lehman S, Bosak A et al 1997 Establishment of behavioral parameters for the evaluation of osteopathic treatment principles in a rat model of arthritis. Journal of the American Osteopathic Association 97(4): 207–214

Hammond A, Lincoln N, Sutcliffe L 1999 A crossover trial evaluating an educational–behavioural joint protection programme for people with rheumatoid arthritis. Patient Education and Counseling 37(1): 19–32

Harrison B J, Symmons D P M, Barrett E M et al 1998 The performance of 1987 ARA classification criteria for rheumatoid arthritis in a population based cohort of patients with early inflammatory polyarthritis. Journal of Rheumatology 25: 2324–2330

Hawley D J, Wolfe F 1993 Depression is not more common in rheumatoid arthritis: A 10 year longitudinal study of 6153 patients with rheumatic disease. Journal of Rheumatology 20: 2025–2031

Heiberg T, Kvien T K 2002 Preferences for improved health examined in 1024 patients with rheumatoid arthritis: Pain has highest priority. Arthritis and Rheumatism 47(4): 391–397

Hider S, Wong M, Oritz M et al 2002 Does a regular exercise program for ankylosing spondylitis influence body image? Scandinavian Journal of Rheumatology 31(3): 168–171

Hogan D B, Campbell N R C, Crutcher R et al 1994 Prescription of nonsteroidal anti-inflammatory drugs for elderly people in Alberta. Canadian Medical Association Journal 151: 315–322

Katz P P, Neugebauer A 2001 Does satisfaction with abilities mediate the relationship between the impact of rheumatoid arthritis on valued activities and depressive symptoms? Arthritis Care and Research 45: 263–269

Katz P P, Yelin E H 1995 The development of depressive symptoms among women with rheumatoid arthritis: The role of function. Arthritis and Rheumatism 38: 49–56

Kavanaugh A 1999 Increasing aggressiveness in rheumatoid arthritis treatment. Paper presented at the annual meeting of the American College of Rheumatology, Boston, MA

Keefe F J, Lefebvre J C, Kerns R D et al 2000 Understanding the adoption of arthritis self-management: Stages of change profiles among arthritis patients. Pain 87: 303–313

Kerns R D, Rosenberg R 2000 Predicting responses to self-management treatments for chronic pain: Application of the pain stages of change model. Pain 84: 49–55

Klippel J H (ed) 1997 Primer on the rheumatic diseases, 11th edn. Arthritis Foundation, Atlanta, GA

Knutson K 1998 Arthroplasty and its complications. In: Brandt K D, Doherty M, Lohmander L S (eds) Osteoarthritis. Oxford University Press, Oxford, p 388–402

Kolt G S 2000 Doing sport psychology with injured athletes. In: Andersen M B (ed) Doing sport psychology. Human Kinetics, Champaign, IL, p 223–236

Kugelmann R 2000 Pain in the vernacular: Psychological and physical. Journal of Health Psychology 5(3): 305–313

Lam P, Horstman J 2002 Overcoming arthritis. Dorling Kindersley, Melbourne, Australia

Lapsley H M, March L M, Tribe K L 2001 Living with osteoarthritis: Patient expenditures, health status, and social impact. Arthritis Care and Research 45: 301–306

Lefebvre J C, Keefe F J, Affleck G et al 1999 The relationship of arthritis self efficacy to daily pain, daily mood, and daily coping in rheumatoid arthritis patients. Pain 80: 425–435

Lister A, Rode, S, Farmer A et al 2002 Does thinking about personal health risk increase anxiety? Journal of Health Psychology 7(4): 409–414

Lorig K 1998 Patient education. In: Brandt K D, Doherty M, Lohmander L S (eds) Osteoarthritis. Oxford University Press, Oxford, p 324–330

Lorig K, Fries J F 2000 The arthritis helpbook, 5th edn. Perseus Books, Cambridge, MA

Lorig K, Holman H 1989 Long-term outcomes of an arthritis self-management study: Effects of reinforcement efforts. Social Science Medicine 29: 221–224

Lorig K, Kraines R G, Holman H 1981 A randomized prospective controlled study of the effects of health education for people with arthritis. Arthritis and Rheumatism 24(4 suppl): S90

Lorig K, Seleznick M, Lubeck D et al 1989 The beneficial outcomes of the arthritis self-management course are inadequately explained by behavior change. Arthritis and Rheumatism 32(1): 91–95

Lorig K, Mazonson P, Holman H 1993 Evidence suggesting that health education for self-management in patients with chronic arthritis has sustained health benefits while reducing health care costs. Arthritis and Rheumatism 36(4): 439–446

Maurer B T, Stern A G, Kinossian B et al 1999 Osteoarthritis of the knee: Isokinetic quadriceps exercise versus an educational intervention. Archives of Physical Medicine and Rehabilitation 80(10): 1293–1299

Meenan R F, Yellin E H, Nevitt M et al 1981 The impact of chronic disease. Arthritis and Rheumatism 24: 544–549

Mitchell A, Cormack M 1998 The therapeutic relationship in complementary health care. Churchill Livingstone, Edinburgh

Morgan W P 1997 Physical activity and mental health. Taylor & Francis, Washington, DC

Multon K D, Parker J C, Smarr K L et al (2001) Effects of stress management on pain behavior in rheumatoid arthritis. Arthritis Care and Research 45: 122–128

Norman P, Bennett P, Smith C et al 1998 Health locus of control and health behavior. Journal of Health Psychology 3(2): 171–180

Oliveria S A, Felson D T, Reed J I et al 1995 Incidence of symptomatic hand, hip, and knee osteoarthritis among patients in a health maintenance organization. Arthritis and Rheumatism 38: 1500–1505

Packham J C, Hall M A 2002 Long-term follow-up of 246 adults with juvenile idiopathic arthritis: Social function, relationships, and sexual activity. Rheumatology (Oxford) 41(12): 1440–1443

Paluska S A, Schwenk T L 2000 Physical activity and mental health: Current concepts. Sports Medicine 29: 167–180

Parr G, Darekar B, Fletcher A et al 1989 Joint pain and quality of life; Results of a randomized trial. British Journal of Clinical Pharmacology 27: 235–242

Petitpas A J, Danish S J, Giges B 1999 The sport-psychologist–athlete relationship: Implications for training. The Sport Psychologist 13: 344–357

Peyron J G, Altman R D 1992 The epidemiology of osteoarthritis. Cited in: Klippel J M (ed) 1997 Primer on the rheumatic diseases, 11th edn. Arthritis Foundation, Atlanta, GA

Philbin E F, Groff G D, Ries M D, Miller T E 1995 Cardiovascular fitness and health in patients with end-stage osteoarthritis. Arthritis and Rheumatism 38: 799–805

Pollard J 2000 Caring for someone with arthritis. Age Concern, London

Prochaska J O, DiClemente C C 1983 Stages and processes of self-change of smoking: Toward an integrative model of change. Journal of Consulting and Clinical Psychology 51: 390–395

Prochaska J O, DiClemente C C 1998 Towards a comprehensive, transtheoretical model of change: States of change and addictive behaviors. In: Miller R W, Heather N (eds) Applied clinical psychology, 2nd edn. Plenum Press, New York, p 3–24

Ramsey S D, Spencer A C, Topoloski T D et al 2001 Use of alternative therapies by older adults with osteoarthritis. Arthritis Care and Research 45: 222–227

Rao J K, Mihaliak K, Kroenke K et al 1999 Use of complementary therapies for arthritis among patients of rheumatologists. Annals of Internal Medicine 131: 409–416

Rejeski W J, Ettinger W H Jr, Martin K et al 1998 Treating disability in knee osteoarthritis with exercise therapy: A central role for self-efficacy and pain. Arthritis Care and Research 11(2): 94–101

Riemsma R P, Taal E, Wiegman O et al 2000 Problematic and positive support in relation to depression in people with rheumatoid arthritis. Journal of Health Psychology 5(2): 221–230

Salaffi F, Cavalieri F, Nolli M et al 1991 Analysis of disability in knee osteoarthritis: Relationship with age and psychological variables, but not with radiographic score. Journal of Rheumatology 18: 1581–1586

Scammell H, Brown T M 1998 The new arthritis breakthrough. M Evans, New York, p 158–163

Shephard R J, Shek P N 1997 Autoimmune disorders, physical activity, and training, with particular reference to rheumatoid arthritis. Exercise Immunology Review 3: 53–67

Simon L S 1999 Osteoarthritis: A review. Clinical Cornerstone 2: 26–34

Simon L S 2000 Treatment strategies in osteoarthritis. Paper presented at the annual meeting of the American College of Rheumatology, Philadelphia, PA

Skevington S M, Blackwell F, Britton N F 1987 Self-esteem and perception of attractiveness: An investigation of early rheumatoid arthritis. British Journal of Medical Psychology 60(1): 45–52

Smalley W E, Griffin M R, Fought R L et al 1996 Excess costs for gastrointestinal disease among nonsteroidal anti-inflammatory drug users. Journal of General Internal Medicine 11: 461–469

Symmons D P M, Jones M A, Scott D L et al 1998 Long-term mortality outcomes in patients with rheumatoid arthritis: Early presenters continue to do well. Journal of Rheumatology 25: 1072–1077

Thomas K S, Muir K R, Doherty M et al 2002 Home based exercise programme for knee pain and knee osteoarthritis: Randomised controlled trial. British Medical Journal 325: 752–757

Tsakonas E, Fitzgerald A A, Fitzcharles M A et al 2000 Consequences of delayed therapy with second-line agents in rheumatoid arthritis: A 3 year followup on hydroxychloroquine in early rheumatoid arthritis (HERA) study. Journal of Rheumatology 27: 623–629

Turner A, Barlow J, Ilbery B 2002 Play hurt, live hurt: Living with and managing osteoarthritis from the perspective of ex-professional footballers. Journal of Health Psychology 7(3): 285–301

Vamos M, White G L, Caughey D E 1990 Body image in rheumatoid arthritis: The relevance of hand appearance to desire for surgery. British Journal of Medical Psychology 63(3): 267–277

Van den Ende C H, Vliet Vlieland T P, Munneke M et al 1998 Dynamic exercise therapy in rheumatoid arthritis: A systematic review. British Journal of Rheumatology 37(6): 677–687

Van den Ende C H, Vliet Vlieland T P, Munneke M et al 2002 Dynamic exercise therapy for treating rheumatoid arthritis (Cochrane Review). The Cochrane Library 4

Van der Heide A, Jacobs J W, Bijlsma J W et al 1996 The effectiveness of early treatment with "second-line" antirheumatic drugs: A randomised, controlled trial. Annals of Internal Medicine 124: 699–707

Van der Heijde D M 1995 Joint erosions and patients with early rheumatoid arthritis. British Journal of Rheumatology 34: 74–78

Visser H, le Cessie S, Vos K et al 2002 How to diagnose rheumatoid arthritis early: A prediction model for persistent (erosive) arthritis. Arthritis and Rheumatism 46: 357–365

Wallston K A, Wallston B S, DeVellis R 1978 Development of multidimensional health locus of control (MHLC) scales. Health Education Monographs 6: 160–170

Wolfe F, Hawley D J 1993 The relationship between clinical activity and depression in rheumatoid arthritis. Journal of Rheumatology 20: 2032–2037

Yelin E H, Such C L, Criswell L A, Epstein W V 1998 Outcomes for persons with rheumatoid arthritis with a rheumatologist versus a non-rheumatologist as the main physician for this condition. Medical Care 36: 513–522

Yellin E, Callahan L F 1995 The economic cost and social and psychological impact of musculoskeletal conditions. Arthritis and Rheumatism 38: 1351–1362

Yochum T R, Rowe L J 1996 Essentials of skeletal radiology, 2nd edn. Williams and Wilkins, Baltimore, MD, p 804–832

Yu D, Kuipers J G 2003 Role of bacteria and HLA-B27 in the pathogenesis of reactive arthritis. Rheumatic Disease Clinics of North America 29(1): 21–36

Chapter 18

Functional somatic syndromes

Rona Moss-Morris, Wendy Wrapson

INTRODUCTION

Physical and manual therapists will often see a patient who presents with an idiosyncratic range of diffuse symptoms such as aches and pains in various joints and muscles, bad headaches, and feelings of weakness and fatigue. Your clinical assessment suggests that there is no particular biomedical explanation for the symptoms, however, as a physical therapist, you feel it is important to provide symptomatic relief. You try a number of different treatment techniques. The effect on the symptoms is minimal and consultations frequently run over the allotted time. Despite these facts the patient keeps coming back demanding further treatment or investigation. You are convinced that neither of these will be particularly beneficial, but in order to appease the patient you either refer on or continue with some form of treatment.

Clinical situations such as this are often extremely frustrating both for the patient and the therapist. The patient is clearly experiencing a number of symptoms that are extremely distressing to them. The therapist may feel that the lack of biomedical findings should reassure the patient, whereas the patient often believes that the actual cause of the disorder has yet to be discovered. The patient is left feeling misunderstood, while the therapist feels that disproportionately heavy demands have been made on him for what appears to be largely medically unexplained symptoms.

The frustration engendered by these patients is due in part to certain underlying attitudes inherent in the practice of Western medicine. Engel & Charles (2000) argued that in our current Western practice, medicine is seen as the reserve of patients whose symptoms are the consequences of clearly defined pathology. Psychiatry, on the other hand, is viewed for patients whose symptoms are not biologically based. Where does that leave patients who present with somatic complaints in whom medical investigations fail to reveal medical pathology? These patients are frequently viewed as the "undeserving sick," the "worried well," or people who are "merely mad" rather than "really ill" (Engel & Charles 2000). It is often implied that these patients are "putting on" or "imagining" their symptoms (Stone et al 2002). These attitudes are maintained by many of the education programs for health professionals, where little information is provided on the etiology and treatment of medically unexplained symptoms. Consequently, many health professionals feel they lack the training or knowledge to deal with these patients.

There is a growing recognition that the attitudes described above are changing. It is becoming increasingly difficult to divide disorders into physical versus psychological, as there now exists a substantial body of research supporting the role of biological factors in explaining psychological disorders, and psychological factors in explaining the level of disability afforded by medical disorders (Engel & Charles 2000). Recent surveys also suggest that a substantial proportion of patients present to healthcare professionals with medically unexplained symptoms. A World Health Organization study found that medically unexplained symptoms were common in all the cultures and countries studied (Gureje et al 1997). These patients made up around 20% of primary care attendees and half remained disabled a year after presentation. The problem is even more extensive in tertiary care, with as many as 50% of new referrals to outpatient specialist clinics presenting with medically unexplained symptoms (Gureje et al 1997, Nimnuan et al 2001a). The cost and impact of these conditions is immense (Lloyd & Pender 1992). There are direct costs associated with increased utilization of healthcare resources and indirect costs related to sick days and cessation or reduction in employment. There are also tremendous personal costs in disability and suffering.

The increasing recognition of the clinical and public health importance of the problem is reflected in the sharp rise in research publications in this area over the past couple of decades. The *British Medical Journal* published an ABC series in 2002 focusing exclusively on disorders that are medically unexplained. Whereas these patients are often given the message that health professionals cannot explain their symptoms, there is in fact a large body of recent literature which helps to provide a coherent understanding of these conditions and how best to manage them.

This chapter will begin by providing an overview of the key functional somatic syndromes (FSS). A biopsychosocial model of the etiology of these syndromes is presented. This is followed by a discussion of the medical and psychological factors that should be taken into account when treating patients with FSS. The final section deals with treatment issues. The treatment of these conditions is primarily focused on the reduction of disability through modification of behavior and environmental contingencies rather than on removing underlying organic pathology.

FUNCTIONAL SOMATIC SYMPTOMS AND SYNDROMES

TERMINOLOGY AND CLASSIFICATION OF FUNCTIONAL SOMATIC SYNDROMES

Several terms are used in the literature to describe the problem of somatic symptoms that cannot adequately be explained by organic findings. These include medically unexplained symptoms, somatization, subjective health complaints, abnormal illness behavior, and functional symptoms. The latter term is preferred, as it assumes a disturbance in bodily functioning rather than a psychological etiology. When patients' functional symptoms are severe enough to significantly interfere with their daily functioning, they may be diagnosed with a FSS (Manu 1998).

A number of different FSS have been described. In fact most specialist areas of medicine have a FSS associated with them. The names of the most commonly occurring syndromes in each area of specialty and a summary of their key features are presented in Table 18.1. Some of the syndromes, such as chronic fatigue syndrome (CFS) (Fukuda et al 1994), fibromyalgia (Wolfe et al 1990), and irritable bowel syndrome (IBS) (Thompson et al 1999), have well-researched, published diagnostic criteria.

These diagnoses are based on a specified symptom profile together with the exclusion of certain medical or psychiatric conditions that may be contributing to the symptoms. Conditions such as non-specific chronic low back pain rely on the clinical decision that the extent of the pain, and disability afforded by the pain, cannot adequately be explained by any organic findings (van Tulder et al 2002). Patients with back pain caused by pathological entities such as vertebral disorders, neoplasms, osteoporosis, rheumatoid arthritis or fractures usually would not be considered to have a FSS.

Table 18.1 Functional somatic syndromes and their key characteristic symptoms

Syndromes by specialty	Key characteristic symptoms
Infectious diseases/endocrinology Chronic fatigue syndrome	Disabling and persistent fatigue Impairment in memory and concentration Muscle and joint pain, headaches, sore throat
Rheumatology Fibromyalgia	Persistent musculoskeletal aches, pains, and stiffness in specified multiple sites
Orthopedics Non-specific chronic low back pain	Persistent pain in the lower back which cannot be adequately explained by an initial injury or musculoskeletal changes
Gastroenterology Irritable bowel syndrome	Abdominal pain that is relieved by defecation and is associated with a change in frequency/consistency of stool Experiencing bloating, urgency, or strain, feeling incomplete after finishing a bowel movement
Dentistry Temporomandibular joint dysfunction	Pain in the face, jaw, or mouth Limitation of jaw movement, pain aggravated by chewing or moving jaw, clicking or popping noises in the jaw on opening or closing
Neurology Tension headache	Headache or neck pain Pain is aggravated by stress, gets worse as day progresses
Cardiology Non-cardiac chest pain	Chest pain, which occurs at rest and is not associated with exertion Pain usually lasts longer than 20 minutes
Respiratory medicine Hyperventilation	Breathing more than normal Associated with two or more of the following: feeling dizzy or faint, heart pounding, numbness or tingling, trembling
Gynecology Premenstrual syndrome	Irritability, mood swings, anxiety, food cravings, increased appetite, fatigue, breast tenderness, and abdominal bloating Symptoms appear just before the period and disappear soon afterwards
Chronic pelvic pain	Pain in the lower abdomen which is not specifically related to the menstrual cycle and has a duration of at least 6 months
Allergy Multiple chemical sensitivity	Adverse reactions to multiple chemically unrelated substances, at lower levels of exposure than commonly tolerated

The diagnosis of other conditions such as hyperventilation syndrome is more controversial, with some researchers insisting it should be diagnosed using physiological tests of hyperventilation, while others suggest a specified symptom profile is more valid (Spinhoven et al 1993, Vansteenkiste et al 1991). At the extreme end of the spectrum are illnesses such as multiple chemical sensitivities, which are not recognized as legitimate syndromes by the international medical organizations despite the fact that the diagnosis is popular with patients and with some healthcare professionals, particularly those who practice alternative medicine (Terr 1998).

FSS are by definition chronic conditions. All the definitions except premenstrual syndrome require that patients must have experienced the symptoms for at least 3 months, with some illnesses such as CFS, tension headache, and chronic pelvic pain having a cut-off of 6 months (Manu 1998, Nimnuan et al 2001a).

Most of the studies on FSS focus on a particular condition. However, there appears to be substantial overlap in the presentations of these illnesses. A recent review of the case definitions of these disorders found that eight definitions contained headache as a core symptom, while six contained fatigue and abdominal distention (Wessely et al 1999). Patients with one FSS frequently meet diagnostic criteria for others (Aaron & Buchwald 2001, Nimnuan et al 2001b). Some authors have suggested that the diagnosis patients receive depends largely on the specialist they are referred to (Shorter 1995, Wessely et al 1999). For example, if a patient seems to be most troubled by fatigue they will be referred to an infectious diseases specialist who may diagnose a postviral CFS. If the same patient is referred to a rheumatologist, they may be more likely to focus on asking questions about painful symptoms or tender points, and the patient could be diagnosed with fibromyalgia. There are certainly some patients who only meet criteria for one disorder, but the overlap is substantial enough to suggest that similar casual factors may be associated with all the FSS (Barsky & Borus 1999).

CAUSAL FACTORS

The cause of FSS has been the subject of significant debate over the past decade. This debate has been anchored by three major postulates: that FSS are an atypical presentation of psychiatric disorders such as anxiety and depression; that FSS represent underlying psychic distress which presents in a somatic fashion; and that FSS are biological disorders reflected in subtle changes to the central nervous, neuroendocrine, and/or immune systems (Manu 1998). These postulates all assume a dualistic stance (i.e., FSS are either psychological or biological in origin). However, there is growing acceptance that these dualistic stances are unhelpful both in explaining the disorder to the patient and in formulating appropriate management strategies (Mayou & Farmer 2002).

Strong evidence now exists to suggest that biological, psychological, and social causes all need to be taken into consideration in understanding the etiology of FSS. It is also useful to understand how each of these causes can operate and interact as predisposing, precipitating, and perpetuating factors (Mayou & Farmer 2002, Surawy et al 1995). Table 18.2 provides a summary of possible causal factors and how these may interact in precipitating and perpetuating a FSS. For example, predisposed people may be highly achievement orientated, basing their self-esteem and the respect from others on their abilities to live up to certain high standards. When these people are faced with precipitating factors that affect their ability to perform, such as a combination of excessive stress and an acute biological illness or injury, their initial reaction is to press on and keep coping. This behavior leads to the experience of ongoing symptoms that may be more closely related to pushing too hard than to the initial insult or injury. However, in making sense of the situation, patients attribute the ongoing symptoms to biological factors. This protects their self-esteem by avoiding the suggestion that their inability to cope might be a sign of personal weakness. The common response to a physical illness is rest. However, reduced activity conflicts with achievement orientation and may result in bursts of activity in an attempt to meet expectations. These periodic bursts of activity inevitably exacerbate symptoms and result in failure, which further reinforces the belief that they have a serious illness. As time goes by, efforts to meet previous standards of achievement are abandoned and patients become increasingly preoccupied with their symptoms and illness. They become fearful of overactivity as this appears to make symptoms worse. This results in chronic disability and the belief that one has an ongoing incurable illness which is eventually diagnosed as one of the FSS.

The interactional model described above has the potential to accommodate both the differences and

Table 18.2 The interaction of possible causal factors in functional somatic syndromes

Causes	Predisposing factors	Precipitating factors	Perpetuating factors
Biological	Genetics Sensitized CNS reactivity	Viral or bacterial illness Injury Allergic reaction	Effects of immobility Lack of fitness Disrupted circadian rhythms CNS arousal and sensitivity Excessive bracing or altered movement patterns
Psychological	History of psychiatric disorder Childhood trauma Achievement-orientated personality	Prolonged stress Negative life events	Interpreting ongoing symptoms as signs of biological disease or trauma Focusing on symptoms Fear that activity will worsen symptoms Catastrophizing about the negative effects of symptoms/exertion
Social	Parental expectations to achieve Society's antipathy towards psychiatry Illness role models	Dissatisfaction with work Employers'/doctors' responses to time off work	Oversolicitous care Litigation processes Support groups

the overlap between the conditions. The factors that precipitate the disorders may be different. It may be a viral or bacterial infection, an adverse reaction to a particular substance, a musculoskeletal overuse pattern, or a specific injury. Patients may also have different predisposing factors such as a genetic propensity for a particular disorder, an achievement-orientated personality, high levels of social desirability, and/or high levels of stress. However, the necessary common features of these disorders appear to be the perpetuating factors. In the following sections a more detailed explanation of how the psychosocial perpetuating factors interact with the biological factors in contributing to the symptoms and disability experienced by patients with FSS is provided.

MEDICAL AND PHYSICAL CONSIDERATIONS

DIAGNOSIS AND ASSESSMENT

There is no specific medical test for FSS. Diagnoses are essentially based on exclusion. In order to be diagnosed with a FSS, patients need to meet specific symptom criteria, and the presence of psychiatric or medical conditions that could explain the symptoms need to be ruled out. For example, patients who present with CFS-like symptoms would need to have thyroid problems, possible malignancies, and sleep apnea ruled out. Patients presenting with

IBS symptoms would need to be assessed for bowel cancer, Crohn's disease, ulcerative colitis, and peptic or duodenal ulcers. Therefore, when a patient is referred to a physical therapist for treatment they need to ensure that all the appropriate steps have been taken to exclude physical disease before commencing treatment (Sharpe et al 1992b).

At the same time, overinvestigation can have negative effects, particularly if it is solely to reassure the patient (Barsky & Borus 1999). Negative findings from diagnostic tests often heighten rather than assuage patients' anxieties (Lucock et al 1997, Weber & Kapoor 1996). Extensive medical testing has been shown to have a number of iatrogenic consequences such as confirming patients' convictions that their illnesses have an "as yet to be discovered" biomedical cause, inappropriate prescription of medications whose side effects cause further symptoms, and misdiagnoses (Kouyanou et al 1997). Therefore, once a FSS diagnosis is confirmed and the therapist feels that appropriate investigations have been made it is important not to refer patients for further testing unless specifically indicated.

SHOULD WE DIAGNOSE FSS AT ALL?

Having briefly discussed methods of diagnosing FSS, it is worth noting that there is a compelling argument in the literature against diagnosing patients with a particular FSS. This is based on the reality that many of the disorders overlap and the possibility that labeling patients with a particular disorder might have negative consequences (Hadler 1993, Shorter 1995). Telling people that they have a chronic disabling syndrome might encourage patients to take a passive role in their recovery, and in so doing, increase their level of disability. However, a recent prospective study showed that the label of fibromyalgia did not adversely affect the clinical outcome of patients with chronic widespread pain (White et al 2002). In fact, patients' satisfaction with their health improved and their major symptoms lessened over time. This finding is consistent with CFS patients' reports that receiving a diagnosis was a great relief as it legitimized their suffering and provided them with something concrete to tackle (Ax et al 1997, Broom & Woodward 1996, Deale & Wessely 2001). Most of these patients had experienced lengthy delays, disputes, or confusion over their diagnosis, which only served to heighten their distress (Ax et al 1997, Broom & Woodward 1996, Deale & Wessely 2001).

Taken together, the above suggestions contest the skepticism of certain authors and practitioners, and suggest that a diagnosis of a FSS has positive rather than negative effects. A diagnosis of a FSS can help patients make sense of their illness and symptoms (Moss-Morris & Wrapson 2003). However, it is important to use the diagnosis in a constructive manner. Many patients will carry a number of misconceptions about the negative consequences of their diagnosis, and these need to be explored so that any unhelpful ideas can be corrected. Patients should also be advised that the popular literature on FSS contains a large amount of inaccurate and unhelpful information such as "the best thing to do is to rest and wait until your symptoms go away." A number of unproven alternative remedies are also promoted on the internet. Web sites from patient support groups and advertisers such as www.Odisease.com and www.cfs-news.org offer solutions such as "magnetic relaxation pads," the "chi machine," and "Gold's remedies." They make dramatic claims about breakthrough discoveries of single causal mechanisms, such as mercury poisoning (www.fibromyalgiacure.com). Presenting a coherent account of the illness that clearly explains the interactions between multiple biopsychosocial factors can help to combat some of these simplistic and inaccurate accounts.

BIOLOGICAL OR "FUNCTIONAL" CHANGES

In explaining the model of the illness to patients it is important to include the possible biological mechanisms. These help to validate the patient's symptom experience and avoid giving the impression that you believe the symptoms are "purely psychological" or even worse "imaginary." It should be stressed to patients that just because biomedical investigations are typically negative does not mean that the illness has no biological basis. A number of potentially relevant physiological or functional abnormalities have been identified in many of the FSS such as sleep disturbance, altered responses to sensory stimuli, and immune and neuroendocrine abnormalities (Mayer 1999, Moss-Morris & Petrie 2000a, Richards & Cleare 2000). Exactly what causes these disturbances is unclear. While some argue that they are primary disturbances, it is likely that many of these changes are related to the behavioral changes that occur when patients become ill (Bortz 1984). In other words, they form part of the perpetuating cycle summarized in Table 18.2. Patients become less active, have altered daily routines, poor sleep/wake cycles, and heightened anxiety. Taken together, these factors can impact on the cardiorespiratory, musculoskeletal, central nervous, neuroendocrine, and immune systems.

The role of deconditioning and disuse

Because patients often become inactive during the course of FSS, they are likely to experience deconditioning, have limited cardiorespiratory function, reduced muscle strength and flexibility, and reduced exercise tolerance. Relatively short periods of bedrest even in healthy individuals can cause orthostatic intolerance, reduced oxygen uptake, reduced heart volume and cardiac output, and decreased aerobic capacity (see review by Powell 2001). These changes can result in symptoms such as dizziness, nausea, fainting, headache, and fatigue. Such symptoms are common to many of the FSS suggesting that inactivity or deconditioning plays an important role in contributing to the ongoing experience of symptoms in FSS.

Other symptoms may be related to the fact that disuse results in loss of muscle tone and bulk, leading to decreased muscle strength particularly in the weight-bearing muscles of the trunk and the locomotive muscles of the leg (Convertino 1986). These changes can result in aching muscles, and feelings of weakness and fatigue in the muscles, all of which are commonly reported by patients with FSS. Patients also describe particular discomfort following exercise, which further reinforces their view that exercise is bad for them. They may be experiencing delayed-onset muscle soreness which is a well-documented postexercise pain following unaccustomed exercise (Edwards et al 1993).

The role of the sleep/wake cycle

Most patients with FSS report that they have good and bad days with regards to their symptoms. Consequently, their levels of activity change from day to day depending on how they are feeling. On a bad day they may decide to spend more time in bed or nap during the day, while on a good day they may be more active. This lack of daily routine has been shown to disrupt patients' circadian rhythms (Williams et al 1996). People who have experienced jetlag after international travel or a change in shift work hours will be familiar with the symptoms of disturbed circadian rhythms, namely tiredness, impaired concentration, and impaired intellectual functioning.

Disruptions to circadian rhythms are often associated with sleep disturbances (Moss-Morris & Petrie 2000b). Sleep disturbances are common in patients with CFS and fibromyalgia and may also play a role in the development of the symptoms. When compared to controls, these patients have higher levels of disruptions to their sleep during the night and significantly less sleep efficiency (Fischler et al 1997, Whelton et al 1992). Alteration in sleep architecture may also contribute to symptoms. Polysomnographic studies have shown that the presence of prominent alpha intrusions in the brain waves during non-REM sleep are related to the classic symptoms of fibromyalgia and CFS including chronic tiredness, unrefreshing sleep, and musculoskeletal discomfort (Macfarlane et al 1996, Whelton et al 1992).

The role of central nervous system alterations

There is evidence that patients with FSS have heightened levels of arousal and sensitized central nervous system responses (Ursin & Erikson 2001). These alterations may be related to genetic predispositions, a past history of traumatic events, recent stressors, and/or fearful beliefs associated with the illness itself (McEwan 1998, Ursin & Erikson 2001). Many patients report that the onset of their symptoms coincided with a particularly stressful time in their lives (Mayer 1999). There is also a high correlation between a history of physical, sex-

ual, or verbal abuse and the development of a FSS (Barsky & Borus 1999). All these factors can activate the body's physiological stress response. In the short term these responses are adaptive and protective, however, in the long term they can have a more damaging effect (McEwan 1998).

The effects of long-term arousal may have both a direct and indirect effect on symptoms. Sympathetic nervous system activity gets the body ready for flight or fight. This directly produces a number of bodily sensations related to increased heart rate, dilated pupils, sweating, muscle tension, alterations to gut motility, and increased respiration. These sensations can be experienced as heart palpitations, hyperventilation or shortness of breath, stomach upsets, and altered vision, which are often interpreted by patients as symptoms or signs of illness (Salkovskis 1992).

Indirect effects on symptoms may occur through the increase in skeletal muscle tone which may set the stage for hyperactive muscle contraction and the possibility of persistence of contraction following conscious muscle activation. Such changes may result in chronic muscle spasm and pain. Flor et al (1992) showed that discussing stressful events with chronic pain patients produces elevated EMG activity localized to the site of the presenting pain problem.

Chronic nervous system activation may also alter the central nervous system mechanisms concerned with antinociceptive responses to sensory stimulation (Mayer 1999). This can result in a hypersensitive response to what would otherwise be a non-noxious stimulus. Brain mechanisms involved with the regulation of attention may determine the site of the hypersensitivity. For example, patients with fibromyalgia have a significantly lower threshold and tolerance to pain and noise stimuli when compared to patients with rheumatoid arthritis and healthy controls (McDermid et al 1996), while patients with IBS show a hypersensitivity to visceral sensations (Naliboff et al 1998). Patients with IBS and fibromyalgia symptoms show both visceral and somatic sensitivities (Mayer 1999).

In summary, the symptoms experienced by patients can be explained, in part, by a number of physiological changes. These changes may be related to predisposing factors such as a past history of stress, or it may be that precipitating events such as a bad virus or injury set off a cycle of autonomic system responses. However, it is likely that many of the changes are related to altered behavioral patterns and increased anxiety that are consequences of the illness itself. As a result, changing some of these behaviors may have a direct effect on physiology and symptoms. In the following section some of the other psychological factors involved in FSS that should be taken into account when treating patients are outlined.

PSYCHOLOGICAL CONSIDERATIONS

PSYCHIATRIC ASSESSMENT

The importance of ruling out the presence of medical disease before diagnosing patients with a FSS has already been discussed. It is equally important to ensure that patients have been assessed for the presence of psychiatric disorders. Some disorders, such as psychotic disorders, eating disorders, or substance abuse problems may rule out a diagnosis of a FSS (Fukuda et al 1994). Other disorders such as anxiety, depression, and somatization disorder are highly prevalent in FSS and are accepted as comorbid conditions rather than exclusionary factors (Barsky & Borus 1999, Manu 1998). These conditions are more common in FSS than in other chronic conditions with similar symptoms such as rheumatoid arthritis and inflammatory bowel disease (Barsky & Borus 1999).

Identifying comorbid psychiatric problems is important for three main reasons. First, comorbidity is associated with higher levels of disability and somatic symptoms (Kroenke et al 1994, Russo et al 1994). Second, depression in particular, is related to a poor response to certain psychological treatments for FSS such as cognitive and behavioral therapy (Bentall et al 2002, Blanchard et al 1992). Third, it may be important to refer patients to a mental health specialist for additional treatment. There is good evidence to suggest that some patients respond well to psychotropic medication (Raine et al 2002). Medication can be used in conjunction with other treatments. At the same time, it is important that patients are reassured that the presence of a psychiatric diagnosis does not call into question the legitimacy of their FSS. It can be explained that the psychiatric disorder is not so much a cause of their FSS, but rather an amplifier of the symptoms that can hinder recovery (Barsky & Borus 1999). In this way physical and manual therapists can still offer treatment while encouraging patients to seek additional help for their psychiatric problem.

THE ROLE OF PATIENTS' ILLNESS AND SYMPTOM BELIEFS

Whereas psychiatric disorders may be relevant to some patients, as discussed earlier the role of patients' illness beliefs is pertinent to all patients with FSS. One of the defining features of this patient group is the way in which they interpret symptoms. Studies that have compared patients with FSS to matched groups with identified medical or psychiatric pathology have found that the functional groups consistently report a significantly higher number of somatic symptoms (Gomborone et al 1995, McGowan et al 1998, Moss-Morris & Petrie 2001, Robbins & Kirmayer 1990). This suggests that the physiological changes discussed in the previous section cannot fully account for the symptoms experienced. One of the reasons FSS patients appear to experience such a wide range of symptoms is their preference for attributing common everyday symptoms, such as headaches or heart palpitations, to biological factors, rather than to psychological or environmental factors (Butler et al 2001, Dendy et al 2001, Robbins & Kirmayer 1991, Stone et al 2002). This attribution is also reflected in their tendency to view the causes of their FSS as largely physical (Gomborone et al 1995, McGowan et al 1998, Moss-Morris & Petrie 2001). The most popular causal beliefs in chronic headache sufferers include heredity factors, menopause or menstrual problems, and overactive lifestyles (Kraaimaat & Van Schevikhoven 1988). Patients with temporomandibular disorders attribute their conditions to injury, dental work, inherent structural problems, and teeth grinding/clenching (Garro et al 1994), while CFS patients attribute their condition to a virus, immune dysfunction, pollution or environmental chemicals, diet, overwork, and stress (Moss-Morris & Petrie 2001). Thus, in making sense of their symptoms patients may reflect back to possible precipitants of the condition. However, as discussed earlier in this chapter, the ongoing symptoms may be more closely associated with the perpetuating factors.

Two other interrelated factors appear to be important in maintaining the degree of symptom experience in FSS. Patients have a tendency to overexaggerate or catastrophize about the possible consequences of experiencing somatic symptoms (Moss-Morris & Petrie 1997), and tend to be more hypervigilant to symptoms. The belief or fear that patients have a serious physical illness may lead them to focus undue attention on somatic information, which in turn may result in a misinterpretation of the symptoms (Naliboff et al 1998). Continually misinterpreting symptoms as signs of illness helps to maintain the chronicity of the condition. Indeed, attributing a wide range of symptoms to the illness, catastrophizing about symptoms, and focusing undue attention on symptoms are all strongly related to ongoing disability in FSS (Moss-Morris & Wrapson 2003).

ILLNESS BELIEFS AND BEHAVIORAL CHANGE

Not only are patients' illness beliefs significant in directly determining disability, but they guide the way in which patients choose to manage their symptoms. Many patients with FSS believe that the best way to control their symptoms is to limit activity levels and exposure to stress (Kraaimaat & Van Schevikhoven 1988, Mello-Goldner & Jackson 1999, Moss-Morris & Petrie 2001, Ray et al 1997). The role of fear in this process, particularly in the development of chronic pain, has received substantial attention from researchers. Vlaeyen (1995b) proposed that when in pain, people avoid doing those activities that they think may cause further pain or discomfort. While such avoidance may assist in preventing exacerbation of symptoms during the early stages of recuperation, the long-term effects of behavioral avoidance have been shown to be negative across a number of syndromes (Moss-Morris & Petrie 2001, Philips & Jahanshahi 1986, Ray et al 1997, Sharpe et al 1992a, Vlaeyen et al 1995b). Of particular clinical relevance is the finding that changes in avoidance behaviors and beliefs are strong predictors of improvement following psychological therapy for FSS, while changes in beliefs about the causes of the illness are not (Deale et al 1998, van Dulman et al 1996). This suggests that it is possible to alter patients' fears and beliefs about the negative consequences of limiting activity without challenging their original beliefs about the cause of the illness. This may help to engage patients by acknowledging that their causal beliefs are precipitators of the illness but that ongoing avoidance may be contributing to the perpetuation of the problem.

PERSONALITY FACTORS

In understanding patients' illness beliefs and behaviors, it is also important to understand personality and social factors that help to shape and maintain these beliefs. At the beginning of this chapter we discussed how an achievement orientation and high personal expectations may predispose people to developing a FSS. These personality features may be a product of underlying assumptions that form part of a person's self-concept. Such assumptions might include an underlying belief that in order to be acceptable to others and oneself one needs to achieve at high levels. There is some evidence to support this idea. Retrospective reports from CFS patients and their spouses suggest that prior to their illness the patients were hard-driving individuals (Van Houdenhove et al 2001). There is also evidence that CFS patients tend to interpret mistakes as equivalent to failure and to believe that failure would mean losing the respect of others (White & Schweitzer 2000), while chronic facial pain patients have an unrealistically high expectation of themselves and a strong sense of obligation to others (Schwartz & Gramling 1997). For these people, integrating their self-concept into a situation where their ability to perform or to help others is threatened, such as an acute illness during a time of stress, is clearly going to pose difficulties. If they attribute their inability to cope to something about themselves this may lead to a perception of failure, self-criticism, and a lowering of self-esteem. One way to protect this from happening is to attribute the symptoms to an external cause. This has the positive effect of protecting the person from feeling they are in any way responsible for failing to live up to expectations. Once again this is important to take into account when treating patients. It reinforces the idea of not being overchallenging of patients' original causal beliefs. These beliefs may be important in maintaining patients' self-esteem.

SOCIAL FACTORS

There are a number of social factors that may help to maintain patients' illness beliefs and consequent behaviors. FSS patient support groups represent a strong political movement sanctioning the organic nature of the condition. The findings from biological studies are overemphasized and patients are often encouraged to rest rather than engage in activity. Active lobbying against psychological research or interventions is not uncommon and may include anonymous denunciations and allegations sent to funding bodies and medical journals (Wessely 1997).

The family also plays an important role, as illness perceptions are not restricted to the person experiencing the illness. The patient's spouse, family, or friends have perceptions that influence the way they respond to the patient. For instance, partners who are very solicitous may encourage the patient to accommodate to their illness by taking on the roles the patient feels they can no longer perform. Indeed, CFS patients who report greater satisfaction in relationships also report higher levels of fatigue and lower levels of activity (Schmaling & DiClementi 1995). Thus, supportive partners may unintentionally collude with patients in maintaining their disability.

In summary FSS patients' tendency to make physical attributions for symptoms may set off a cycle of responses, which leads to the ongoing symptoms. These include both the belief that rest is an effective way of controlling the symptoms and a fear that overexertion may have negative consequences. Behavioral avoidance of overexertion results. These factors, in combination with a tendency to focus on bodily symptoms and to catastrophize about the consequences of symptoms, leads to the development of a strong illness identity, and the beliefs that one has a chronic serious illness. Social and personality factors may maintain these beliefs and behaviors, which are associated with ongoing disability in these conditions. In the remainder of this chapter how different treatment methods can break this cycle of responses and lead to symptom reduction and improved quality of life for patients with FSS will be discussed.

PSYCHOLOGICAL INTERVENTIONS

There are few effective medical interventions for FSS. Consequently psychological interventions are often the treatment of choice. These treatments focus on reducing symptoms and disability rather than providing a cure. There are four main approaches. Cognitive therapy focuses on modifying patients' maladaptive beliefs about their symptoms and encourages associated behavioral changes. The focus is on helping patients to make the link between thoughts, feelings, behaviors, and symptoms. Behavioral or operant therapies focus on changing behavior through rewarding "healthy" behaviors so that they occur more frequently and withdrawing attention from "illness" behaviors so that they occur less frequently. The focus is on gradually increasing physical exercise, social, and work-related activities. Respondent treatments are aimed at direct modification of the physiological system

(e.g., decreasing muscle tension by the use of relaxation and biofeedback techniques; van Tulder et al 2002). These three therapies focus on modifying either the cognitive or behavioral processes involved in the perpetuation of FSS, or both. The final form of therapy, interpersonal therapy, focuses on resolving difficulties in interpersonal relationships that underlie or exacerbate somatic symptoms. The focus is on areas of conflict such as unresolved grief, role transitions, and relationship discord.

UTILIZING PSYCHOLOGICAL METHODS IN EXERCISE PROGRAMS

Exercise programs for FSS based on operant methods of behavior change are frequently implemented by physical therapists. Such programs also appear to be a particularly effective method of treating FSS. Consequently we have made these the focus of the remainder of this chapter. At the end of this section we also provide a brief overview of the effectiveness of respondent, cognitive, and interpersonal therapy. The former is often used by physical therapists, but the latter two methods usually require specialist psychological training in these areas.

General considerations when designing exercise programs for FSS patients

Exercise may not be the treatment of choice for many patients with FSS and a number of factors may create difficulties in engaging these patients in active forms of physical therapy. We have already seen that FSS patients often hold strong beliefs about the cause of their illness. As a result they may reject treatment that is incongruent with these illness beliefs. For example, CFS patients commonly attribute the cause of their illness to a virus or to environmental factors such as chemical toxicity. It may be difficult to encourage such patients to undertake an exercise program when this treatment does not appear to directly treat the perceived cause of their condition. They may also resist treatment because they feel it important to have a specific diagnosis before embarking on treatment that in effect seems to be merely treating symptoms rather than the condition itself.

A further consideration is that many FSS patients believe that rest is an essential part of their treatment program (Ray et al 1997, Wigers et al 1996). Exercise, therefore, is often perceived as harmful rather than beneficial. In one study, patients were asked before they were randomized into treatment groups how effective they expected each intervention to be. Eighty-two percent expected stress management treatment to improve their condition, while only 50% thought they would improve from aerobic exercise. Indeed, 30% of participants believed that aerobic exercise would make them worse (Wigers et al 1996). Patients may also prefer to undertake passive treatments aimed at alleviating discomfort such as transcutaneous electrical neuromuscular stimulation, hot-packs, or acupuncture, where they perceive little risk of adverse consequences. In the Wigers et al (1996) study, when participants were asked how they would feel if they were allocated to the standard medical care group, 70% of participants responded favorably.

Getting the patient on-side

The initial challenge for the physical therapist, then, is to present a model of the patient's illness that makes sense to the patient according to their own illness beliefs. Incorporating the factors discussed in the sections on physical and psychological considerations can help engage patients in seeing the need to change their behavior. The initial approach should focus on the physiological changes and de-emphasize the psychological factors. If the patient believes their illness started with a factor such as a virus this can be incorporated into the description as a precipitating factor. The behavioral changes which may be perpetuating the condition can be presented as natural responses to having a chronic illness, to avoid blame or the suggestion that the patients have done the wrong thing. However, it can be emphasized that these changes are reversible and that by working together these changes can occur in a carefully controlled environment. It is also worth noting that not all the behavioral factors may be important. For example, if your history-taking uncovers that the patient sleeps well but tends to be very inactive, your explanation would focus on deconditioning and disuse rather than alterations to circadian rhythms. Patients will often more readily accept explanations that involve psychosocial factors if the therapist acknowledges the genuineness of their symptoms first (Mayou & Farmer 2002). Exercise can then be suggested as one way of increasing the patient's fitness and, in turn, increasing the patient's ability to cope with the stresses and strains of everyday life (Peters et al 2002).

Use of operant methods in exercise trials

The use of graded exercise, reinforcement of appropriate behavior, and activity-contingent pain management form the backbone of an operant method of illness behavior change (Fordyce 1976). This section will start with a brief description of these ingredients. A description of a specific exercise program conducted according to operant principles of behavior change is outlined in Lindström et al (1992).

Graded exercise Due to the limited tolerance to exercise or activity that many FSS patients have, it is clearly unrealistic for these patients to suddenly undertake unaccustomed exertion without experiencing adverse consequences. It is recommended, therefore, that an exercise program commences at a level below that which a patient can comfortably achieve, and builds up the duration and intensity of exercise over a period of time so that the patient's success in reaching one level encourages an increase in performance to the next level.

As patients' symptomatology varies widely even across the same FSS, exercise programs are generally tailored to the individual's physical capacity. To establish a baseline, the patient is asked to perform specific exercises until pain or discomfort prevents them from continuing. During the program, patients increase their participation in each exercise at a rate established by the patient and physical therapist (Fulcher & White 1998). Expectations are kept realistic so that there is a high probability of the set goals being reached.

Reinforcement One of the underlying principles of behavior modification is that the consequences of behavior determine its future occurrence. For example, if when a person performs an action it is followed by a pleasant consequence (positive reinforcement), they are likely to perform the same action in the future. In exercise trials the physical therapist offers encouragement to the patient and praise when a set quota of exercise is achieved or when functional gains are made. Feedback of performance can also be provided by patients checking their pulse rate at regular intervals with portable pulse monitors to ensure they are exercising at the prescribed intensity. In a study conducted by Peters et al (2002), at the end of some exercise sessions patients were able to view a graphic display on a laptop computer of their individual pulse readings. Assignments such as keeping a diary of prescribed exercises undertaken at home provide a useful record for the physical therapist and can also be used as a means of reinforcement. Targets for future sessions are often based on the activity levels recorded in homework diaries.

Activity–contingent symptom management   When the patient starts the program they are used to their symptoms or discomfort telling them when to rest. In an operant treatment program, however, the patient is encouraged to keep to the targets set and to rest only once the quota is met. The quota is always set in collaboration with the patient. A standard rule is that they should never do more on a "good" day or less on a "bad" day. If they have a particularly bad day, patients can be encouraged to perform at the same level as the day before and forgo increasing their daily target. The use of biofeedback, such as heart rate monitors, can also be useful here (Fulcher & White 1998). Patients can be given a set heart rate to achieve. They can be reassured that this level of intensity is safe and to use the heart rate monitor as the measure of intensity rather than their symptoms. Reinforcement from the physical therapist is given when the patient performs the quota agreed. It is important not to be punitive when targets are not met, but rather to explore with the patient the reasons for not meeting these. New goals can then be set accordingly.

TREATMENT TRIALS OF EXERCISE THERAPY IN FSS

In this section the evidence for the effectiveness of exercise as a behavioral therapy in FSS will be reviewed. From a clinical point of view it is important to look at the evidence base in order to determine how to use exercise therapy in an optimal manner. Research in this area has tended to target some FSS more than others. There are many studies investigating the effect of exercise on patients with fibromyalgia (see review by Busch et al 2002); in contrast, research into other FSS has relied on medically oriented or multifaceted interventions. For example, treatment for premenstrual syndrome has traditionally relied on pharmacological interventions and interventions for non-cardiac chest pain patients have favored cognitive behavioral therapy (CBT).

We have reviewed the key exercise trials conducted in this area (only studies with a minimum of 20 participants in each condition at the commencement of the program). Specifically, we looked at chronic fatigue syndrome, fibromyalgia, and chronic low back pain, as these are the FSS most commonly treated with an operant-behavioral approach (see

Table 18.3). One study also involved patients with a range of FSS diagnoses (Peters et al 2002). Of the 18 trials reviewed (Burckhardt et al 1994, Frost et al 1995, Fulcher & White 1997, Jentoft et al 2001, Kole-Snijders et al 1999, McCain et al 1988, Mannerkorpi et al 2000, Martin et al 1996, Peters et al 2002, Powell et al 2001, Ramsay et al 2000, Reilly et al 1989, Richards & Scott 2002, Turner & Clancy 1988, Turner et al 1990, van Santen et al 2002, Wearden et al 1998, Wigers et al 1996), six compared a behavioral physical therapy program with an alternative form of exercise, relaxation, or biofeedback, eight with normal medical care, one with a pharmaceutical intervention, six with other types of treatment such as education or cognitive behavioral treatment, and three with a similar type of physical therapy but in a different form or setting (i.e. pool-based versus land-based aerobic exercise, supervised versus unsupervised programs). Some studies had a number of intervention groups.

Exercise programs ranged from 6 weeks to 6 months in length, and generally consisted of supervised group or individual sessions comprising a total of 1 or 2 hours per week. A few programs comprised an unsupervised self-managed program at home according to specific instructions. A program might incorporate a range of exercise including aerobic, flexibility and balance, muscle strengthening, and relaxation exercises (van Santen et al 2002), or consist entirely of aerobic exercise with patients using treadmills and exercise bicycles (Richards & Scott 2002). There was little standardization among programs as to the type, intensity, duration, and frequency of exercise.

In the 18 studies identified above, clinical examination or medical assessment was used to measure physiological fitness and, in the case of patients with fibromyalgia, the number of tender points. Measurements of other variables were obtained by the participants completing questionnaires at each assessment point and thus reflected their subjective perceptions of their symptoms and disability. A brief summary of the outcomes in the intervention groups is given in Table 18.3. Due to the wide variety of variables used across studies, where possible we have categorized variables into four main areas: physical function (e.g., cardiovascular fitness, strength, walking time), physical symptoms (e.g., number of tender points, pain, fatigue), disability (e.g., health perception, interference of FSS on life, self-efficacy), and emotional state (e.g., anxiety, depression). As the patient's perception of improvement following treatment seemed to war-

Table 18.3 Functional somatic syndrome randomized controlled exercise trials

Study	No. of participants/ selection criteria	Treatment (no. of participants at time of randomization)	Type and number of sessions/ duration of training	Additional treatment elements	Improvements At treatment completion	Improvements At long term follow-up (≥ 6 months)	Percentage completing program*
			FSS – General				
Peters et al (2002)	228 Unexplained physical symptoms for ≥ 12 months	1. Aerobic exercise (114) 2. Stretching exercises (114)	1 & 2: Group sessions, 20 × 1 h over 10 weeks	1 & 2: Between session exercises (20 min 3 × weekly) guided by written and pictorial information, recorded in a homework diary	*Between groups:* No significant differences *Within groups:* 1 & 2: Health care use, disability, emotional state	*Within groups:* Generally maintained in both groups together with some further improvement in disability	Groups 1 & 2: 34% overall attended ≥ 15 sessions
			Chronic fatigue syndrome				
Powell et al (2001)	148 Oxford	1–3. Graded exercise (37, 39, 38) 4. Medical care (34)	1–3: Self-managed exercise program over 3 months	1–3: Educational pack containing explanations for symptoms to encourage graded activity, supported by verbal explanations (minimum, telephone and maximum intervention groups) 4: Information booklet to encourage graded activity but no explanation for symptoms	Not reported	*Between groups:* 1–3 > 4: Disability, physical symptoms, emotional state, impression of overall change	Groups 1–3: 92%, 95%, 95% Group 4: 94%

Continued

Table 18.3 Functional somatic syndrome randomized controlled exercise trials — cont'd

Study	No. of participants/ selection criteria	Treatment (no. of participants at time of randomization)	Type and number of sessions/ duration of training	Additional treatment elements	Improvements At treatment completion	Improvements At long term follow-up (≥ 6 months)	Percentage completing program*
			Chronic fatigue syndrome – cont'd				
Wearden et al (1998)	136 Oxford	1. Graded aerobic exercise and fluoxetine (33) 2. Graded aerobic exercise and drug placebo (34) 3. Fluoxetine and exercise placebo (35) 4. Exercise placebo and drug placebo (34)	1 & 2: Self-managed exercise program, 20 min 3 × weekly over 26 weeks and 8 sessions with physiotherapist to monitor progress 3 & 4: 8 sessions with physiotherapist and recommendation to exercise but no specific advice on exercise quantity	Keeping activity diary for 1 week every 4 weeks	*Between groups:* 1 & 2 > 3 & 4: (completers only) physical symptoms *Within groups:* 1 & 2: Work capacity, (completers only) physical symptoms, disability		Group 1: 85% Group 2: 79% Group 3: 86% Group 4: 94%
Fulcher & White (1997)	66 Oxford	1. Graded aerobic exercise (33) 2. Flexibility and relaxation exercises (33)	1 & 2: Supervised sessions, 12 × 1 h over 12 weeks	1 & 2: Between session exercises (5–15 min increasing to 30 min, 5 × weekly); keeping weekly activity diary	*Between groups:* 1 > 2: Disability, physical fitness, impression of overall change		Group 1: 88% Group 2: 91%
			Fibromyalgia				
Richards & Scott (2002)	136 ACR	1. Graded aerobic exercise (69) 2. Relaxation (67)	1 & 2: Group sessions, 24 × 1 h over 12 weeks	Weekly information leaflets	*Between groups:* 1 > 2: Impression of overall change *Within groups:* 1 & 2: Physical symptoms, disability	*Between groups:* 1 > 2 Physical symptoms, number of patients meeting ACR criteria *Within groups:* 1 & 2: mprovement lin disability maintained	Groups 1 & 2: 79% attended at least one class, 53% attended > 8 classes

van Santen et al (2002)	143 ACR	1. Fitness training (58) 2. Biofeedback (56) 3. Medical care (29)	1: Group sessions, 1 h 2 × weekly over 24 weeks with an optional unsupervised third session 2: Individual sessions, 30 min 2 × weekly over 8 weeks and encouragement to practise relaxation 2 × daily at home	1 & 2: Keeping activity diary Half of the participants in Groups 1 & 2 also received an educational program of 6 × 1½ h sessions over 24 weeks	Based on completers only Between groups: No significant improvement. Physical fitness worsened in all groups although the decrease was significantly less in the fitness training group compared to the control group Within groups: No significant differences	Group 1: 81% Group 2: 77% Group 3: 97%
Jentoft et al (2001)	42 ACR	1. Pool-based aerobic exercise (22) 2. Land-based aerobic exercise (20)	1 & 2: Group sessions, 40 × 1 h over 20 weeks		Based on completers only Between groups: 2 > 1: Physical fitness (grip strength only) Within groups: 1 & 2: Physical fitness, physical symptoms, disability 1 only: Emotional state	Maintained apart from some loss of physical fitness in both groups
Mannerkorpi et al (2000)	69 ACR	1. Pool-based aerobic exercise (37) 2. Medical care (32)	1: Group sessions, 35 min weekly over 6 months	Education program of 6 × 1 h sessions	Between groups: 1 > 2: Physical fitness, physical symptoms, disability, emotional state	Attended ≥ 50% sessions – Group 1: 82% Group 2: 80% Group 1: 77% Group 2: 94%

Continued

Table 18.3 Functional somatic syndrome randomized controlled exercise trials – cont'd

Study	No. of participants/ selection criteria	Treatment (no. of participants at time of randomization)	Type and number of sessions/ duration of training	Additional treatment elements	Improvements		Percentage completing program*
					At treatment completion	At long term follow-up (≥ 6 months)	
			Fibromyalgia – cont'd				
Ramsay et al (2000)	74 ACR	1. Supervised aerobic exercise (37) 2. Unsupervised aerobic exercise (37)	1: Group sessions, 12 × 1 h over 12 weeks 2: Group sessions, 1 × 1 h to demonstrate exercises to be undertaken at home	1 & 2: Stretching and relaxation techniques Written advice and encouragement to continue and increase exercises at home	Between groups: 1 > 2: Emotional state		Group 1: 41% attended ≥ 75% of classes Group 2: 95% attended the single session
Martin et al (1996)	60 ACR	1. Aerobic/ strengthening/ flexibility exercise (30) 2. Relaxation (30)	1 & 2: Group sessions, 18 × 1 h over 6 weeks		Between groups: 1 > 2: Physical symptoms, physical fitness		Group 1: 60% Group 2: 67%
Wigers et al (1996) Smythe (1979) and Yunus et al (1981)	60	1. Aerobic exercise (20) 2. Stress management (cognitive therapy and relaxation) (20) 3. Medical care (20)	1: Group sessions 40 × 45 min over 14 weeks 2: Group sessions 20 × 1½ h over 14 weeks	2 only: Audiotape containing relaxation procedures for use at home, registration sheets for noting compliance, and a thermal biofeedback measure as an aid for monitoring arousal	Between groups: 1 > 2: (Completers) physical symptoms, disability 1 > 3: Physical symptoms, work capacity; (completers) overall subjective improvement, additional improvements in physical symptoms disability and 2 > 3: Physical symptoms; (completers) additional	4 years: Between groups: 2 > 3: Physical symptoms 6 patients (Group 1: 3, Group 2: 1, Group 3: 2) no longer fulfilled the ACR criteria	Group 1: 80% Group 2: 75%

Study	Sample	Intervention	Sessions	Outcomes	Results
Burckhardt et al (1994)	99 ACR	1. Physical therapy and education (33) 2. Education (31) 3. Medical care (35)	1: Group sessions, 6 × 2½ h over 6 weeks (1½ h education and 1 h physical therapy) 2: Group sessions, 6 × 1½ h over 6 weeks (education component only)	improvements in physical symptoms, and emotional state *Between groups:* 1 & 2 > 3: Disability (self-efficacy – for function only) 1 > 3: Disability (self-efficacy – for pain and for other symptoms)	Over all groups: 87%
McCain et al (1988)	42 Smythe (1981)	1. Graded cardiovascular fitness training (20) 2. Flexibility exercise (22)	1 & 2: Group sessions, 60 × 1 h over 20 weeks	*Between groups:* 1 > 2: Physical fitness, physical symptoms, patients' and physicians' assessment of disease activity *Within groups:* 1 & 2: Emotional state	Group 1: 90% Group 2: 91%

Chronic low back pain

Study	Sample	Intervention	Sessions	Outcomes	Results
Kole-Snijders et al (1999)	148 Low back pain for ≥6 months	1. Graded physical therapy program and cognitive coping skills training (59) 2. Graded physical therapy program and group discussion (58) 3. Medical care (31)	1 & 2: Individual and group sessions, 5 weeks inpatient treatment and 3 weeks outpatient treatment (3 × weekly) 1 & 2: Spouse group training. Homework assignments	*Between groups:* 1 & 2 > 3: Negative affect, motoric behavior, disability 1 > 2:Disability	Over all groups: 90%

Continued

Table 18.3   Functional somatic syndrome randomized controlled exercise trials — cont'd

Study	No. of participants/ selection criteria	Treatment (no. of participants at time of randomization)	Type and number of sessions/ duration of training	Additional treatment elements	Improvements — At treatment completion	Improvements — At long term follow-up (≥ 6 months)	Percentage completing program*
			Chronic low back pain – cont'd				
Frost et al (1995)	81 Low back pain for ≥ 6 months	1. Exercise program and backschool (41) 2. Backschool (40)	1. Group sessions, 8 × 1 h over 4 weeks 2. Group sessions (number not reported)	1 & 2: Advice on exercises to undertake at home, keeping a pain diary for 1 week before and after treatment	*Between groups:* 1 > 2: Physical fitness, physical symptoms, disability, perceived benefit of treatment *Within groups* 1 & 2: General health	No between group comparison as Group 2 crossed over to exercise intervention	Groups 1 & 2: 88%
Turner et al (1990)	96 Low back pain for > 6 months	1. Graded aerobic exercise (24) 2. Operant-behavioral therapy (25) 3. Operant-behavioral therapy and graded aerobic exercise (24) 4. Medical care (23)	1–3: Group sessions, 8 × 2 h over 8 weeks 1 & 3: Self-managed exercise program (10 min increasing to 20 min, 5 × weekly)	1. Keeping activity diary. Spouses took part in 5 sessions 2. Homework assignments 3. Same as for Groups 1 & 2	*Between groups:* 3 > 1 & 4: Physical symptoms, disability, observer ratings of pain behaviors *Within groups:* All groups: Physical fitness	(No follow-ups of Group 4 undertaken) *Between groups:* No significant differences *Within groups:* 1–3: Physical symptoms, disability, observer ratings of pain behaviors	Group 1: 88% Group 2: 72% Group 3: 75% Group 4: 83%
Reilly et al (1989)	40 Diagnosis of chronic lumbosacral strain	1. Supervised exercise (aerobic/ strengthening/ flexibility) (20) 2. Unsupervised exercise (20)	1. Individual supervised sessions, 4 × weekly over 6 months (session duration not reported) 2. Individual unsupervised sessions with compliance monitored by health club staff		*Between groups:* 1 > 2: Physical fitness, physical symptoms		All participants completed their program. Sessions attended on average: Group 1: 95% Group 2: 33%

| Turner & Clancy (1988) | 81 Low back pain for ≥ 6 months | 1. Operant-behavioral therapy and graded aerobic exercise (30) 2. Cognitive-behavioral therapy and relaxation/ imagery (26) 3. Medical care (25) | 1 & 2: Group sessions, 8 × 2 h over 8 weeks 1 only: Self-managed exercise program (10 min increasing to 20 min, 5 × weekly) | 1. Keeping activity diary and diary of pain behavior and spouse responses. Spouses took part in 4 sessions 2. Daily practice with audiotapes; keeping diary of cognitions | *Between groups:* 1 > 3: Disability, patient and spouse reports of pain behavior | (No follow-ups of Group 3 undertaken) *Between groups:* No significant differences *Within groups:* 1 & 2: General improvement across all measures | Group 1: 97% Group 2: 92% Group 3: 84% |

*The percentage reported relates to those participants undertaking the first assessment following completion of treatment. Where this is not reported, some measure of attendance is reported if available.

rant particular recognition, this variable is identified separately.

On the whole, exercise therapy appears to have positive outcomes for FSS patients. Most exercise groups improved on one or more variables in each category but the variable(s) on which there were positive outcomes varied across studies. A key outcome measure in four of the studies was the amount of improvement the patient felt they had experienced following treatment compared to baseline. In one study 55% of CFS patients who completed their graded aerobic exercise program considered themselves to be "much" or "very much" better at the completion of the program compared to 27% of the control group who undertook a relaxation program (Fulcher & White 1997). This study excluded patients with comorbid depression and anxiety. A study which included a broader range of patients with fibromyalgia found that after treatment, 35% of the exercise group rated themselves as "very much better" or "much better" compared with 18% of the relaxation arm (Richards & Scott 2002).

Larger differences were reported in studies that did a completer rather than an intention to treat analysis. A study on fibromyalgia found that 75% of the exercise group rated themselves as "better" or "much better" compared to 12% who received standard medical care (Wigers et al 1996). A CFS study conducted in Liverpool had a particularly impressive treatment effect with 84% of the patients in the exercise group reporting that they felt "very much better" or "much better" compared with 12% of control patients (Powell et al 2001).

Maximizing the treatment effect

One of the reasons for the large treatment effect in the Powell et al (2001) study could be the inclusion of a comprehensive education package with the exercise program. The package included a detailed physiological model to explain the symptoms experienced by patients and to motivate for the need to exercise. Patients were also given advice on challenging negative or fearful thoughts about exercise and symptoms as well as advice about managing stress and anxiety.

The education package appears to have been effective in altering patients' illness beliefs. Powell et al (2001) found that 81% of the intervention groups believed their condition was caused by a persistent virus before treatment with only 15% relating it to deconditioning. At 12-month follow-up only 23% maintained the belief that their condition was

related to a virus and 81% now believed it was related to physical deconditioning. Eighty-two percent reported avoidance of physical activity prior to treatment compared to 6% following treatment. These findings suggest that incorporating simple cognitive strategies within an exercise intervention may be an effective way of altering maladaptive beliefs and maximizing the treatment effect.

The inclusion of simple education packages may also help change patients' self-efficacy beliefs (beliefs in their ability to carry out certain functions). Burckhardt et al (1994) found that self-efficacy for physical functioning improved in both a group that undertook an exercise and education intervention and a group that received the education component only.

One question that has yet to be answered definitively is whether an increase in fitness is necessary for a positive outcome for patients. A number of studies found that aerobic exercise resulted in greater improvement in physical status than non-aerobic exercise (Fulcher & White 1997, McCain et al 1988, Mannerkorpi et al 2000, Martin et al 1996). However, objective improvements often occurred in only one out of several measures, while self-reported improvements occurred over a number of measures. Two studies found no difference in physical fitness before and after the exercise program, but found that patients did improve on a number of self-report measures (Moss-Morris et al submitted, Peters et al 2002). Furthermore, Fulcher & White (1997) found that self-reported improvement following exercise was unrelated to improvements in physical fitness. These results suggest that subjective improvement may be relatively independent of improvement in cardiovascular fitness. Rather, the psychological processes such as reducing the fear of exercise and symptom focusing may be more important in reducing disability and symptoms. Support for this idea comes from a CFS study where patients in the graded exercise group reported a substantial decrease in the tendency to focus on symptoms (Moss-Morris et al submitted). This change in symptom focusing was highly correlated with positive changes in disability and fatigue.

As one of the factors responsible for maintaining a preoccupation with symptoms is the attention significant others and family members bestow on the patient, it may also be important to involve the patient's immediate family in the treatment process where possible. In one study an important component of the graded exercise program was the "partner group instruction program" which taught patients' spouses to recognize the difference between pain behavior and health behavior, and to respond more to health behaviors than pain behaviors (Vlaeyen et al 1995a).

Although increased fitness does not appear to be paramount in improvement, encouraging participants to keep to the duration and intensity of their planned program is an important element. In one program the exercise intensity was left up to the participants, allowing them to stop when they felt too tired or were experiencing too much pain (van Santen et al 2002). No improvements on any outcomes were found. This supports the concept of activity-contingent rather than symptom-contingent exercise programs.

A recent study investigated predictors of response to exercise treatment in CFS (Bentall et al 2002). The extent of symptoms and the chronicity of the illness were unrelated to treatment response, suggesting that all ambulatory patients can potentially benefit from exercise therapy regardless of the severity of their condition. However, poor treatment response was predicted by membership of a self-help group, receipt of a sickness benefit, and concurrent emotional difficulties. These findings suggest that patients should be screened for psychological disorders before engaging in exercise treatment. These patients may benefit from psychotropic medications or other forms of therapy such as cognitive or interpersonal therapy. Membership of a support group may reinforce the belief that exercise is harmful as many of these groups advise against exercise as a form of therapy. Liaising with local support groups may help to combat some of these negative effects.

Compliance and retention

One of the problems with exercise treatment is that there is often a high dropout rate. On the whole the retention rates in the exercise trials reviewed were good with most studies reporting retention rates upwards of 75%. One study which retained only 60% of participants in the exercise group reported that patients dropped out because of "lack of efficacy by their own assessment," lack of time, and illness (unrelated to the treatment) (Martin et al 1996). This provides further support for including specific information in the program regarding self-efficacy. There is little known about motivating factors in program compliance but the social dimension in group exercise sessions was considered by patients in one trial to be one of the most positive aspects of treatment (Wigers et al 1996), suggesting that group treatment may suit some patients better than individual therapy. Working with patients on incorporating exercise into their daily schedule may also improve retention.

Whereas retention rates were generally good across studies, attendance at all the sessions and adherence to the protocol posed greater difficulties. As expected, attendance is generally related to better outcome. Peters et al (2002) found that attendance at exercise sessions was related to a reduction in health care use in the 6 months following an aerobic exercise program. In another study there was a strong relationship between the number of sessions completed and a reduction in pain (Reilly et al 1989).

Adherence to treatment was reported in a few studies and tended to be rather low. Adherence did not appear to be related to type of intervention. Peters et al (2002) found that only 34% of participants attended at least 15 out of 20 sessions with 53% attending at least ten sessions. There was no difference in attendance between the exercise group and relaxation group. Richards & Scott (2002) found that only 53% of all participants attended over one-third of the 24 exercise sessions.

How do we improve adherence to exercise treatment? It seems likely that a supervised program that closely monitors and encourages patients' activities would result in greater rates of adherence than an unsupervised program. However, Powell et al (2001) compared three different "dosages" (defined in terms of therapist contact time and follow-up telephone contacts) of an educational intervention where patients were given physiological explanations of their symptoms and were encouraged to undertake home-based graded exercise programs. The minimum intervention group received only two individual treatment sessions plus two follow-up telephone calls. The maximum group received nine face-to-face sessions over a 4-month period. The improvement rates in all three groups were equivalent and significantly greater than a control group. This trial had particularly high retention rates. This suggests that the important ingredients for adherence may be engaging the patients in the process of exercise and validating their symptoms.

Another study specifically investigated the effect of supervision by designing the same fitness program for two groups of chronic low back pain patients but assigning a trainer to work with and monitor the patients in the experimental group (Reilly et al 1989). The control group attended a health club. The experimental group on average attended 95% of sessions compared to 33% in the control group. The experimental group also reported a significantly greater reduction in symptoms. In this study there were clearly beneficial effects of increased exposure to the physical therapist. It may be, however, that the rationale for the treatment was not strong enough to maintain the patients in the low-supervision group.

A number of programs have given patients advice at the end of the training program on continuing to exercise at an appropriate level taking into account their individual circumstances and access to exercise resources. In one study, at treatment completion all participants in aerobic exercise and stress management training intended to continue with their training although most of the exercise group intended reducing from three to two sessions per week (Wigers et al 1996). Despite these intentions, only one-fifth of the exercise group members were doing aerobic exercise at follow-up 4 years later while nearly half the stress management training group were still practicing relaxation regularly. However, three out of the four exercise group continuers no longer fulfilled the American College of Rheumatology (ACR) criteria for fibromyalgia compared to one member of the stress management training group. In another study, although there were no improvements in any of the outcome measures, the majority of the exercise group patients continued training weekly with the same trainer but at their own expense for several years after the treatment program ended (van Santen et al 2002). The authors concluded that the participants valued the opportunity of sharing experiences with each other and the invigorating environment provided by the instructor.

In summary, the evidence suggests that coherently laid out exercise programs with a clear rationale and a good educational component are effective in increasing adherence and improving outcome. Programs that incorporate simple cognitive elements may also enhance the efficacy of the programs. If finances allow, one-on-one supervision can also be an effective way of improving compliance and outcome. More work needs to be done on helping patients to maintain their exercise programs after treatment has been completed. Including a social element in the ongoing exercise may act as a reinforcer for continuation.

LIMITATIONS TO CURRENT RESEARCH

One of the difficulties in interpreting the results from exercise studies is that there is a lack of consistency of program design across studies, making it difficult to draw conclusions regarding the efficacy of any particular component or components of each exercise program. Although most exercise groups improved on one or more variables in each category, the variable(s) on which there were positive outcomes varied across studies.

Whereas exercise appears to be an effective intervention for FSS patients, and may compare favorably to other interventions such as CBT, it should be remembered that many of the exercise trials have excluded patients with comorbid psychiatric disorders or have included these patients once they have received appropriate treatment for the psychiatric disorder. CBT on the other hand is generally used to treat all of the patient's symptoms and disorders and therefore those patients with a more severe disability may be more likely to undergo CBT than exercise therapy (Reid et al 2000). It is therefore difficult to make a direct comparison between the effectiveness of different therapies.

More work needs to be done on looking at responders versus non-responders to treatment. Predictors of the mechanisms of change during exercise programs should also be explored further in order to maximize the treatment effect. Little is also known about the necessary intensity, frequency, and duration of a program to ensure optimum treatment outcomes. At this stage it is also unclear as to whether a group or individual approach is more effective. Research suggests compliance is an important factor in a positive outcome yet we still know little about the respective contributions that grading of exercise, feedback and contingent reinforcement, and addressing illness and symptom beliefs make to the treatment outcome.

GRADED EXPOSURE THERAPY

A promising new form of exercise therapy has recently been developed around the concept of fear-avoidance (Vlaeyen et al 2001). As was mentioned earlier in this chapter, when people have ongoing pain or symptoms they often start to avoid activity for fear of exacerbating their pain or causing injury to the site of the pain. For these patients, graded exposure therapy, a form of treatment that gradually exposes people to the specific movements and activities that give rise to their fears, and allows them to confront their fears without adverse consequences, may be warranted.

"Graded exposure therapy" has long been used with phobic patients but in a recent single subjects design study it was used to treat four chronic low back pain patients who reported substantial fear of movement (Vlaeyen et al 2001). Patients were asked to imagine performing various physical activities and movements from daily life and to rate them according to the extent they felt the movement would be harmful to their back. A hierarchy of fear stimuli was then established starting off with activities that arouse little fear at the bottom of the hierarchy, working up to activities that the patient was convinced would do them irreparable harm. The patient was then asked to perform tasks at the very bottom of the hierarchy and to engage in these activities as much as possible until their anxiety levels with respect to these tasks decreased. A gradual progression onto tasks further up the hierarchy was then undertaken. A comparison of graded exposure and graded exercise in reducing pain-related fears in the Vlaeyen et al (2001) study found that improvements in pain-related fear only occurred during the graded exposure treatment, suggesting that this may be a useful pretreatment for some patients prior to a more mainstream exercise program.

RESPONDENT THERAPY

The most common forms of respondent therapy are electromyographic (EMG) biofeedback, and applied and progressive relaxation techniques. Biofeedback is a widely used therapy for treating many stress-related problems. In biofeedback a bodily function is monitored and information is fed back to a patient to facilitate improved control of the physiological process. EMG feedback is intended to enhance relaxation and is commonly used in the treatment of FSS. In a typical treatment a patient is hooked up to an EMG device and its recordings of the patient's muscle tension are transformed into an auditory signal or digital readings. The physical therapist teaches the patient to alternately tighten and relax different groups of muscles and to recognize changes in muscle tension by the signals or readings from the biofeedback equipment.

The evidence base for the effectiveness of biofeedback and relaxation techniques is unclear.

A recent review of behavioral treatments for chronic low back pain concluded that these forms of respondent therapy were equivalent in effectiveness to cognitive therapy and CBT (van Tulder et al 2002). However, all the reviewed studies were rated as low quality making it difficult to draw firm conclusions. A high-quality study comparing CBT with relaxation for CFS patients found CBT to be significantly more effective in reducing fatigue and disability than relaxation (Deale et al 1997).

INTEGRATED MANAGEMENT APPROACHES

The most common integrated approach to treatment for FSS is CBT. The advantage of CBT is that it not only addresses patients' inappropriate beliefs and behaviors but it also involves teaching the patient strategies for managing symptoms. Therapists in most CBT treatment trials are mental health specialists, either psychologists or psychiatrists. However, in clinical settings CBT approaches often require input from a number of different therapists. A psychiatrist or psychologist may teach patients how to take control over their pain and how to manage their anxiety and mood, while a physical therapist may be required to encourage a graded increase in activity/exercise and also to teach relaxation techniques.

A recent review of controlled clinical trials of CBT as a treatment for FSS found that patients' physical symptoms were most responsive to treatment (Kroenke & Swindle 2000). Symptoms in patients treated with CBT improved more than in control subjects in 71% of the studies reviewed and a trend towards improvement was evident in a further 11%. The positive effects for functional improvement were more modest, with CBT-related improvements in 47% of the studies and a further 28% showing a trend. Almost all of the studies reviewed maintained their improvement at 12-month follow-up. For six of the studies there was a "sleeper" effect, whereby patients continued to improve during the follow-up period. Both individual and group formats of CBT appear to be equally effective.

An interesting finding in the Kroenke & Swindle (2000) study was that only 38% of the CBT studies reviewed showed a positive effect for psychological distress (Kroenke & Swindle 2000). Consequently, symptom reduction itself is not solely dependent on improvements in mood. However, these findings may mean that additional treatments should be used to treat mood disorder or high levels of distress in these patients. Psychotropic medication has been shown to be an effective treatment in a number of FSS including fibromyalgia, IBS, premenstrual syndrome, and tension headache (O'Malley et al 1999, Raine et al 2002). However, they appear to be ineffective in CFS (Raine et al 2002). Few studies have investigated more psychodynamic forms of therapy such as interpersonal therapy, although there is evidence that this is an effective form of therapy for patients with IBS (Raine et al 2002). It is possible that interpersonal therapy may be more effective in addressing dysphoria in patients with FSS.

SUMMARY

Patients with FSS have a variety of somatic symptoms that cannot be explained by observable biomedical pathology. A biopsychosocial model that incorporates predisposing, precipitating, and perpetuating factors has been proposed to explain the occurrence and maintenance of FSS. There are few effective medical interventions for FSS and psychological interventions, aimed at reducing symptoms and disability rather than providing a cure, are often the treatment of choice. One of these approaches,

operant-behavioral therapy, uses a number of strategies to encourage "healthy" behaviors as opposed to "illness behaviors." Although many patients believe rest is the most effective form of treatment, operant therapy usually includes an exercise component to encourage increased activity. The challenge that faces physical and manual therapists, therefore, is to present a model of the patient's illness and the benefits of the proposed treatment that fits in with the patient's own illness beliefs.

A review of exercise trials used with FSS patients suggests that physical therapy is a valuable treatment addition to the range of available psychological interventions that include cognitive therapy and interpersonal therapy. Nevertheless, the empirical literature leaves many questions unanswered. We know little about what treatment components contribute most to the effectiveness of an exercise program, and whether physical therapy is a sufficient treatment on its own or whether it is more useful as an integral part of other treatment regimes. What is needed now are more studies that can tell us who is likely to benefit from exercise programs, how programs should be designed to ensure they do benefit, and how to maintain those benefits once they occur.

References

Aaron L A, Buchwald D 2001 A review of the evidence for overlap among unexplained clinical conditions. Annals of Internal Medicine 134(9 Part 2 Suppl S): 868–881

Ax S, Greg V H, Jones D 1997 Chronic fatigue syndrome: Sufferers' evaluation of medical support. Journal of the Royal Society of Medicine 90: 250–254

Barsky A J, Borus J F 1999 Functional somatic syndromes. Annals of Internal Medicine 130(11): 910–921

Bentall R P, Powell P, Nye F J et al 2002 Predictors of response to treatment for chronic fatigue syndrome. British Journal of Psychiatry 181: 248–252

Blanchard E B, Scharff L, Payne A et al 1992 Prediction of outcome from cognitive-behavioral treatment of irritable bowel syndrome. Behaviour Research & Therapy 30(6): 647–650

Bortz W M 1984 The disuse syndrome. Western Journal of Medicine 141(5): 691–694

Broom D H, Woodward R V 1996 Medicalisation reconsidered: Toward a collaborative approach to care. Sociology of Health and Illness 18: 357–378

Burckhardt C S, Mannerkorpi K, Hedenberg L et al 1994 A randomized, controlled clinical trial of education and physical training for women with fibromyalgia. Journal of Rheumatology 21(4): 714–720

Busch A, Schachter C L, Peloso P M et al 2002 Exercise for treating fibromyalgia syndrome. Cochrane Database of Systematic Reviews 3: CD003786

Butler J A, Chalder T, Wessely S 2001 Causal attributions for somatic sensations in patients with chronic fatigue syndrome and their partners. Psychological Medicine 31(1): 97–105

Convertino, V 1986 Exercise responses after inactivity. In Sandler H, Vernikos J (eds) Inactivity: Physiological effects. Academic Press, Orlando, p 149–191

Deale A, Wessely S 2001 Patients' perceptions of medical care in chronic fatigue syndrome. Social Science & Medicine 52(12): 1859–1864

Deale A, Chalder T, Marks I et al 1997 Cognitive behavior therapy for chronic fatigue syndrome: A randomized controlled trial. American Journal of Psychiatry 154(3): 408–414

Deale A, Chalder T, Wessely S 1998 Illness beliefs and treatment outcome in chronic fatigue syndrome. Journal of Psychosomatic Research 45(1): 77–83

Dendy C, Cooper M, Sharpe M 2001 Interpretation of symptoms in chronic fatigue syndrome. Behaviour Research and Therapy 39: 1369–1380

Edwards R H, Gibson H, Clague J E et al 1993 Muscle histopathology and physiology in chronic fatigue syndrome. Ciba Foundation Symposium 173: 102–117; discussion 117–131

Engel Jr C C, Charles C 2000 Unexplained physical symptoms: Medicine's "dirty little secret" and the need for prospective studies that start in childhood. Psychiatry 63(2): 153–159

Fischler B, Le Bon O, Hoffmann G et al 1997 Sleep anomalies in the chronic fatigue syndrome. A comorbidity study. Neuropsychobiology 35(3): 115–122

Flor H, Birbaumer N, Schugens M M et al 1992 Symptom-specific psychophysiological responses in chronic pain patients. Psychophysiology 29: 452–460

Fordyce W E 1976 Behavioral methods for chronic pain and illness. Mosby, St Louis, MO

Frost H, Klaber Moffett J A, Moser J S et al 1995 Randomised controlled trial for evaluation of fitness programme for patients with chronic low back pain. British Medical Journal 310(6973): 151–154

Fukuda K, Straus S E, Hickie I et al 1994 The chronic fatigue syndrome: A comprehensive approach to its definition and study. Annals of Internal Medicine 121(12): 953–959

Fulcher K Y, White P D 1997 Randomised controlled trial of graded exercise in patients with the chronic fatigue syndrome. British Medical Journal 314(7095): 1647–1652

Fulcher K Y, White P D 1998 Chronic fatigue syndrome: A description of graded exercise treatment. Physiotherapy 84(5): 223–226

Garro L G, Stephenson K A, Good B J 1994 Chronic illness of the temporomandibular joints as experienced by support-group members. Journal of General Internal Medicine 9: 372–377

Gomborone J, Dewsnap P, Libby G et al 1995 Abnormal illness attitudes in patients with irritable bowel syndrome. Journal of Psychosomatic Research 39: 227–230

Gureje O, Simon G E, Ustun T B et al 1997 Somatization in cross-cultural perspective: A World Health Organization study in primary care. American Journal of Psychiatry 154: 989–995

Hadler N M 1993 The danger of the diagnostic process. In: Hadler N M (ed) Occupational musculoskeletal disorders. Raven, New York, p 16–33

Jentoft E S, Kvalvik A G, Mengshoel A M 2001 Effects of pool-based and land-based aerobic exercise on women with fibromyalgia/chronic widespread muscle pain. Arthritis & Rheumatism 45(1): 42–47

Kole-Snijders A M J, Vlaeyen J W S, Goossens M E J B et al 1999 Chronic low-back pain: What does cognitive coping skills training add to operant behavioral treatment? Results of a randomized clinical trial. Journal of Consulting & Clinical Psychology 67(6): 931–944

Kouyanou K, Pither C E, Wessely S 1997 Iatrogenic factors and chronic pain. Psychosomatic Medicine 59: 597–604

Kraaimaat F W, Van Schevikhoven R E O 1988 Causal attributions and coping with pain in chronic headache sufferers. Journal of Behavioral Medicine 11(3): 293–302

Kroenke K, Swindle R 2000 Cognitive-behavioral therapy for somatization and symptom syndromes: A critical review of controlled clinical trials. Psychotherapy and Psychosomatics 69: 205–215

Kroenke K, Spitzer R L, Williams J B et al 1994 Physical symptoms in primary care. Predictors of psychiatric disorders and functional impairment. Archives of Family Medicine 3(9): 774–779

Lindström I, Öhlund C, Eek C et al 1992 The effect of graded activity on patients with subacute low back pain: A randomized prospective clinical study with an operant-conditioning behavioral approach. Physical Therapy 72(4): 279–290

Lloyd A R, Pender H 1992 The economic impact of chronic fatigue syndrome. The Medical Journal of Australia 157: 599–601

Lucock M P, Morley S, White C et al 1997 Responses of consecutive patients to reassurance after gastroscopy: results of a self-administered questionnaire survey. British Medical Journal 315: 572–575

McCain G A, Bell D A, Mai F M et al 1988 A controlled study of the effects of a supervised cardiovascular fitness training program on the manifestations of primary fibromyalgia. Arthritis & Rheumatism 31(9): 1135–1141

McDermid A J, Rollman G B, McCain G A 1996 Generalized hypervigilance in fibromyalgia: Evidence of perceptual amplification. Pain 66: 133–144

McEwan B S 1998 Protective and damaging effects of stress mediators. The New England Journal of Medicine 338: 171–179

Macfarlane J G, Shahal B, Mously C et al 1996 Periodic K-alpha sleep EEG activity and periodic limb movements during sleep – comparisons of clinical features and sleep parameters. Sleep 19(3): 200–204

McGowan L P A, Clark-Carter D D, Pitts M K 1998 Chronic pelvic pain: A meta-analytic review. Psychology and Health 13: 937–951

Mannerkorpi K, Nyberg B, Ahlmen M et al 2000 Pool exercise combined with an education program for patients with fibromyalgia syndrome. A prospective, randomized study. Journal of Rheumatology 27(10): 2473–2481

Manu P 1998 Functional somatic syndromes: Etiology, diagnosis and treatment. Cambridge University Press, Cambridge

Martin L, Nutting A, MacIntosh B R et al 1996 An exercise program in the treatment of fibromyalgia. Journal of Rheumatology 23(6): 1050–1053

Mayer E A 1999 Emerging disease model for functional gastrointestinal disorders. American Journal of Medicine 107: 12S–19S

Mayou R, Farmer A 2002 Functional somatic symptoms and syndromes. British Medical Journal 325: 265–268

Mello-Goldner D, Jackson J 1999 Premenstrual syndrome (PMS) as a self-handicapping strategy among college women. Journal of Social Behavior and Personality 14(4): 607–616

Moss-Morris R, Petrie K J 1997 Cognitive distortions of somatic experiences: Revision and validation of a measure. Journal of Psychosomatic Research 43(3): 293–306

Moss-Morris R, Petrie K J 2000a Chronic fatigue as a biomedical illness: Objective findings and the patient's perspective. In: Moss-Morris R, Petrie K J (eds) Chronic fatigue syndrome. Routledge, London, p 29–54

Moss-Morris R, Petrie K J 2000b Chronic fatigue syndrome. Routledge, London

Moss-Morris R, Petrie K J 2001 Discriminating between chronic fatigue syndrome and depression: A cognitive analysis. Psychological Medicine 31: 469–479

Moss-Morris R, Wrapson W 2003 Representational beliefs about functional somatic syndromes. In Cameron L D, Leventhal H (eds) The self regulation of health and illness behavior. Routledge, London, p 119–137

Moss-Morris R, Wash C, Tobin R, Baldi JC Submitted Mechanisms of change during a randomised controlled graded exercise trial for chronic fatigue syndrome.

Naliboff B D, Munakata J, Chang L et al 1998 Toward a biobehavioural model of visceral hypersensitivity in irritable bowel syndrome. Journal of Psychosomatic Research 45: 485–492

Nimnuan C, Hotopf M, Wessely S 2001a Medically unexplained symptoms: An epidemiological study in seven specialities. Journal of Psychosomatic Research 51: 361–367

Nimnuan C, Rabe-Hesketh S, Wessely S et al 2001b How many functional somatic syndromes? Journal of Psychosomatic Research 51: 549–557

O'Malley P G, Jackson J L, Kroenke K et al 1999 Efficacy of antidepressants for physical symptoms: A critical review of the literature. Journal of Family Practice 48: 980–990

Peters S, Stanley I, Rose M et al 2002 A randomized controlled trial of group aerobic exercise in primary care patients with persistent, unexplained physical symptoms. Family Practice 19(6): 665–674

Philips H C, Jahanshahi M 1986 The components of pain behaviour report. Behaviour Research & Therapy 24(2): 117–125

Powell P 2001 An educational intervention treatment using physiological explanation of symptoms to encourage graded exercise in chronic fatigue syndrome. Liverpool University, Liverpool

Powell P, Bentall R P, Nye F J et al 2001 Randomised controlled trial of patient education to encourage graded exercise in chronic fatigue syndrome. British Medical Journal 322(7283): 387–390

Raine R, Haines A, Sensky T et al 2002 Systematic review of mental health interventions for patients with common somatic symptoms: Can research evidence from secondary care be extrapolated to primary care? British Medical Journal 325(7372): 1082–1085

Ramsay C, Moreland J, Ho M et al 2000 An observer-blinded comparison of supervised and unsupervised aerobic exercise regimens in fibromyalgia. Rheumatology 39(5): 501–505

Ray C, Jefferies S, Weir W R C 1997 Coping and other predictors of outcome in chronic fatigue syndrome – A 1-year follow-up. Journal of Psychosomatic Research 43(4): 405–415

Reid S, Chalder T, Cleare A et al 2000 Extracts from "clinical evidence" – Chronic fatigue syndrome. British Medical Journal 320(7230): 292–296

Reilly K, Lovejoy B, Williams R et al 1989 Differences between a supervised and independent strength and conditioning program with chronic low back

syndromes. Journal of Occupational Medicine 31(6): 547–550

Richards S, Cleare A 2000 Fibromyalgia: Biological correlates. Current Opinion in Psychiatry 13: 623–628

Richards S C, Scott D L 2002 Prescribed exercise in people with fibromyalgia: Parallel group randomised controlled trial. British Medical Journal 325(7357): 185

Robbins J M, Kirmayer L J 1990 Illness worry and disability in fibromyalgia syndrome. International Journal of Psychiatry in Medicine 20(1): 49–63

Robbins J M, Kirmayer L J 1991 Attributions of common somatic symptoms. Psychological Medicine 21: 1029–1045

Russo J, Katon W, Sullivan M et al 1994 Severity of somatization and its relationship to psychiatric disorders and personality. Psychosomatics 35(6): 546–556

Salkovskis P M 1992 Somatic problems. In Hawton K, Salkovskis P M, Kirk J, Clark D M (eds) Cognitive behaviour therapy for psychiatric problems: A practical guide. Oxford University Press, Oxford, p 235–276

Schmaling K B, DiClementi J D 1995 Interpersonal stressors in chronic fatigue syndrome: A pilot study. Journal of Chronic Fatigue Syndrome 1: 153–158

Schwartz S M, Gramling S E 1997 Cognitive factors associated with facial pain. Cranio – The Journal of Craniomandibular Practice 15(3): 261–266

Sharpe M, Hawton K, Seagroatt V et al 1992a Follow up of patients presenting with fatigue to an infectious diseases clinic. British Medical Journal 305: 147–152

Sharpe M, Peveler R, Mayou R 1992b The psychological treatment of patients with a functional somatic syndrome: A practical guide. Journal of Psychosomatic Research 36: 515–529

Shorter E 1995 Sucker-punched again: Physicians meet the disease-of-the-month syndrome. Journal of Psychosomatic Research 39(2): 115–118

Smythe H A 1979 Non-articular rheumatism and psychogenic musculoskeletal syndromes. In McCarty D J (ed) Arthritis and allied conditions. Lea and Febiger, Philadelphia, p 881–891

Smythe H A 1981 Fibrositis and other diffuse musculoskeletal syndromes. In Kelley W N, Harris E D Jr, Ruddy S, Sledge C B (eds) Textbook of Rheumatology. W B Saunders, Philadelphia

Spinhoven P, Onstein E J, Sterk P J et al 1993 Discordance between symptom and physiological criteria for the hyperventilation syndrome. Journal of Psychosomatic Research 37: 281–289

Stone J, Wojcik W, Durrance D et al 2002 What should we say to patients with symptoms unexplained by disease? The "number needed to offend". British Medical Journal 325: 1449–1450

Surawy C, Hackmann A, Hawton K et al 1995 Chronic fatigue syndrome: A cognitive approach. Behaviour Research & Therapy 33(5): 535–544

Terr A I 1998 Multiple chemical sensitivities. In Manu P (ed) Functional somatic syndromes: Etiology, diagnosis and treatment. Cambridge University Press, Cambridge, p 202–218

Thompson W G, Longstreth G F, Drossman D A et al 1999 Functional bowel disorders and functional abdominal pain. Gut 45(Suppl II): 1143–1147

Turner J A, Clancy S 1988 Comparison of operant behavioral and cognitive-behavioral group treatment for chronic low back pain. Journal of Consulting & Clinical Psychology 56(2): 261–266

Turner J A, Clancy S, McQuade K J et al 1990 Effectiveness of behavioral therapy for chronic low back pain: A component analysis. Journal of Consulting & Clinical Psychology 58(5): 573–579

Ursin H, Erikson H R 2001 Sensitization, subjective health complaints, and sustained arousal. Annals of the New York Academy of Sciences 933: 119–129

Van Dulman A M, Fennis J F M, Bleijenberg G 1996 Cognitive-behavioural group therapy for irritable bowel syndrome: Effects and long term follow-up. Psychosomatic Medicine 58(5): 508–514

Van Houdenhove B, Neerinckx E, Lysens R et al 2001 Victimization in chronic fatigue syndrome and fibromyalgia in tertiary care – A controlled study on prevalence and characteristics. Psychosomatics 42(1): 21–28

van Santen S M, Bolwijn P, Verstappen F et al 2002 A randomized clinical trial comparing fitness and biofeedback training versus basic treatment in patients with fibromyalgia. Journal of Rheumatology 29(3): 575–581

van Tulder M W, Ostelo R W J G, Vlaeyen J W S et al 2002 Behavioural treatment for chronic low back pain (Cochrane Review). Cochrane Database of Systematic Reviews 4

Vansteenkiste J, Rochette F, Demedts M 1991 Diagnostic tests of hyperventilation syndrome. European Respiratory Journal 4: 393–399

Vlaeyen J W S, Haazen I W C J, Schuerman J A et al 1995a Behavioural rehabilitation of chronic low back pain: Comparison of an operant treatment, an operant-cognitive treatment and an operant-respondent treatment. British Journal of Clinical Psychology 34: 95–118

Vlaeyen J W S, Kole-Snijders A M J, Boeren R G B et al 1995b Fear of movement/(re)injury in chronic low back pain and its relation to behavioral performance. Pain 62: 363–372

Vlaeyen J W S, de Jong J, Geilen M et al 2001 Graded exposure in vivo in the treatment of pain-related fear: A replicated single-case experimental design in four patients with chronic low back pain. Behaviour Research & Therapy 39(2): 151–166

Wearden A J, Morriss R K, Mullis R et al 1998 Randomised, double-blind, placebo-controlled treatment trial of fluoxetine and graded exercise for chronic fatigue syndrome. British Journal of Psychiatry 172: 485–490

Weber B E, Kapoor W N 1996 Evaluation and outcomes of patients with palpitations. American Journal of Medicine 100: 138–148

Wessely S 1997 Chronic fatigue syndrome: A 20th century illness? Scandinavian Journal of Work, Environment & Health 23(Suppl 3): 17–34

Wessely S, Nimnuan C, Sharpe M 1999 Functional somatic syndromes: One or many? The Lancet 354: 936–939

Whelton C L, Salit I, Moldofsky H 1992 Sleep, Epstein–Barr virus infection, musculoskeletal pain, and depressive symptoms in chronic fatigue syndrome. Journal of Rheumatology 19(6): 939–943

White C, Schweitzer R 2000 The role of personality in the development and perpetuation of chronic fatigue syndrome. Journal of Psychosomatic Research 48: 515–524

White K P, Nielson W R, Harth M et al 2002 Does the label "fibromyalgia" alter health status, function, and health service utilization? A prospective, within group comparison in a community cohort of adults with chronic widespread pain. Arthritis & Rheumatism 47: 260–265

Wigers S H, Stiles T C, Vogel P A 1996 Effects of aerobic exercise versus stress management treatment in fibromyalgia. A 4.5 year prospective study. Scandinavian Journal of Rheumatology 25(2): 77–86

Williams G, Pirohamed J, Minors D et al 1996 Dissociation of body-temperature and melatonin secretion circadian rhythms in patients with chronic fatigue syndrome. Clinical Physiology 16: 327–337

Wolfe F, Smythe H A, Yunus M B et al 1990 The American College of Rheumatology 1990 criteria for the classification of fibromyalgia. Report of the multicenter criteria committee. Arthritis & Rheumatism 33: 160–172

Yunus M B, Masi A T, Calabro J J, Miller K A, Feigenbaum S L 1981 Primary fibromyalgia (fibrositis): clinical study of 50 patients with matched normal controls. Seminars in Arthritis and Rheumatism 11: 151–171

Chapter **19**

Personality disorders

Mark B. Andersen

INTRODUCTION

This chapter will be similar to Chapter 7 in that it will be another primer on psychopathology. This time, however, the focus will be on Axis II of the Diagnostic and Statistical Manual of Mental Disorders (DSM-IV-TR, 4th edition, Text Revision) (American Psychiatric Association 2000). All of Axis II will be covered with the exception of mental retardation. The complete list of disorders on Axis II can be found in Box 19.1. As in Chapter 7, there will be no review of theory and research into physical and manual therapists working with people with personality disorders. Such a literature is virtually non-existent. Rather, the goals of this chapter are to describe all the personality disorders in the DSM-IV-TR, and the behaviors those individuals might manifest in a physical or manual therapy setting. People with personality disorders have behaviors and perceptions that are difficult to change, and most are resistant to the idea of entering formal psychological treatment. There will be, however, a few words about referral in most sections and at the end of the chapter.

GENERAL PERSONALITY DISORDERS

Before discussing specific disorders of personality, it is important to examine what it is that psychologists and psychiatrists mean when they use the word "personality." That answer is going to vary depending on what school of psychology or psychiatry one embraces. At one extreme, Freudians will talk about personality structures (id, ego, superego) and fixations at various psychosexual stages (oral,

Box 19.1 Diagnostic and Statistical Manual of Mental Disorders Axis II Disorders

- Paranoid personality disorder
- Schizoid personality disorder
- Schizotypal personality disorder
- Antisocial personality disorder
- Borderline personality disorder
- Histrionic personality disorder
- Narcissistic personality disorder
- Avoidant personality disorder
- Dependent personality disorder
- Obsessive-compulsive personality disorder
- Personality disorders not otherwise specified
- Mental retardation

anal, phallic, genital), and some general Freudian formulations will be present in some of the sections below. At the other end, radical behaviorists will deny any internal construct of personality and talk about overt behavior and the history of reinforcement as constituting what we believe to be personality. For the purposes of this chapter, personality will be considered the sum of those consistent patterns of thinking, feeling, behaving, and desiring that are unique (at least in the patterning) to each individual. It is when these patterns, or traits, become rigid and inflexible, and begin to cause some personal distress, impair social functioning, or are at odds with social norms that a personality disorder may be suspected. Personality disorders show up in two or more of the following areas:

- thinking (e.g., consistent, but irrational or delusional processes)
- emotions (e.g., radical swings in affect)
- interactions with others (e.g., aggression, exploitation of others)
- impulsivity (e.g., acting out, substance use).

The dysfunctional patterns found in those with personality disorders are long term and may be present as early as childhood, but certainly appear by late adolescence or early adulthood.

The DSM-IV-TR (American Psychiatric Association 2000) groups the personality disorders into three clusters:

- Cluster A personality disorders show odd or eccentric features (paranoid, schizoid, schizotypal)

- Cluster B personality disorders show emotional or dramatic features (antisocial, borderline, histrionic, narcissistic)
- Cluster C personality disorders show fear or anxiety-like features (avoidant, dependent, obsessive-compulsive).

These groupings may be useful from a heuristic point of view, but they are not mutually exclusive (e.g., people with paranoid personality disorders may experience considerable anxiety). Also, people may have features of more than one personality disorder that cross clusters (e.g., individuals meeting diagnostic criteria for both schizotypal and histrionic disorders).

An essential feature of personality disorders is that they are longstanding patterns, and not the result of some recent stressor or trauma. Another feature of many personality disorders is that individuals often "don't see a problem" with themselves, and if there is a problem with how they see the world and behave, they believe it lies within others, not themselves. Such a viewpoint makes successful referral a difficult, if not impossible, task.

This chapter will cover the personality disorders by cluster, followed by some suggestions for referral. Finally, a case study of a client with a personality disorder seeking treatment in a physical and manual therapy clinic will be presented and discussed.

CLUSTER A PERSONALITY DISORDERS

The following Cluster A personality disorders will be discussed: schizoid personality disorders, schizotypal personality disorders, and paranoid personality disorders.

SCHIZOID PERSONALITY DISORDER

There is much confusion in the media (television, movies), and in popular conception, about the terms "schizo" and "schizophrenia." Because "schizo," from which we get the word "schism," means to split or separate, many people mistakenly believe that schizophrenia means "split (or multiple) personality." People with schizophrenia do not have more than one personality within them; the "splitting" has more to do with thoughts being separated from emotion, and thoughts themselves being fragmented and disorganized. It is more like one personality breaking into pieces. Schizoid personality disorder also has much to do with splitting and separating, but it occurs not so much in the intrapsychic world as in the social realm.

People with schizoid personality disorder are "split" away from intimate, or even casual and friendly, human interaction. They generally avoid most social interaction, and this pattern of being "a loner" usually begins to manifest by late adolescence or early adulthood. Most people have encountered a person with this disorder. In social situations, this person is the one sitting away from others, the one who shows little emotion or interest when one tries to engage in conversation, and the one who may prefer the computer and computer games to talking with anyone.

People with schizoid personality disorder seem to have low hedonic tone and do not appear to derive pleasure from many activities. They usually have little interest in sex or other sensory experiences that many people enjoy. Because intimacy and social contact are not important, and even shunned by these individuals, they are not usually sensitive to what others think or say about them. They often appear detached and aloof. In terms of employment, positions that involve a minimum of interpersonal contact, and allow the individual to work in relative isolation, are ideal. As more companies and work organizations allow for working at a distance and "telecommuting" through computers and email, people with this disorder may be finding more jobs that suit their personal needs.

In the physical and manual therapies, a person with schizoid personality disorder may seem quite flat emotionally as they go through treatment. They will most likely not express any good feelings from interventions that most others enjoy (e.g., massage). They will be difficult to engage in conversations, and may even become irritated if a physical or manual therapist keeps probing for personal information. These individuals are the ones who go through therapy cool, distant, and aloof, and for the physical or manual therapist who enjoys human contact, these people can be quite frustrating. The major danger from the therapists' view is that in response to the coldness of such clients, they too become distant and aloof, further depersonalizing the therapy situation.

As mentioned above, many people with personality disorders do not perceive that anything is wrong, so making a referral would most often be met with a blank stare or a response such as "I don't see how that would be of any use." I guess the advice to physical and manual therapists who encounter people with schizoid personality disorders is to remain as pleasant as possible, do not keep probing about their personal lives, and let them be. The problem with treating these people is that sympathetic and sensitive therapists often want to reach out and connect with these individuals because they seem so alone and detached. Such reaching out will most likely be met with greater detachment. That response may make the therapist try even harder to connect, and further alienate the person. The best advice is probably to offer competent care and leave them alone.

SCHIZOTYPAL PERSONALITY DISORDER

Schizotypal personality disorder is another "schizo" disorder, and in this case the schizotypal personality has features of schizoid personality disorders, plus there are generally milder features of some symptoms of schizophrenia. Schizotypal individuals, like schizoid persons, are socially detached and often become uncomfortable in social situations. A feature that distinguishes these individuals from schizoid types is that they are often overtly and distinctly "odd" (by usual Western cultural standards). Their dress may be eccentric or unkempt or both. They may communicate a "specialness" to others in that they have magical powers or extrasensory perceptions. They often have "ideas of reference" where some normal event (e.g., raining on one's birthday) has some special personal meaning.

People with schizotypal personality disorders also often experience psychotic-like symptoms (e.g., hearing voices, paranoid delusions, loose thought patterns and associations), but these features are not as extreme or as long lasting as they are with schizophrenia. This disorder is relatively common (approximately 3% of the population), and physical and manual therapists will certainly come into contact with such persons. Schizotypal symptoms (e.g., social withdrawal, weird thoughts, odd fantasies, lack of close similar-age friends) may begin to appear in childhood and early adolescence. In therapy, they may tell tales of being able to read the therapist's mind, or of how they have special powers to heal themselves, or how they are intimately involved in the paranormal.

Referral may be an option for these individuals, but not necessarily for the personality disorder. Unlike the schizoid pattern, people with schizotypal personalities often experience anxiety (especially in social situations), depression, and even brief psychotic episodes. These experiences are distressing, and they may seek help because of them. If a physical and manual therapist suspects that a client has a schizotypal personality disorder, then probing gently for stories about anxiety, depression, or odd distressing experiences (e.g., brief psychotic episodes) may help the client talk about problems, and prepare the client to be receptive to a referral to a mental health specialist for those symptoms.

As part of the rapport-building process, physical and manual therapists should not try to contradict the claims of special powers, extrasensory perception, and so forth, but rather engage the person in talking about their experiences. Often the stories they will tell will be quite interesting, if a bit vague and hard to follow at times.

PARANOID PERSONALITY DISORDER

Individuals with paranoid personality disorders are profoundly distrustful of others and suspect that people are out to exploit them or hurt them in some way. There is, of course, no objective evidence that any harm is coming their way. These individuals harbor grudges for imagined betrayals or injuries from others. For example, if someone had to break a lunch date, the person with the paranoid personality would read all sorts of meaning into that event and consider it a major betrayal of friendship. Individuals with this disorder have difficulty holding on to friends because of their suspicions and irrational thinking. Early symptoms of paranoid personality disorder are similar to schizotypal features (e.g., social withdrawal, hypersensitivity, strange thoughts and fantasies) and may appear in childhood or early adolescence. This disorder is also more common in males.

If partnered, people with paranoid personalities may be suspicious of the partner's faithfulness, suspect that the partner has been cheating on them, and try to control all aspects of the relationship. They may psychologically badger their partners with demands to know where they have been, who they were with, and what they have been doing.

Paranoid individuals do not have a tendency to disclose information to others because that information could be used against them. If a physical or manual therapist begins to make lots of casual inquiries about how things are going in their lives, people with paranoid personality disorder may begin to become suspicious and more withdrawn. Further questioning by the therapist will probably only increase the suspicions and paranoia. Even a simple intake interview about past medical conditions could be an occasion for stimulating the person's paranoid world view.

A referral to a mental health professional will most likely be met with extreme resistance, and could easily backfire on the physical or manual therapist in that the client would suspect that the therapist was out to have them locked up or committed to an institution. So in most cases, referral is often counterproductive to the working relationship between the therapist and the client who is paranoid. It is probably best for physical and manual therapists to just listen and acknowledge stories of betrayal, suspicions, and unfaithfulness, if they arise in conversation during treatment. They often will not, because disclosing information to others gives them too much power to use against one. But if stories do emerge of a paranoid flavor, then it would be wise not to contradict or challenge them. Such a response may stimulate a paranoid reaction and the physical or manual therapist may become part of the world that is against the client.

CLUSTER B PERSONALITY DISORDERS

The following Cluster B personality disorders will be discussed: narcissistic personality disorder, borderline personality disorder, histrionic personality disorder, and antisocial personality disorder.

NARCISSISTIC PERSONALITY DISORDER

Individuals with narcissistic personality disorder are entranced with the image they have of themselves. They believe themselves to be special, worthy of great admiration, and bound for great success in life. They also have a strong sense of entitlement (e.g., good things should come their way automatically) and are often exploitative of others. People with this disorder are so wrapped up in themselves and the (often fragile) image they have of themselves that they lack empathy and cannot see the world from another's viewpoint. They are often arrogant and envious of the success of others. In the case study example in Chapter 7 on transference and countertransference, the character Evelyn has some features of narcissistic personality disorder (e.g., imperious manner, wanting only the best physical therapist, dismissive of others "beneath" her), but does not fit enough criteria for a true diagnosis.

Most of us have come across this "conceited" type. The "friends" they have are mainly there to admire the individual and serve to bolster the already inflated ego. The "state" of the person with a narcissistic personality disorder is that at the core they know (at some level) they are empty and fatuous. Their self-esteem is usually extremely fragile, and their responses to criticism are exaggerated. The successful, competent, lovable, charming, desirable, deserving image they have built is often in response to an upbringing filled with psychological abuse, being told they were not worthy and not lovable, with possibly even experiences of public humiliation. In defensive response to that psychological abuse, individuals with this disorder may have built up fantasy worlds where everyone loved them, and they were great successes.

When seeking services in the healthcare professions (or any other professions), people with narcissistic personality disorder often demand having "the best in the business" as their physicians or therapists. If the therapist does not meet their expectations, they can be quite dismissive. Not meeting expectations is a common problem for people with this disorder. They believe their situations and their needs are special, and cannot be understood and appreciated by just anybody. Only other really special, intelligent, and gifted others can understand what they are going through. Such a world view, of course, is going to come up against reality often, especially in some medical fields. The person with this disorder, when seeking medical treatment, is looking for status (the best in the business), but is also looking for an ally in their world view of their own uniqueness and specialness. If such a person does not find that ally and admirer, the individual may cease treatment, disparage the practitioner, and go on to try and find another high status professional who will join the "fan club."

Narcissistic personality disorder may not be obvious when people first meet. These individuals, especially if rather intelligent, can be extremely charming, and even complimentary and attentive to others. Their compliments and attention, however, are often hollow and insincere. They know how to get people on their side, and can use social graces to good effect. They can use their charm to get what they need, and that charm can be used as a tool to accomplish a series of sexual conquests.

For practitioners in the physical and manual therapies, experiences with such individuals may initially be "charming," but as time and treatment go by, the person begins to manifest entitlement and self-absorption. So what is a physical and manual therapist to do? Contradicting the person's world view (e.g., "Well, this condition is really quite common, and it's just like 100 other cases I have treated") will not endear them to the therapist. Referral to a mental health professional will invariably be met with incredulity, expressions of disappointment in the professional, and often termination (by the client) of treatment. So that is really not an option in most cases. Possibly the best course of action is to listen to their stories of future success and specialness, and nod one's head. The physical therapist may not become an active ally of the client, but if the client perceives that the therapist is at least sympathetic, then the likelihood of remaining in therapy is increased. There are dangers here also for the physical or manual therapist, especially those with hero worship tendencies and weak ego boundaries. Some people with narcissistic personality disorders can be quite seductive, and a therapist with personal problems could easily be ensnared in an exploitative web.

BORDERLINE PERSONALITY DISORDER

The individual with a borderline personality disorder is on a behavioral, emotional, and cognitive rollercoaster. Their instability and ups and downs cross many areas of their lives including interpersonal relationships, how they view themselves, their emotional reactions to situations, and their problems controling impulses. One of the major, and often all-pervasive, features of borderline personality disorder is the fear of abandonment. If this fear is triggered strongly enough, depression, self-mutilation, and even suicide may eventuate. Abandonment anxiety can happen in response to something as simple as having to change an appointment with a therapist to later in the week. If a person with a borderline personality disorder was scheduled for six sessions with a physical or manual therapist, then it would be quite common for the fifth (and especially the sixth) session to be one where the client seems to have regressed, or gotten worse. The sixth and final session would trigger abandonment anxiety, and getting worse would be a way to extend treatment and avoid that anxiety.

People with borderline disorders have tendencies to have stormy interpersonal relationships. They often fall in love hard, even after only one or two meetings with the other person. The process usually involves the projection of an idealized lover onto the person, and then falling in love with that projection. Inevitably, the other person cannot live up to that image, and disappointment sets in; the borderline person may then begin to disparage the now deficient ex-lover. This falling in and out of love rapidly and dramatically is a common feature. Physical and manual therapists who have clients with borderline personality disorders are likely to hear such stories of turbulent relationships. And herein lies a danger for therapists. People with borderline personality disorders often have difficulty interpreting social signals. Professional interest and courtesy from a therapist may be interpreted as romantic interest. Couple this misinterpretation of social encounters with the therapist touching the client's body (as a normal part of treatment), and there is the potential for serious client–therapist relationship problems. It is quite common for clients with borderline personalities to "fall in love" with their therapists, and the process of rejecting that "love" can be painful, embarrassing, and may even involve legal issues. A client with a borderline personality, romantically rejected by a therapist, may, in revenge for the rejection, accuse the therapist of inappropriate sexual behavior.

People with borderline personality disorders have mercurial self-images. Sometimes they see themselves as "bad" people while other times they may see themselves as quite virtuous. They may change plans for their futures often and may shift (or at least experiment) with other sexual orientations. In terms of body image, borderline personality disorder is not an uncommon comorbidity with eating disorders (see Chapter 7).

Impulsivity is often a central feature of borderline personalities. Substance abuse, irresponsible spending, engaging in dangerous thrill seeking (e.g., reckless driving), and so forth are common and self-destructive patterns for these people. Self-mutilation and suicidal gestures and attempts are also common. Such actions are likely to occur when imagined or real abandonment looms closely. For

the physical and manual therapist, especially towards the end of the course of treatment, any reference to hopelessness (e.g., "it seems all so pointless," "I really don't see much future") should be taken seriously, and questions should be asked about intentions to self-harm. One way to approach this problem will be illustrated in the case study example at the end of this chapter.

The person with borderline personality disorder may have a history of abuse (physical, sexual, psychological) or may have lost a parent early in life through death or separation. Clients with this disorder will probably be some of the most challenging physical and manual therapists will face in their careers.

HISTRIONIC PERSONALITY DISORDER

People with histrionic personality disorders have features in common with borderline and narcissistic disorders, but the central features of abandonment anxiety, self-destructiveness, and grandiosity are not present. What people with this disorder do have in common with those other disorders is extreme emotional lability and a craving of attention. The person with a histrionic personality needs to be the center of attention. They tend to be flamboyant and are often the life of the party. The classic stereotype of the opera "Diva" fits this personality disorder well. They are often effusive, flirtatious, and dramatic, and can be quite entertaining and a lot of fun. But their demands to be in the spotlight all the time become, after a time, irritating and alienating.

Their behavior with physical and manual therapists may involve flirting, the telling of dramatic stories, displays of affection (e.g., hugs before or after treatment), and even the bringing of gifts. A central concern of people with histrionic personalities is how they look. They often dress in a provocative manner or in other ways that draw attention to them. They may spend an inordinate amount of money on clothes and makeup. In females with this disorder, stereotypic feminine traits may be exaggerated, and in males, stereotypic "macho" behaviors and posturing may be present.

These individuals have difficulties with sexual and other intimate relationships. They are often emotional manipulators and dependent on their romantic partners. They often have elaborate romantic fantasies, and the physical and manual therapist may become the object of such fantasies. Rejection by others may result in suicidal ideation or gestures as a means of gaining more attention and manipulating others.

After a while physical and manual therapists may become frustrated and irritated at clients with this disorder. If the therapist becomes reserved and more distant, the person with a histrionic personality may escalate that attention seeking behavior, often leading to further withdrawal by the therapist, and thus begins a cycle of mutual alienation and risk of leaving treatment. Patience and good humor, although difficult to display, may help keep the client in therapy.

ANTISOCIAL PERSONALITY DISORDER

People with antisocial personality disorder can present in a variety of ways. The main feature of this disorder is a violation of the rights of others with no shame or guilt attached. In Freudian terms, these individuals seem to lack a superego or moral conscience, and are mainly interested in the gratification of their own desires regardless of whether they hurt others or not. This disorder often begins in childhood or early adolescence. Many playground bullies develop into people with this disorder.

Some people with antisocial personality disorder have considerable problems with impulse control, and often those impulses can be violent. They may engage in physical violence if their desires are thwarted, especially if substance use (e.g., alcohol) is involved. They are often in conflict with social norms, and may have histories of arrest and incarceration. Some people with this disorder find niches in society where their aggressive and violent behaviors are actually rewarded (e.g., in violent sports such as American football).

Individuals with this disorder who are in the higher ranges of intelligence may be able to manipulate and intimidate others for gratification in different ways than violence. The heartless, but charming and seductive "con man" is a good example of an intelligent antisocial personality. Prisons are filled with people with this disorder. As with most personality disorders, these individuals do not learn well, and keep repeating patterns of destructive behavior.

It is unlikely that a physical or manual therapist would be the victim of a violent outburst from a client with this disorder. More likely, a client of the "con man" variety might use his charm and seductive skills (the "he" was intentional because this disorder appears much more common in males) to seduce a therapist, make requests for psychoactive drugs, or try to engage a therapist in a "really exciting business adventure" (ultimately a con). Red flags should begin to fly when a therapist begins to feel "charmed" by a client's compliments and attention. That charm is a first step in getting a therapist to comply with the client's manipulations.

Many people with antisocial personality disorders have been abused physically, psychologically, or sexually in childhood. They have learned that the world is an awful place, full of pain, and in order to survive, they have to look out for number one, and take what they can get. Referral is not usually an option, because these individuals do not see a problem. The major warning to physical and manual therapists is to watch that one does not get caught up in their charm, or ensnared in their manipulations.

CLUSTER C PERSONALITY DISORDERS

The following Cluster C personality disorders will be discussed: obsessive-compulsive personality disorder, avoidant personality disorder, and dependent personality disorder.

OBSESSIVE-COMPULSIVE PERSONALITY DISORDER

The main distinction between obsessive-compulsive personality disorder and obsessive-compulsive anxiety disorder (see Chapter 7) is the absence of clinical obsessions (e.g., intrusive, repetitive thoughts) and compulsions (e.g., excessive handwashing). Individuals with this disorder are perfectionistic, extremely orderly, and require a huge measure of control. They are often sticklers for rules and procedures. In Freudian terms, they have anal-retentive personalities. They are inflexible, up-tight, and often miserly. Their perfectionism and attention to detail often work against them in that nothing is ever good enough, and projects they engage in often do not come to completion because they have to be reworked over and over again. Their "tightness" often extends to issues of morality, and they are often quite rigid when it comes to ethics and correct behavior. They are often overly dedicated to work, and may not engage in many leisure time activities. In group settings, or when involved in group tasks, theirs is the only way that they want the group to pursue. They have difficulty trusting others to complete work, and often take on huge tasks rather than delegate parts of those tasks to others.

People with obsessive-compulsive personality disorder may also be high achievers in the realms of business and sport. These two realms actually may reinforce their personality traits, and high success in these areas often requires a good measure of single-mindedness. Interviews with elite sportspeople often reveal obsessive-compulsive tendencies and perfectionism. Their perfectionism, however, is also a source of distress, and they may seek some counseling and advice on how better to handle their time and commitments. Referral for psychological assistance may be an option for physical and manual therapists to make for some of these individuals. An initial referral for learning time management skills may be the most palatable, and once in counseling or psychotherapy, other issues of control may be addressed.

In physical and manual therapy, these individuals may be difficult clients. Their attention to detail and perfectionism may lead to frustration in their progress or in their completing home exercises. They will often want to know the specific course of treatment, and the markers of progress, in detail. If the time course of treatment does not go to schedule, then they may experience substantial frustration. Also, if they prescribe to the principle "more is better" then the possibility of overdoing rehabilitation exercises increases. That overdoing it will often lead to setbacks in therapy and further frustration. The physical or manual therapist can use these clients' desires for order and concern for rules in carefully laying out treatment plans with strong emphasis on doing the treatments at home (e.g., stretching, cryotherapy) in a very precise and controlled manner, with nothing over and above the "rules." On the positive side, these individuals will usually be good and compliant clients, wanting to get through therapy in the most orderly and efficient manner.

AVOIDANT PERSONALITY DISORDER

Most people have met individuals who retreat from social situations, seem awkward when interacting with others, and generally steer clear of social encounters. These people are often labeled "painfully shy," and many may fit the diagnostic criteria for avoidant personality disorder. These individuals feel inferior to others, avoid social interactions, and are hypersensitive to what others think of them. Unlike the schizoid type, these individuals want human contact, but they have inordinate fears of rejection and disapproval. They have trouble making intimate connections with others and are afraid to disclose their feelings and risk ridicule. Their hypersensitivity leads them to exaggerate what might be slight disapproval from others into global condemnation, and their low self-esteem is all-pervasive.

People with avoidant personalities often do have strong desires for affection and human contact, but their behaviors and sensitivities almost ensure that they will not achieve these desired interactions. They often behave in awkward ways that confirm that they are inadequate and inferior (at least in their perceptions).

Physical and manual therapists, when engaging people who are obviously extremely shy and anxious, need to be careful of how they communicate in order not to stimulate the client's fears of negative evaluation. Constant reassurance that they are doing well in therapy may be helpful, and when a client does not seem to be progressing, the blame should not be directly focused on them. For example, if a client has not been completing home exercises, instead of saying "You really need to be more attentive to those exercises and get them done" an alternative might be "Oh, I am sorry, I probably put too much on your plate. Let's go back and see if we can adjust those exercises so you'll have time to get them done." That approach keeps negative evaluation at bay, and may help the person with an avoidant personality feel more comfortable and less inferior to a therapist. As the name of the disorder implies, these people do a lot of avoiding. If the therapy environment has a considerable evaluative atmosphere, then the client may end up avoiding the clinic altogether. These individuals desire human contact, and with these clients, maybe more than others, the therapeutic trait of the practitioner having unconditional positive regard will go a long way to helping them successfully complete their courses of treatment.

Referral for psychological intervention may be a possibility, but must be handled with utmost sensitivity and only after a strong alliance has been formed. The suggestion that one see a mental health professional could easily be interpreted as serious criticism and further evidence that one is inferior. The suggestion should sound something like the following: "You know, you are doing so well here in rehab. I am really pleased with how things are going. I did notice that at times you seem a bit shy, and may be a little uncomfortable in some social situations, like here in the clinic at times. I have a good friend and colleague and he (she) is an expert at helping people who are shy get more comfortable around others. If you would like, we could have him (her) come in and have a chat with us." This soft and gentle, hand-holding approach would likely be more successful than a more direct referral to a psychologist.

DEPENDENT PERSONALITY DISORDER

The person with a dependent personality disorder has an extremely strong need to be taken care of, to be protected, and to submit to others. These people cling desperately to others and can feel like a burden to family and friends. Their helpless behaviors stem from feelings of being unable to get along without the aid of others, and are aimed at getting people to do things for them and make decisions. They are generally quite passive, and will even agree to do things that they know are not in their best interests in order not to offend those they are dependent upon. They can easily become victims of unscrupulous others, such as those with antisocial personality disorders. They may even go so far as to tolerate psychological or physical abuse as long as they can remain dependent on the abuser. They may have fears of becoming competent and independent, because that could mean abandonment by those on whom they depend. They are convinced that they cannot function alone, and the fear of abandonment is all-pervasive. They have little confidence in their skills and positive traits, and will often refer to themselves in disparaging ways (e.g., "I am not smart, I am stupid").

People with dependent personality disorder are at substantial risk of anxiety and mood disorders, and some predisposing factors may include loss of a loved one early in life or a long childhood illness where they were dependent for extended periods of time. This disorder is one of the more common personality disorders found in the mental health field and may be more common in females than males, but some research says it is relatively common in both genders.

For the physical and manual therapist, clients with this disorder will, at least in the beginning, be compliant and motivated. These clients usually will do anything the therapist asks and be conscientious with home exercises and put out considerable effort during time in the clinic or office. They will want to please the therapist, and may show signs of dependence early (e.g., asking for more time, calling between appointments to ask questions). Similar to borderline personality disorder, these clients have a strong fear of abandonment, and may regress when therapy is coming to a close in order to keep contact with the therapist. If the client is in an exploitative or abusive relationship, their connection to the therapist may become particularly strong, because the therapist may represent the idealized and fantasized benevolent dominant other that the client desires over the current abusive one. The major problem a physical or manual therapist may face with such a client is the termination of services. The client is likely to cling and not want to let go. Probably the best course of action, if circumstances, insurance payments, and so forth will allow is to slowly wean the dependent client away from the therapist, moving the client from weekly to fortnightly to monthly appointments over the course of several months.

A FINAL WORD ON PERSONALITY DISORDERS

The above descriptions of people with personality disorders are based on the diagnostic criteria in the DSM-IV-TR (American Psychiatric Association 2000), and they represent the "pure" types. In reality, such pure types may actually be relatively rare. Often it is the case that people with personality disorders manifest symptoms and patterns of behavior and thought that cross different disorders and different clusters of disorders. So these descriptions are meant to be rough guidelines for practitioners. In the real world things are not so simple and clear cut.

REFERRAL FOR FORMAL PSYCHOLOGICAL ASSISTANCE

As noted above, for several personality disorders, a referral to a mental health professional will be met with substantial resistance, and it is not the job of the physical and manual therapist to make sure all clients with psychopathology get treatment. One of the problems is that physical and manual therapists are in the helping professions, and they want to help. With more and more emphasis on holistic approaches and team treatment of clients, therapists may desire to get problematic clients, such as those with personality disorders, into psychotherapy. For many, it just is not going to work.

For those where a referral may work (avoidant, dependent personality disorders), the process needs to be sensitive. I have found over the years that instead of referring "out" to some other helping professional a good first move with many clients is to refer "in." That is, bring the new psychologist (or nutritionist) into the physical or manual therapy session, introduce them to the client, and all three parties start talking.

In working with clients in the physical and manual therapies, the following scenario is quite common. Therapy is progressing well. The therapist and client have had several sessions together, and the client has become quite comfortable with the therapist to the point of revealing some serious anxieties, or an eating disorder, or a growing social phobia. It has taken several weeks or months for the client to get comfortable enough, and to get up enough nerve to talk about a worrisome personal concern. To say at this point "That stuff is beyond my area of expertise, here's the address and telephone number of a psychologist" is not an optimal way to proceed. It has a rejecting flavor to it, something to be devoutly avoided. Something more along the lines of what was said in the section with the avoidant personality would be a lot more salubrious.

Physical and manual therapists need to cultivate a referral circle of experts in a variety of fields, not just psychology, and not just names from the phone book, but real contacts that they know personally. Being able to say "I have a great colleague who I know well, and she is . . ." will help instil confidence in the referral for the client, and for a referral to be successful, the client needs to be secure in the process.

A CASE EXAMPLE

A case study example will now be presented to illustrate the impact that a personality disorder can have on the rehabilitation process. This case example demonstrates the dialogue between a physical therapist and a client with intermittent commentary on and analysis of that dialogue.

Thomas (a physical therapist) has been working with Rebecca for some months. Rebecca was involved in a motor vehicle accident and had sustained serious damage to her shoulder that required surgery. Her scars from the surgery were quite visible. She had progressed well in rehabilitation and was getting near completion. Thomas had noticed that her moods were erratic, one day she would be cheerful and effusive, and the next appointment she would be moody and even angry. Thomas was not well-trained in personality disorders, but he knew something was a bit strange about Rebecca. Following is the dialogue from the beginning of the session.

Thomas (T): So how are you doing today?
Rebecca (R): Crappy, why do you ask?
T: I was just concerned about how you were getting along.
R: What do you care?
T: I care for you and want you to get better.
R: So you think of me between sessions? Are you sure I am not "out of sight, out of mind"?
T: Of course I think about you, I am concerned about all my clients.
R: So I am not special, just another body to work on?
T: Rebecca, all my clients get my full attention, and I want them all to get better, you know that.

Thomas cannot win here. Rebecca is wanting to hear that she is a special person in his world, and that he cares for her more than others. She throws such mean comments towards him in an effort to elicit what she wants to hear, but he does not respond as she would like. A little later she says:

R: It is all so worthless.
T: What is worthless?
R: Coming here, rehab, working with you.
T: Why do you believe that?
R: Well look at me! Look at these scars! I'll never be able to wear a sleeveless dress, and when guys get a look at these scars, they will head for the hills.
T: (trying to be helpful) Well, some guys might find them interesting, and they could make for great conversation starters.
R: Yeah, right (dismissively). "Let's talk to the cut-up chick."
T: They are not that bad.
R: Well, would you date someone who was all sliced up like me?

T: Rebecca, I am a physical therapist. I see this sort of thing all the time, of course I would.

R: Well would you go out with me then?

T: You know I can't do that professionally.

Thomas is trying to be helpful, but is floundering a bit, and actually falling into Rebecca's borderline trap of confirming that he would reject her. His rejection triggers her abandonment anxiety, and escalates her dysphoria.

R: I just don't see any point any more.

T: What do you mean?

R: What's the use of going on? I am damaged goods. It would be better if it was just all over.

Often, direct threats of suicide are not made, but rather vague statements such as the above allude to suicidal ideation. Fortunately, Thomas has had some background in working with clients who start to manifest self-destructive thoughts and gently confronts her about what she is saying.

T: Rebecca, when you say things like that you start to make me anxious. It is like you don't feel life is worth living.

R: Well it isn't! Just look at me!

An acronym for assessing suicide risk is PAL: P is for do they have a plan, A is for their ready availability to carry out the plan, and L is for the lethality of the plan (see Cogan 2000 for more information about working with a suicidal client). Thomas is worried and moves into a concerned suicide assessment mode.

T: Now you have me really worried, have you made any plans for doing harm to yourself.

R: What do you mean? Like killing myself?

T: Yes, have you had those ideas, and have you thought about how you might do it.

R: Hell, I have those thoughts twice a day.

T: And when those thoughts come, what do you think about? How would you do it?

R: Well, I could take a truckload of Tylenol.

That response has just answered all three of the PAL questions. Yes, she does have a plan, a drug overdose. The availability of the materials needed for the plan is in any grocery store or pharmacy. The lethality of the plan is not extremely high, but an overdose of Tylenol could easily cause serious liver damage. Her risk of a suicide attempt seems fairly high, but given that she has a borderline personality

disorder, her talk may be more to gain attention. Thomas, however, cannot take the risk of considering her thoughts as merely attention seeking.

T: Now you have me really scared. I don't want to lose you, and I am really worried about what you will do when you leave here today.

R: So you do care about me?

T: Of course I do.

R: You would miss me if I was gone?

T: Yes, Rebecca, I would hate to lose a client.

R: So I am just another client, poor you if you lost a client, bad for your reputation.

Rebecca is weaving borderline traps for Thomas, and this sort of interchange is not going to be helpful. Her pattern of response to Thomas is one of seeking reassurance that she is loved and special, coupled with aggressiveness when she gets information that she is, in her mind, "just another client". Thomas needs to switch gears.

T: I don't care about my reputation; I care about you, and right now I am really concerned about your welfare. You have to promise me something.

R: What is that?

T: You have to promise me that you will not do anything to harm yourself between now and our next appointment.

R: I don't know if I can promise that.

T: Then I am going to have to do everything I can to get that promise before you leave here. This is just too serious to just let go. What if I say that between now and our next appointment, if you feel like harming yourself, that you will call me, and we will talk. Can you give me that promise?

R: Maybe.

T: I can't take a maybe, I need a yes.

R: OK, alright, yes, I won't do anything, and I'll call.

T: Thanks so much. I feel a lot better, but this is not over. I really want you to talk to a friend and colleague of mine about your thoughts. I could call her now, if you would like.

R: What? You mean a shrink? I don't want to see a shrink by myself.

T: Not to worry, I will not leave you. I will see her with you and we three can talk. Will that be OK?

R: I guess so.

T: Should I call now, or should we wait until Thursday for you next appointment?

R: Let's wait.

T: And you will keep your promise.

R: Yes, yes.

T: Good, that's a great relief.

Thomas has done a good job in an extremely difficult situation, even though he has played into Rebecca's borderline world view (i.e., she is special; she can call him anytime; he will be thinking about her a lot). But in this case, his actions are aimed at preserving life, and so using her pathology to keep her from harm seems justified. He has gained a promise of no action of harm and has set the stage for a referral for further treatment. Such a case is taxing and exhausting for physical and manual therapists and illustrates how important it is to have some training in how to work with difficult clients at risk. Physical and manual therapists are often not trained for dealing with borderline or suicidal clients, and I hope in the future such training (e.g., readings on suicide, class discussions, role plays) will become a part of standard curricula.

SUMMARY

This chapter serves as a primer for physical and manual therapists to help them recognize another class of psychopathologies, the Axis II disorders in the DSM-IV-TR (American Psychiatric Association 2000). Personality disorders are characterized by inflexible, long-lasting, and generally maladaptive patterns of thinking, feeling, perceiving, and behaving that are often at odds with social norms and may cause some level of distress. Many people with personality disorders do not recognize (as is the case with many anxiety disorders) that there is a problem, and are resistant to referral to mental health practitioners.

Personality disorders have been grouped into three clusters: those with strange or odd features (schizoid, schizotypal, paranoid), those with dramatic or fluxuating features (antisocial, borderline, histrionic, narcissistic), and those with anxiety-like features (avoidant, dependent, obsessive-compulsive). The disorders in this chapter were presented by cluster. These clusters, however, are primarily a convenience, and there is probably a lot of overlap between disorders with some people manifesting features of two or three disorders at the same time.

Each section described the features of the personality disorder in general terms. Then there was a part of each section that contained descriptions of how a person with that personality disorder might behave in a physical or manual therapy setting. Each section then addressed the possibility of referral, and if referral was possible, how one might go about it.

The chapter concluded with some comments about referral and a case example of a therapist working with a client with a borderline personality disorder who was reporting suicidal ideation. People with personality disorders make interesting clients, but are often challenging, frustrating, and demanding. Learning how to work with such people will have substantial benefits for both practitioners and the clients they serve.

References

American Psychiatric Association 2000 Diagnostic and statistical manual of mental disorders, 4th edn (text revision). American Psychiatric Association, Washington, DC

Cogan K D 2000 The sadness in sport: Working with a depressed and suicidal athlete. In: Andersen M B (ed) Doing sport psychology. Human Kinetics, Champaign IL, p 107–119

Chapter 20

Terminal illness

Stephen A. Gudas

INTRODUCTION

Although the concept of terminal illness is not at all new to medicine, the management approaches used to deal with patients and families facing life-ending illness have evolved under the concept and specialty of palliative medicine. As an example, traditionally medical oncology and palliative care have been considered two distinct and separate disciplines, but more recently, the former encompasses care that ranges from primary prevention to terminal phases (Maltoni & Amadori 2001). Well-managed terminal care may be described as rehabilitation of the dying; it has comfort as its primary objective, and requires the healthcare professional to support the patient in the face of decreased physical health and function (Twycross 1981).

Terminal care for patients is multifaceted, and necessitates the intervention of a multidisciplinary team (Robertson 2002). In this chapter, the role of those in the physical therapies and other health professionals, will be explored within the context of life-ending illness. The chapter will describe the physical and medical considerations that are encountered in terminal illness, including pain and symptom control, and comfort care principles. Major psychological considerations will be outlined, exploring therapist–patient relationships, the emotional aspects of terminal illness, and the psychology of the dying process. Lastly, integrated management approaches to terminal care will be described, emphasizing patients and families, hospice care and concept, and specific location of care issues.

PHYSICAL AND MEDICAL CONSIDERATIONS

PHYSICAL ASPECTS OF TERMINAL ILLNESS

The physical decline of the patient in terminal illness is almost inevitable and embraces many different aspects of the patient's function (Leahy 2000). In addition to weight loss, strength decrease, change in cosmetic appearance, and loss of function, physical symptoms may occur which can appreciably affect the patient's suffering. Pain occurs in approximately 66% of patients with terminal illness. Nausea, vomiting, and constipation occur in 50% of patients, and respiratory symptoms (mainly dyspnea) occur in a further 30–40% (Driscoll 1987). The fatigue, weight loss, and anorexia that ensue can be perplexing to both patient and therapist alike. Although many people think of cancer as synonymous with terminal illness, there are many other medical conditions (e.g., kidney failure, progressive heart disease, progressive neurological disorders) that can be classified as terminal. Each disease will manifest in different physical changes that accompany the dying process. However, the major physical characteristics of terminal illness (cachexia, decreased strength and function, and cosmetic loss of appearance and body image) may be common to many if not most terminal illnesses. If the physical aspects of terminal illness, and the physical symptoms that occur concomitantly to the dying process are not relieved, the possibility of alleviating psychological, social, and spiritual experiences, improving quality of life, or completing any life closure that may be possible, becomes difficult (Paolini 2001).

Cancer as a disease entity is frequently used as an example of where terminal care is paramount, since the majority of people with cancer are not cured of their disease, and terminal care and its encompassing issues need to be administered and evaluated. Management for people with cancer, and their families, extends throughout their illness, and includes the care provided at the end of life (McCahill et al 2001). Although major reform is largely needed to improve relief of pain and other symptoms in cancer care, major educational efforts are required to ensure that rehabilitation professionals can respond to this need.

In some cultures, notably American, the dominant value on orientation and self-reliance, physical ability, and individualism places a very high premium on the self-determination and control of one's own destiny (Pacquino 2001). However, this value is not always consistent with the dominant cultural views of the particular sick or dying individual, and might not be at all congruous with the physical decline of the patient. When the patient accepts the physical deterioration of his/her body, whatever be the cause, and moves toward the acceptance and inevitability of ensuing terminality, there will be a move toward things ahead rather than behind. Particularly if the family/significant others desire that the patient struggle on against these physical changes, the discrepancy between the patient's wishes and the expectations of those in the environment can be the source of great grief and turmoil. The well-trained therapist should acknowledge this common phenomenon when it transpires, and offer assistance in guiding the patient and family toward a mutual understanding beneficial to both the patient and family.

Family members may react more strongly than the patient to the physical changes encountered, such as weight loss and appearance change, and the clinician should be cognizant of this fact and be supportive where necessary. It might help to think of the patient as someone's intimate family member, the latter individual often not being able to think or act clearly or appropriately in the face of the significance of these physical changes. Death has a different meaning for everyone and this impacts greatly on how people communicate with each other as they deal with it together (McQuellon & Cowan 2000). The physical changes of impending death propel a patient into a psychological state referred to as "mortal time," and terminal illness is a powerful force that can lead a patient to this period. Typically, one encounters anxiety, pain, nausea and vomiting, and respiratory symptoms in the patient with terminal illness (Driscoll 1987). The therapist's relationship with a patient can have the effect of increasing coping, understanding, and acceptance of the physical changes that accompany dying. This relationship can very well enrich the meaning of life for patients and caregivers alike (McQuellon & Cowan 2000).

PAIN AND SYMPTOM CONTROL

Appropriate and successful management of the common symptoms of the terminally ill is tantamount to good care (Ross & Alexander 2001). Although uncontrolled pain is usually the patient's greatest fear, many physical symptoms other than pain can contribute to suffering at the end of life. Fatigue, anorexia, weight loss, nausea and vomiting, constipation, dyspnea, and site-specific symptoms can all occur in terminal illness, and need the attention of the appropriate professional to alleviate. Management involving a diagnostic evaluation of the cause of each symptom is paramount, so that skilled intervention by the appropriate professional can commence. Unfortunately, little is known of the pathophysiology of some of these terminal symptoms, especially fatigue (Ross & Alexander 2001). Education of both patient and family is the foundation of treatment.

Pain

As dying progresses, symptoms may accumulate which are progressively more difficult to manage, and may become refractory to standard medical intervention (Wein 2000). The literature on pain control is extensive (see Chapter 11), and there are specific protocols for alleviating the pain associated with terminal illness (Ross & Alexander 2001, Stevens et al 1994, Wein 2000). The therapist, in treating the patient, should be aware that in addition to pain and other physical symptoms, there may be agitated delirium, and existential or psychological distress. Terminal sedation (i.e., opioid or other drug induced somnolence employed to completely relieve the abject symptoms of death) is argued by some to hasten death, and therefore is a type of physician-assisted suicide (Wein 2000). Although a moral distinction can be made between the intention of relieving symptoms and unintended consequences, this double effect must be kept in mind in the pharmacological control of pain and other terminal symptomatology. Sedation, therefore, can be viewed as a risk-laden, but at times, necessary procedure. Regarding pain control, special populations such as children should be evaluated carefully (Stevens et al 1994). Differences occur in cancer-related pain between children and adults; the assessment of pain in the preverbal child is generally inadequate. The clinician can use gentle palpation, pointing to a painful body part, and asking simple "yes" or "no" questions to enhance pain evaluation in a very young child who cannot adequately verbalize his or her discomfort (Stevens et al 1994). Localizing signs are not as prominent in children. A multidisciplinary approach is recommended, and sedation may produce tolerance, constipation, and involuntary movements as side effects.

Nausea, vomiting, and dyspnea

The causes of nausea and vomiting in the terminal patient are complex, but these symptoms can usually be controlled with the proper and scheduled use of antiemetic pharmaceutical agents. The symptom of dyspnea, occurring in from one-third to one-half of terminal patients, can be frightening to both patient and family, and has received recent attention in the literature (Bruera et al 2000a, Jennings et al 2001, Webb et al 2000). Dyspnea is a devastating symptom in patients with advanced cancer, and the intensity of its manifestation is correlated with lung involvement, fatigue, and anxiety (Bruera et al 2000a). Jennings et al (2001) found that nonnebulized (i.e., oral or parenteral) medications designed to relax the patient and control dyspnea had a significant positive effect. Webb et al (2000) emphasized that accurate assessment and management of dyspnea are essential in the provision of increased quality of life for patients. In addition to inhalants, oxygen therapy, positioning, and steroids, other therapies should be considered, such as relaxation (see Chapter 9), guided imagery (see Chapter 10), and controlled breathing (Webb et al 2000).

Dehydration and nutrition

Dehydration can be a painful and uncomfortable occurrence for the dying patient. Hydration via intravenous fluids can relieve stress and aid comfort in the patients' final days (McCauley 2001). In addition, adequate support mechanisms should be employed. The anorexia that is so pervasive in cancer and other terminal illnesses can be particularly distressing, perhaps even more so to the family than patient (Hughes & Neal 2000). Food refusal can be a source of conflict between the patient and caregivers. Anthropologists have examined the role of food in human societies extensively, but the knowledge gained is not often utilized in healthcare practice, and there is little work regarding social transactions between dying people and their caregivers regarding food (Hughes & Neal 2000). Since a good deal of the patient–caregiver interaction is in the institutional setting, studies which explore the organizational processes to maximize food intake as it relates to autonomy and comfort are recommended.

Other symptoms

Other problems in the terminally ill include malignant bowel obstruction and malignant cutaneous wounds. Malignant bowel obstruction is common in terminal colorectal and gynecological cancer, and patients may experience distressing symptoms that can be difficult to manage (William & Bailey 2001). Little has been written regarding the patient's perceptions and quality of life with this event. It is well to remember that the meaning of being unable to eat may be more significant to the patient than the nutritional/biological loss of food, and that the bowel obstruction may mark a transition to social disengagement and disrupted identity (William & Bailey 2001). Malignant cutaneous wounds can be seen in the terminally ill patient; the presence of a fungating, painful wound, whatever the cause, is a constant visible reminder of their disease (Schiech 2002). Patients may have to cope with bleeding, exudates, odor, and infection, and the care is challenging. Physical therapists and other health professionals trained in wound care management will find the care of these patients rewarding, as such management enables the patient to maintain or even improve quality of life.

Spinal cord compression, once a relatively uncommon result of cancer spreading to the epidural space, is more common now, as a result of better treatment of patients with lung, breast, and prostate cancer (Hicks et al 1993). Although this complication has been studied extensively from a medical and surgical perspective, its exact relation to hospice or terminal care is less well documented. The outcomes are related to the performance status prior to the complication; survival is shorter for those non-ambulatory after treatment, and those patients who remain non-ambulatory will require intensive palliative care. Motor paralysis at the end of life is an added stressor for the patient and the effects can be overwhelming (Hicks et al 1993).

Lung cancer presents some special issues in symptom control, as this disease, with its frequent aggressive nature, widespread metastatic potential, and distressing symptomatology, can rapidly lead to a debilitated status (Brescia 2001). Bony mestatases are frequent, leading to fractures and immobility, further compromising function and control. Decision making for this condition requires prioritizing values much beyond medical knowledge alone, and there may be guilt and anger on the part of the patient and family respectively since a potentially controllable behavior (e.g., smoking) is causative in the majority of cases. End of life issues may become more important sooner than in other cancer diagnoses (Brescia 2001).

Physical and occupational therapy can be utilized to ease symptoms in the terminally ill patient. Soft tissue massage, for example, has been found successful in managing symptoms in patients with cancer (Briggs 1997, 2000, Smith et al 2002). Phototherapy was used in one study of terminal illness, as there is a clear link between mood and symptomatology and light exposure (Cohen et al 1994). The mobility of terminally ill patients may be seriously reduced, resulting in little exposure to direct sunlight. Phototherapy can be used in terminally ill patients to alleviate the depression and heightened physical symptomatology that may occur. Hypnosis is a neglected and available resource for patients with terminal illness, and may well be part of the misconceptions of psychiatric care in terminal patients (Douglas 1999). Hypnosis has been shown to assist in relaxation, help insomnia, and aid pain relief, and is an affirmed complementary or alternative therapy for terminally ill patients (Douglas 1997, Genuis 1995, Katz et al 1987).

In summary, a wide variety of techniques can be used to control pain and other symptoms in the terminally ill. The therapist should offer skills to alleviate the distressing symptoms that make the dying process difficult for the patient and family, and should work collaboratively with the other members of the multidisciplinary team for this purpose.

COMFORT CARE OF THE TERMINALLY ILL

Individuals react to terminal illness or imminent death in various ways, depending upon their lifestyles, previous experience, and the disease itself. Generally, personality structures and ways of coping do not change much in the face of terminal illness (Teno 1999), and the clinician can expect patients to react to the environment much as they did prior to becoming terminally ill. Nonetheless, comfort care of the terminally ill has risen to the forefront with increased awareness of the physical and psychosocial variables that affect and accompany the process.

McDonnell et al (2002) studied 263 nurses and found that 70% of them felt that managing comfort care of the dying is an integral part of hospital care. However, only 8% of the sample felt that the hospital setting was the ideal environment for the dying patient. Barriers to optimum comfort care reported were lack of education and training in comfort care, work pressures, and lack of support. Despite this, palliative care education is of better quality compared to 20 years ago (Field & Wee 2002). Over this period, there has been an increase in training related to the management of symptoms of the terminally ill, and in comfort care that reflects the establishment of palliative care as a specialty.

There is a pervasive belief that terminally ill people receive a great deal of healthcare. A recent Canadian study (Wilson & Truman 2002) found that hospital use varied, but was low, and that the last hospital stay for the patient was only infrequently resource intensive. In the Wilson & Truman (2002) study, age, gender, and illness did not distinguish use of institutional resources in the dying process.

Measuring the quality of comfort care in the terminally ill is difficult. There is a lack of valid and reliable measurement tools, and existing quality of care measures do not attend to the changes in priorities and dimensions that acquire new significance in the terminally ill (Teno 1999). It is clear that development of measurement tools should utilize both patient and family perspective to assess the quality of care rendered to the terminally ill.

Interesting issues arise in comfort care, and the question of resuscitation is one that deserves some thought. Hinkka et al (2001) studied the issue of the clinician performing cardiopulmonary resuscitation (CPR) in the unexpected death of a young terminal cancer patient. Although this is a very specific hypothetical situation, those in favor of CPR were found to be younger physicians with no or little experience in terminal care, and valued life to a much greater extent. The findings of the Hinkka et al (2001) study of course are not generalizable to the larger population of all physicians attending terminally ill individuals, but they do underscore the need for advanced directive and enhanced communication with the patient and family.

Comfort care of the dying is multidimensional, and necessitates a mature and integrated approach to ensure that all patients' needs are met in a timely and appropriate manner. Physical therapists and other healthcare workers can do much to alleviate the suffering of these individuals. Focused training on this manner of care, however, is lacking somewhat in professional curricula. Comfort care encompasses appropriate positioning of the patient, maintenance of range of motion, massage where indicated, meticulous hygiene, and attention to fungating wounds if present. At this time, gentle reassurance to the family, and just the mere presence of a trusted healthcare worker (one who has developed and maintained a good relationship with the patient) can mean the difference between a "good death" and one that occurs in isolation.

Patients deserve access to optimal care at the end of life. Clinicians that have a longstanding relationship with the patient throughout the course of terminal illness, who are responsive to the patient's wishes, and who exhibit sensitive empathetic communication can be paramount in comprehensive and quality end of life care (Asco 1998). There are several obstacles that can hinder delivery of high-quality end of life care, but they are not insurmountable. Healthcare workers committing themselves to informing colleagues and the public about these significant barriers to optimal comfort care in terminal illness is an important first step.

PSYCHOLOGICAL CONSIDERATIONS

THERAPIST–PATIENT RELATIONSHIPS

The relationship between the patient and physical, occupational, or other therapist is crucial to the delivery of optimal terminal care. It is important to recognize when and where to intervene with the patient exhibiting one of many emotional and psychological aspects of terminal illness. The ability to identify physical waypoints along the continuum of illness may give end-stage patients and their families opportunities for goal reframing and psychological incorporation (Doyle-Brown 2000).

The transitional phase refers to the period between active participation in activities of daily living and the bedbound status, and is characterized by anorexia, increased sleep, weakness, and confusion, and may be a period of heightened anxiety for families. It is at this point that the therapist–patient relationship becomes increasingly important. To identify these behaviors as part of a definable and finite phase allows the healthcare worker to educate the family and relieve any undue anxiety. Understanding this transitional phase may prevent unnecessary placement outside the home for terminal care, especially prematurely.

It is during the transitional time that the patient may need special assessment and intervention, as the passage toward a bedbound status can be modified or delayed; at the least the family can be prepared for the event. Openness on the part of the therapist is extremely important. The dying experience is ultimately a complex one, and one that the caregiver cannot fully understand (Boston et al 2001). It is apparent that empathy is an important therapeutic skill that requires vulnerability and personal risk within the patient–caregiver relationship.

Competence in end of life care requires skill in communication, decision-making, and building relationships (VonGunten et al 2000). Steps that a therapist should consider are to establish an appropriate environment, establish what the patient knows and expects, determine how information is to be handled, respond to emotions, establish goals, and set an overall management plan that incorporates both physical and psychosocial components. This process can be used for goal setting, resolving conflict, and in guiding the patient through the last hours of living. One study found that occupational therapists needed to discover and respond to their own inner needs in delivering appropriate and effective terminal care (Dawson 1993). The occupational therapist should not feel conflicted in supporting the dual statuses of living and dying in patients with terminal illness; the occupational therapists were found to be holistic, addressing physical, social, emotional, and spiritual aspects of care (Rahman 2000). Also, experiential education-simulation teaching using patient scenarios can be a successful model for increasing student comfort in responding to difficult clinical communication tasks during their training (Rosenbaum & Kreiter 2002). This approach can be applied to the therapist in training.

Cultures will differ greatly in how terminal illness and its ramifications are approached with a patient. One study (Bruera et al 2002b) compared physicians in Europe, South America, and Canada on attitudes to terminal care. South American physicians were more likely to support beneficence and justice compared to autonomy, while the Canadian physicians felt the opposite. More research is needed regarding attitudes and beliefs on the part of healthcare workers, and the effect of these concepts on terminal care and the therapist–patient relationship.

The relationship between therapist and patient is close and often involves physical touch, and patients may feel comfortable in communicating with their therapist regarding end of life issues (Dawson 1993). Therapists should develop and foster their communication and care skills as they apply to the terminal patient. Since death is a universal experience, all therapists need to tap their own emotional resources and reserves, and be ready to apply their attributes successfully to the patient.

EMOTIONAL ASPECTS OF TERMINAL ILLNESS

The reality of a terminal diagnosis can be overwhelming to a patient and family. Many factors interact in a patient's will to live. A recent study found anxiety, dyspnea, nausea, colon cancer, and having no religion to cause variance in the will to live or lack thereof (Tataryn & Chochinov 2002). As mentioned previously, patients will tend to keep with their premorbid personality and coping strategies during the course of the terminal illness. McCarthy et al (2000), in studying patients with lung and colon cancer at terminal stages, found that there was more pain and confusion as death approached, but that patients were only moderately depressed and anxious during the last 3 days of life. The authors of this study highlighted opportunities to improve the quality of life at the end of life in patients dying of cancer. Such opportunities included careful evaluation and discernment regarding symptoms, comprehensive attention and treatment of psychosocial distress, and sustained contact with families of the patient.

A study by Fernsler et al (1999) found that the demands of colorectal cancer and the associated stress were perceived to be greater in men, younger patients, and those who reported a decrease in activity or metastatic disease. A greater degree of psychosocial and spiritual well-being may help to mitigate the demands of such illness in the terminal stages, and therapists can foster efforts to facilitate the acquisition of such well-being as appropriate. Throughout terminal illness, and particularly at end stage, therapists need to respect the uncertainty that the patient feels regarding the possible course that the illness may take or length of life that can be expected (Penson 2000). Hope is part of the emotional response to dying, and can be fostered and supported during the palliative phase, paying attention to the potential problems that may arise from false or unrealistic hope. Perhaps specific emphasis is needed on capturing the intangible, inner experience of hope, and to validate the strategies that develop/maintain hope in patients and families (Herth & Cutcliffe 2002).

At the terminal stages of life, there may be multifaceted suffering, as the uncontrolled deterioration of one's body can be significant (Finucane 2002). Nearly all patients want companionship in the face of death (Penson 2000, Robertson 2002). The choice between certain death, even if comfortable and dignified, and hope, is a difficult and painful choice that patients may have to make. Certainly a gentle, unhurried healthcare worker who can act with soothing advocacy and humility can be of great assistance to the patient (Finucane 2002).

Terminally ill patients usually experience the five stages of grief first described by Kubler-Ross in her pioneering work on death and dying (Forman 1998). They are denial, anger, bargaining, depression, and acceptance. Not all patients go sequentially through the five stages. Often people pass back and forth through the stages, and not all patients will exhibit all stages. Denial can be healthy and even beneficial, preventing psychological health from unnecessary or premature deterioration. Connor (1992) examined the effects of a psychosocial intervention on denial-related coping ability in the terminally ill, and found that it preserves relationships important to the patient. Some patients may benefit from intervention only after developing additional adaptive coping strategies.

The skilled therapist will recognize that there is a vast array of emotional responses to a life-threatening illness, and that patients will progress toward acceptance at different rates, or not at all. It is inappropriate for a therapist to force patients to come to grips with their dying in a manner that the therapist thinks they should. The emotional aspects of the actual terminal stages of illness can also vary tremendously among patients. Clinicians should listen carefully and support the patient through his/her emotional reactions without being judgmental. The clinician who examines his/her own feelings and beliefs regarding terminal illness will be better equipped to respond to the needs of the patient.

Special populations, such as the mentally ill, and children and adolescents, sometimes need additional support and care in approaching terminal illness. In adolescents who are terminally ill, the therapist should understand that many of the completion tasks usually associated with aging are suddenly thrust to the forefront in this population, and the illness may catapult the younger terminal patient into more mature stages of life for which they may be unprepared (Rancour 2002). It is indeed no small task to "complete the gestalt of one's life tapestry," so to speak, especially when young (Rancour 2002). The medical profession has an obligation to decrease the impact of loss in the adolescent with terminal illness, and prepare the family to facilitate the adolescent's mastery of adaptive tasks posed by terminal illness and death (Christ et al 2002). Therapist training programs are only beginning to approach these extremely delicate matters.

PSYCHOLOGY OF THE DYING PROCESS

Psychological aspects of the dying process are complex and broad. Psychological reactions are generally closely tied to the emotional aspects of terminal illness, but many factors may be contributory. Despite multiple efforts, researchers still struggle to identify outcome measures that adequately assess patients' and families' exact experience in dying (Steinhauser et al 2002). To improve care, health workers should assess the quality of these experiences and interventions.

It is important to note that during the dying process the patient is experiencing multiple losses: job, function, role in the family, daily routines, etc. There is loss of what might have occurred, loss of a career in its prime, or loss of the ability to see ones' children grow and mature. There may be the inability of the patient to see many of his/her life goals come to fruition. Since lifestyles vary considerably, these are only examples of the losses that a patient will have to endure. The therapist needs to be cognizant of these multiple losses, and at the same time give the patient some tangible goals toward which to work. In this respect, therapists with their emphasis on practical, basic functioning and mobility, can often play a significant role in the patient's care. Assistance can be offered to the patient in realizing some of these basic goals, and the rewards of such intervention can be substantial. The creative therapist can constantly summon a repertoire of interventions that can be applicable, and therefore useful in the terminally ill. In this way, some of the more painful losses can be attenuated.

Four major areas of ethics apply to the dying patient: general ethical principles, patient decision-making, conflict of interests, and management of risks associated with terminal care (Smith 1997). Each clinician should be aware of these ethical concepts, and allow the patient laterality in choosing therapist intervention. The right of a patient to make decisions regarding his or her care is paramount, and should be respected at all times. The dying process can take on many different ramifications. For example, for terminally ill people still active within the community, an altered body image can pose significant problems (Price 2000). The patient may be unsure how to present a positive image to others, and lay people may be equally unsure how to react to the changed appearance. Although it is likely to remain a difficult matter to facilitate, the patient usually eventually learns to manage such social encounters.

Much has been written of the depression that accompanies terminal illness. Some degree of depression is expected in most patients during the course of their illness (Craig & Abeloff 1974, Lander et al 2000, Valente et al 1994). Depression remains a considerable source of suffering among older dying patients (Lander et al 2000), and is often overlooked. Major depression occurs in approximately 25% of patients dying from cancer (Valente et al 1994). However, fewer than half of patients suffering from depression are offered treatment. Clinicians should detect the subtle signs of depression, offer cognitive strategies during management, and detect and evaluate the risk of suicide, if present. A higher incidence of depression has been correlated with advanced disease (Craig & Abeloff 1974), and there is a greater incidence in those with lower Karnofsky scores. Karnofsky severity ratings are ratings by the clinician of the patient's overall functioning level (Box 20.1). Scores of 0 represent minimal functioning (death) while scores of 100 represent unimpaired functioning (The Measurement Group 2003). Therapists and others should keep in mind that mood disorders may be due to electrolyte disturbances, endocrinopathies, or nutritional imbalances. In approaching the patient, it is advisable to remind the patient of the legitimization of the difficulty of the situation (i.e., advanced cancer) and of the right to be upset to reduce the fear of being judged weak or inappropriate (Greenstein & Breitbart 2000).

The psychology of dying can impact on many areas of life (Greenstein & Breitbart 2000). Life's meanings, including responsibility towards others, creativity, transcendence, and ascertaining one's values and priorities are all examples. Patients usually want to have goals on which to focus, and feel part of a larger whole. These goals are generated by a sense of temporal continuity of one's life despite the disruption of serious illness. Greisinger et al (1997) studied 120 terminally ill cancer patients, and

---

Box 20.1 Karnofsky Performance Scale

100 Able to work, normal, no complaints, no evidence of disease
90 Able to work, able to carry on normal activity, minor symptoms
80 Able to work, normal activity with effort, some symptoms
70 Independent, not able to work, cares for self, unable to carry on normal activity
60 Disabled, dependent, requires occasional assistance, cares for most needs
50 Moderately disabled, dependent, requires considerable assistance and frequent care
40 Severely disabled, dependent, requires special care and assistance
30 Severely disabled, hospitalized, death not imminent
20 Very sick, active supportive treatment needed
10 Moribund, fatal processes are rapidly progressing

Accessed from The Measurement Group 2003.

---

found that their concerns included existential, spiritual, familial, physical, and emotional domains. Unfortunately many of these domains were not the focus of their care as the disease was assessed and treated. Therapists should endeavor to create an atmosphere where the patient feels comfortable exploring the quality of life issues within each of the domains.

Yedida and MacGregor (2001) recently conducted serial in-depth interviews with 30 patients confronting the prospects of dying, and found that their feelings about dying were grounded in their frames of reference, enabling them to give meaning and consistency to other major events in their lives. Healthcare workers should be aware of patient's thoughts regarding death in order to understand their preferences for care and responses to treatment recommendations. It is also true that the end of life can offer opportunities for personal growth and the deepening of relationships (Block 2001). Optimal end of life care requires willingness to address families, the patient's psychological integrity, and meaning. This enhanced understanding of the common psychological concerns of patients can improve care but also allow the caregiver to develop a sense of satisfaction and meaning in caring for the dying (Block 2001).

Chochinov et al (2002) developed a model of dignity in the terminally ill. Three categories emerged from their study: illness-related concerns, a dignity-conserving repertoire, and social dignity inventory. The patients' concept of their own dignity was a difficult item to comprehend, but the model offers a way of understanding how patients face advancing terminal illness. Rarely are the biomedical, clinical, and psychosocial data considered simultaneously as influences on cancer patients' outcomes. One group found that the psychosocial milieu made an independent contribution to survival time estimation (Clipp et al 2001) underscoring the importance of psychological variables in terminal illness.

Some patients with terminal illness will desire an early death, and this is usually associated with depression (Tiernan et al 2002). Better recognition of depression might improve the lives of people with terminal illness, and possibly decrease the desire for early death. Some terminal illnesses carry their own particular psychological ramifications. Pancreatic cancer, for example, is usually diagnosed in late stages and often secondary to severe pain (Alter 1996). There is a higher incidence of depression in patients with pancreatic cancer than other forms of cancer, and palliative considerations are central. An aggressive evaluation and treatment of pain, mood, and emotional symptoms is necessary in this subpopulation of terminally ill individuals (Alter 1996).

Finally, the risk of suicide in the terminally ill needs to be addressed by clinicians caring for the patient. Cancer of the brain and central nervous system, AIDS, and multiple sclerosis are associated with an increased risk of suicide (Kleepsies et al 2000). Depression and suicide ideation are undertreated, and there is currently great concern in the United States regarding the ethics of physician assisted suicide. An aspect of this issue might be the apparent acceptance on the part of some psychologists and others, of assisted suicide under certain conditions. Filiberti et al (2001) studied a small sample of patients, interviewing family and staff after a suicide. They reported that patients tended to exhibit concern for loss of autonomy and independence, depression, physical impairments, fear of suffering, and a fear of being a burden on others. Interestingly, 60% of patients showed aggressiveness toward the family during the terminal illness.

Therapists and other clinicians involved with the patient need to recognize that despite all preventative efforts, some terminally ill patients will succeed in killing themselves. In these cases, tender and sustained support of surviving family members is crucial. A nonjudgmental approach is best, putting aside any personal feelings about suicide, and viewing the patient and family within their framework is necessary to afford complete closure for all concerned.

PSYCHOLOGICAL INTERVENTIONS

PSYCHOSOCIAL SUPPORT

Offering psychosocial support to the terminally ill individual is a task that many therapists will be called upon to do at some time in their career. The skills necessary for this to transpire are not extensive, sometimes a good listener is all that is needed to calm and comfort the patient. However, there are many impediments to being present and actively listening to people in difficult times (Stevens & Katsekas 1999). There are many suggestions on how to "be" with patients in a terminal illness. The therapist should eliminate external intrusions, and facilitate the creation of a therapeutic milieu so that the patient can feel comfortable in sharing their thoughts and fears (Stevens & Katsekas 1999). Just listening to the patient, and often just simply being present, can be comforting.

The experience of a terminal illness is something that we can only fully imagine if it faces us directly. Responses to the patient along the lines of "I know how you feel" generally should be avoided. Although well meant, statements such as these can be upsetting to the patient because it is obvious that one does not really know how a dying person feels. Psychosocial support can be offered in a variety of ways and in a variety of settings, and there is no one manner of intervention or location where the support can be proven to be superlative. There are problems in isolating the effect of one intervention from the changing dimensions of the environment surrounding the progress of terminal illness (Maddocks 2002). Often the clinician is more adept at studying the disease than understanding the patient.

During psychosocial support, the physician in particular may often censor information given to patients, which is a well intentioned but misguided assumption about human behavior (Fallowfield et al 2002). Desiring to shield patients from reality can cause problems, creating an increased state of fear, anxiety, and confusion (Fallowfield et al 2002). This may also have the effect of denying patients and the family opportunities to re-organize and re-adapt their lives toward attainment of more achievable goals. This ripple effect may spread into many areas of the patients' lives, and limited time should not be wasted in supporting denial, for example, when it is destructive. Making the distinction of when and where to intervene and offer support and counseling is an art and is learned through practice and experience.

All healthcare workers can participate in the psychosocial care of the terminal patient. Physical therapists often spend more time with their patients than other healthcare workers, by nature of their evaluation and treatment procedures (Briggs 2000). The skilled therapist can capitalize on this fact, and recognize that the patient may feel more comfortable with him or her than some of the other staff. Gently listening to the patient's concerns during the therapy session can be helpful to both patient and therapist, as goals can be re-evaluated and reformulated as necessary. This will also give the therapist insight and knowledge concerning the patient's reaction to the terminal illness. Open lines of communication in these situations help considerably. At the time of death, families will vary in their ability to receive emotional support and/or information, and the therapist should look for an abnormal grief response. Sustained, uncontrollable weeping, refusal to plan or participate in a memorial service, and public hostility between family members are examples. Each grief reaction will be personal, and in some cases, private. At all times the wishes of the patient's family should be respected.

PSYCHIATRIC CARE IN TERMINAL PATIENTS

There are many myths concerning psychiatric care in terminally ill patients. It should be remembered that many patients and families consider psychiatric intervention as a sign of weakness in the face of a universal experience (death). Since major depression, among other symptoms, may be neglected in the terminally ill, many patients face increased isolation and anxiety as the disease progresses. Although psychiatric illness may be present in the patient prior to the diagnosis of a terminal illness,

this can usually be ascertained, and psychiatric care, if ongoing prior to the illness, will likely continue. It is the patient who presents with psychiatric symptoms after the terminal illness diagnosis who sometimes requires difficult management decisions.

Many symptoms of terminal illness can be controlled with specific diagnosis and treatment. Delirium in the terminally ill cancer patient can have a variety of causes, and its multiple dimensions make definition, measurement, and assessment difficult (Brown & Degner 2001). Use of a delirium assessment instrument that involves all caregivers would be important so that early detection can be implemented. Often the cause is metabolic, and can be reversed with immediate treatment (Brown & Degner 2001). Some of the more common causes of delirium in cancer patients are cerebral metastases, pharmacological agents (e.g., opiates or sedatives), cranial irradiation, organ failure, and paraneoplastic syndromes (Lawler et al 2000). In about half of patients, the delirium can be reversed. Reversible causes of delerium include dehydration, renal function, infections, metabolic causes, drug withdrawal, psychoactive medications, and accumulation of opioid metabolites (Lawler et al 2000). It should be noted that delirium in its full floridity can be particularly distressing for families, especially in terminal stages. Families want their loved ones conscious and communicative as long as possible, and that goal should be facilitated if at all possible.

Derogatis et al (1983) studied the prevalence of psychiatric disorders among cancer patients, and found that 53% of a sample of 215 patients were adjusting "normally" to the stress of cancer, and 47% had some type of psychiatric disorder. Of the latter group, two-thirds had reactive or situational anxiety and depression, 13% a major depression, 8% organic medical disorder, 7% personality disorder, and 4% a pre-existing anxiety disorder (Derogatis et al 1983). In these patients, a higher incidence of mixed anxiety and depressive symptoms than anxiety alone was seen. Depression can be manifest as a range of presentations including despair, agitation, irritability, anorexia, fatigue, weight loss, and sleep disorders. All these symptoms can be addressed by competent psychiatric care and intervention.

Lloyd-Williams (2001) advocated psychiatric intervention when necessary, and reported that for 25% of patients in a palliative care ward, depression was a major problem. There are misconceptions that erroneously report a low mood as being a normal facet of terminal illness. It may be difficult to distinguish between appropriate sadness over the end of one's life, and treatable depressive illness, and the tools to assess depression may not be applicable to the palliative care population. There is a strong role for both cognitive therapies and medication in serious depression (Lloyd-Williams 2000). Up to 80% of both psychological and psychiatric morbidity in patients with cancer goes unrecognized and untreated. Therefore, the ability of healthcare workers to recognize the existence of such symptoms is paramount to successful care of patients with terminal illness.

In summary, the psychiatric care of the patient with terminal illness is an important area for continued research. It is important to be able to discern which psychiatric symptomatology is treatable. For example, personality disorders are an example where behavioral modification can be attempted, but not much change in the patient is to be expected (Derogatis et al 1983). Supportive care in patients with pre-existing, refractory psychiatric syndromes is tantamount to effective overall patient care. When more clinicians are able to distinguish between appropriate sadness and clinical depression in terminal illness, appropriate care can be ordered and administered. Patients and families who are reticent to psychiatric intervention and/or stigmata associated with psychiatric disorders should be appropriately educated.

SUPPORT SYSTEMS FOR CAREGIVERS

With an increasing literature on burnout in the health profession, many caregivers now recognize their limitations as they render care to the terminally ill. Gribich et al (2001) documented the emotional experiences and coping strategies of caregivers from diagnosis of terminal illness through caring to bereavement. They found strong positive emotions of caregivers regarding the opportunity given them to express their love through care of dying individuals. However, there was a lack of emotional support from other healthcare professionals, particularly during the bereavement phase (after the patient's death), when perhaps the need for support is greatest (Gribich et al 2001). All therapists have experienced the sadness, sometimes intensely, over the death of a special patient, and this grief should be recognized as normal and healthy.

Individuals involved in the death of a patient often rate the death as "good" or "bad" (Kristjansen et al 2001). Many factors are assessed when determining the success or failure of a caregiver or staff. There may be feelings of failure, unmet expectations, and feelings of regret. Many caregivers will have specific expectations of themselves, and that they believe others hold for them, in assisting patients in the terminal phases of their illness (Jones 1999). It is important to note that the emotional issues of the patient and family can saturate the healthcare giver, and that the emotional trauma of others can be assimilated into physical symptoms. Caregivers can benefit from making some sense of their experiences and integrate them into a meaningful life continuum (Jones 1999).

Predeath depressive symptomatology, overall health, setting of the death, and age and gender of the patient have all been shown to be predictors of postdeath depression and feelings of sadness (Kurtz et al 1997). Optimism, effective social support, and staff support are all predictors of good recovery from such depression. Healthcare workers are advised to keep a strong social support system ongoing, and separate their personal and professional lives through compartmentalization (Kurtz et al 1997). Staff support group meetings have been reported as beneficial for caregivers. Healthcare workers should build and nurture a strong personal life and pursue activities outside of their professional occupation. Keeping in touch periodically with family caregivers after the death of the patient can also help the healthcare worker assimilate the death experience of the patient.

PSYCHOLOGICAL INVOLVEMENT

The use of psychological skills in terminal illness is not as extensive as it possibly could be. A skilled and experienced psychologist with training in palliative care can be invaluable in the care of the terminal patient. Involvement can be of many types: psychoeducational, behavioral, cognitive behavioral, or group interventions (Fawzy et al 1995). Clinicians can choose which method would be most appropriate for the individual patient. Relaxation techniques (see Chapter 9), guided imagery (see Chapter 10), and hypnotherapy are often used. It has been found that adjuvant psychological therapy is better at reducing anxiety than supportive counseling alone (Stedeford 1979). It must not be forgotten that physical and manual therapists can incorporate basic psychological skills (e.g., cognitive behavioral techniques) into the physical management of their patients.

The clinician may be reluctant to bring in the services of a psychologist in the care of the terminally ill patient for a variety of reasons, including lack of patient desire, fear of upsetting the family, and lack of availability (Stedeford 1979). One of the major obstacles in effectively managing terminal illness is getting the patient to relax enough to accept the intervention, without feeling weak or stigmatized. Many patients will feel a lack of control over the experience, and there may be self anger in their perceived inability to cope with the demands of the illness. This barrier can be broken through gentle education, and psychological intervention can be used throughout the disease continuum.

A range of psychological strategies should be employed, and with careful assessment and evaluation, a successful method of intervention can be found for any particular patient. Therapists working with the terminally ill should familiarize themselves with basic knowledge of psychological skills, not so much to become competent psychologists, but rather to be able to recognize when psychological intervention can be of value in the terminally ill. As with all interventions, psychological management in the dying patient must be individualized, and patient confidentiality respected. Therapists may witness significant changes from such interventions, and a taciturn, uncooperative and depressed patient may become much more affable and reachable when relieved of the distressing burden placed on him by the event of a terminal illness.

INTEGRATED MANAGEMENT APPROACHES

PATIENTS AND FAMILIES IN TERMINAL ILLNESS

Each terminally ill patient is someone's mother or father, sister or brother, or friend. Some families are enmeshed (high cohesion) and demand excessive amounts of time from the healthcare team, and find it difficult to follow simple medical directions (Andershead & Ternestedt 2001). Family members may show anger, fear, powerlessness, survivor guilt, and confusion as they attempt to care for the patient (Hockley 2000). At times, family members give all the care and attention to the patient to the point of exhaustion. It is both appropriate and necessary to assess the impact of terminal illness and its treatment on the lives of the family.

Not all families are supportive throughout the course of a terminal illness. Especially toward the end, anticipatory grief and emotional withdrawal from the dying patient, occurring more commonly than thought, can create confusion and concern in the patient (Patterson & Dorfman 2002). Some family structures may be unable to tolerate the influence of external forces, and others with severe dysfunction isolate and protect themselves from the outside world with rigid outer boundaries. These latter families may be inaccessible for any assistance in caring for their dying family member. A nonjudgmental approach is always best, recognizing that there will be a continuum of family participation and integration during the course of terminal illness.

Strange et al (2002) reported that end of life care is an intense, exhausting, and singular experience, and its setting is a world apart from everyday life. Family members need to take cognitive as well as physical breaks from the situation, but often respite means staying engaged in living life with the dying family member. A significant proportion of families will not be knowledgeable concerning options at the end of life, and any advanced care planning should be preceded by education (Silveira et al 2000). Carter & Chang (2000) studied 51 family caregivers who rendered care for a terminally ill patient, and found that 95% had severe sleep problems, and more than 50% had depressive symptoms at a level that would suggest risk for clinical depression.

There are complex dynamics surrounding a patient and family during terminal illness (Hockley 2000). Aspects of communication, openness within the family, and factors that enable the family to function under the stress of a loved one's terminal illness are all integrative. The healthcare worker should piece together the family dynamics as best as possible, thereby gaining knowledge that can be helpful in care. The manner in which staff interact with the patient and relatives will influence the relatives' possibilities for involvement, and facilitate an appropriate death (Andershead & Ternestedt 2001).

Patterson & Dorfman (2002) studied family support, conducting interviews before and after death, and found that not only did the primary caregiver in the family offer the most care, but also at times needed the most support from others. The experience was positive for most of the sample with emotional support described as being good, the frequency of assistance appropriate, and the families growing closer throughout the experience. Patterson & Dorfman (2002) reported less agreement regarding family communication during the process. For the special case of a dying child, Steele (2000) found that relationships with healthcare workers, availability of information, the gender of the child, and communication between parents were all important factors in assuring optimal terminal care in children.

The common thread through much of the above literature is the importance of good communication within the family and patient, family and staff, and staff and patient. Care of the terminally ill, regardless of setting, can be strenuous, exhausting, and tax the family beyond its capacity. Signs of poor coping should be identified and the therapist working closely with families of terminally ill patients must respect the importance of those families to their patients. Far too many people die alone and efforts to prevent this unfortunate occurrence should always be implemented where possible. Finally, family support immediately after death is of the utmost importance, and when possible, the therapist involved with the patient should be in attendance for this purpose.

HOSPICE CONCEPT AND CARE

Early efforts to develop hospice care were the result of a reaction to and against the impersonalization of dying. The concepts of hospice are simple: pain relief and symptom control are paramount; psychological, spiritual, and physical pain are all addressed; patients and families are the unit of care; bereavement care is important; and it is provided regardless of the ability of the patient or family to pay for the service. The evidence base for the distinct possibility of dying with symptom control, psychosocial support, the attention of caregivers, and spiritual attention, is mounting (Abrahm & Hansen-Flaschen 2002, Crawley et al 2002, Dupee 1982).

Hospice care is physician directed, multidisciplinary, and can occur in a variety of settings (Dupee 1982). Such care is designed to meet the emotional and physical needs of patients, and the primary goal is to maintain the highest quality of life attainable for as long as possible. It is thought by one author (Dupee 1982), that the increased enthusiasm for the hospice concept reflects deficiencies in other

care of terminally ill patients. The concept of "prehospice" (i.e., preparing a patient for entry into a formal hospice program) is new and exciting. This would involve careful patient selection, and introduction of the hospice concept to both patient and family. At this stage the healthcare worker may discover that the patient may not be psychologically ready to make the transition to hospice care. There is evidence that suggests that hospice programs are still underutilized, especially for some classes of patients (e.g., patients without insurance, those in rural areas). Abrahm & Hansen-Flaschen (2002) studied hospice care for advanced lung disease patients and found that the unpredictability of death from lung disease (noncancer) was a factor in this underutilization.

In using a hospice service, the differences in beliefs, values, and traditional healthcare practices are all of particular relevance at the end of life (Crawley et al 2002). Care in a hospice can be complicated by the fact that even in this specialized center designed to care for the terminally ill, the healthcare worker and patient/family may not have a shared understanding of the meaning of illness/death. Therapists should be sensitive to cultural differences, and develop skills to work with patients from diverse backgrounds. Attention to this enables the clinician to provide comprehensive, compassionate and effective palliative care.

Healthcare workers who experience loss will often find the event painful and emotionally charged, but it can provide opportunity for growth and healing (Zerber & Steinberg 2000). In the hospice setting, staying open to feelings promotes a greater connection to our patients and their families. On a practical side, Briggs (2000) described several practice patterns for physical therapists in the hospice setting. "Rehab light" is a concept where more gradual therapy is offered and adjusted as strength/motor function improves. Rehabilitation "in reverse" adjusts to the decline in the patient (Briggs 2000). Skilled maintenance is used when a patient needs help to stand or ambulate on an intermittent basis. Lastly, "supportive care," with all its implications, is another pattern of practice. A peaceful death at home, surrounded by a loving family who were able to assist in many aspects of care, completes this process.

In the hospice setting, patients differ markedly in their level of disease acceptance, expectations for the future, and in dimensions of life that are meaningful to them (Cheville 2000). During hospice care, the role of rehabilitation at the end of life remains somewhat unclear, but the rehabilitation process can attenuate cancer's assaults on functional autonomy.

Gentle range of motion, massage, positioning, problem solving, and bed mobility can all be employed to maintain maximum function despite increasing loss (Briggs 1997). The hospice therapist gives the patient permission and support in letting go of the life-long functions of walking and getting out of bed. At this time, the supportive care is as important as the medical care.

Hospice, which started as an alternative for those during the dying process, now provides comprehensive palliative and supportive care in patient oriented settings (Milch 2000). Challenges of hospice care go beyond the philosophic, and include the organizational, demographic, and pragmatic difficulties of providing care in various settings. Hospice is a concept, not a location. Whether the care is delivered in a free-standing hospice, a palliative care unit, in a general hospital, or at home, the hospice concept remains the same. Pain control and relief of symptoms are the most important facets, and comfort care procedures that are instituted are appropriate to the individual. As the concept of a good death in the presence of family and trusted caregivers takes hold, more patients will be seeking hospice services and will choose to end their lives in such settings.

THE PALLIATIVE CARE UNIT

The primary goal of palliative care is to improve the quality of life in people with a terminal illness (Cohen et al 2001). Separate palliative care units are now being started in general or specialized hospitals, and the goals are simple: allowing the disease to progress and the patient to end their life in a specialized setting designed to heighten the attention to symptom control and comfort care (Cohen et al 2001). Units tend to be quieter and less busy than general hospital wards, and the staff receive special training in supporting the palliative care concept. Cohen et al (2001) were the first to demonstrate that the palliative care unit can be instrumental in improving existential well-being, in addition to psychological and physical well-being.

The palliative care unit, or if one is not available, the general hospital ward, can do much for the dying patient. Although shortcomings in end of life

care in hospitals are endemic (Cohen et al 2001), distressing symptoms can be relieved, and communication with patients and families can be clear. A general hospital can increase the number and timeliness of referrals to a formal hospice. Although dying well in the United States in particular may not yet be the standard of care, the barriers of staff shortage, lack of knowledge, and lack of hospice or palliative settings can be overcome (Campbell 2002). Ideally, patients not expected to survive a critical illness will experience compassionate and comprehensive care that is both family- and patient-focused, all directed to allow them to die well (Pantilat 2002)

Many therapeutic interventions may still be employed in the palliative unit setting. One example of such an intervention is music therapy (Hartley 2001, Mramor 2001). The three phases of the music therapy process in terminal illness (engagement, relationship building, and actively dying) can be carried out in the palliative care setting, and assist a patient during this difficult time. Music enables one to achieve what may not be achievable in other ways (Hartley 2001). The general use of physical therapy in palliative care has several benefits. These relate to social relationships, spirituality, outlook on mortality, meaningful physical activity, and possibly spirituality (McKey & Sparling 2000).

In summary, the palliative care unit in the general hospital can do much to allow the patient to die with dignity, and efforts of these units should be directed toward that purpose. As in other settings, the multidisciplinary team is utilized, and skilled intervention offered and given when requested and appropriate. Research is needed to determine the success of palliative care units, a relatively new concept in the milieu surrounding terminal care.

CARE FOR THE TERMINALLY ILL AT HOME

In 1983, approximately 76–80% of patients died in medical institutions, 10–14% died in hospices, and only 5–10% of patients died at home (McCusker 1983). These figures have not changed much over the past few decades, with about 20% dying in hospice programs, and about 12–15% at home (Smith 1997). Home care can offer a rich and compelling opportunity to learn about the patient's and family's experience with terminal illness, the impact on culture and environment, and have a broad and humanizing effect on staff who tend to people at home (Billings et al 2001). Academic medical centers and hospice/home health agencies should work together and collaborate to develop effective programs that allow the patient to die at home.

It is unclear, however, whether people with terminal illnesses living in their own homes have access to the services that they need (Beaver et al 2000). Lay caregivers (e.g., the family) may not always receive all the information and support that they need in order to be effective caregivers. In home care, the caregiver may have no formal training and has to learn all aspects of providing for all needs of the patient (Thielmann 2000). The needs of such caregivers fall into three categories: physical needs of the patient, community resources, and the patient's illness. Further research is needed to build comprehensive educational programs that maximize the role of caregivers.

In Canada, there is increased fiscal pressure for patients to be cared for at home during terminal illness (Dudgeon & Kristjanson 1995). However, the health problems of spouses, responsibilities of family members, and the mere physical, financial, and psychological strain of providing care at home can make it difficult to honor a terminally ill person's desire to die at home. There is a pressing need to examine more closely the type and intensity of services needed to support patients and their families in the final stages of terminal illness. If a patient and the family request death at home, intensive efforts should be directed toward this goal (Smeenk et al 1998).

Advanced care planning can be done in the home setting, and should be a part of patient management (Ratner et al 2001). Even with the best management, requests to return to the hospital to die may be made by patients and their families who initially wanted to die at home. The reasons for changes in their decision may vary from those that are obvious and practical (e.g., medical emergency) to those which are irrational and unconscious (e.g., sudden fear of the patient's impending death) (McCusker 1983). It is unkind to force a family to have the patient die at home when they are not prepared, or even if they change their mind at a later stage. Likewise, when a family member communicates to the therapist or other clinician that they cannot perform some or all of the necessary home care, this must be respected, as there are always reasons for such refusals to render care.

Healthcare professionals in the home setting will find extensive opportunities for care giving, personal growth, and satisfaction in the task of assisting a patient in dying in familiar, comforting, settings. Efforts that make this possible should be facilitated and promoted where possible. Many families report intense satisfaction that they cared for their loved one at home, and that they did all they could to make the last days of the patient meaningful. In this way, staff that support this concept will also know that they contributed to the patient's requests.

SUMMARY

This chapter described the physical and medical considerations of terminal illness, and addressed pain and symptom control, as well as comfort care. The psychological and social ramifications of terminal illness were explored, and the psychology of the dying process was outlined. Various psychological interventions were discussed, with the emphasis on intense psychosocial support throughout the terminal illness. Lastly, integrated management approaches, which included the all-important role of the family in terminal care, were summarized in the context of location of terminal care (i.e., hospice, palliative care unit, and the home setting).

Although rehabilitation may seem paradoxical or unwarranted in terminal care, this is hardly the case. The therapist who has the strength of character to face his/her own mortality, and is secure in beliefs, attitudes, and knowledge of terminal illness, can offer a rich and appreciated form of specialized care to the dying.

References

Abrahm J L, Hansen-Flaschen J 2002 Hospice for patients with advanced lung disease. Chest 121(1): 220–229

Alter C L 1996 Palliative and supportive care of patients with pancreatic cancer. Seminars in Oncology 213(2): 229–240

Andershead B, Ternestedt B M 2001 Development of a theoretical framework describing relative's involvement in palliative care. Journal of Advanced Nursing 34(4): 554–562

Asco J 1998 Cancer care during the last phase of life. Journal of Clinical Oncology 16(5): 1986–1996

Beaver K, Luker K, Woods S 2000 Primary care services received during terminal illness. International Journal of Palliative Nursing 6(5): 220–227

Block S D 2001 Perspectives on care at the close of life. Psychological considerations, growth, and transcendence at the end of life: The art of the possible. Journal of the American Medical Association 285(22): 2898–2905

Billings J A, Ferris F D, MacDonald N et al 2001 The role of palliative care in the home in medical education: Report from a national consensus conference. Journal of Palliative Medicine 4(3): 361–371

Boston P, Towers A, Barnard D 2001 Embracing vulnerability: Risk and empathy in palliative care. Journal of Palliative Care 17(4): 248–253

Brescia F J 2001 Lung cancer – a philosophical, ethical, and personal perspective. Critical Reviews in Oncology and Hematology 40(2): 139–148

Briggs R W 1997 Physical therapy in hospice care. Rehabilitation Oncology 15(3): 16–17

Briggs R W 2000 Models for physical therapy practice in palliative medicine. Rehabilitation Oncology 18(2): 18–19, 21

Brown S, Degner L 2001 Delirium in the terminally ill cancer patient: Aetiology, symptoms, and management. International Journal of Palliative Nursing 7(6): 266–272

Bruera E, Schmitz B, Pither J, Neumann C M 2000a Frequency and correlates of dyspnea in patients with advanced cancer. Journal of Pain and Symptom Management 19(5): 357–362

Bruera E, Neumann C M, Mazzacato C et al 2000b Attitudes and beliefs of palliative care physicians regarding communication with terminally ill cancer patients. Palliative Medicine 14(4): 287–298

Campbell M L 2002 End of life care in the ICU: Current practice and future hopes. Critical Care Nursing Clinics of North America 14(2): 197–200

Carter P A, Chang B L 2000 Sleep and depression in cancer caregivers. Cancer Nursing 23(6): 410–415

Cheville A L 2000 Cancer rehabilitation and palliative care. Rehabilitation Oncology 18(1): 19–20

Chochinov H M, Hacke J, McClement S et al 2002 Dignity in the terminally ill: A developing empirical model. Society of Science and Medicine 54(3): 433–443

Christ G M, Siegal K, Christi A E 2002 Adolescent grief – "It never really hit me until it actually happened". Journal of the American Medical Association 288(10): 1269–1278

Clipp E C, Hollis D R, Cohen H J 2001 Considerations of psychosocial illness phase in cancer survival. Psychooncology 10(2): 166–178

Cohen J R, Steiber W, Mount B M 1994 Phototherapy in the treatment of depression in the terminally ill. Journal of Pain and Symptom Management 9(8): 534–536

Cohen S R, Boston P, Mount B M et al 2001 Changes in quality of life following admission to palliative care units. Palliative Medicine 15(5): 363–371

Connor S R 1992 Denial in terminal illness: To intervene or not to intervene. Hospital Journal 8(4): 1–15

Craig J, Abeloff M D 1974 Psychiatric symptomatology among hospitalized cancer patients. American Journal of Psychiatry 131: 1323–1327

Crawley L M, Marshall P A, Lo B et al 2002 Strategies for culturally effective end of life care. Annals of Internal Medicine 136(9): 673–679

Dawson S 1993 The role of OT groups in an Australian hospice. American Journal of Hospice and Palliative Care 10(4): 13–17

Derogatis L R, Morrow G R, Fetting J et al 1983 The prevalence of psychiatric disorders among cancer patients. Journal of the American Medical Association 249: 751–755

Douglas D B 1997 Patient and close person, relationship, and hypnosis in pain management. Hypnosis 24(4): 196–199

Douglas D B 1999 Hypnosis: Useful, neglected, available. American Journal of Hospice and Palliative Care 16(5): 665–670

Doyle-Brown M 2000 The transitional phase: The closing journey for patients and family caregivers. American Journal of Hospice and Palliative Care 17(5): 354–357

Driscoll C E 1987 Symptom control in terminal illness. Principles of Care 14(2): 353–363

Dudgeon D J, Kristjanson L 1995 Home vs. hospital death: Assessment of preferences and clinical challenges. Canadian Medical Association Journal 152(3): 337–340

Dupee R M 1982 Hospice – compassionate, comprehensive approach to terminal care. Postgraduate Medicine 72(3): 239–241, 244–246

Fallowfield L S, Jenkins V A, Beveridge H 2002 Truth may hurt but deceit hurts more: Communication in palliative care. Palliative Medicine 16(4): 297–303

Fawzy F, Fawzy N, Arndt T L 1995 Critical review of psychosocial interventions in cancer care. Archives of General Psychiatry 52: 100–108

Fernsler J I, Klemm P, Miller M M 1999 Spiritual well-being and demands of illness in people with colorectal cancer. Cancer Nursing 22(2): 134–135

Field D, Wee B 2002 Preparation for palliative care: Teaching about death, dying, and bereavement in the UK medical schools 2000–2001. Medical Education 36(6): 561–567

Filiberti A, Ripamontic C, Totis A et al 2001 Characteristics of terminal cancer patients who committed suicide during a home palliative care program. Journal of Pain and Symptom Management 22(1): 544–553

Finucane T E 2002 Care of the patients nearing death: Another view. Journal of the American Geriatric Society 50(3): 551–553

Forman W 1998 The evolution of hospice and palliative medicine. In: Berger A, Portenoy R, Weissman D (eds) Principles and practice of supportive oncology. Lippincott-Raven, Philadelphia, p 735–739

Genuis M 1995 The use of hypnosis in helping cancer patients control anxiety, pain, and emesis: A review of recent empirical studies. American Journal of Clinical Hypnosis 37(4): 196–199

Greenstein M, Breitbart W 2000 Cancer and the experience of meaning: A group psychotherapy program for people with cancer. American Journal of Psychotherapy 54(4): 486–500

Greisinger A J, Lorimore R J, Aday L A et al 1997 Terminally ill cancer patients. Their most important concerns. Cancer Practice 5(3): 147–154

Gribich C Parker D, Maddocks I 2001 The emotions and coping strategies of caregivers of family members with a terminal cancer. Journal of Palliative Care 17(1): 30–36

Hartley N J 2001 On a personal note: A music therapist's reflections on working with those who are living with a terminal illness. Journal of Palliative Care 17(3): 135–141

Herth K A, Cutcliffe J R 2002 The concept of hope in nursing 3: Hope and palliative care nursing. British Journal of Nursing 11(14): 977–983

Hicks F, Thorn V, Alison D et al 1993 Spinal cord compression: The hospice perspective. Journal of Palliative Care 9(3): 9–13

Hinkka H, Kosunen E, Metsnoi R et al 2001 CPR in young terminal cancer patients. Resuscitation 49(3): 289–297

Hockley J 2000 Psychosocial aspects in palliative care – communicating with the patient and family. Acta Oncologica 39(8): 905–910

Hughes N, Neal R D 2000 Adults with terminal illness: A literature review of their needs and wishes for food. Journal of Advanced Nursing 32(5): 1101–1107

Jennings A L, Davies A N, Higgins J P et al 2001 Opioids for the palliating of breathlessness in terminal illness. Cochrane Database Systems and Development 4: CD00–2066

Jones A 1999 A heavy and blessed experience: A psychoanalytical study of community MacMillan nurses and their roles in serious illness and palliative care. Journal of Advanced Nursing 30(6): 1297–1303

Katz E, Kellerman J, Ellenberg L 1987 Hypnosis in the reduction of acute pain and distress in children with cancer. Journal of Pediatric Psychology 12: 379–394

Kleepsies P M, Hughes D H, Gallacher F P 2000 Suicide in the medically and terminally ill: Psychological and ethical considerations. Journal of Clinical Psychology 56(9): 1153–1171

Kristjanson L, McPhee T, Pickstock S et al 2001 Palliative nurses' perceptions of good and bad deaths and care expectations: A qualitative analysis. International Journal of Palliative Nursing 7(3): 129–139

Kurtz M E, Kurtz J C, Given C W et al 1997 Predictors of post bereavement depressive symptomatology among family caregivers of cancer patients. Support and Care for Cancer 5(1): 53–60

Lander M, Wilson K, Chochinov H M 2000 Depression and the dying older patient. Clinics in Geriatric Medicine 16(2): 335–336

Lawler P O, Gagnon B, Mancini I L 2000 Occurrence, causes, and outcome of delirium in patients with advanced cancer: A prospective study. Archives of Internal Medicine 160: 786–794

Leahy M E 2000 Factors effecting end stage disease quality of life. Patient and caregiver burdens. Clinical Journal of Oncology Nursing 4(6): 285–286

Lloyd-Williams M 2000 Difficulty in diagnosing and treating depression in the terminally ill cancer patient. Postgraduate Medicine Journal 76: 555–558

Lloyd-Williams M 2001 Screening for depression in palliative care patients: A review. European Journal of Cancer Care 10(1): 31–35

McCahill L, Ferrell BR, Virani R 2001 Improving cancer care at the end of life. Lancet Oncology 2(2): 103–108

McCarthy E P, Phillips R S, Zhong Z et al 2000 Dying with cancer: Patient's function, symptoms, and care preferences as death approaches. Journal of the American Geriatric Society 48(5 suppl): S110–121

McCaulay D 2001 Dehydration in the terminally ill patient. Nursing Standards 16(4): 33–37

McCusker J 1983 Where cancer patients die: An epidemiological study. Public Health Reports 98: 170–176

McDonnell M, Johnson G, Gallagher A G et al 2002 Palliative care in district general hospitals: The nurse's perspective. International Journal of Palliative Nursing 8(4): 169–175

McKey K M, Sparling J W 2000 Experiences of older women with cancer receiving hospice care: Significance for physical therapy. Physical Therapy 80(5): 459–468

McQuellon R P, Cowan M A 2000 Turning toward death together: Conversation in mortal time. American Journal of Hospice and Palliative Care 17(5): 312–318

Maddocks I 2002 Issues in the conduct of therapeutic trials in palliative care: An Australian perspective. Drugs and Aging 19(7): 495–502

Maltoni M, Amadori D 2001 Palliative medicine and medical oncology. Annals of Oncology 12(4): 443–450

Milch RA 2000 The dying patient: Pain management at the hospice level. Current Reviews of Pain 4(3): 215–218

Mramor K M 2001 Music therapy with persons who are indigent and terminally ill. Journal of Palliative Care 17(3): 182–187

Pacquino D 2001 Addressing cultural incongruities of advanced directives. Bioethics Forum 17(1): 27–31

Pantilat S Z 2002 End of life care for the hospitalized patient. Medical Clinics of North America 86(4): 749–770

Paolini C A 2001 Management at the end of life. Journal of the American Osteopathic Association 101(10): 609–615

Patterson L B, Dorfman L T 2002 Family support for hospice caregivers. American Journal of Hospice and Palliative Care 19(5): 315–323

Penson J 2000 A hope is not a promise: Fostering hope within palliative care. International Journal of Palliative Nursing 6(2): 94–98

Price B 2000 Altered body image: Managing social encounters. International Journal of Palliative Nursing 6(4): 179–185

Rahman H 2000 Journey of providing care in hospice: Perspectives of occupational therapists. Quality Health Reports 10(6): 806–818

Rancour P 2002 Catapulting through life stages. When younger adults are diagnosed with life-threatening illnesses. Journal of Psychosocial Nursing and Mental Health Services 40(2): 32–37

Ratner E, Norlander L, McSteen K 2001 Death at home following a targeted advance care planning process at home: The kitchen table discussion. Journal of the American Geriatric Society 49(6): 833–844

Robertson R G 2002 End of life care. American Family Physician 65(5): 787–788

Rosenbaum M E, Kreiter C 2002 Teaching delivery of bad news using experiential sessions with standardized patients. Teaching and Learning in Medicine 14(3): 144–149

Ross D D, Alexander C S 2001 Management of common symptoms in terminally ill patients: Part I. Fatigue, anorexia, cachexia, nausea, and vomiting. American Family Physician 64(5): 807–814

Schiech L 2002 Malignant cutaneous wounds. Clinical Journal of Oncology Nursing 6(5): 305–309

Silveira M J, DiPiero A, Gerrity M S et al 2000 Patient's knowledge of options at the end of life: Ignorance in the face of death. Journal of the American Medical Association 284(19): 1483–1488

Smeenk F W, deWittle L P, VanHagstregt J C et al 1998 Transmural care – a new approach in the care for terminal cancer patients: Its effect on rehospitalization and quality of life. Patient Education and Counseling 35(3): 189–199

Smith T 1997 Medical care of the dying patient. Rehabilitation Oncology 15(1): 20–25

Smith M C, Kemp J, Hemphill L et al 2002 Outcomes of therapeutic massage for hospitalized cancer patients. Journal of Nursing Scholarship 34(3): 257–262

Stedeford A 1979 Psychotherapy of the dying patient. British Journal of Psychiatry 135: 7–14

Steele R G 2000 Trajectory of certain death at an unknown time: Children with neurodegenerative life threatening illness. Canadian Journal of Nursing Research 32(3): 49–67

Steinhauser K E, Clipp E C, Tulsky J A 2002 Evolution in measuring the quality of dying. Journal of Palliative Medicine 5(3): 407–414

Stevens R D, Katsekas B S 1999 Nursing the terminally ill. Being with people at difficult times. Home Health Nurse 17(8): 504–510

Stevens M M, PallaPozza L, Cavalletto B et al 1994 Pain control in children with cancer. Cancer Survivor 21: 211–231

Strange V R, Koop D M, Peden J 2002 The experience of respite during home based family caregiving for persons with advanced cancer. Journal of Palliative Care 18(2): 97–104

Tataryn D, Chochinov H M 2002 Predicting the trajectory of will to live in terminally ill patients. Psychosomatics 43(5): 370–377

Teno J M 1999 Putting patient and family voice back into measuring quality of care for the dying. Hospital Journal 14(3–4): 167–176

The Measurement Group 2003 Karnofsky Severity Rating. Retrieved May 6, 2003, from http://www.themeasurementgroup.com/Definitions/Karnofsky.htm

Thielmann P 2000 Educational needs of home caregivers of terminally ill patients: Literature review. American Journal of Hospice and Palliative Care 17(4): 253–257

Tiernan E, Casey P, O'Boyule C et al 2002 Relations between desire for early death, depressive symptoms, and antidepressant prescribing in terminally ill patients with cancer. Journal of the Royal Society of Medicine 95(8): 386–390

Twycross R G 1981 Rehabilitation in terminal cancer patients. International Journal of Rehabilitation Medicine 3(3): 135–144

Valente S M, Saunders J M, Cohen M I 1994 Evaluating depression among patients with cancer. Cancer Practice 2(1): 65–71

VonGunten C F, Ferris F D, Emanuel L L 2000 The patient–physician relationship. Ensuring competency in end of life care: Communication and relational skills. Journal of the American Medical Association 284(23): 3051–3057

Webb M, Moody L E, Marin L A 2000 Dyspnea assessment and management in hospice patients with pulmonary disorders. American Journal of Hospice and Palliative Care 17(4): 259–264

Wein S 2000 Sedation in the imminently dying patient. Oncology 14(4): 585–592, 597–598, 600

William B, Bailey C 2001 The nature of terminal malignant bowel obstruction and its impact on patients with advanced cancer. International Journal of Palliative Nursing 7(10): 474–481

Wilson D M, Truman C D 2002 Addressing myths about end of life care: Research into the use of acute care hospitals over the last five years of life. Journal of Palliative Care 18(1): 29–38

Yedida M J, MacGregor B 2001 Confronting the prospect of dying. Reports of terminally ill patients. Journal of Pain and Symptom Management 22(4): 807–819

Zerber J, Steinnberg D L 2000 Coming to grips with grief and loss. Can skills for dealing with bereavement be learned? Postgraduate Medicine 108(6): 97–98

Author index

Subject index